TEACHING IN NURSING

TEACHING IN NURSING

A Guide for Faculty

Fifth EDITION

Diane M. Billings, EdD, RN, FAAN, ANEF
Chancellor's Professor Emeritus
Indiana University School of Nursing
Indianapolis, Indiana

Judith A. Halstead, PhD, RN, ANEF, FAAN
Executive Director, Commission for Nursing Education Accreditation
National League for Nursing
Washington, DC
Professor Emeritus
Indiana University School of Nursing
Indianapolis, Indiana

ELSEVIER

ELSEVIER

3251 Riverport Lane
St. Louis, Missouri 63043

TEACHING IN NURSING, FIFTH EDITION ISBN: 978-0-323-29054-8

Notices

Knowledge and best practice in this field are constantly changing. As new research and experience broaden our understanding, changes in research methods, professional practices, or medical treatment may become necessary.

Practitioners and researchers must always rely on their own experience and knowledge in evaluating and using any information, methods, compounds, or experiments described herein. In using such information or methods they should be mindful of their own safety and the safety of others, including parties for whom they have a professional responsibility.

With respect to any drug or pharmaceutical products identified, readers are advised to check the most current information provided (i) on procedures featured or (ii) by the manufacturer of each product to be administered, to verify the recommended dose or formula, the method and duration of administration, and contraindications. It is the responsibility of practitioners, relying on their own experience and knowledge of their patients, to make diagnoses, to determine dosages and the best treatment for each individual patient, and to take all appropriate safety precautions.

To the fullest extent of the law, neither the Publisher nor the authors, contributors, or editors, assume any liability for any injury and/or damage to persons or property as a matter of products liability, negligence or otherwise, or from any use or operation of any methods, products, instructions, or ideas contained in the material herein.

International Standard Book Number: 978-0-323-29054-8

Content Strategist: Lee Henderson
Content Development Manager: Laurie Gower
Content Development Specialist: Laura Goodrich
Marketing Manager: Kate Odem
Publishing Services Manager: Hemamalini Rajendrababu
Senior Project Manager: Divya Krishna Kumar
Designer: XiaoPei Chen

Printed in the United States of America

Last digit is the print number: 9 8 7 6 5 4 3 2 1

To all nurse educators who, through their teaching,
influence the future of the nursing profession

Contributors

Bimbola Akintade, PhD, MBA, MHA, ACNP-BC, CCRN
Assistant Professor and Specialty Director, Adult Gerontology Acute Care Nurse Practitioner/Clinical Nurse Specialist DNP Specialty
University of Maryland, Baltimore
Baltimore Maryland,
Chapter 18

G. Rumay Alexander, EdD, MSN, BSN, FAAN
Clinical Professor and Director, Office of Multicultural Affairs
University of North Carolina at Chapel Hill School of Nursing
Chapel Hill, North Carolina
Chapter 16

Halina Barber, PhD, MS, RN
Assistant Professor
University of Portland
Portland, Oregon
Chapter 5

Diane M. Billings, EdD, RN, FAAN, ANEF
Chancellor's Professor Emeritus
Indiana University School of Nursing
Indianapolis, Indiana
Chapter 24

Wanda Bonnel, PhD, RN, APRN, ANEF
Associate Professor
University of Kansas School of Nursing
Kansas City, Kansas
Chapter 25

Mary P. Bourke, PhD, MSN, RN
Assistant Dean, Associate Professor
Indiana University
Kokomo, Indiana
Chapter 22

Lori Candela, EdD, RN, APRN, FNP-BC, CNE
Associate Professor
School of Nursing University of Nevada, Las Vegas
Las Vegas, Nevada
Chapter 13

Linda S. Christensen, EdD, JD, MSN, RN, CNE
Chief Administration Officer
National League for Nursing
Washington, DC
Chapter 3

Jeanne R. Conner, MN, APRN, FNP-C
Nursing Instructor/Course Coordinator
Montana State University-Bozeman
Billings, Montana
Chapter 14

Diann A. DeWitt, PhD, RN, CNE
Professor/Director RN-BSN Option
Colorado Christian University
Lakewood, Colorado
Chapter 23

Peggy Ellis, PhD, RN, FNP-BC
Dean, School of Nursing and Allied a Health Sciences
Lindenwood University
St. Charles, Missouri,
Chapter 26

Mary L. Fisher, PhD, MSN, RN
Professor Emeritus, Indiana University
Clinical Professor, University of Florida
Sun City Center, Florida
Chapter 1

Betsy Frank, PhD, RN, ANEF
Professor Emerita
School of Nursing, Indiana State University
Terre Haute, Indiana
Chapter 4

Joan L. Frey, EdD, MSN, RN
Interim Vice President for Academic Affairs, Dean—Louisville Campus
Interim Dean—Cincinnati Campus
Galen College of Nursing
Louisville, Kentucky
Chapter 2

Barbara Manz Friesth, PhD, RN
Clinical Associate Professor/Assistant Dean of Learning Resources
Co-Director of the ELITE Center—Encouraging Learning, Innovation and Technology
Excellence
Indiana University School of Nursing
Indianapolis, Indiana
Chapter 20

Karen Grigsby, PhD, RN
Associate Professor, Interim Director MSN Program
College of Nursing
University of Nebraska Medical Center
Omaha, Nebraska
Chapter 9

Paula Gubrud, EdD, RN, FAAN
Senior Associate Dean for Education
Oregon Health & Science University
School of Nursing
Portland, Oregon
Chapter 17

Susan M. Hendricks, EdD, RN, CNE
Associate Professor
Associate Dean for Undergraduate Programs
Indiana University School of Nursing
Indianapolis, Indiana
Chapter 8

Betty J. Horton, PhD, CRNA, FAAN
Manager for the International Federation of Nurse Anaesthetists'
Anaesthesia Program Approval Process (IFNA–APAP)
Tower Hill, Illinois
Chapter 27

Barbara A. Ihrke, PhD, RN
Vice President of Academic Affairs, School of Nursing
Indiana Wesleyan University
Marion, Indiana
Chapter 22

Pamela R. Jeffries, PhD, MSN, RN, FAAN, ANEF
Dean and Professor of Nursing
George Washington University
Washington, DC
Chapter 18

Jane M. Kirkpatrick, PhD, RNC-OB, ANEF
Head, School of Nursing
Associate Dean, College of Health and Human Sciences
Purdue University
West Lafayette, Indiana
Chapter 23

Michael J. Kremer, PhD, CRNA, FNAP, FAAN
Professor & Director
Nurse Anesthesia Program
Rush University College of Nursing & Co-Director
Rush Center for Clinical Skills and Simulation
Chapter 27

Susan Luparell, PhD, APRN, ACNS-BC, CNE, ANEF
Associate Professor/Faculty
Montana State University
Bozeman, Montana
Chapter 14

Julie McAfooes, MS, RN-BC, CNE, ANEF
Web Development Manager
Chamberlain College of Nursing
Downers Grove, Illinois
Chapter 21

Carla Mueller, PhD, RN
Professor, Department of Nursing
University of Saint Francis
Fort Wayne, Indiana
Chapter 12

Janet M. Phillips, PhD, RN, ANEF
Director RN to BSN Degree Completion Program
Clinical Assistant Professor, Indiana University School of Nursing
Governor-at-large, National League for Nursing
Indianapolis, Indiana
Chapter 15

Ann M. Popkess, PhD, RN, CNE
Assistant Professor
Southern Illinois University Edwardsville
Edwardsville, Illinois
Chapter 2

Martha Scheckel, PhD, RN
Professor and Chairperson
Winona State University Department of Nursing
Winona, Minnesota
Chapter 10

Elizabeth Speakman, EdD, RN, ANEF, FNAP
Co-Director, Jefferson Center for Interprofessional Education, Associate Professor of Nursing
Thomas Jefferson University
Philadelphia, Pennsylvania
Chapter 11

Dori Taylor Sullivan, PhD, RN, NE-BC, CPHQ, FAAN
Principal Consultant
Leadership/Education/Quality Consulting
Stuart, Florida
Chapter 6

Sandra M. Swoboda, RN, MS, FCCM
Research Program Coordinator/Simulation Educator, Simulation Team Coordinator
Johns Hopkins University Schools of Medicine and Nursing
Baltimore, Maryland
Chapter 18

Theresa M. "Terry" Valiga, EdD, RN, CNE, ANEF, FAAN
Professor and Director, Institute for Educational Excellence
Duke University School of Nursing
Durham, North Carolina
Chapter 7

Brent W. Thompson, PhD, RN
Associate Professor, Department of Nursing
West Chester University of Pennsylvania
West Chester, Pennsylvania
Chapter 19

Linda M. Veltri, PHD, RN
Clinical Assistant Professor
Oregon Health and Science University
Ashland, Oregon
Chapter 5

Reviewers

Amanda Alonzo, PhD, RN
Faculty, School of Nursing
Ohio University
Athens, Ohio

Mary Barrow, PhD, RN
Interim Coordinator
Delgado Community College—Charity School of Nursing
New Orleans, Louisiana

Suzanne M. Clark, RN, MS
Trauma Critical Care Clinical Nurse Specialist
Commander, Nurse Corps, U.S. Navy (Retired)
Adjunct Professor
California Baptist University
Riverside, California

Tina Covington, RN, MN, CCRN, CNE
Professor, Nursing Faculty
Delgado Community College—Charity School of Nursing
New Orleans, Louisiana

Lisa Davis, PhD, RN, NC-BC
Professor
West Texas A&M University
Canyon, Texas

Michelle De Lima, DNP, APRN, CNOR, CNE
Assistant Professor
Delgado Community College—Charity School of Nursing
New Orleans, Louisiana

Michelle Dellaria Doas, EdD, MSN, RN
Associate Professor
Chatham University
Pittsburgh, Pennsylvania

Kristina Thomas Dreifuerst, PhD, RN, CNE, ANEF
Assistant Professor
Indiana University
Indianapolis, Indiana

Michelle L. Edmonds, PhD, FNP-BC, CNE
Professor of Nursing
Jacksonville University
Jacksonville, Florida

Ruth Fiedler, EdD, PMH-CNS, CNE
Assistant Professor
Rush University College of Nursing
Chicago, Illinois

Cris Finn, PhD, FNP, RN
Associate Professor
Regis University
Denver, Colorado

Sandy Forrest, PhD, MSN, MEd, LPC
Professor and Master of Science in Nursing Program Director
Colorado Mesa University
Grand Junction, Colorado

Wendy Garretson, MN, RN, CCRN, CNE
Associate Professor
Delgado Community College—Charity School of Nursing
New Orleans, Louisiana

Suzanne Kim Genovese, PhD, MSN, MSA, RN-BC, CNE
Associate Professor, Coordinator of International Students, MHA and HCL Program
Valparaiso University
Valparaiso, Indiana

Lynn George, PhD, RN, CNE
Inaugural Dean
Carlow University's College of Health and Wellness
Pittsburgh, Pennsylvania

Linda Gibson-Young, PhD, ARNP, FNP-BC, CNE
Assistant Professor
University of Central Florida
Orlando, Florida

Joannie S. Hebert, PhD, RN, CNE
Instructor, Southeastern University School of Nursing, Baton Rouge Campus
Southeastern Louisiana University
Hammond, Louisiana

Sarah Jackson, RDH, MS
Associate Professor of Dental Hygiene
Eastern Washington University
Spokane, Washington

Maria Lauer-Pfrommer, PhD, RN, APN-C, CNE
Doctor of Nursing Practice (DNP) Learner
Duke University
Durham, North Carolina

Frances D. Monahan, PhD, RN, ANEF
Consultant Faculty
Excelsior College
Albany, New York
Adjunct Faculty
University of Arkansas at Little Rock
Little Rock, Arkansas

Bridget K. Parsh, RN, CNS, EdD
Associate Professor
Sacramento State University
Sacramento, California

Patricia M. Price, EdD, MSN, RN
Assistant Professor Rowan University
Rowan University
Glassboro, New Jersey

Margaret Reneau, PhD, MSN, RN
Online Nursing Faculty
Saint Xavier University School of Nursing
Chicago, Illinois

Rachel Spector, RN, PhD, CTN-A, FAAN
Associate Professor, Capstone Program
Boston College
Chestnut Hill, Massachusetts

Jason T. Spratt, PhD
Dean of Students
Indiana University–Purdue University Indianapolis
Indianapolis, Indiana

Anita M. Stineman, PhD, RN
Associate Clinical Professor
College of Nursing, University of Iowa
Iowa City, Iowa

Kimberly Kilpatrick Uddo, RN, DNP, CNE, CCRN
Professor
Delgado Community College—Charity School of Nursing
New Orleans, Louisiana

Ethel Ulrich, DNP, APRN, ANP-BC
Assistant Professor, Division of Nursing
Molloy College
Rockville Centre, New York

Francene Weatherby, RN, PhD, ANEF
Professor
University of Oklahoma, College of Nursing
Oklahoma City, Oklahoma

Peggy A. Weissinger, EdD, MBA
Associate Dean of Evaluation and Educational Scholarship
Georgetown University School of Medicine
Washington DC, Maryland

Diane M. Wink, EdD, FNP-BC, FAANP
Family Nurse Practitioner
Professor, College of Nursing
University of Central Florida
Orlando, Florida

Preface

As we reflect on the nearly 20 years that this book has been serving as a teaching guide for faculty, we are amazed at how much has changed in nursing education and practice, and marvel about how nurse educators continue to strive to develop the science of nursing education and improve their teaching practice. We note nursing education's earlier reliance on theories and practices from higher education and educational psychology, and remark on how the evidence for best practice in nursing education is now increasingly derived from our own science. We note, too, how changes in health care with the emphasis on patient-centered care, shifts from acute care to community-based settings, and the emerging era of connected health are changing the role of the nurse, thus requiring nurse educators to carefully consider the educational experiences they design for learners, so future graduates are prepared for practice in a changing health care system. The nurse of the future must be able to access, evaluate, and synthesize vast amounts of information, use clinical decision support tools, communicate effectively with patients as a member of an interdisciplinary health care team, and make clinical decisions for safe patient care. Preparing this nurse requires educators to guide students to higher-order learning, the deep and applied learning that prepares students for the complex health care settings in which they will be employed. The role of the nurse educator is changing as well, as we promote active learning in a "connected classroom," develop learning activities for interprofessional education, modify strategies for the increasingly culturally and linguistically diverse student body, and design curricula to facilitate academic progression across nursing programs. The variety of educational programs, designed to prepare graduates for system changes in health care, require savvy leaders who can guide curriculum development and program evaluation, collaborate with our colleagues in practice and from multiple disciplines, and advocate on behalf of nursing education to funding and policymaking agencies.

We have developed this edition of *Teaching in Nursing* to prepare nurse educators to address these changes in both academic and practice settings. For example:

- The scope and standards of the advanced practice role of the nurse educator have been more clearly defined and supported with the development of evidence-based core competencies. Certification as a nurse educator is now a credential that is possible to achieve. The chapter on faculty role reflects this recent emphasis on evidence-based faculty competencies and how the faculty role is evolving. As the educational environment continues to transform in response to multiple influences, novice and experienced faculty alike share a need for continuing development in the role throughout their career.
- Educators must be prepared to teach in classrooms that are "flipped," "connected," and global. Our classrooms are composed of students of diverse ages, generations, genders, ethnic backgrounds, races, religions, languages, and learning styles. Faculty must be able to respond to a variety of student needs, engage in inclusive teaching, choose learning strategies to appeal to a variety of groups and individuals, integrate technology into their teaching, and manage classes with larger numbers of students. To prepare faculty for these classrooms, we have substantively updated chapters on meeting the diverse needs of students, proactively managing the classroom learning environment, and engaging in multicultural education, and we have added a new chapter on connected learning.
- Students will be practicing in a changed health care environment and in settings in which interprofessional practice and collaborative practice will be the norm. New clinical models, such as the dedicated educational unit and residency programs, are used with the goal of more closely aligning nursing education with the realities of the practice setting. At the

same time there is a dramatic increase in the use of preceptors and adjunct and part-time faculty to support clinical teaching, all of whom must be oriented and welcomed as they transition to faculty roles. The shortage of clinical placements and clinical faculty and the shift of clinical placements from acute care to the community will challenge faculty to develop new and focused clinical models that ensure connecting classroom learning to clinical practice. Strategies such as simulation and unfolding case studies will complement clinical experiences. Chapters related to clinical learning experiences and simulation have been dramatically revised, and we have added a new chapter on interprofessional education.

- As nurse educators respond to the need for new types of academic programs, most notably the proliferation of doctorate in nursing practice (DNP) degrees, chapters on curriculum development and program evaluation assume new importance. Faculty must be able to establish dynamic and fluid curriculum structures and processes that can rapidly address changes in health care delivery. Developing academic progression models that foster seamless transition between program curricula will continue to be an area of curriculum development on which faculty must focus their attention. The complexities of developing prelicensure and graduate curricula have become more marked, and to this end we have included updated and expanded information on curriculum design and development in two distinct chapters, as well as an updated chapter overview on curriculum development. Recognizing the importance of continuous quality improvement and meeting standards for quality established by state boards and national accrediting agencies, we also have updated the chapter on program accreditation.
- As nurse educators respond to national calls for increasing the number of graduates with baccalaureate and doctoral degrees and to become lifelong learners, there will be increasing numbers of nursing programs and continuing education courses offered at a distance. Students and faculty are seeking educational experiences that are accessible, engaging, and interactive, and educators now find themselves in high-tech campus classrooms with multimedia projection capabilities, using electronic response systems and integrating smart phone and other social media applications into the lesson plan. Educators will find themselves equally teaching online and hybrid courses and using webinars and video conferencing to reach learners worldwide. We have extensively updated the chapters on teaching in the connected classroom and in distance education and online learning environments. All faculty must be prepared to promote active learning through the effective use of the now pervasive information technologies that make education accessible and convenient.

This edition of *Teaching in Nursing* has been written for nurses who are preparing to teach, for nurses who have recently become faculty members or staff educators and who are searching for answers to the daily challenges presented in their role as educators, as well as for experienced faculty members who are transforming teaching practices for the future. This book is also written for nurses who are combining clinical practice and teaching as preceptors or part-time or adjunct faculty and for graduate students or teaching assistants who aspire to assume a full-time teaching role. Given the current shortage of nurse educators, it is crucial that we continue to prepare and mentor future nursing faculty now. It is our hope that this book can help influence that preparation by providing guidance on the competencies essential to the effective implementation of the educator role.

This edition continues to draw on foundational work while integrating findings from recent research in nursing, education, and related fields. We have attempted to provide a balance of the practical and the theoretical, and urge readers to not only seek new evidence, but also test its application in their classrooms.

We continue to consider this book to be a guide, bringing under one cover an overview of models and approaches for assuming the faculty role; interacting with students; developing curricula; designing learning experiences; using technology and learning resources; and evaluating students, faculty, courses, and programs. Although the book is organized in five units, teaching in nursing is an integrative process and we encourage readers to select chapters as appropriate for their needs and teaching practice.

We suggest that readers use the book as a guide and resource but recognize that implementation must be adapted to the values and missions of the institutional settings and the personal style and philosophy of the faculty. We intend for this book to stimulate faculty to engage in the scholarship of teaching and learning by reflecting on their own teaching practices, implementing and evaluating new approaches to creating an interactive and inclusive learning community, and conducting their own educational research in classroom and clinical settings.

When we wrote the first edition of this book almost 20 years ago, we did so because we believed that the role of the nurse educator was an exciting and rewarding role, one that required nurturing and development over time. It was our goal to provide a comprehensive resource for faculty that would help guide them as they developed their practice as nurse educators. We still believe this is an exciting time to embrace a career in nursing education and teach nursing—a time that is filled with many challenges, opportunities, and rewards for those who step forward to accept the responsibility. It is our hope that this book provides those who engage in the rewarding activity of teaching the future of our profession—our students—with a resource that will lead to greater fulfillment of the teaching role.

Diane M. Billings
Judith A. Halstead
October, 2015

Acknowledgments

We thank the contributors to this edition of this book who shared their experience and expertise with us and the readers. We continue to value and build on the work of the original chapter authors, recognize the work of sustaining contributors, and welcome contributors who are new to the book. We also thank those who served as reviewers of the book for their insightful comments, as well as the many nurse educators who have used the book over the past few years. *Teaching in Nursing* is a public and peer-reviewed work and we appreciate the feedback from a variety of readers.

Many thanks, as well, to those who made the production process easier. We especially thank Louise Clendenen for her administrative support—her organizational skills were a tremendous assistance to us in the preparation of the manuscript. We also acknowledge the editorial support at Elsevier: Robin Carter, Laura Goodrich, and Lee Henderson.

As always, we thank our families and colleagues for their continued support and encouragement throughout this project. We also offer special thanks to our students, who continue to be our own guides to teaching in nursing.

Diane M. Billings
Judith A. Halstead

1 Teaching in Nursing*

The Faculty Role

Mary L. Fisher, PhD, MSN, RN

Over time, as nursing education has moved from the service sector to college and university campuses, the role of nursing faculty has evolved, becoming increasingly complex. As higher education and the science of nursing have developed, the effect on nursing education has been tremendous.

Nursing education is enmeshed in sweeping changes. The forces driving these changes are numerous and difficult to isolate; they include the severe nursing faculty shortage, the increasing multiculturalism of society, the decreasing financial resources in education and health care, changes in the delivery of health care through health care reform, the integration of evidence-based practice and the need for more nurses with higher degrees, expanding technology and the accompanying knowledge explosion, the need for lifelong learning, a shifting emphasis to learning instead of teaching, and the increasing public demand for accountability of educational outcomes. There has been a call by the federal government and others to build more points of student assessment into postsecondary education to provide evidence that outcomes are being met in an effort to hold colleges and universities accountable for the learning experiences they provide (Dwyer, Millett, & Payne, 2006). These are just a few of the issues that educators must consider as they fulfill the responsibilities of their role.

The need to maintain strong clinical skills within the context of a continuing critical shortage of nurses that is projected to last for decades has created an additional challenge for nurse educators (Beck & Ruth-Sahd, 2013). The requirement to maintain certification qualifications in their specialties is another factor contributing to work strain for nurse educators. In addition to clinical certifications, nurse educators now have the additional option of seeking credentialing as a certified nurse educator (CNE) through the National League for Nursing's (NLN) Academic Nurse Educator Certification Program (National League for Nursing (NLN), 2014). This additional affirmation of teaching expertise helps to close the widening practice–education gap. As of 2013, more than 3800 nurse educators had achieved CNE certification (Hagler, Poindexter, & Lindell, 2014), and it is estimated the number will reach 5000 by 2016.

To meet projected demands for registered nurses, nursing programs must increase their graduation rates, especially for nurses with higher degrees (Institute of Medicine [IOM], 2010; US Department of Health and Human Services, 2010). According to the American Association of Colleges of Nursing (AACN), 78,089 qualified applicants were turned away from baccalaureate and graduate nursing programs because of lack of available faculty and clinical resources (American Association of Colleges of Nursing (AACN), 2014). The *Future of Nursing* report released by the Institute of Medicine (2010) issued a call for a nursing workforce in which 80% of nurses will have a bachelor's degree in nursing by 2020 as well as doubling the number of nurses prepared with a doctorate. At the same time, the Tri-Council for Nursing (2010)—made up of the AACN, the American Nurses Association, the American Organization of Nurse Executives, and the NLN—reports a scarcity of prepared nursing faculty. Only one in four full-time nursing faculty held a doctoral degree in 2009, whereas two-thirds were masters prepared (Kaufman, 2010).

The demand for more nurses in service settings with advanced degrees and a scarcity of prepared

*The author acknowledges the work of Linda M Finke, PhD, RN, in the previous editions of the chapter.

nursing faculty have placed a tremendous burden on nursing education and the faculty trying to meet the growing needs. Nursing education is in a crisis, overloaded by the demand to teach more students with fewer faculty members.

The faculty shortage is being exacerbated by the projection that 500,000 nursing faculty will retire in the next 10 years (Aiken, 2011). Nearly 76% of full-time nursing faculty were older than 45 in 2009 (Kaufman, 2010). According to the AACN, "The average ages of doctorally prepared nurse faculty holding the ranks of professor, associate professor, and assistant professor were 61.6, 57.6, and 51.4 years, respectively. For master's degree–prepared nurse faculty, the average ages for professors, associate professors, and assistant professors were 57.1, 56.8, and 51.2 years, respectively" (Nursing Faculty Shortage Fact Sheet, 2015, http://www.aacn.nche.edu/media-relations/FacultyShortageFS.pdf)). The AACN found that, on average, nearly two full-time positions go unfilled in nursing schools annually.

In addition to losing nursing faculty to retirements, faculty leave academia at an alarming rate for other reasons. Factors identified that influence faculty turnover include workload, demand of a tenure-track position, perceived lack of collegiality, and noncompetitive salaries. Areas of satisfaction that enhance faculty retention include faculty identity (autonomy and role), research satisfaction, and sense of belonging to an academic community (Tracy & Fang, 2011).

As faculty in higher education face these challenges, they need to find new ways to teach and implement their role. Benner, Sutphen, Leonard, and Day (2010) call for a radical change in how nursing students are educated. As a result of their study of selected nursing programs, they concluded that nursing programs have many deficits, including weak classroom pedagogy, failure to integrate classroom and clinical content and experiences, and poor development of students' clinical reasoning and inquiry skills. They made 26 recommendations to transform nursing education, calling for a major paradigm shift. Nursing faculty of the future will need to embrace innovation and be advocates for change and forward movement if these goals are to be met.

This chapter provides a brief historical perspective of the faculty role; outlines future trends; identifies faculty rights and responsibilities; and describes the process of faculty appointment, promotion, and tenure (APT) within the current context. In addition, faculty development of the competencies related to teaching as a scholarly endeavor is discussed, and implications for change in the faculty role needed to meet current and future expectations and demands are addressed.

Historical Perspective of Faculty Role in Higher Education

The role of the faculty member in academia has developed through time as the role of higher education in America has evolved. Three phases of overlapping development can be identified in the history of American higher education (Boyer, 1990).

The first phase of development occurred during colonial times. Heavily influenced by British tradition, the role of faculty in the colonial college was a singular one: that of teaching. The educational system "was expected to educate and morally uplift the coming generation" (Boyer, 1990, p. 4). Teaching was considered an honored vocation with the intended purpose of developing student character and preparing students for leadership in civic and religious roles. This focus on teaching as the central mission of the university continued well into the nineteenth century.

Gradually, the focus of education began to shift from development of the individual to development of a nation, signaling the beginning of the second phase of development within higher education. Legislation such as the Morrill Act of 1862 and the Hatch Act of 1887 helped create public expectations that added the responsibility of service to the traditional faculty role of teaching. This legislation provided each state with land and funding to support the education of leaders for agriculture and industry. Universities and colleges accepted the mission to educate for the common good (Boyer, 1990). Educational systems were expected to provide service to the states, businesses, and industries.

In the 1870s the first formal schools of nursing began to appear in the United States. Diploma nursing programs were established in hospitals to help meet the service needs of the hospitals. Nursing faculty were expected to provide service to the institution and to teach new nurses along the way. Nursing students were expected to learn while they helped staff the hospitals.

In the mid-nineteenth century, a commitment to the development of science began in many universities on the East Coast (Boyer, 1990), thus beginning the third phase of development in higher education. Scholarship through research was added as an expectation to the role of faculty. This emphasis on research was greatly enhanced in later years by federal support for academic research that began during World War II and continued after the war.

Gradually, as expectations for faculty to seek funding for and to conduct research spread throughout institutions across the nation, teaching and service began to be viewed with less importance as a measurement tool for academic prestige and productivity within institutions. Faculty found it increasingly difficult to achieve tenure without a record of funded research and publication, despite accomplishments in teaching and service. As nursing education entered the university setting, nursing faculty began to be held to the same standards of research productivity as faculty in other more traditionally academia-based disciplines. It is important to understand that, while the emphasis on research continues, institutions vary greatly in this regard based on their missions and strategic plans. Potential faculty should seek opportunities in nursing education in institutions whose missions fit their interests and credentials.

Future of Faculty Role in Higher Education

A rapidly changing political environment and health care reform are now having a dramatic effect on the role of nursing faculty. Diminishing resources, increasing public scrutiny, and heightened expectations place a heavy burden on faculty in higher education. Changes in health care brought on by the Patient Protection and Affordable Care Act (2010) require that nursing curricula be updated to ensure that nursing graduates achieve competencies needed for the future. There is increasing emphasis on the teaching role of faculty without a concomitant reduction in scholarly requirements. Nursing faculty are also responsible to assess the outcomes of the educational process. The balance among teaching, research, and service is being reexamined in many institutions for its congruence with the institution's mission.

A revolution in teaching strategies is also happening as universities and colleges change the focus from teaching to learning. Sole reliance on the use of lecture is no longer an accepted teaching method. Faculty integrate the use of technology into their teaching and promote the active involvement of students in the learning process. Computer-mediated courses and the use of simulation technology are the future of higher education, as movement is made away from the structured classroom to the much larger learning environments of the home, community, and clinical setting. Because today's students, with their complex lives, demand convenience and flexibility in their educational endeavors, distance education strategies play an increasingly important role in the education of learners.

Furthermore, the future of nursing care delivery will be changing to a community-based, consumer-driven system. The shift in emphasis from acute care to an enhanced role for primary care must have an effect on the undergraduate and graduate nursing curricula.

There also is a continuing gap in the representation of minorities in nursing education programs, with the percentage holding at 10% for decades. There is a need to expand the number of nursing graduates from underrepresented populations. Even with this emphasis on minority nurse recruitment, all nurses must increase their cultural competence skills to meet the needs of growing underserved populations as the United States minority population continues to grow.

The American Association of Colleges of Nursing (2010) reports that there is a growing need for increased numbers of nurses prepared at the doctoral level, not only to teach but also to collect and analyze data necessary to evaluate the effectiveness of health care and to identify trends of future development. The clinical movement toward advanced practice nurses holding the Doctor of Nursing Practice degree creates an overwhelming need for nurses prepared with a doctorate. The majority of nursing programs (61.4%) reported not being able to accept more students because of the need for qualified faculty, with the programs predicting a growing need. All of these issues place nursing faculty at the heart of the nursing shortage.

Faculty Rights and Responsibilities in Academia

The professoriate in the United States has traditionally enjoyed a number of rights, including the right to self-governance within the university setting.

Governance includes participation on department and university committees focusing on academic and workplace issues of concern to faculty such as faculty affairs, student affairs, curriculum and program evaluation, and providing consultation to administrators. Faculty, in cooperation with administrators, share in addressing issues that face the university and the community it serves. Faculty are evaluated as "university citizens," in part, on their service on committees or task forces at the department, school, or university level. Leadership in national nursing organizations is also a component of the service expectation.

As constituents place more and more expectations on faculty for productivity, faculty governance is not as highly valued by those outside of academia (Plater, 1995). Methods must be instituted to maintain the participation of faculty in governance while allowing for less of a time commitment.

The core responsibility of faculty is the teaching and learning that takes place in the institution. Boards and administrators delegate decisions about most aspects of the teaching–learning process to faculty. This responsibility includes not only the delivery of content but also curriculum development and evaluation, development of student evaluation methods, and graduation requirements. (Trower & Gitenstein, 2013).

Intellectual property, copyright, and fair-use laws govern faculty and student use of works developed by faculty, students, and others. The easy online access of course content has added to this complicated issue by making plagiarism more common and easily revealed with the use of software. Most academic settings have policies that guide the development of "works for hire," which may include course content, written works, and products. Many universities now enter into ownership agreements, with some financial split of any profits related to works developed by faculty. A wise faculty member is well informed about these institutional policies so that there is no misunderstanding about ownership of course materials and other works developed by the faculty member.

Evaluation is a major responsibility of faculty. Faculty engage in the evaluation of students and of colleagues. Peer evaluation is a vital aspect of faculty development and is part of the documentation data considered in the decision-making process for promotion and tenure. Tenured faculty are involved in the development of fair and equitable evaluation criteria on which to base these judgments. Another responsibility of faculty is mentoring. Nursing faculty mentor not only nursing students but also other faculty members in their development as teachers and scholars. The mentoring of students includes formal academic advisement as well as coaching, supporting, and guiding protégés through the academic system and into their professional careers. The mentoring of faculty members also involves coaching, supporting, and guiding as they develop in their role as faculty (Jackobson & Sherrod, 2012). When starting at a new institution, even an experienced faculty member requires mentoring relative to specific institutional norms.

Providing mentoring to new faculty members is an especially important responsibility of senior faculty, because nurses are not usually prepared in graduate nursing programs for a role in academia. Faculty are dropped into an environment with unspoken rules and expectations that can be markedly different from those of their previous practice environment. Faculty know the role of the student from experience but have only seen the faculty role from a distance. Mentoring is needed to assist new faculty members as they learn to balance all aspects of their complex role.

The responsibilities of nursing faculty include teaching and scholarship, as well as service to the school, university, community, and the profession of nursing. Nursing faculty have the responsibility to expand their service beyond the university and local community to include active leadership in professional nursing organizations at local, regional, and national levels where they often influence national public policy agendas. As a faculty member climbs the promotion and tenure ladder, service responsibilities increase and leadership at the national and international levels is required. In a recent study, Young, Stiles, Nelson, & Horton-Deutsch (2011) found that most nurse leaders had stumbled into leadership without seeking such responsibilities and often felt unprepared. Their own way of being—acting as advocates, speaking their truths, and building consensus—put them into positions where others sought their leadership and they responded to those needs.

True success as a faculty member is measured by the person's ability to juggle all aspects of the faculty role—teaching, research, and service. Most institutions require a tenure candidate to declare one "area of excellence" on which their tenure will focus. It is important that faculty choose this area carefully and early in their tenure track. With careful planning and selection of activities, nursing faculty can integrate their clinical interests into teaching, scholarship and service, thus meeting the expectations of the role in the most efficient manner. On initial appointment to a faculty position, the faculty member will be well served by the development of a 5- to 6-year career plan designed to ensure that the candidate will meet the criteria for all aspects of the role.

Some faculty work in an environment where they are represented by a union. The American Association of University Professors (AAUP) is probably the best-known faculty union. Faculty can also be members of AAUP, as a professional organization, without belonging to a union. In a setting that has a union, faculty rights and responsibilities are affected by the negotiated contract.

Faculty Appointment, Promotion, and Tenure

Faculty are appointed by the governing body of the college or university and are responsible, in cooperation with the administration of the institution, for teaching, scholarship, and service (Association of Governing Boards of Universities and Colleges, 1996). Faculty are appointed to fulfill various responsibilities to meet the mission and goals of the college or university and the school of nursing and, according to their degrees and experience, are promoted and tenured on the basis of achievement of specified criteria. Faculty may hold appointments in more than one unit of the institution, including other academic units or service units. Criteria for promotion and tenure are based on the institution's overall mission and thus vary among institutions.

Appointment Tracks

Faculty may be appointed to a variety of full-time or part-time positions within tracks. The tracks may include tenure, clinical, research scientist, or lecturer/instructor. Within each track, faculty have the possibility for promotion through ranks: assistant professor, associate professor, and professor. Each rank has its own criteria for teaching, scholarship, and service, and for promotion within the rank.

Appointment in the tenure track may lead to tenure after a successful probationary period, often of seven years' length. The awarding of tenure results in a permanent position at the school of nursing. Reappointment and review of continued service in tenured positions are based on the evaluation of teaching, research, service components of the faculty role, and is termed *post-tenure review.* Non-tenure track positions require reappointment at specific intervals (e.g., yearly or every 3 to 5 years).

The *tenure* track is established for faculty whose primary responsibilities are teaching and research. A doctoral degree or near completion of the degree is required for appointment to the tenure track at most schools of nursing. A promise of excellence and the ability to be promoted to senior ranks is required for a tenure track appointment. Faculty appointment to this rank is considered *tenure probationary* until tenure is obtained after an extensive review process, generally concluding in the seventh year of appointment.

The *clinical* track, which does not have the protection of tenure, has been developed at many institutions as an educator track, clinical educator track, or educator–practitioner track, depending on the primary focus of assigned responsibilities. Appointment to this track is based on teaching and service (clinical skills or clinical joint appointments). Because this track allows for possible promotion through the ranks of assistant, associate, and full professor, a doctoral degree often is required for appointment to a clinical track. Although research is not the focus of this track, clinical or educational scholarly dissemination are required for promotions in this track. The increased use of clinical faculty is a growing trend as universities and colleges reduce their reliance on tenure.

The *research scientist* track is for faculty whose primary responsibility is funded research and research dissemination through publications and presentations. Although research scientists may have responsibilities for working with students; serving on dissertation committees; teaching in the area of their expertise; or providing service to the school, campus, or profession, their time is protected for research through their securing of research grants from external agencies. Appointment is based on evidence of or promise of a funded program of research. A doctoral degree and at least beginning research experience are prerequisites for appointment to this track.

Each school of nursing defines the criteria for appointment and promotion to ranks (assistant, associate, and full professor). These criteria specify the responsibilities associated with teaching, scholarship, and service. Schools of nursing also develop temporary positions to which faculty can be appointed.

Visiting positions may be appointed at any rank and designate someone who has a limited appointment (1 or 2 years), who is on leave from another institution, who is employed on a temporary basis, or who may be under consideration for a permanent position within the school.

The *lecturer* (sometimes called *instructor*) position is considered to be a pre-rank position. It is used for faculty who lack the necessary credentials (usually a terminal degree) for appointment to a ranked position. Some institutions have an additional level within this track (Senior Lecturer), allowing for at least a small avenue for advancement in this track.

Adjunct faculty are courtesy appointments for individuals whose primary employment is outside the school of nursing but who have responsibility as clinical preceptors or working with students on research projects. Adjunct faculty may be appointed at any appropriate rank.

Emeritus is an honorific title that may be conferred on faculty who are retired after significant service to an institution. Faculty with emeritus status may be granted specific privileges, such as use of the library, or computing services, or an office and secretarial support.

Students may be employed in limited teaching positions. These appointments, such as *teaching assistant* and *associate instructor,* are temporary and usually part-time. Student employees are responsible only for teaching or assisting faculty with teaching. They do not have the same level of responsibility as full- or part-time faculty. Teaching assistants must be assigned to work with a faculty member who assumes responsibility for the quality of their work. Student employees with teaching responsibilities often receive a level of tuition waiver as part of their compensation.

The Appointment Process

The appointment process in universities and colleges is somewhat different from positions in nursing service, and nurses who are applying for teaching positions in schools of nursing should understand the differences. A search and screen committee, appointed by the dean or another university administrator, manages the interview process. Interested applicants submit an application and curriculum vitae that are screened by this committee. Potential candidates are invited for an interview with the search committee, faculty and administrators at the school of nursing, and others at the college or university as appropriate. Depending on the requirements of the position for which they are applying, applicants may be asked to make a presentation of their research or to demonstrate their teaching skills. At the time of appointment, the applicant's records are reviewed by the APT committee, or other appropriate committee, which recommends a hiring rank to the dean.

Tenure and Promotion

Tenure

Tenure to the university is a reciprocal responsibility on the part of both the university and the faculty. The faculty member is expected to remain competent and productive: maintaining high standards of teaching, research, service, and professional conduct. Tenure also assumes that the faculty member is promotable at the time of tenure, and typically promotion to the next level and tenure occur at the same time. Tenure, then, provides the faculty member the protection of academic freedom. Academic freedom has been affirmed since 1940 by more than 200 institutions of higher education. It guarantees protection against efforts by government, university administration, students, and even public opinion to restrain faculties' free expression in teaching or the free exercise of their research interests (American Association of University Professors (AAUP), 1989).

On the other hand, academic freedom does not give faculty unbounded rights. For example, an individual faculty member does not have the right to alter the curriculum, the sequence of courses, or the content of established courses, or to subject students to discussions that are irrelevant to the course. Tenure can be withdrawn for reasons of financial exigency on the part of the university and for unprofessional faculty behavior. Finally, tenure does not relieve faculty from participating in performance review. Many institutions have instituted a post-tenure review process.

Tenure is granted after an extensive review, using published criteria, of the evidence submitted by the faculty member (a curriculum vitae and dossier). Most institutions affirm excellence through the use of additional reviewers from external peer institutions. The tenure or promotion review is typically held in the faculty member's sixth year, with tenure granted in the seventh year for successful candidates. Unsuccessful candidates are usually given a 1-year notice of non-reappointment (often referred to as "up or out"). At appointment, faculty with a record of significant achievement may be granted a specific number of years toward tenure, thus shortening the time for the tenure review. Faculty who have achieved tenure at a comparably ranked institution may be hired with tenure already conferred.

The tenure process is specific to each school of nursing and institution, and faculty who are appointed to a tenure track position should familiarize themselves with the criteria and process before appointment. Although the tenure and promotion process may seem mysterious, there are clear and specified criteria. The current attitude is to employ faculty who show high promise for attaining tenure and being promoted and to provide support and mentoring that will facilitate their developing into successful and fully capable members of the academic community. Although at one time tenure was an unquestioned right of faculty, critics are now questioning its true benefit, and some institutions of higher education have abandoned the notion altogether.

Promotion

Promotion refers to advancement in rank. As with the tenure review process, faculty must submit evidence of excellence in teaching, scholarship, and/or service, as well as other criteria established by the school and be judged by a committee of peers, external reviewers, school and university administrators, and governing bodies. Criteria and processes for promotion, like those for tenure, are established by faculty committees and are made public.

Faculty should familiarize themselves with promotion criteria and processes at the time of appointment and establish a relationship with the primary APT committee and the department chair, whose role it is to inform faculty about APT policies and procedures. As noted earlier, an expectation of senior faculty is to guide and mentor junior faculty through the tenure and promotion process. Some schools of nursing assign mentors at the time of appointment. If a mentor is not assigned, the newly appointed faculty member should seek one.

Mentoring for Faculty

The faculty role is a multifaceted one with multiple demands. Faculty, especially those new to the role, find that having a mentor, or mentors, is beneficial to establishing and succeeding in an academic career. Mentors are helpful for the career development of senior faculty as well as novice faculty (Halstead and Frank, 2011). Singh, Pilkington, and Patrick (2014) studied the orientation and mentoring needs of nursing faculty. Mentoring related to "establishing a program of research included how to plan a program of research, creating partnerships, developing an awareness of funding mechanisms, hiring research and graduate assistants, grant writing, publishing, and time management to balance demands of teaching, research, service, and a personal life" (p. 7). As can be seen from this brief description related to developing a research program, many aspects of the process could benefit from the input of a more experienced faculty and researcher. Faculty should carefully reflect on their career development needs and seek out mentors who can help them achieve their career goals.

Teaching as a Scholarly Endeavor

Boyer (1990) first proposed a new paradigm for scholarship that encompassed all aspects of the faculty role but placed a renewed emphasis on teaching as a scholarly endeavor. In *Scholarship, Reconsidered: Priorities of the Professorate,* Boyer called for the development of a balance between research and teaching when measuring the faculty member's success in academia. He described four types of scholarship in which faculty engage: the scholarship of *discovery,* the scholarship of *integration,* the scholarship of *application,* and the scholarship of *teaching.* In these four types of scholarship, the previously narrow view of scholarly productivity that rested only on the careful discovery of new knowledge through research has been greatly expanded. Boyer's model supports the practice model of nursing, which calls for more than the discovery of knowledge; it also calls for the application and integration of knowledge into professional practice. As Boyer stated:

> We believe the time has come to move beyond the tired old "teaching versus research" debate and give the familiar and honorable term "scholarship" a broader, more capacious meaning, one that brings legitimacy to the full scope of academic work. Surely, scholarship means engaging in original research. But the work of the scholar also means stepping

> back from one's investigation, looking for connections, building bridges between theory and practice, and communicating one's knowledge effectively to students. Specifically, we conclude that the work of the professorate might be thought of as having four separate, yet overlapping, functions. These are: the scholarship of discovery; the scholarship of integration; the scholarship of application; and the scholarship of teaching. (p. 16)

The Scholarship of Discovery

The scholarship of discovery is the traditional definition of original research or discovery of new knowledge (Boyer, 1990). The scholarship of discovery may be considered the foundation of the other three aspects of scholarship because new knowledge is generated for application and integration into the discipline, as well as for teaching.

It is through the scholarship of discovery that scientific methods are used to develop a strong knowledge base for the discipline. Evidence-based practice in nursing builds on the knowledge generated by the scholarship of discovery. Most federal funding traditionally has been appropriated for the scholarship of discovery, and until recently tenure decisions in many universities have been based primarily on the faculty member's engagement in the generation of new knowledge. The scholarship of discovery remains an important aspect of the role of many faculties, including nursing faculties. At the federal level, research efforts in nursing are supported by the National Institute of Nursing Research and content-specific institutes such as the National Institutes of Health and the National Institute of Mental Health, as well as private philanthropic foundations.

The Scholarship of Integration

The scholarship of integration involves the interpretation and synthesis of knowledge within and across discipline boundaries in a manner that provides a larger context for the knowledge and the development of new insights (Boyer, 1990). The scholarship of integration requires communication among colleagues from various disciplines who work together to develop a more holistic view of a common concern. The combined expertise of all who are involved leads to a more comprehensive understanding of the issue and results in more thorough recommendations for solutions to the phenomena of concern.

Nursing faculty have long integrated knowledge from various disciplines into their practice, and have many competencies that enable them to be productive members of interdisciplinary teams that study a variety of health problems and issues. With the emphasis in today's world on the development of collaborative, team-building, and knowledge-sharing efforts across disciplines, the scholarship of integration assumes an ever-increasing importance for faculty who must remain at the forefront of the information age. Nursing content often builds on the knowledge students have learned from other disciplines such as the biological and social sciences. The scholarship of integration involves designing learning models that guide the students to apply their previously learned knowledge to clinical situations such as with the use of high-amplitude patient simulation. Much scholarship of integration is being published in the area of patient simulation at this time.

The Scholarship of Application

The scholarship of application, which connects theory and practice, is an area of scholarship in which nursing faculty should also excel. In the scholarship of application, faculty must ask themselves, "How can knowledge be responsibly applied to consequential problems?" (Boyer, 1990, p. 21). Service activities that are directly connected to a faculty member's areas of expertise warrant consideration as application scholarship. It is in the performance of service activities that practice and theory interact, thus leading to the potential development of new knowledge.

For example, in nursing, clinical practice and expertise that result in the development of examples of nursing interventions and positive patient care outcomes meet the definition of scholarship of application (Paskiewicz, 2003; Riley, Beal, Levi, & McCausland, 2002). Activities that encourage students to use critical decision making, self-reflection, and self-evaluation are examples of the scholarship of application in teaching. Faculty practice in nursing centers is another example. Faculty should disseminate the knowledge gathered through practice and service activities by publishing in professional journals.

The scholarship of application, which includes service to the profession of nursing at the local, regional, national, and international levels, also involves developing policies and practices for nursing and health care. Nursing faculty often provide leadership in professional organizations and on community or national panels and boards.

The Scholarship of Teaching

The heart of the faculty role can be found in the scholarship of teaching. An important attribute of any scholar is having the ability to effectively communicate the knowledge he or she possesses to students. Boyer's (1990) definition of scholarship provides a model through which the special competencies and skills that are an integral part of the scholarly endeavor of teaching are acknowledged. Developing innovative curricula, using a variety of teaching methods that actively involve students in the learning process, collaborating with students on learning projects, and exploring the most effective means of meeting the learning needs of diverse populations of students are all examples of the scholarship of teaching.

The scholarship of teaching requires evidence of effective teaching and dissemination of the knowledge that is acquired as a result of teaching. Faculty should share their teaching expertise with their colleagues through publication and presentation of their innovative teaching methods and the outcomes of their working with students.

The scholarship of teaching brings many exciting opportunities for nursing faculty in classroom and clinical settings. It is based on the scholarship of discovery, integration, and practice (Shoffner, Davis, & Bowen, 1994). At a time when health care practice arenas are rapidly changing, curriculum models are being designed to meet the needs of a global society. The use of technology in education is increasing, and perspectives on teaching and learning are changing. The scholarship of teaching provides nursing faculty with the opportunity to demonstrate their innovation and creativity. It also provides a means for recognizing the effort spent preparing students to be competent health care providers for the future.

Summary

Although the role of the faculty member remains complex, Boyer's (1990) broad description of scholarship provides a model that legitimizes all aspects of the faculty role. Boyer has given credibility to aspects of the faculty role that extend beyond the creation of new knowledge through research to include teaching and service to the university, community, and profession. As a scholarly endeavor, teaching is the synthesis of all types of scholarship described by Boyer. Faculty can combine the role of researcher with the integration, application, and dissemination of knowledge. Boyer has provided a model for nursing faculty to use to develop their expertise in teaching as a scholarly endeavor (Shoffner et al., 1994). Nursing education has moved from the notion that there is only one way to do something to a broader perspective that recognizes the creativity and uniqueness of each student. The teacher is no longer the only expert but instead is someone who joins with the student in the learning process and evaluates the results of the teaching–learning process in a scholarly manner.

National League for Nursing Core Competencies of Nurse Educators

Teaching in nursing is a complex activity that integrates the art and science of nursing and clinical practice into the teaching–learning process. Specifically, teaching involves a set of skills, or competencies, that are essential to facilitating student-learning outcomes. The NLN (2005; 2012) published eight Core Competencies of Nurse Educators (see Box 1-1). These competencies encompass the entirety of the nurse faculty role (teaching, research, and service) that can be developed through educational preparation, faculty orientation programs, and faculty development opportunities. Most graduate programs in nursing, unless they are specifically preparation for the educator role, do not prepare the graduate to teach. Therefore mentoring of new faculty and strong professional development programs are essential for the preparation of nursing faculty.

Orientation Programs and Faculty Development

Orientation to the teaching role and the school of nursing for newly appointed faculty, as well as ongoing faculty development for all faculty, is assuming renewed importance as rapid changes in higher education and health care and the use of information technologies are creating new environments

BOX 1-1 National League for Nursing Nurse Educator Competencies (2012)

COMPETENCY 1: FACILITATE LEARNING

To facilitate learning effectively, the nurse educator:

- Implements a variety of teaching strategies appropriate to learner needs, desired learner outcomes, content, and context
- Grounds teaching strategies in educational theory and evidence-based teaching practices
- Recognizes multicultural, gender, and experiential influences on teaching and learning
- Engages in self-reflection and continued learning to improve teaching practices that facilitate learning
- Uses information technologies skillfully to support the teaching–learning process
- Practices skilled oral, written, and electronic communication that reflects an awareness of self and others, along with an ability to convey ideas in a variety of contexts
- Models critical and reflective thinking
- Creates opportunities for learners to develop their critical thinking and critical reasoning skills
- Shows enthusiasm for teaching, learning, and nursing that inspires and motivates students
- Demonstrates interest in and respect for learners
- Uses personal attributes (e.g., caring, confidence, patience, integrity, and flexibility) that facilitate learning
- Develops collegial working relationships with students, faculty colleagues, and clinical agency personnel to promote positive learning environments
- Maintains the professional practice knowledge base needed to help prepare learners for contemporary nursing practice
- Serves as a role model of professional nursing

COMPETENCY 2: FACILITATE LEARNER DEVELOPMENT AND SOCIALIZATION

To facilitate learner development and socialization effectively, the nurse educator:

- Identifies individual learning styles and unique learning needs of international, adult, multicultural, educationally disadvantaged, physically challenged, at-risk, and second-degree learners
- Provides resources to diverse learners that help meet their individual learning needs
- Engages in effective advisement and counseling strategies that help learners meet their professional goals
- Creates learning environments that are focused on socialization to the role of the nurse and facilitate learners' self-reflection and personal goal setting
- Fosters the cognitive, psychomotor, and affective development of learners
- Recognizes the influence of teaching styles and interpersonal interactions on learner outcomes
- Assists learners to develop the ability to engage in thoughtful and constructive self and peer evaluation
- Models professional behaviors for learners including, but not limited to, involvement in professional organizations, engagement in lifelong learning activities, dissemination of information through publications and presentations, and advocacy

COMPETENCY 3: USE ASSESSMENT AND EVALUATION STRATEGIES

To use assessment and evaluation strategies effectively, the nurse educator:

- Uses extant literature to develop evidence-based assessment and evaluation practices
- Uses a variety of strategies to assess and evaluate learning in the cognitive, psychomotor, and affective domains
- Implements evidence-based assessment and evaluation strategies that are appropriate to the learner and to learning goals
- Uses assessment and evaluation data to enhance the teaching–learning process
- Provides timely, constructive, and thoughtful feedback to learners
- Demonstrates skill in the design and use of tools for assessing clinical practice

COMPETENCY 4: PARTICIPATE IN CURRICULUM DESIGN AND EVALUATION OF PROGRAM OUTCOMES

To participate effectively in curriculum design and evaluation of program outcomes, the nurse educator:

- Ensures the curriculum reflects institutional philosophy and mission, current nursing and health care trends, and community and societal needs, so as to prepare graduates for practice in a complex, dynamic, multicultural health care environment
- Demonstrates knowledge of curriculum development including identifying program outcomes, developing competency statements, writing learning objectives, and selecting appropriate learning activities and evaluation strategies
- Bases curriculum design and implementation decisions on sound educational principles, theory, and research
- Revises the curriculum based on assessment of program outcomes, learner needs, and societal and health care trends
- Implements curricular revisions using appropriate change theories and strategies

BOX 1-1 National League for Nursing Nurse Educator Competencies (2012)—cont'd

- Creates and maintains community and clinical partnerships that support educational goals
- Collaborates with external constituencies throughout the process of curriculum revision
- Designs and implements program assessment models that promote continuous quality improvement of all aspects of the program

COMPETENCY 5: FUNCTION AS A CHANGE AGENT AND LEADER

To function effectively as a change agent and leader, the nurse educator:

- Models cultural sensitivity when advocating for change
- Integrates a long-term, innovative, and creative perspective into the nurse educator role
- Participates in interdisciplinary efforts to address health care and educational needs regionally, nationally, or internationally
- Evaluates organizational effectiveness in nursing education
- Implements strategies for organizational change
- Provides leadership in the parent institution as well as in the nursing program to enhance the visibility of nursing and its contributions to the academic community
- Promotes innovative practices in educational environments
- Develops leadership skills to shape and implement change

COMPETENCY 6: PURSUE CONTINUOUS QUALITY IMPROVEMENT IN THE NURSE EDUCATOR ROLE

To develop the educator role effectively, the nurse educator:

- Demonstrates commitment to lifelong learning
- Recognizes that career enhancement needs and activities change as experience is gained in the role
- Participates in professional development opportunities that increase one's effectiveness in the role
- Balances the teaching, scholarship, and service demands inherent in the role of educator and member of an academic institution
- Uses feedback gained from self, peer, student, and administrative evaluation to improve role effectiveness
- Engages in activities that promote one's socialization to the role
- Uses knowledge of the legal and ethical issues relevant to higher education and nursing education as a basis for influencing, designing, and implementing policies and procedures related to students, faculty, and the educational environment
- Mentors and supports faculty colleagues

COMPETENCY 7: ENGAGE IN SCHOLARSHIP

To engage effectively in scholarship, the nurse educator:

- Draws on extant literature to design evidence-based teaching and evaluation practices
- Exhibits a spirit of inquiry about teaching and learning, student development, evaluation methods, and other aspects of the role
- Designs and implements scholarly activities in an established area of expertise
- Disseminates nursing and teaching knowledge to a variety of audiences through various means
- Demonstrates skill in proposal writing for initiatives that include, but are not limited to, research, resource acquisition, program development, and policy development
- Demonstrates qualities of a scholar: integrity, courage, perseverance, vitality, and creativity

COMPETENCY 8: FUNCTION WITHIN THE EDUCATIONAL ENVIRONMENT

To function as a good "citizen of the academy," the nurse educator:

- Uses knowledge of history and current trends and issues in higher education as a basis for making recommendations and decisions on educational issues
- Identifies how social, economic, political, and institutional forces influence higher education in general and nursing education in particular
- Develops networks, collaborations, and partnerships to enhance nursing's influence within the academic community
- Determines own professional goals within the context of academic nursing and the mission of the parent institution and nursing program
- Integrates the values of respect, collegiality, professionalism, and caring to build an organizational climate that fosters the development of students and teachers
- Incorporates the goals of the nursing program and the mission of the parent institution when proposing a change or managing issues
- Assumes a leadership role in various levels of institutional governance
- Advocates for nursing and nursing education in the political arena

From: National League for Nursing. (2012). *The scope of practice for academic nurse educators, 2012 Revision.* New York: National League for Nursing. Included with the permission of the National League for Nursing, Washington, D.C.

for teaching and changes in the faculty role. Most schools of nursing have established orientation programs and instituted mechanisms for faculty development and renewal.

Orientation Programs

Comprehensive orientation programs are necessary to assist new faculty to acquire teaching competencies, facilitate socialization to the teaching role, and support faculty members as they develop as fully participating members of the faculty. Orientation programs should include information about the rights and responsibilities of the faculty and institution, information about school- and department-specific policies and procedures, an overview of the curriculum with an orientation to the instructional technologies and computer-mediated instruction used at the school, and orientation to teaching assignments and clinical facilities. Orientation is particularly important for part-time faculty members, who have fewer opportunities for contact with the school and faculty colleagues.

Orientation programs are most effective when they occur over time and provide for ongoing support. Some schools of nursing have school-, department-, or course-developed programs. Orientation to the teaching aspect of the faculty role also can be facilitated through a mentor relationship. Many schools of nursing have formal mentor programs in which each new faculty member is assigned to a senior faculty member, who guides the new faculty member. Other mentoring relationships can occur on an informal basis.

Faculty Development

Faculty development refers to a planned course of action to develop all faculty members, not only those newly appointed for current and future teaching positions. Faculty development is assuming new importance as faculty prepare for teaching in new and reformed health care environments and community-based settings, delivering instruction in new ways, and using new teaching and learning technologies.

Faculty development is a shared responsibility of individual faculty members, the department chair and other academic officers, and the school or university. It may include the school providing formal and informal workshops and sessions, credit courses, and informal "brown bag lunches," and encouraging faculty to attend local and national conferences related to teaching, as well as providing the financial support to do so. Because effective teaching also requires clinical competence, faculty are encouraged to maintain clinical expertise through faculty practice and by keeping abreast of changes in the field through literature review and attending professional meetings related to the practice area. Sabbatical leaves provide another opportunity for faculty renewal for tenured faculty, and are approved based on submission of an acceptable project plan for research or publication during the sabbatical leave. The university supports sabbatical leaves when the proposed project meets both the individual's and institution's goals. Specific outcome deliverables are required for sabbaticals.

Evaluation of Teaching Performance

To ensure competent teaching, the faculty members themselves, as well as administrators, peers, colleagues, and students, regularly review their teaching performance. Evaluation of teaching is a critical component of tenure review and reappointment for non–tenure track faculty. Results of this evaluation may also be used in making decisions about reappointment, merit raises, and awards that recognize and honor excellence in teaching.

Evidence for review of teaching effectiveness can be provided by a number of sources, including student evaluations of teaching, peer and colleague observations of teaching and teaching products (e.g., syllabi, case studies, publications, videotapes, computer-mediated lessons, Internet-based courses, study guides), letters from former students, success of graduates in employment, publications of students, teaching awards, administrative review, and self-evaluation. Methods for gathering data for evaluation include promotion and tenure review, peer and colleague review, post-tenure review, and the use of a teaching portfolio or dossier (Halstead & Frank, 2011).

Summary

Because of the multiple aspects of the faculty role, the demands of a career in academia can be challenging and require the ability to develop and change with the needs of the learner. To be successful, individuals aspiring to the role of a faculty member must be clear about the expectations of the role. This chapter described the various competencies expected of faculty members, as well as their rights and responsibilities.

Many nursing faculty have found that the rewards of the role greatly outweigh the demands and expectations. The challenges of the role provide many creative and innovative opportunities for faculty, leading to a career filled with diversity and productivity. Whether it be through teaching a new generation of nurses the art and science of nursing; providing service and consultation to constituents within a local, regional, national, or even international community; or generating new knowledge that influences the delivery of quality patient care through evidence-based nursing, being a member of the academic community provides faculty with stimulation and the opportunity to debate and collaborate with colleagues from their own discipline and others. Faculty are given a "laboratory" to explore new technology and solutions to the problems found in society and health care, while meeting an important societal need. In what other role could a nurse touch the lives of patients and future generations of nurses while developing a knowledge base that will assist in the further evolution of nursing and health care? The career of a faculty member is indeed a rewarding one.

REFLECTING ON THE EVIDENCE

1. Describe the teaching philosophy that would guide your implementation of the nursing faculty role.
2. Describe innovative teaching strategies you could use to prepare students for their future roles as nurses.
3. Compare the faculty role expectations for tenure in a college or university that has a primary focus on research and in one that has a primary focus on teaching.
4. Describe a project that would fit into the Boyer model as an example of the scholarship of teaching.

REFERENCES

Aiken, L. H. (2011). Nurses for the future. *New England Journal of Medicine, 364*(3), 196–198.

American Association of Colleges of Nursing. (2010). *Final data from 2009 survey*. Washington, DC: Author.

American Association of Colleges of Nursing (AACN). (2014). *2013–2014 enrollment and graduation in baccalaureate and graduate programs in nursing*. Washington, DC: Author.

American Association of Colleges of Nursing (AACN). (2015). *Nursing faculty shortage fact sheet*. Washington, DC: Author. From, http://www.aacn.nche.edu/media-relations/FacultyShortageFS.pdf.

American Association of University Professors (AAUP). (1989). *1940 statement on academic freedom and tenure (Updated 1989)*. Washington, DC: Author. Accessed 03.09.14., from, http://www.aaup.org/report/1940-statement-principles-academic-freedom-and-tenure.

Benner, P., Sutphen, M., Leonard, V., & Day, V. (2010). *Educating nurses: A call for radical transformation*. Princeton, NJ: The Carnegie Foundation for the Advancement of Teaching.

Beck, J., & Ruth-Sahd, L. (2013). The lived experience of seeking tenure while practicing clinically: Finding balance in academia. *Dimensions of Critical Care Nursing, 32*(10), 37–45.

Boyer, E. (1990). *Scholarship reconsidered: priorities of the professorate*. Princeton, NJ: The Carnegie Foundation for the Advancement of Teaching.

Dwyer, C., Millett, C., & Payne, C. (2006). *A culture of evidence: postsecondary assessment and learning outcomes*. Princeton, NJ: ETS.

Hagler, D., Poindexter, K., & Lindell, D. (2014). Integrating your experience and opportunities to prepare for nurse educator certification. *Nurse Educator, 39*(1), 45–48.

Halstead, J., & Frank, B. (2011). Planning your career trajectory. In J. Halstead & B. Frank (Eds.), *Pathways to a nursing education career* (pp. 161–181). New York: Springer Publishing Company.

Institute of Medicine (IOM). (2010). *The future of nursing: leading change, advancing health*. Washington, DC: The National Academies Press.

Jacobson, S. L., & Sherrod, D. R. (2012). Transformational mentorship models for nurse educators. *Nursing Science Quarterly, 25*(3), 279–284.

Kaufman, K. A. (2010). Findings from the 2009 faculty census: study confirms reported demographic trends and inequities in faculty. *Nursing Education Perspectives, 31*(6), 404–405.

National League for Nursing (NLN) Task Group on Nurse Educator Competencies. (2005). *Competencies for nurse educators*. New York: Author.

National League for Nursing (NLN). (2012). *The scope of practice for academic nurse educators: 2012 revision*. New York: Author.

National League for Nursing (NLN). (2014). Certification for nurse educators, Accessed 07.11.14., from http://www.nln.org/certification/index.htm.

Paskiewicz, L. (2003). Clinical practice: an emphasis strategy for promotion and tenure. *Nursing Forum, 38*(4), 21–26.

Plater, W. (1995). Future work: faculty time in the 21st century. *Change, 27*(3), 23–33.

Riley, J., Beal, J., Levi, P., & McCausland, M. (2002). Revisioning nursing scholarship. *Journal of Nursing Scholarship, 34*(4), 383–389.

Shoffner, D. H., Davis, M. W., & Bowen, S. M. (1994). A model for clinical teaching as a scholarly endeavor. *IMAGE: Journal of Nursing Scholarship, 26*(3), 181–184.

Singh, M. D., Pilkington, F. B., & Linda Patrick, L. (2014). Empowerment and mentoring in nursing academia. *International Journal of Nursing Education Scholarship, 11*(1), 1–11.

Tracy, C., & Fang, D. (2011). *Special survey on vacant faculty positions for the academic year 2010–2011.* American Association of Colleges of Nursing. Accessed 01.09.14., from, http://www.aacn.nche.edu/IDS/pdf/vacancy10.pdf.

Tri-Council for Nursing. (2010). *New consensus policy statement on the educational advancement of registered nurses.* New York: Author.

Trower, C. A., & Gitenstein, R. B. (2013). *What board members need to know about faculty.* Washington, D.C.: Association of Governing Boards of Universities & Colleges.

U.S. Department of Health and Human Services. (2010). *The registered nurse population: Initial findings from the 2008 national sample survey of registered nurses.* Washington, DC: Author.

Young, P. K., Stiles, K. A., Nelson, K. A., & Horton-Deutsch, S. (2011). Becoming a nurse faculty leader. *Nursing Education Perspective, 32*(4), 222–228.

2 Strategies to Support Diverse Learning Needs of Students*

Ann M. Popkess, PhD, RN, CNE
Joan L. Frey, EdD, MSN, RN

Students in today's college classrooms represent a wide array of diversity in learning needs and expectations. Nursing faculty are not only faced with the challenges of teaching students from varied backgrounds, of varied ages, and with an array of life experiences, but also are faced with the challenges of teaching students with significant technological experiences and demands on their time. Faculty must continually think creatively as they develop interactive learning environments to foster students' successful integration into an ever-changing and increasingly diverse health care system. This chapter presents a brief profile of today's nursing students and describes the unique demographic characteristics of students, along with strategies to improve success in nursing programs (see Chapter 16 for an in-depth discussion of multicultural education in nursing). Also, the chapter provides information about students' learning styles, thinking skills, and cognitive abilities. Specific teaching and learning strategies related to students' diverse needs are presented to enable faculty to plan for effective and successful learning experiences for all students and help prepare them for transition into practice.

A Nation's Health Care Needs Coupled with Population Projections

The rapid growth of older populations and a significant increase in ethnic and racial diversity will be realized in the United States from now to 2060 (National Population Projections, 2014). Although the actual rate of growth can only be predicated based on an estimate of net international migration, census trends depict growing diversity in the composition of our many communities. In fact, more than 76 nationalities are represented in the United States' 307 million households, and more than 40 languages are spoken (U. S. Census Bureau, 2011). With increasing data collection regarding the nation's diverse populations there has been special, and necessary, interest paid to meeting the diverse health care needs of its citizens, not the least of which is the shortage of diversity in the health care workforce (American Association of Colleges of Nursing, 2014b). Overall, the definitive Institute of Medicine's (IOM) extensive report, *In the Nation's Compelling Interest: Ensuring Diversity in the Health Care Workforce* (2004), paints a broad picture of the benefits of greater diversity among health professionals, the need for strategies to increase diversity in all the health professions, the promotion of both quality and quantity of interactions across diverse groups, the importance of an educational culture that promotes the exchange of diverse ideas, the challenge to reframe our thinking about unbalanced education representations, the reduction of financial barriers for minority health care education, and the promotion to all stakeholders for comprehensive support of diversification strategies.

Profile of Contemporary Nursing Students

The profile of nursing students in the twenty-first century is markedly different from that of the prior century. There are disparities in secondary education preparation for higher learning, student demographic differences, gender shifts, generational differences, and increasing racial and ethnic diversity. Meanwhile student and faculty age differentials are widening and faculty composition is

*The author acknowledges the work of Nancy Burruss, PhD, RN, CNE in the previous editions of the chapter.

less representative of the wider population demographic. Planning effective learning experiences to meet the needs of students has implications for nursing programs as the development of curricula is contemplated and necessary resources are determined to support the academic performance of all students.

Enrollment Demographics

The Bureau of Labor Statistics (2014) reports that the registered nurse (RN) employment opportunities are expected to grow more than the average for all occupations at a rate of 19% from 2012 to 2022. Therefore there can be little doubt that nursing is a sought-after career, even as a second or late career choice. Findings from the National League for Nursing (NLN) Annual Survey of Schools for Academic Year 2011–2012 (2013) provide assurance that the goal of a nursing degree continues to grow for all age groups, genders, minorities, and program types. The percentage of baccalaureate students older than 30 were enrolled at the rate of 16%, whereas the percentage of other prelicensure students older than 30 enrolled in associate degree and diploma programs remains high at 50% and 33%, respectively. Degree transition and graduate programs in nursing are also well represented by students older than 30: RN bachelor of science in nursing students were 71% of enrollees, master of science in nursing students were 67%, and doctoral students were 83% of enrollees. This wide age diversity among students in nursing offers unique challenges to nurse educators when these students are mixed in classrooms.

The college student population is also becoming more representative of the increasing cultural diversity that exists in American society. The percentage of minority students enrolled in prelicensure RN programs as reported to the National League for Nursing (2013) by race and ethnicity increased from a total of 15.7% in 1993 to 32.5% in 2012. Also, because of the positive career outlook, more men are enrolling in basic prelicensure programs with reported increases from 1992 to 2012 of 10% to 15% (National League for Nursing, 2013).

Competition for admission into baccalaureate, associate, and master's degree nursing schools remains significant, which also shifts the demographic profile of the student nurse. Of all qualified applications submitted to prelicensure nursing schools in fall 2012, only 39% were accepted (NLN, 2012). In a 2014 report, the American Association of Colleges of Nursing (AACN) stated that "though nursing student enrollment inched forward, … more than 53,000 qualified applicants to entry-level nursing programs were turned away" (American Association of Colleges of Nursing, 2014a). The major reasons for turning away qualified applicants, as reported by nursing schools, include a shortage of faculty, insufficient clinical teaching sites, limited classroom space, lack of preceptors, limited funding, and budget cuts (American Association of Colleges of Nursing, 2014a; NLN, 2012). At the same time, faculty and administrators are challenged to continue to recruit qualified, diverse student bodies and to maintain high academic standards and outcomes despite a critical shortage of resources.

The IOM report (2011), *The Future of Nursing: Leading Change, Advancing Health,* has been hailed as a landmark reference that directs vital attention to the development of a diverse nursing workforce to prepare the nation to meet present and future health care challenges. To achieve this goal, nursing programs need to recruit and retain students who represent the increasing diversity of the U.S. population.

Bridging Differences in Generations

Nursing students have a singular goal to graduate and enter practice as a nursing professional; nursing faculty are similarly focused on preparing and graduating *competent* nurses to enter the profession of nursing. Although students and faculty can agree on a similar focus, the lens through which each group views the teaching and learning experience is often considered based on subjective differences, such as age and generation cohort, gender, education level and background, economic resources, race, ethnicity, or lived experiences.

Age and generation cohort differences can create both implicit and explicit disconnects between students and faculty. With information extrapolated from enrollment in all types of nursing programs (National League for Nursing, 2013), we find that 50% or more of enrolled students are 30 years of age or younger. Contrast these younger student age groups with results from the 2013 Human Resources and Services Administration (HRSA) report where faculty older than 30 represent 97% of the nursing education workforce; 72% of nurse faculty respondents to the HRSA 2013 study were 50 years of age or older.

Students in nursing classrooms represent a variety of generations, each with unique perspectives and learning needs. Hence, the generation of the student will likely be different from that of the faculty. Aside from distinct age comparisons, generational differences present challenges for nursing students and the faculty alike. Although it is easy for both groups to make quick judgments concerning differences in values, attitudes, beliefs, and role expectations, a commitment by faculty to facilitate dialogue and initiatives to close the gap in value orientations create a professional commitment to support learning for all students (Bonaduce & Quigley, 2011; Hutchison, Brown, & Longworth, 2012). Students in education environments where generational diversity is accepted and supported will find themselves prepared to create better health care work environments. These workplaces will benefit from the graduates' comprehensive exposure to multiple generations and diverse backgrounds as they work with peers, health care team members, and patients (Hendricks & Cope, 2012).

Generation X or "Baby Busters"

Generation X represents a smaller cohort (50 million) of people born between 1965 and 1976 (U. S. Census Bureau, 2011). They are more diverse in race and ethnicity than previous generations, but not as diverse as their counterpart Millennials. These are children of Baby Boomers and their work ethics and loyalties differ from those of their parents. Many are children of divorced parents or working parents, and are referred to as *latchkey kids.* This cohort "has learned how to manage their own time, set their own limits and get their work completed without supervision" (Hendricks & Cope, 2012, p. 719). This generation was the first to demonstrate a need for work–life balance and self-sufficiency, coining the phrase "what's in it for me?" Generation Xers are comfortable with change and technology, as their members have participated in the development of Google, YouTube, and Amazon (Hendricks & Cope, 2012).

Millennials or Generation Y

Millennials, or Generation Y, are persons born between the late 1970s and middle to late 1990s. They are described as "the next great generation" and outnumber any previous generation at around 76 million strong (U. S. Census Bureau, 2011). Millennials grew up as highly valued children of the Generation X "baby busters" and are generally described as optimistic, team-oriented, high-achieving rule-followers. Aptitude test scores among this group have risen across all grade levels, and the pressure to succeed has risen likewise (Dols, Landrum, & Wieck, 2010). Millennials characteristically have good relationships with their parents and families and share their interests in music and travel. Parents of Millennials involved their children in academic and sports activities at younger ages to prepare them for success. Millennials are accustomed to living highly structured lives planned by their parents and have had very little free time. By the time they reach college, they have learned how to work with others and be a member of a team (Dols et al., 2010; Hendricks & Cope, 2012; Howe, 2010; Stanley, 2010).

Implications for nurse educators in teaching this generation include providing immediate feedback and structure in the classroom, providing for the safety of the students on campus and in clinical sites, and providing opportunities for service and giving back to their communities. Millennial learners are technologically savvy and comfortable with multitasking, and value doing rather than knowing. They are "digital natives," having grown up with technology (Wolff, Ratner, Robinson, Oliffe, & Hall, 2010); however, this can sometimes be a barrier to critical thinking, as students may have difficulties refining their abilities to focus on priority issues. Millennials as a group are more diverse than previous generations, with 36% being nonwhite or Hispanic (U. S. Census Bureau, 2011; Wolff et al., 2010). The parents of this generation expect that their children's schools and universities will reflect diversity and thus provide a richer learning experience.

Generation Z

The newest cohort of people born after the Millennial Generation is Generation Z, which represents those born from the middle to late 1990s to the present day. Other names proposed for this cohort include but are not limited to the *iGeneration, Gen Tech, Gen Wii, Gen Next,* and *Plurals.* Most important to note is that this cohort is coming of age and advancing into college programs and careers, thereby presenting yet another group of distinctly technologically focused students with contexts for learning different from educators (McCrindle & Wolfinger, 2014; Raphelson, 2014).

The implications of such generational demographics should be significant to nursing faculty and the profession as a whole. Teaching strategies that successfully engage the Millennial learner need to be interactive, group focused, objective, and experiential (Baker, 2010; Hutchison et al., 2012; Igbo et al., 2011; Wolff et al., 2010). Older students who are returning to school with multiple role responsibilities may require support resources such as tutoring, remediation, day care, and the opportunity for part-time study and entirely different learning strategies. Students may find that online courses help facilitate their ability to meet multiple responsibilities while seeking their education.

Incorporating a variety of teaching strategies, such as the selectively used teacher-centered lecture as well as entertaining, interactive, web-based media that appeals to multigenerational students recognizes both groups' learning needs and preferences. Faculty can benefit from the diverse generational component in their classes, and draw on the diverse perspectives represented among learners. Faculty must prepare for an increasingly diverse student body by closely examining the changing demographics of their student body, the adequacy of support services for the adult learner in their institution, and the flexibility of nursing curricula in their program (Baker, 2010; Hutchison et al., 2012; Igbo et al., 2011; Wolff et al., 2010).

Racial and Ethnic Diversity

There continues to be lack of ethnic and racial diversity in the nursing profession. Even with concerted efforts to increase the diversity of the U.S. nursing workforce, at 75% it still remains predominately White in composition (Human Resources and Services Administration, 2013b). According to the Human Resources and Services Administration (2013a), 9.9% of the nursing workforce reported themselves as African American; 4.8%, Hispanic; and 8.2%, Asian.

Similarly, despite an emphasis on recruitment of ethnically diverse students, minority students enrolled in schools of nursing continue to be underrepresented. The NLN (2012) reported that of all nursing students enrolled in prelicensure nursing programs, 12.9% reported themselves as African American; 6.8%, Hispanic; 5.6%, Asian; and 0.8%, American Indian, meaning approximately 26% of the students in prelicensure programs represented racial and ethnic diversity. These numbers remained relatively stable for the following 2 years. The nursing profession is challenged to recruit and retain students representing diversity. Chapter 16 provides an in-depth discussion on creating an inclusive learning environment and supporting the learning needs of diverse students.

Men in Nursing

According to the Annual Survey of Schools (NLN, 2013), men compose 11.4% of students in baccalaureate programs, 9.9% of master's students, and 9% of students in doctoral programs. Men in doctoral nursing programs compose 6.8% of students in research-focused programs and 9.4% of students in practice-focused programs (American Association of College of Nursing, 2012). While the data shows encouraging trends, there remains an imbalance in gender enrollment in nursing programs as well as evidence of male students not completing their respective educational programs. Various studies indicate the possibility of barriers in the professional schools that lead male students to feel marginalized and, in some cases, even to abandon their career choice before graduating (Burke, 2011; Rajacich, Kane, Williston, & Cameron, 2013).

Men in nursing currently represent approximately 7% of the nurse population according to the National Nursing Workforce Survey of Registered Nurses (Budden, Zhong, Moulton, & Cimiotti, 2013) and nearly 15% of the prelicensure student population (NLN, 2013). Numbers of men choosing to pursue nursing continue to grow through increased enrollment in schools of nursing because of the job flexibility and varied career opportunities (Burke, 2011; Rajacich et al., 2013). As previously noted, male students may feel marginalized and may abandon the field before graduation (Burke, 2011; Rajacich et al., 2013; MacWilliams, Schmidt, & Bleich, 2013). Given the paucity of current references, newer research in the study of men in nursing is needed to highlight the issues and inherent continued struggles of male nursing students. Nursing faculty should be compelled to recognize barriers perceived by men in schools of nursing and seek to rectify them.

Male nursing students present with their own perceptions and needs, whereby the use of sexist language in the classroom and textbooks creates a less inviting classroom for male students, including the determination that curricula in nursing programs are designed for female learners (Burke, 2011;

Rajacich et al., 2013; MacWilliams et al., 2013), especially in relation to testing, classroom lecture and discussion, and course structure. Tape-recorded interviews and diaries written by the participants to identify factors influencing male nursing students' course completion determined that the presence of male role models in nursing education was important for student support and inspiration. However, a lack of these role models creates self-doubt and social isolation in male students, potentially contributing to increased dropout rates.

The use of sexist language, lack of role models, and a biased curriculum all present barriers to the successful recruitment and retention of male students in schools of nursing and, subsequently, the profession. Challenges to public perceptions regarding men in nursing, dedicated initiatives to increase the number of men in all levels of nursing academia, promotion of scholarly articles on gender diversity enrichment in nursing, and mentorship promotion in schools of nursing and workplaces are but a few of the efforts recommended to dispel barriers, perceived or real, to men entering the nursing profession (MacWilliams et al., 2013). Faculty need to be sensitive to the learning environment they create within the classroom, and ensure that it is inviting to all students. Avoiding sexist language in textbooks, tests, and lectures is essential. Male students can benefit from peer support groups and exposure to male nurse role models.

Veterans Entering Nursing

Veterans who want to apply their Military Occupational Specialty after completing service to their nation have been faced with difficulties in transferring prior knowledge and skills into a professional nursing career. The Veterans Administration and HRSA have recently joined forces with schools of nursing to help make the transition from military service to nursing school a smoother and rewarding process. The Helping Veterans Become Nurses Initiative is the result of a partnership between HRSA and several branches of the military (Army, Navy, Air Force) to align curriculum requirements in nursing programs with corpsmen and medics' enlisted medical training to receive academic credit for military service in health care–related fields (American Association of Colleges of Nursing, 2014c). Additional and specific initiatives and funding have been developed to transition veterans' skills into nursing careers. Nine geographically distinct colleges and universities have been award grants totaling $2.8 million over 4 years to enable up to 1000 veterans to enroll in and complete baccalaureate nursing degrees (HRSA, 2013a).

In addition to the barriers researched and catalogued regarding men in nursing, veterans and the schools that enroll them are faced with additional potential issues that confront men and women as a result of military service. Prior traumatic mental and physical experiences require veterans to recreate themselves in a civilian world that has little insight into the challenges they may face entering college, deflecting beliefs toward the military, making personal connections to academic rigor and study requirements, or accessing resources to assist the former veterans to successfully complete their nursing program and transition into a professional career. Faculty can best help veteran-students by their availability and mentorship, willingness to listen, helpfulness in navigating a "foreign" academic system, and guiding them to liaisons and others positioned to provide the additional assistance to success (Bowman, 2014; HRSA, 2013a).

First Generation College Students

Many students experience the stressors of being a college freshman during their first year in postsecondary academic studies. Traditional students who enter college directly from high school to college discover an environment vastly different from the one they experienced over the preceding 4 years. In college, they need to create their own futures through self-directed academic activities amid a new social milieu. Some are easily dazed by the campus size, locating classes, purchasing books, arranging financial aid, understanding complex syllabi, balancing assignment calendars, and locating campus resources (Baker, 2010; Cohen, 2013; Shelton, 2012; Wright, 2012).

During that first year, freshmen need to fine-tune study habits, develop time-management and test-taking skills, and generally adjust to the workload of college studies. However, the most significant transformation for students is their change in classic theory approaches to learning from dualism to multiplicity to relativism (Erickson & Strommer, 1991). Initially, students see learning as either right or wrong (dualism), resulting in the belief that faculty know the truth and students merely absorb information to display knowledge during tests. As students progress in their studies, multiplicity in thinking develops whereby virtual truth in right or wrong gives way to opinion: faculty implant theoretical beliefs and students begin to think and respond to learning differently. The successful student eventually and, one hopes quickly, understands that thinking needs to be transformed by evidence and reasoning; hence, relativism.

Imagine the same development as experienced by students who are the first in their families to attend a postsecondary institution. They have no family member or close relative who can mentor or counsel them through these different and difficult scenarios; they do not have family members who developed the self-confidence to navigate the college experience and can relay that same confidence to them. Postsecondary nursing programs and faculty can best assist first-generation students by developing student-centered environments that not only identify at-risk students but dedicate resources and personnel to assist them to successful program completion (Baker, 2010; Cohen, 2013; Shelton, 2012; Wright, 2012).

Barriers That Affect the Success of Diverse Students

Students with diverse backgrounds can face a number of barriers that hamper their ability to succeed in college. Cultural differences between and within student and faculty groups, the previously discussed gender and generational differences, and a lack of rigorous academic preparation are thought to contribute to the difficulty of teaching a diverse student body (Bednarz, Schim, & Doorenbos, 2010). The most common barriers are the lack of financial resources, academic preparedness, language skills, and role models among ethnically diverse faculty (Condon et al., 2013; Dapremont, 2014; Davis, Davis, & Williams, 2010; Igbo et al., 2011; Loftin, Newman, Dumas, Gilden, & Bond, 2012; Loftin, Newman, Gilden, Bond, & Dumas, 2013).

Lack of Financial Resources

Financial problems are a major stressor for students. Rising tuition costs and other fees, coupled with a reduction in government support for higher education, affect all students. Financial concerns may be particularly difficult for minority students who are often the first in their family to seek higher education. They often come from low-income households and therefore their families may lack the necessary financial resources to support their education. Financial aid in the form of loans or scholarships is becoming more competitive, and less money is available (Condon et al., 2013; Loftin et al., 2012).

Lack of Rigorous Academic Preparation

Insufficient academic preparation and lack of support can also prevent students from completing their program of study. Many Latino youth attend elementary and secondary schools with few academic and physical resources and are thus not prepared for the academic challenges of a nursing program (Condon et al., 2013; Donnell, 2015; Shinn & Ofiesh, 2012; Torregosa, Ynalvez, Schiffman, & Morin, 2015). Many colleges offer special enrichment programs to help students achieve basic academic skills, as well as adjust to the college learning environment. Through academic advisement, skills assessment, and assistance with developing study skills, instructors can help students achieve a better academic record. Through programs such as that of Lehman College in New York City (Georges, 2012), opportunities are created for individuals from disadvantaged backgrounds for precollege preparation, enrollment, retention, and student scholarships. Opportunities have included (1) improvement in recruitment of disadvantaged students into health care careers; (2) development of a rigorous retention program; (3) provision of scholarships and education technologies to support academic success; and (4) an increase of culturally competent, quality health care through the graduation of diverse nurses to provide services to diverse populations.

Another project, called Bring Diversity to Nursing (BDN), is supported by the University of Massachusetts–Lowell Department of Nursing and Bureau of Health Professions funding. BDN developed entrance requirement initiatives and middle and high school workshops; employed minority nurse recruiters; developed retention activities, including sociocultural activities; and summarized retention and success data (Devereaux-Melillo, Dowling, Qbdallah, Findeisen, & Knight, 2013).

Lack of Language Skills

For many students, English is an additional language (EAL), and the students may speak English at school and another language at home. Most studies of EAL have examined Hispanic, Asian, and American Indian students, but ignored other significant immigrant African students. Several studies have found that EAL students experience several barriers such as lack of self-confidence; reading, writing, and learning difficulties; isolation; prejudice; and lack of family and financial support (Shinn & Ofiesh, 2012).

Lack of Diverse Faculty

There is a need to recruit more faculty from diverse racial, ethnic, and gender minorities. According to data from AACN member schools (2014b), only 12.3% of full-time nursing faculty members come from minority backgrounds. A lack of racial, ethnic, and gender diversity among faculty represented in nursing is a reflection of the failure to recruit and retain the same diversity in the undergraduate and graduate student population. Furthermore, the lack of ethnically diverse faculty can perpetuate a culture of insensitivity to the needs of those ethnically diverse students.

Faculty need to embrace the cultural differences of their students and use available resources to foster a successful learning environment. Collaboration with ethnic student associations on campus could assist faculty to promote learning among their culturally diverse student population. Furthermore, faculty could work to promote student success by offering access to role models, peer support and encouragement, tutoring opportunities, and communication strategies (Condon et al., 2013; Devereaux-Melillo et al., 2013; Donnell, 2015; Shinn & Ofiesh, 2012; Torregosa et al., 2015).

Strategies to Increase the Success of Diverse Students

Many nursing programs have created academic success initiatives that include strategies specific to course learning, retention, and progression. Although recent reports (American Association of Colleges of Nursing, 2014b; Institute of Medicine (IOM), 2011; National League for Nursing, 2013) cite the need for increasing diversity in the nursing workforce, nursing leaders and nurse educators need to enhance programs and strategies to promote the success of diverse students. Minority students from diverse backgrounds and varying levels of secondary school preparation generally experience continuing disadvantages in the postsecondary nursing education environments (Condon et al., 2013; Dapremont, 2014; Hockings, Brett, & Terentjevs, 2012; Loftin et al., 2012; Saunders & Kardia, 2014).

Role Models and Mentors

Although the recruitment and retention of racially and ethnically diverse students in the nursing profession is an important issue, and many nursing programs are directing considerable efforts and resources to recruit and admit diverse student bodies, equal, if not elevated, efforts must be dedicated to assist these students toward academic success (Baker, 2010; Coddington & Karsten, 2014; Loftin et al., 2012; Shelton, 2012). It is important to acknowledge that many nursing programs rely on standardized tests and GPAs as criteria for admission. These types of recruitment strategies do not take into account the educational experience of many minority students and constitute incomplete efforts to strategize for success for diversity students beyond admission quotas. It is painfully obvious to potential applicants who are socially or economically disadvantaged, particularly when a limited number of admission slots are available, that they may be excluded when admissions are determined by GPA alone. Such selection processes reap outcomes where only a few diverse students are admitted, and many of those tend to be labeled "high-risk" (Baker, 2010; Coddington & Karsten, 2014; Loftin et al., 2012; Shelton, 2012).

Practicing minority nurses can be encouraged to function as role models and mentors. Many nursing students plan to practice in a hospital or community setting after graduation, and matching them with a practicing nurse is a way to instill the confidence that they can be successful (Payton, Howe, Timmons, & Richardson, 2013). Nursing school faculty could work with their school's alumni association and with diverse nursing groups to provide role models for students.

Faculty commitment is crucial to the success of all students, and those students who must also overcome barriers need a student faculty relationship with a faculty member who is not responsible for assigning a grade. Students report that mentoring by faculty is the single most important strategy for success to aid in retention (Baker, 2010). Other highly effective student–faculty–centered strategies include faculty availability, faculty tutoring, and timely feedback on clinical performance and test performance (Baker, 2010). It is essential for all faculty members and administrators to develop sensitivity with regard to the diversity of the students on their campus and awareness of the needs of these students. Faculty commitment to student success results in more successful students.

Faculty members who represent the dominant race at the school can also assist in the recruitment and retention of minority students by modeling a commitment to developing cultural competence among the faculty (Campinha-Bacote, 2012). Assessment of faculty cultural competence is an important step in gaining commitment and support of the value of working with racially and ethnically diverse students and colleagues. Campinha-Bacote (2012) developed a cultural competence assessment tool based upon her model of cultural competence, the Inventory for Assessing the Process of Cultural Competence Among Healthcare Professionals in Mentoring (IAPCC-M), to assist in developing a culturally competent mentoring program for faculty. Use of culturally conscious mentoring programs can help improve the success of minority and other diverse students in nursing programs. In the model, cultural competence is viewed as a process that involves the integration of cultural awareness to achieve competence in mentoring. Using the Awareness, Skill, Knowledge, Encounters, and Cultural Desire (ASKED) model as a basis for developing a mentoring program could help address the critical need for increasing and retaining diverse students in nursing programs (see Chapter 16 for additional information on multicultural education).

Faculty can also advocate for policies, procedures, and support services that assist students and support an institutional faculty "mix" that is diverse. Faculty members need to remember that many students feel isolated in their educational experience and therefore faculty may need to be more assertive in establishing and maintaining open lines of communication with minority students. Helping students access campus support services will help students feel more connected to the institution.

Support Systems

Participating in special support programs can increase the chance of academic success for culturally diverse students. Many schools of nursing have identified and implemented strategies focused on securing the success of the culturally diverse student. At California State University, a Minority Retention Project (MRP) was developed to improve the retention and success of its minority students (Gardner, 2005). The MRP was designed based on Tinto's Theory of Student Retention (1993) that those students who felt connected and committed to their educational institution were more likely to be successful in their academic pursuits and achieve graduation. Building upon that premise, California State University then identified the role that faculty played in providing a safe, warm, and nurturing learning environment, both in the didactic and clinical settings (Gardner, 2005).

Support for improved English language proficiency has been provided in the form of language evaluation, academic networking, faculty interventions, and social activities to enhance student ability to be successful in nursing school (Torregosa et al., 2015). Preliminary results of the program indicated that academic networks provided the significant mediation role between entrance grade point averages (GPAs) and academic success of students (Torregosa et al., 2015). Support for English as an additional language (EAL) students was provided at one historically black university in the form of language, academic, faculty, and social activities to enhance a student's ability to be successful in nursing school (Brown & Marshall, 2008). Preliminary results of the program indicated increased retention of EAL students along with higher scores in standardized exit and first-time NCLEX exam scores and improved perceptions of the learning environment (Brown & Marshall, 2008).

Meeting the Challenge of Inclusivity

Although faculty may believe that their classrooms embrace cultural and societal neutrality, given all the discussion and research devoted to the needs of diverse learners, nurse educators need to embark on an honest assessment of institutional support for inclusive teaching and individual classroom strategies that engage in inclusive teaching. It is one thing to gain an understanding of students' social identities and to acknowledge the important role that nursing programs and faculty have in the recruitment, retention, and success of diverse and at-risk students. It is quite another to be proactive and incorporate diversity into classrooms and curricula.

Inclusive classrooms are ones in which students and educators work together to create and sustain an environment where students feel safe to express views, course content can be viewed from multiple perspectives, opinions can be expressed to the greater understanding of all concerned, and all lived experiences (student and faculty) can be shared and valued with equanimity (Saunders & Kardia, 2014).

First and foremost, nursing educators need to recognize their own tendencies to stereotype students or to hold biases. This important step is of primary importance to create an inclusive environment for student and faculty interactions. Only after this initial self-examination can faculty (and institutions) proceed to consider multiple other factors for the establishment of inclusive classroom strategies, including an understanding as to what degree class interactions are affected by course content; prior assumptions and awareness of potential cultural issues in classroom settings; plans for class sessions, including student learning groups; knowledge of diverse student backgrounds; and evolving issues, comments, and interactions during class processes (Saunders & Kardia, 2014).

Teaching Strategies to Promote Success

If nurse educators in nursing programs continue to teach in the same way that they have always approached the classroom and student learning, there will be very little value and progress achieved in the transformation of nursing education for the twenty-first century. Teaching with presentation slides must be put aside to develop new ways of teaching and learning such that innovative teaching strategies, the employment of new technologies, and risk taking can lead the way to creative methodologies for learning for all students. Simulations, gaming, art, narrative, reflection, and problem- and context-based teaching and learning strategies have been successfully implemented to meet the diverse learning needs of students (Crookes, Crookes, & Walsh, 2013).

Summary

The recruitment of an academically qualified and diverse student body has been an emphasis of many nursing schools. The data are beginning to show that, although recruitment is effective, there is concern that minority students appear to be less successful than white students in graduating from nursing programs. It is important for nurse educators to reexamine their minority student recruitment efforts as well as the teaching and learning methods and support services available for these students. Recruiting diverse faculty and developing them as role models and mentors is essential to the successful recruitment and retention of diverse students.

Understanding Student Learning Style Preferences

The definition of *learning* depends on the theoretical lens used to view the process. Learning in nursing is derived from several theoretical models including cognitive–constructivist and experiential. From a cognitive perspective, learning is an active mental process in which the learner constructs meaning based on prior knowledge and his or her view of the world (Kolb, 1984). The focus is on the acquisition of knowledge rather than on the resulting behavior change. In contrast, learning from the experiential framework results from a concrete experience, reflection on the experience, and subsequent construction of meaning from the experience. Finally, the learner actively experiments or applies the meaning that he or she has created (Kolb, 1984). Promoting learning through the use of cognitive development, experiential learning, and other teaching strategies is the primary responsibility of nurse educators. Further explanation of other learning theories can be found in Chapter 13; they are not detailed here. The plethora of learning theories that exist give rise to the discussion of a variety of learning strategies a student may enlist to achieve academic success.

Within the educational program itself, fostering the development of cognitive abilities in students requires faculty to shift the major focus of concern from content to the student. It will be imperative that faculty continually "rethink" their approach to "teaching" and use varied learning methods to meet the needs of all students. The following discussion provides a description of a variety of learning styles, the assessments of those learning styles, and their implications for faculty.

Assessment of Diverse Learning Style Preferences

Competency 2 of The NLN's *Core Competencies for Nurse Educators with Task Statements* in the *Scope of Practice for Nurse Educators* (National League for Nursing, 2012a) states that educators must facilitate current student development and socialization by identifying individual learning style preferences and the unique learning needs of students who are culturally diverse (including international), traditional versus nontraditional, and at risk (e.g., those who are educationally disadvantaged, learning or physically challenged, or experiencing social and economic issues; NLN, 2012a). Over the years, learning styles and preferences have been discussed and measured profusely in the literature. Learning style preference is the manner in which a learner perceives, interacts with, and responds most effectively to the learning environment (Kolb & Kolb, 2005). Components of learning style are the cognitive, affective, and physiologic elements, all of which may be influenced by a person's cultural background.

The literature supports the existence of learning styles or, more aptly, *learner preferences* (Kolb & Kolb, 2005). However, because of a lack of evidence connecting outcomes to learning preferences, some researchers assert that there is no strong evidence that a teacher should tailor instruction to a particular learning style (Pashler, McDaniel, Rohrer, & Bjork, 2008). Instead, these researchers argue that faculty should put effort into matching instruction to the content they are teaching and the expected learning outcomes. Nurse educators are challenged to identify learning-style preferences and develop appropriate learning experiences to match content that will meet the complex needs of the current nursing student (Fountain & Alfred, 2009; Pettigrew, Dienger, & O'Brien King, 2011). Learning style preferences and strategies should be identified early in the undergraduate nursing curriculum with the intent to empower individual students to use their knowledge of learning style preferences to achieve positive outcomes (Dapremont, 2014).

As a group, underrepresented minority students and nontraditional students have diverse learning style and cultural learning preferences (Bednarz et al., 2010). Acknowledgment of diverse students' learning styles enhances the learning environment while supporting academic achievement (Choi, Lee, & Jung, 2008). Advocates of learning style models posit that students learn in different ways; however, there is a lack of evidence to support that students *only* learn in those preferred ways (Pashler et al., 2008). Therefore the use of learning style inventories should be tempered and used as one guide to better understand students' learning needs. The following discussion briefly describes several widely used learning style models.

Learning Style Frameworks and Models

Several learning style models guide faculty in their understanding of student preferences. The Witkin (Witkin & Goodenough, 1981) and Myers-Briggs (McCauley, 1990) models are described as the innermost personality factors models.

The Witkin model is a measure of field-dependent/field-independent cognitive style that assesses the manner in which students perceive and process information and classifies students along a continuum of field dependence to field independence. The field dependence–independence model describes individuals' approach to the perception, acquisition, processing organization, and application of information. These instruments distinguish field-independent from field-dependent cognitive styles. Field-independent people tend to be more autonomous when it comes to the development of unfamiliar technical skills and problem solving, and less autonomous in development of interpersonal skills. Field-dependent students prefer a more structured social learning environment and require feedback for success (Witkin & Goodenough, 1981). Noble, Miller, and Heckman (2008) reported nursing students were classified as more field dependent than students in other health-related disciplines. Because of their cognitive processing requirements, field-dependent nursing students may be at risk for academic failure. Therefore instructional strategies tailored to students' needs should be incorporated into the nursing curriculum. The Myers-Briggs Type Indicator defines 16 personality types via the use of four factors. The factors used by this model are extroversion (focus on people)–introversion (ideas); sensors (detail oriented)–intuitors (imagination oriented); thinkers–feelers; and judgers–perceivers (Hirsh, Hirsh, & Hirsh, 2009). It is a helpful tool, as it encourages individuals to recognize their strengths and understand their areas to improve.

The Kolb Model of Experiential Learning (1978) is an information processing model that classifies students in one of four learning style preferences based upon how they perceive information and learn information. Kolb believed that learning required different abilities that include concrete experience (CE), abstract conceptualization (AC), active experimentation (AE) or reflective observation (RO) (Hauer, Straub, & Wolf, 2005). The learning style preferences are diverging (CE/RO), assimilating (AC/RO), converging (AC/AE), and accommodating (CE/AE). This model states that students use any of the four styles some of the time by claiming that the classification is a preferred method, not an exclusive one. Kolb's Learning Style Inventory (LSI) categorizes students according to this model

(Willcoxson & Prosser, 1996). The Kolb LSI-IIa Survey is developed from Kolb's (1978) four-stage model of experiential learning. The Kolb LSI (www.learningfromexperience.com) is one of the most commonly used LSIs in nursing education, as well as in other disciplines. Table 2-1 describes learning activities corresponding to various types of learning styles according to Kolb's LSI.

Gregorc's (1982) mind style model identifies two dimensions to how the mind processes information: a perceptual quality ranging from concrete to abstract and an ordering quality ranging from sequential to random. The learner is classified according to one of four styles using the Gregorc Style Delineator (GSD). The four learning styles are abstract sequential, concrete sequential, abstract random, and concrete random. The GSD is commercially available (www.gregorc.com). The instrument asks the respondent to rank 10 sets of four words that correspond to the four poles. Students and faculty can self-administer, self-score, and self-interpret the GSD (Hawk & Shah, 2007). Examples of teaching learning strategies corresponding to the Gregorc learning styles are in Table 2-2.

The Dunn, Dunn, and Price (1996) Productivity Environmental Preference Survey (PEPS) provides information about patterns through which learning occurs. The theory underpinning development of the PEPS is that students possess biologically based physical and environmental learning preferences that, along with well-established traitlike emotional and sociological preferences, combine to form an individual learning style profile.

An adaptation of the PEPS (Dunn et al., 1996), the Self-Assessment Inventory (SAI) was created by the Assessment Technologies Institute (2000). The SAI assesses students' personal characteristics and attitudes as they relate to the qualities of a successful nursing candidate. The SAI is composed of a number of subscales designed to measure the individual in four areas: critical thinking, learning styles, professional characteristics, and work values. The learning styles content area has a subscale with factors such as physical (visual, auditory, tactile) and sociological (individual and group) that parallel the PEPS elements.

TABLE 2-2 Teaching and Learning Strategies Corresponding to Gregorc Learning Styles

Concrete Sequential	**Abstract Sequential**	**Abstract Random**	**Concrete Random**
Worksheets	Lectures	Mapping	Brainstorming
Outlines	Outlines	Group work	Case studies (unfolding)
Charts	Readings	Music	Hands on experience
Demonstrations	Audio tapes	Humor	Simulations
Field trips	Writing reports	Role Play	Problem solving
Diagrams	Doing research	Interviewing	Investigations
Flowcharts	Term papers	Journaling	Mapping

Source: Adapted from Hawk, Thomas, Shah, Amit. Using Learning Style Instruments to Enhance Student Learning. Vol 5, 1. January 2007, Wiley.

Fleming's (2001) model suggests four categories that reflect the experiences of the students. The acronym *VARK* is used to indicate the following categories: visual (V), auditory (A), read and write (R), and kinesthetic (K). The VARK questions and results focus on the ways in which people like to receive information and the ways in which they like to deliver their communication.

TABLE 2-1 Teaching and Learning Strategies Corresponding to Kolb Learning Style Preferences

Concrete Experience	**Reflective Observation**	**Abstract Conceptualization**	**Active Experimentation**
Lecture	Thought questions	Lecture	Lecture examples
Problem sets	Brainstorming	Papers	Laboratories
Readings	Discussions	Text reading	Case studies
Films	Logs	Projects	Homework
Simulations	Personal journals	Model building	Projects
Laboratories			
Field work, observations	Reflective writing	Model critiques	Field work, observations

Source: Adapted from Hawk, Thomas, Shah, Amit. Using Learning Style Instruments to Enhance Student Learning. Vol 5, 1. January 2007, Wiley.

The VARK Inventory provides metrics in each of the four perceptual modes, with individuals having preferences for anywhere from one to all four. The free VARK questionnaire (http://vark-learn.com/the-vark-questionnaire/) offers thirteen statements that describe a situation and ask the respondent to pick one or more of three or four actions that the respondent could take. Each corresponds with a VARK learning style preference. Fleming (2001) reported that 41% of the general population has a single style preference, whereas 21% demonstrates a preference for all four styles. Only 27% of the population has a preference for two styles and 9% has a preference for three styles. Recommended teaching strategies that correspond to VARK learning styles are in Table 2-3.

Implications of Learning Style Preferences

Currently, obtaining knowledge of the learner and his or her characteristics is a vastly underused but complex approach to improving teaching and learning strategies. To address this concern, faculty should be encouraged to assess student learning style preferences using one of the many instruments available to help students develop an awareness of their preferred learning styles (Fleming, Mckee, & Huntley-Moore, 2011; Hallin, 2014; Robinson, Scollan-Koliopoulos, Kamienski, & Burke, 2012). The results would also enhance faculty ability to select and design learning activities that appeal to a broad range of student learner preferences, rather than to narrow teaching strategies to specific learning styles.

TABLE 2-3 Teaching and Learning Strategies Corresponding with VARK Learning Styles

Visual	Aural	Read/Write	Kinesthetic
Diagrams and graphs	Debates	Books and texts	Real-life examples
Charts	Discussions	Reading	Demonstrations
Written text with varied fonts	Audio tapes	Note taking	Simulations and role play
Designs	Seminars Music	Multiple choice Essays	Working models Physical activity

VARK, Visual, auditory, read and write, and kinesthetic.
Source: Adapted from Hawk, Thomas, Shah, Amit. Using Learning Style Instruments to Enhance Student Learning. Vol 5, 1. January 2007, Wiley.

Of further concern are achievement gaps that-continue to exist for diverse students. In programs with high numbers of adult students, there may be a larger number of students who leave the program because of family problems or job-related issues (Sauter, Johnson, & Gillespie, 2009). There are lower graduation rates among institutions serving high proportions of minority, low-income, and first-generation college students. Current students are striving to reduce achievement gaps, and it is important that educators augment their efforts (Brown & Marshall, 2008). Students are diverse in their experiences, cultural backgrounds, and traditional versus nontraditional and at-risk status. A one-size-fits-all educational accommodation is likely to stress and discomfort many students who might otherwise perform well if their individual uniqueness were recognized and responded to instructionally (Li, Yu, Liu, Shieh, & Yang, 2014).

As a result of this diversity, it is unlikely that any single teaching style would be effective for all or most students in a class of 25 or more. Students may experience a difficult transition caused by the loss of individuality in large classes in which personal recognition is absent. Faculty must employ a variety of creative teaching approaches to engage the diversity of learners in larger classes, such as personal response systems ("clickers") (Bachman & Bachman, 2011), short writing assignments (Boyd, 2010), and interactive assignments (Hourigan, 2013).

Faculty should assist individual students to identify their learning style preferences, help them to improve study habits, and aid them in the selection of courses or work environments that are compatible with their learning styles (Fleming et al., 2011). Students of varying generations might profit substantially from knowledge on how to accommodate their own learning style (Robinson et al., 2012). In class and clinical settings, faculty can use learning style preferences to create a learning environment where different types of learner preferences are valued.

Developing Cognitive Skills in Students

The increased complexity of the health care system requires nurses to problem solve and collaborate across the disciplines. The nursing student is challenged to develop cognitive skills that foster reasoning, remembering, and deep learning, and that ultimately leads to the development of clinical reasoning skills. Designing curricula that foster critical thinking in students has long been a desired program outcome in nursing programs. In more recent years, emphasis has been placed on clinical judgment, decision making, and reasoning, which are the desired outcomes of critical thinking applied to nursing.

Because of this changing emphasis in nursing education, critical thinking is often associated with problem solving, clinical decision making, and clinical reasoning. Problem solving focuses on identification and resolution, whereas critical thinking incorporates questioning and critiquing solutions. Clinical reasoning is critical thinking applied to the decision-making process related to patients and their diagnoses (Alfaro-LeFevre, 2012).

Students vary in the way they approach thinking and problem solving. The ability to think critically and make individualized but safe clinical judgments is a significant outcome in nursing programs. Benner, Sutphen, Leonard, and Day (2010) recommend that students develop a variety of thinking skills, including critical thinking, clinical reasoning, and clinical imagination. Faculty can assess students' cognitive development as well as their dispositions and abilities to think critically and make clinical decisions to guide students to think like a nurse.

Critical Thinking

Professional nursing practice requires using multiple ways of thinking and problem-solving abilities. The emphasis of nursing curriculum has shifted toward guiding students to become lifelong, independent critical thinkers (Kalisch & Begeny, 2010; Oliver, 2010). Nurse educators remain accountable for creating and implementing curricula that produce graduate nurses who are able to use critical thinking as a component of clinical reasoning to formulate appropriate clinical judgments (Mann, 2012).

Despite many years of discussing critical thinking in the nursing education literature, experts on critical thinking cannot agree on a definition for it, nor is there any effective way to measure critical thinking and the effect it has on patient care. Some research suggests a link between critical thinking and learning style preferences; however, the evidence lacks rigor and is not generalizable (Andreou, Papastavrou, & Merkouris, 2013). Critical thinking underlies independent and interdependent decision making. The critical thinker must have the attitude or desire to approach the problem and to accept that the problem needs to be solved. The critical thinker must also have knowledge of the problem's subject matter and the necessary skills to use and manipulate this knowledge in the problem-solving process (Bradshaw & Lowenstein, 2011).

Despite the difficulty of defining critical thinking, several critical thinking inventories have been developed and are frequently used to assess critical thinking skills in nursing students. These inventories include the Watson-Glaser Critical Thinking Appraisal (Watson & Glaser, 1980), the California Critical Thinking Skills Test (Facione, Blohm, Howard, & Giancarlo, 1998); and the California Critical Thinking Disposition Inventory (Facione, Facione, & Sanchez, 1994). For a brief description of each, see Table 2-4.

Clinical Reasoning

Clinical reasoning is the process of gathering and thinking about patient information, analyzing the options, and evaluating alternatives. This cognitive process precedes the decision to act. Reasoning is a cyclical process that depends on results of prior experience, and is the hallmark of the experienced nurse (Simmons, 2010). In one systematic review of 24 studies of educational interventions to improve nurses' clinical reasoning, there was a lack of consistency in defining successful interventions because of a general lack of study quality (Thompson & Stapley, 2011).

Strategies to Develop Cognitive Skills

Developing cognitive skills in students requires nursing faculty to implement a variety of teaching strategies appropriate to content, setting, learner needs, learning style, and desired learner outcomes (NLN, 2005). The following are examples of teaching strategies that have been associated with fostering the development of cognitive skills and clinical decision making.

Reflection

In the nursing literature, there is an emphasis on the use of reflection to develop and engage in critical thinking. Critical thinking is an attribute that enhances one's skill in problem solving and decision making (Romeo, 2010). Critical thinking is not a single way of thinking but rather a complex process.

TABLE 2-4 Critical Thinking Inventory Instruments

Instrument	Forms	Subscales	Considerations
Watson Glaser Critical Thinking Appraisal (WGCTA) http://us.talentlens.com/watson-glaser-original 2015 Pearson Education, Inc. Cognitive asssessment contains statements, arguments, and interpretations, requiring the application of analytic reasoning skills. Normed for 14 groups based on occupation/industry type. Use of "holistic score" for hiring, development and promotion of individuals. Tool available in multiple languages and forms (online/paper)	WG Form A 80 items WG Form S–Short Form 40 items WGTA II–Form D 40 items	Inference Recognition of assumptions Deduction Interpretation Evaluation of arguments	Form D includes more difficult items with improved differentiation Face validity of form D higher than others; items validated in six countries and United States. Available online. Reliable in health professions students. Passing rates in Form A, Form S tend to be high overall with limited differentiation.
California Critical Thinking Skills Test (CCTST) College Level Designed to be objective measure of the core reasoning skills needed for reflective decision making concerning what to believe or what to do. Numeracy form assesses quantitative reasoning skills	CCTST 34 items and CCTST with Numeracy	Scores are provided on seven scales: analysis, inference, evaluation, deduction, induction, and overall reasoning ability	Used with many health professions students. Available in 17 translations; online delivery. Studies in nursing demonstrate inconsistent results; lacks sufficient power and has inherent design flaws.
California Critical Thinking Disposition Inventory (CCTDI) http://www.insightassessment.com Measures beliefs, values, and attitudes and intentions on seven dispositions that move one toward critical thinking.	Companion instrument to assess the learners' willingness to think critically on seven scales 75 items.	Truth seeking or bias Open-mindedness or tolerance Anticipating consequences or heedlessness Systematic or unsystematic Confident in reasoning or mistrustful Inquisitiveness Mature judgment	Targets college undergraduates. Available in 17 translations.
Health Sciences Reasoning Test (HSRT) http://www.insightassessment.com The HSRT is specifically calibrated for trainees in health sciences educational programs (undergraduate and graduate) and for professional health science practitioners. Scores on this instrument have been found to predict successful professional licensure and high clinical performance ratings. Numeracy test adds quantitative reasoning	HSRT 33 items HSRT with Numeracy	Scores are provided on seven scales: analysis, inference, evaluation, deduction, induction, and overall reasoning ability	Similar to the CCTST. Can be delivered online. Items are written in the context of the health sciences workplace. Test has been normed in the masters' level, undergraduate, and 2-year college health professions students. No published reliability data available; relatively new test; few published studies with pharmacy students used as an admissions test.

Moore (2013) identified seven concepts among the various process descriptions of critical thinking. These seven concepts include self-reflexivity, judgment, skepticism, simple originality, engagement with knowledge, rationality, and sensitive readings. As nursing educators seek to assess their students' knowledge and critical-thinking abilities, providing opportunities for reflective learning on evidence-based practice can be an effective strategy. See Chapter 15 for further discussion of reflection as a teaching strategy.

Simulation

A systematic review of literature including eight simulation studies found that simulation improved critical thinking, skills performance, and knowledge of subject matter, although evidence of improved clinical reasoning was inconclusive (Lapkin, Levett-Jones, Bellchambers, & Fernandez, 2010). Researchers found that providing nursing students with practice scenarios using a human patient simulator increased their critical thinking skills, and that those who were assigned more simulated scenarios demonstrated a greater increase in critical thinking (Sullivan-Mann, Perron, & Fellner, 2009). Recently, the National Council State Board of Nursing published the first national simulation study with results suggesting that well-designed simulation experiences could be substituted for up to half of traditional clinical hours with comparable end-of-program outcomes (Hayden, Smiley, Alexander, Kardong-Edgren, & Jeffries, 2014). The effective use of simulation in nursing education continues to be researched; however, early findings suggest that when faculty are prepared and resources are available to design and deliver high-quality simulation, the critical thinking skills, clinical reasoning, and knowledge of students are enhanced. The use of simulation as a teaching strategy is discussed in depth in Chapter 18.

Assessing the Learning Outcomes of Diverse Students

Nurse educators have a responsibility to prepare students to successfully meet established learning outcomes and achieve licensure. Faculty use a variety of methods to assess learning outcomes such as mind maps, simulation events and demonstration, essays and reflective writing, and presentations. By far the most used assessment technique is objective and standardized testing. Entire course grades, progression, and graduation are based solely on results of objective or standardized exams. These "high-stakes tests" are defined by the American Education Research Association (2014) as tests that have significant consequences for the test takers, curricula, or institution. Nurse educators therefore must adopt a thoughtful approach to test development and policies surrounding standardized test use and the effect these exams have on all students who must take them.

Use of High-Stakes Testing

There is abundant use of high-stakes testing in nursing curricula. High-stakes exams in nursing have several defining characteristics: (1) they hold students, schools, and programs accountable by virtue of serious consequences for failure; (2) there is a clear distinction between pass and fail; and (3) test takers have a vested personal, monetary, or emotional interest in the exam outcome (Sullivan, 2014). High-stakes tests are designed to measure curricular strengths and weaknesses, as well as students' preparedness for the National Council Licensure Examination (NCLEX), and to provide recommendations for students' remediation. These exams provide critical information to schools of nursing where the first-time test taker rate is used as an outcome indicator of program quality and effectiveness by state boards and the public.

Literature on the ability of these exit tests to reliably predict student success or failure on NCLEX is prolific and not without controversy (Harding, 2010; Santo, Frander, & Hawkins, 2013). Faculty in nursing programs have implemented progression and remediation policies that use these exit exams as benchmarks that affect a student's eligibility for graduation and taking the licensure exam. There are also legal and ethical concerns with administration of a single high-stakes, predictive test that may restrict a student from completing a program and licensing by exam (Santo et al., 2013). As a result, the NLN has published a document to guide faculty in their decision making with regard to high-stakes tests and the policies generated (National League for Nursing, 2012b). See Chapter 3 for a further discussion of the possible legal and ethical issues associated with high-stakes testing.

How the use of high-stakes tests and the policies associated with them can affect diverse students in nursing programs has not been extensively studied. A review of the literature related to English as an

Additional Language (EAL) or English language learner nursing students included 25 articles citing cultural, language, and academic barriers to success for these students (Olson, 2012). Specific barriers includes reading speed and translation (Amaro, Abriam-Yago, & Yoder, 2006), lack of faculty cultural awareness (Starr, 2009), and use of grammar and language in multiple-choice test questions (Bosher & Bowles, 2008; Lampe & Tsaouse, 2010).

Faculty are challenged to incorporate strategies to promote student success on high-stakes exams by reducing barriers that inherently exist within a diverse student body. The literature suggests a number of strategies that students and faculty may employ to encourage success in students of diverse cultural, racial, and ethnic backgrounds. EAL students should be encouraged to keep vocabulary cards, to access native English and medical dictionaries regularly, to study in mixed (native speaker and EAL) groups, and to practice explaining the information in their native language (Coddington & Karsten, 2014; Hansen & Beaver, 2012). Faculty can also provide copies of lecture slides and class notes, and can allow audiotaping of lectures (Sanner & Wilson, 2008). Early identification of EAL students for referral to language support programs and tutoring is also essential.

Several studies have demonstrated success building test-taking skills of under-represented minorities through the use of peer and faculty tutorial support as well as supplemental instruction (Brown & Marshall, 2008; Sutherland, Hamilton, & Goodman, 2007; Swinney & Dobal, 2008). Providing EAL students an alternative testing environment as a way to reduce anxiety is also recommended (Abel, 2009) as EAL students often require extended testing time for reading and processing test items (Caputi, Engelmann, & Stasinopoulos, 2006). Encouraging students to practice many multiple-choice test items throughout the program and teaching students how to read and analyze items is critical to success (Lujan, 2008).

Testing bias also affects a student's ability to perform well on an exam. Testing bias occurs when a test or items on a test are "not readily understood by all cultural groups" (Dudas, 2011). It is incumbent on faculty to write and review exam questions to ensure they are free of cultural, structural, and linguistic bias (Bosher & Bowles, 2008; Hicks, 2011). One study of 664 items revealed a 47.3% rate of flawed test items on teacher-made, high-stakes assessments (Tarrant & Ware, 2008). Please see Chapter 24 for further information on item and test construction.

"Learning to Fly": Preparing Diverse Learners for Practice

The transition from education to practice is fraught with challenges for the new graduate. New graduates are faced with integrating their "anticipatory socialization" experience, the perceived expectations of their new role, into the reality of "organization socialization" (Scott, Engelke, & Swanson, 2008, p. 76)—in other words, what actually occurs on the job. New graduates report heightened work stress caused by feelings of inability to prioritize, delegate, and manage care of a group of patients; inadequate staffing; and a lack of communication and collaboration skills with physicians (Lin, Viscardi, & McHugh, 2014). Surprisingly little literature exists about the transition to practice experience of the minority new graduate. Since The Sullivan Commission (2004) on the contribution of a diverse workforce was published, there has been little progress toward increasing diversity in nursing to reflect the population. This may in part be due to a decline in the funding of the Title VII Nursing Workforce Development Grants Program, a government program designed to address these same goals (American Association of Colleges of Nursing, 2014d). In one descriptive study of 111 Latino and Latina nurses, fewer than 20% of whom were described as novice or beginners, 74% of the participants reported they had experienced bias in the workplace (Moceri, 2012). Recent work from the National Council State Board of Nursing on the Transition to Practice Model development indicates that employers report new graduates are not ready to practice (Spector & Echternacht, 2010) and that there is a widening gap between experienced nurses and new graduates (Orsolini-Hain & Malone, 2007). The efforts of the AACN, the Robert Wood Johnson Foundation, and other private funding sources are vital to the continued support of diverse student recruitment and retention.

Benner et al. (2010) recommend developing clinical residencies for all new graduates. Transition-to-practice residency programs are extended (6 months to 1 year) formal and informal learning opportunities focused on developing the new nurses' understanding of policy, standards, and structures of the work environment. The residency should include time for reflection and connection with other professionals as well as an extension of communication, confidence, and critical thinking competencies (Bleich, 2012).

Models of transition programs exist in a partnership created by the AACN and the University HealthSystem Consortium (http://www.aacn.nche.edu/education-resources/nurse-residency-program). The model incorporates five modules based on the IOM and Quality Safety in Nursing Education competencies and incorporates preceptor as well as classroom experiences (Spector & Echternacht, 2010). Further recommendations to specifically address issues affecting new graduates of color include the promotion of nonbiased interactions in communication as well as inclusion of discussions about cultural sensitivity and perceived language bias among staff and other disciplines (Moceri, 2012). A program at Coppin State University pairs students with professional nurses in a workplace mentoring situation, providing students with real-world exposure to the nursing profession (Gordon & Copes, 2010).

Summary

This chapter describes the demographic characteristics of the current population of nursing students and the unique needs of students from varied generations, men in nursing, and students who are not in the racial or ethnic majority in their classrooms. The chapter also provides information related to understanding learning styles and the cognitive abilities of students. Faculty are responsible for creating an environment that is conducive to learning. Likewise, students are responsible for identifying environments that will best help them to learn. Understanding students' diverse learning needs will help faculty and students develop collaborative partnerships that will foster the acquisition of the attitudes, knowledge, and skills necessary to become a nurse.

REFLECTING ON THE EVIDENCE

1. Assess learning style preferences with instruments that fit the needs of your students. How would you share the results of the learning style preference assessment with the students? How would you assist the students to use their learning style preference information and counsel them on learning strategies that will help them to be successful in their studies?
2. Engage students in creative learning environments that appeal to their diverse needs and learning styles by redesigning a course module to stimulate critical thinking through active learning. Consider how you could provide the students with a choice of learning strategies that would stimulate higher-order thinking.
3. Reflect on one of the courses you teach. What teaching and learning strategies can you incorporate into the course that will lead to a greater emphasis on clinical reasoning and clinical judgment? How can you create opportunities for students to develop their clinical reasoning and clinical judgment skills?

REFERENCES

Abel, J. V. (2009). The role of intentional caring in ameliorating incapacitating test anxiety. In S. Bosher & M. Pharris (Eds.), *Transforming nursing education: The culturally inclusive environment* (pp. 231–258). New York: Springer.

Alfaro-LeFevre, R. (2012). Nursing process and clinical reasoning. *Nursing Education Perspectives, 33*(1), 7.

Amaro, D., Abriam-Yago, K., & Yoder, M. (2006). Perceived barriers for ethnically diverse students in nursing programs. *Journal of Nursing Education, 45*(7), 247–254.

American Association of College of Nursing. (2012). *Annual survey report of schools*. Retrieved from, http://www.aacn.nche.edu/research-data/standard-data-reports.

American Association of Colleges of Nursing. (2014a). *AACN finds slow enrollment growth at schools of nursing*. Retrieved from, http://www.aacn.nche.edu/Media/Annualreport.htm.

American Association of Colleges of Nursing. (2014b). *Enhancing diversity in the workforce*. Retrieved from, http://www.aacn.nche.edu/media-relations/fact-sheets/enhancing-diversity.htm.

American Association of Colleges of Nursing. (2014c). *Joining forces: Enhancing veterans' care tool kit: Veteran/active military nursing students*. Retrieved from, http://www.aacn.nche.edu/downloads/joining-forces-tool-kit/veteran-nursing-students.

American Association of Colleges of Nursing. (2014d). *The changing landscape: Nursing student diversity on the rise policy brief*. Retrieved from, http://www.aacn.nche.edu/government-affairs/Student-Diversity-FS.pdf.

American Education Research Association. (2014). *Standards for educational and psychological testing*. Washington, D.C: American Education Research Association.

Andreou, C., Papastavrou, E., & Merkouris, A. (2013). Learning styles and critical thinking relationship in baccalaureate nursing education: A systematic review. *Nurse Education Today*, *34*, 362–371.

Assessment Technologies Institute. (2000). *Technical manual for the self assessment inventory*. Overland Park, KS: Author.

Bachman, L., & Bachman, C. (2011). A study of classroom response system clickers: Increasing student engagement and performance in a large undergraduate lecture class on architectural research. *Journal of Interactive Learning Research*, *22*(1), 5–21.

Baker, B. H. (2010). Faculty ratings of retention strategies for minority nursing students. *Nursing Education Perspectives*, *31*(4), 216–220.

Bednarz, H., Schim, S., & Doorenbos, A. (2010). Cultural diversity in nursing education: Perils, pitfalls, and pearls. *Journal of Nursing Education*, *49*(5), 253–260.

Benner, P., Sutphen, M., Leonard, V., & Day, L. (2010). *Educating nurses: A call for radical transformation*. San Francisco, CA: Jossey-Bass.

Bleich, M. R. (2012). In praise of nursing residency programs. *American Nurse Today*, *7*(5), 47–49.

Bonaduce, J., & Quigley, B. (2011). Florence's candle: Educating the millennial nursing student. *Nursing Forum*, *46*(3), 157–159.

Bosher, S., & Bowles, M. (2008). The effects of linguistic modification on ESL students' comprehension of nursing course test items. *Nursing Education Perspective*, *29*(3), 165–172.

Bowman, K. (2014). From combat to the classroom: Serving military students. *Public Purpose*. Winter 2014. Retrieved November 2014 from, www.aascu.org/workarea/DownloadAsset.uspx?id=8012.

Boyd, J. (2010). The best of both worlds: The large lecture, writing-intensive course. *Communication Teacher*, *24*(4), 229–237.

Bradshaw, M., & Lowenstein, A. (2011). *Innovative teaching strategies in nursing and related health professions* (5th ed.). Sudbury, MA: Jones and Bartlett.

Brown, J., & Marshall, B. (2008). A historically Black university's baccalaureate enrollment and success tactics for registered nurses. *Journal of Professional Nursing*, *24*(1), 21–29.

Budden, J., Zhong, E., Moulton, P., & Cimiotti, J. (2013). The national council of state boards of nursing and the forum of state nursing workforce centers 2013 national workforce survey of registered nurses. *Journal of Nursing Regulation*, *4*(2), S8. July 2013 Supplement.

Bureau of Labor Statistics, U.S. Department of Labor. (2014). *Occupational outlook handbook* (2014–15 ed.). Registered Nurses. Retrieved September 1, 2014, from, http://www.bls.gov/ooh/healthcare/registered-nurses.htm.

Burke, J. (2011). Men in nursing. *Registered Nurse Journal*, May/June, 12–16.

Campinha-Bacote, J. (2012). The process of cultural competence in the delivery of healthcare services. In P. L. Sagar (Ed.), *Transcultural nursing theory and models: Application in nursing education, practice, and administration* (pp. 39–51). New York: Spring Pub. Co.

Caputi, L., Engelmann, L., & Stasinopoulos, J. (2006). An interdisciplinary approach to the needs of non-native speaking nursing students: Conversation circles. *Nurse Educator*, *31*(3), 107–111.

Choi, I., Lee, S., & Jung, J. (2008). Designing multimedia case-based instruction accommodating students' diverse learning styles. *Journal of Educational Multimedia and Hypermedia*, *17*(1), 5–25.

Coddington, D. M., & Karsten, K. (2014). Eliminating cultural bias in nursing examinations. *Teaching and Learning in Nursing*, *9*, 134–138.

Cohen, S. (2013). Recruitment and retention: How to get them and how to keep them. *Nursing Management*, *44*(4), 11–14.

Condon, V. M., Morgan, C. J., Miller, E. W., Mamier, I., Zimmerman, G. J., & Mazhar, W. (2013). A program to enhance recruitment and retention of disadvantaged and ethnically diverse baccalaureate nursing students. *Journal of Transcultural Nursing*, *24*(4), 397–407.

Crookes, K., Crookes, P. A., & Walsh, K. (2013). Meaningful and engaging teaching techniques for student nurses: A literature review. *Nurse Education in Practice*, *13*, 239–243.

Dapremont, J. (2014). Black nursing students: Strategies for academic success. *Nursing Education Perspectives*, *35*(3), 157–161.

Davis, S., Davis, D., & Williams, D. (2010). Challenges and issues facing the future of nursing education: Implications for ethnic minority faculty and students. *Journal of Cultural Diversity*, *17*(4), 122–126.

Devereaux-Melillo, K., Dowling, J., Qbdallah, L., Findeisen, M., & Knight, M. (2013). Bring diversity to nursing: Recruitment, retention, and graduation of nursing students. *Journal of Cultural Diversity*, *20*(2), 100–104.

Dols, J., Landrum, P., & Wieck, K. (2010). Leading and managing an intergenerational workforce. *Creative Nursing*, *16*(2), 1–8.

Donnell, W. (2015). A correlational study of a reading comprehension program and attrition rates of ESL nursing students in Texas. *Nursing Education Perspectives*, *36*(1), 16–21.

Dudas, K. (2011). Strategies to improve NLCEX style testing in student who speak English as an additional language. *The Online Journal of Cultural Competence in Nursing and Healthcare*, *1*(2), 14–23.

Dunn, R., Dunn, K., & Price, G. (1996). *Productivity environmental preference survey*. Lawrence, KS: Price Systems, Inc.

Erickson, B., & Strommer, D. (1991). *Teaching college freshmen*. San Francisco: Josey-Bass.

Facione, N., Blohm, S., Howard, K., & Giancarlo, C. (1998). *California critical thinking skills test manual*. Millrae, CA: California Academic Press.

Facione, N. C., Facione, P. A., & Sanchez, C. A. (1994). Critical thinking disposition as a measure of competent clinical judgment: The development of the California Critical Thinking Disposition Inventory. *Journal of Nursing Education*, *33*(8), 345–350.

Fleming, N. (2001). *Teaching and learning styles: VARK strategies*. Christchurch, New Zealand: Neil D. Fleming.

Fleming, S., Mckee, G., & Huntley-Moore, S. (2011). Undergraduate nursing students' learning styles: A longitudinal study. *Nursing Education Today*, *31*, 444–449.

Fountain, R., & Alfred, D. (2009). Student satisfaction with high-fidelity simulation: Does it correlate with learning styles? *Nursing Education Perspectives*, *30*(2), 96–98.

Gardner, J. D. (2005). A successful minority retention project. *Journal of Nursing Education*, *44*(12), 566–568.

Georges, C. (2012). Project to expand diversity in the nursing workforce. *Nursing Management*, *19*(2), 22–26.

Gordon, F. C., & Copes, M. A. (2010). The Coppin academy for pre-nursing success: A model for the recruitment and retention of minority students. *ABNF Journal*, *21*(1), 11–13.

Gregorc, A. (1982). *Gregorc style delineator: Development, technical and administrative manual*. Maynard, MA: Gabriel Systems, Inc.

Hallin, K. (2014). Nursing students at a university—A study about learning style preference. *Nurse Education Today, 34*(12), 1443–1449.

Hansen, E., & Beaver, S. (2012). Faculty support for ESL nursing students: Action plan for success. *Nursing Education Perspectives, 33*(4), 246–250.

Harding, M. (2010). Predictability associated with the exit examinations: A literature review. *Journal of Nursing Education, 49*(9), 493–497.

Hauer, P., Straub, C., & Wolf, S. (2005). Learning styles of allied health students using Kolb's LSI-IIa. *Journal of Allied Health, 34*(3), 177–182.

Hawk, T. F., & Shah, A. J. (2007). Using learning style instruments to enhance student learning. *Decision Sciences Journal of Innovative Education, 5*(1), 1–19.

Hayden, J. K., Smiley, R. A., Alexander, M., Kardong-Edgren, S., & Jeffries, P. R. (2014). The NCSBN national simulation study: A longitudinal, randomized, controlled study replacing clinical hours with simulation in prelicensure education. *Journal of Nursing Regulation, 5*(2). Supplement S3–S64.

Hendricks, J., & Cope, V. (2012). Generational diversity: What nurse managers need to know. *Journal of Advanced Nursing*, 717–725. May 2012.

Hicks, N. (2011). Guidelines for identifying and revising culturally biased multiple-choice nursing examination items. *Nurse Educator, 36*(6), 266–270.

Hirsh, E., Hirsh, K. W., & Hirsh, S. K. (2009). *MBTI teambuilding program*. Sunnyvale, CA: CPP, Inc.

Hockings, C., Brett, P., & Terentjevs, M. (2012). Making a difference—Inclusive learning and teaching in higher education through open educational resources. *Distance Education, 33*(2), 237–252.

Hourigan, K. L. (2013). Increasing student engagement in large classes: The ARC model of application, response, and collaboration. *Teaching Sociology, 41*(4), 353–359.

Howe, N. (2010). *Millennials in the workplace: Human resource strategies for a new generation*. New York: Lifecourse Associates, Inc..

Human Resources and Services Administration. (2013a). *HHS awards $2.8 million to transition veterans' skills into nursing careers*. Retrieved from, http://hhs.gov/news/press/2013pres/09/20130919c.html.

Human Resources and Services Administration. (2013b). *The U.S. nursing workforce: Trends in supply and education*. Retrieved from, http://bhpr.hrsa.gov/healthworkforce/reports/nursingworkforce/.

Hutchison, D., Brown, J., & Longworth, K. (2012). Attracting and maintaining the Y generation in nursing: A literature review. *Journal of Nursing Management, 20*(4), 444–450.

Igbo, I. N., Straker, K. C., Landson, M. J., Symes, L., Bernard, L. F., Hughes, L. A., et al. (2011). An innovative, multidisciplinary strategy to improve retention of nursing students from disadvantaged backgrounds. *Nursing Education Perspectives, 31*(3), 375–379.

Institute of Medicine (IOM). (2004). *In the nation's compelling interest: Ensuring diversity in the health care workforce*. Retrieved April 27, 2015, from, https://www.iom.edu/Reports/2004/In-the-Nations-Compelling-Interest-Ensuring-Diversity-in-the-Health-Care-Workforce.aspx.

Institute of Medicine (IOM). (2011). *The future of nursing: Leading change, advancing health*. Washington, DC: National Academies Press.

Kalisch, B., & Begeny, S. (2010). Preparation of nursing students for change and innovation. *Western Journal of Nursing Research, 32*(2), 157–167.

Kolb, D. (1978). *Learning style inventory: Technical* (rev. ed.). Boston, MA: William McBee.

Kolb, D. (1984). *Experiential learning: Experience as the source of learning and development*. Englewood Cliffs, NJ: Prentice Hall.

Kolb, A. Y., & Kolb, D. A. (2005). *The Kolb learning style inventory: Version 3.1 2005 technical specifications*. Experience Based Learning Systems, Inc.

Lampe, S., & Tsaouse, B. (2010). Linguistic bias in multiple choice questions. *Creative Nursing, 16*(2), 63–67.

Lapkin, Levett-Jones, Bellchambers, & Fernandez. (2010). Effectiveness of patient simulation manikins in teaching clinical reasoning skills to undergraduate nursing students: A systematic review. *Clinical Simulation in Nursing, 6*(6), e207–e222.

Li, Y., Yu, W., Liu, C., Shieh, S., & Yang, B. (2014). An exploratory study of the relationship between learning styles and academic performance among students in different nursing programs. *Contemporary Nurse: A Journal for the Australian Nursing Profession, 48*(2), 229–239.

Lin, P. S., Viscardi, M. K., & McHugh, M. D. (2014). Factors influencing job satisfaction of new graduate nurses participating in nurse residency programs: A systematic review. *Journal of Continuing Education in Nursing, 45*(10), 439–450.

Loftin, C., Newman, S., Dumas, B., Gilden, G., & Bond, M. (2012). Perceived barriers to success for minority students: An integrative review. *International Scholarly Research Network ISRN Nursing, 2012*. Article ID 806543, 9 pages.

Loftin, C., Newman, S. D., Gilden, G., Bond, M. L., & Dumas, B. P. (2013). Moving toward greater diversity: A review of interventions to increase diversity in nursing education. *Journal of Transcultural Nursing, 24*(4), 387–396.

Lujan, J. (2008). Linguistic and cultural adaptation needs of Mexican American nursing students related to multiple-choice tests. *Journal of Nursing Education, 47*(7), 327–330.

MacWilliams, B., Schmidt, B., & Bleich, R. (2013). Men in nursing. *American Journal of Nursing, 113*(1), 38–44.

Mann. (2012). Critical thinking and clinical judgment skill development in baccalaureate nursing students. *The Kansas Nurse, 87*(1), 26–30.

McCauley, M. H. (1990). The Myers-Briggs type indicator: A measure for individuals and groups. *Measurement and Evaluation in Counseling & Development, 22*(4), 181.

McCrindle, M., & Wolfinger, E. (2014). *The ABC of XYZ: Understanding the global generations*. Retrieved from, http://www.theabcofxyz.com.

Moceri, J. T. (2012). Bias in the nursing workplace: Implications for Latino(a) nurses. *Journal of Cultural Diversity, 19*(3), 94–101.

Moore, T. (2013). Critical thinking: Seven definitions in search of a concept. *Studies in Higher Education, 38*(4), 506–522.

National League for Nursing. (2012a). *The scope of practice for academic nurse educators 2012 revision*. Philadelphia: Wolters Kluwer.

National League for Nursing. (2012b). *The fair testing imperative in nursing education*. NLN Board of Governors. Retrieved from, http://www.nln.org/docs/default-source/about/nln-vision-series-%28position-statements%29/nlnvision_4.pdf.

National League for Nursing. (2013). *Annual Survey of Schools of Nursing, academic year 2011–2012*. www.nln.org/research/slides/index.htm.

National Population Projections. (2014). *United States population projections: 2000 to 2060*. Retrieved from, http://www.census.gov/population/www.projections/2009projections.html.

Noble, K., Miller, S., & Heckman, J. (2008). The cognitive style of nursing students: Educational implications for teaching and learning. *Journal of Nursing Education, 47*, 245–253.

Oliver, G. M. (2010). Wanted: Creative thinkers. *Western Journal of Nursing Research, 32*(2), 155–156.

Olson, M. A. (2012). English as a second language (ESL) nursing student success: A critical review of the literature. *Journal of Cultural Diversity, 19*(1), 26–31.

Orsolini-Hain, & Malone. (2007). Examining the impending gap in clinical nursing expertise. *Policy, Politic, & Nursing Practice, 8*(3), 158–169.

Pashler, H., McDaniel, M., Rohrer, D., & Bjork, R. (2008). Learning styles: Concepts and evidence. *Psychological Science in the Public Interest, 9*(3), 106–116.

Payton, T. D., Howe, L. A., Timmons, S. M., & Richardson, M. E. (2013). African American nursing students' perceptions about mentoring. *Nursing Education Perspectives, 34*(3), 171–177.

Pettigrew, A. C., Dienger, M. J., & O'Brien King, M. (2011). Nursing student today: Who are they and what are their learning preferences? *Journal of Professional Nursing, 27*(4), 227–236.

Rajacich, D., Kane, D., Williston, C., & Cameron, S. (2013). If they do call you a nurse, it is always a "male nurse": Experiences of man in the nursing profession. *Nursing Forum, 48*(1), 71–80.

Raphelson, S. (2014). *From Gis to Gen Z: How generations get nicknames.* Retrieved from, http://www.npr.org/2014/10/06/349316543/don-t-label-me-origins-of-generaltional-names-and-why-we-use-them.html.

Robinson, J., Scollan-Koliopoulos, M., Kamienski, M., & Burke, K. (2012). Generational differences and learning style preferences in nurses from a large metropolitan medical center. *Journal for Nurses in Staff Development, 28*(4), 166–171.

Romeo, E. (2010). Quantitative research on critical thinking and predicting nursing students' NCLEX-RN performance. *Journal of Nursing Education, 49*, 378–386.

Sanner, S., & Wilson, A. (2008). The experience of students with English as a second language in a baccalaureate nursing program. *Nurse Education Today, 28*(7), 807–813.

Santo, L., Frander, E., & Hawkins, A. (2013). The use of standardized exit examinations in baccalaureate nursing education. *Nurse Educator, 38*(2), 81–84.

Saunders, S., & Kardia, D. (2014). *Creating inclusive college classrooms.* Retrieved from, http://crit.umich.edu.gsis/p3_1. 1–7.

Sauter, M., Johnson, D., & Gillespie, N. (2009). *Educational program evaluation.* St Louis, MO: Saunders Elsevier.

Scott. (2008). New graduate nurse transitioning: Necessary or nice? *Applied Nursing Research, 21*(2), 75–83.

Shelton, E. (2012). A model of nursing student retention. *International Journal of Nursing Education Scholarship, 9*(1), 1–16.

Shinn, E., & Ofiesh, N. (2012). Cognitive diversity and the design of classroom tests for all learners. *Journal of Postsecondary Education and Disability, 25*(3), 227–245.

Simmons, B. (2010). Clinical reasoning: Concept analysis. *Journal of Advanced Nursing, 66*(5), 1151–1158.

Spector, N., & Echternacht, M. (2010). A regulatory model for transitioning newly licensed nurses to practice. *Journal of Nursing Regulation, 1*(2), 18–25.

Stanley, D. (2010). Multigenerational workforce issues and their implications for leadership in nursing. *Journal of Nursing Management, 18*(2), 846–852.

Starr, K. (2009). Nursing education challenges: Students with English as an additional language. *Journal of Nursing Education, 48*, 478–487.

Sullivan, D. (2014). A concept analysis of "high stakes testing". *Nurse Educator, 39*(2), 72–76.

Sullivan-Mann, J., Perron, C. A., & Fellner, A. N. (2009). The effects of simulation on nursing students' critical thinking study. *Newborn and Infant Nursing Reviews, 9*(2), 111–116.

Sutherland, J. A., Hamilton, M. J., & Goodman, N. (2007). Affirming at-risk minorities for success (ARMS): Retention, graduation, and success on the NCLEX-RN. *Journal of Nursing Education, 46*(8), 347–353.

Swinney, J. E., & Dobal, M. T. (2008). Embracing the challenge: Increasing workforce diversity in nursing. *Hispanic Healthcare International, 6*(4), 200–204.

Tarrant, M., & Ware, J. (2008). Impact of item-writing flaws in multiple-choice questions on student achievement in high-stakes nursing assessments. *Medical Education, 42*, 198–206.

The Sullivan Commission. (2004). *Missing persons: Minorities in the health professions.* Retrieved January 20, 2015, from, http://www.aacn.nche.edu/media-relations/SullivanReport.pdf.

Thompson, C., & Stapley, S. (2011). Do educational interventions improve nurses' clinical judgment and decision making? *International Journal of Nursing Studies, 48*, 881–893.

Tinto, V. (1993). *Leaving college: Rethinking the causes and cures of student attrition.* Chicago: University of Chicago Press.

Torregosa, M., Ynalvez, M., Schiffman, R., & Morin, K. (2015). English-language proficiency, academic networks, and academic performance of Mexican American baccalaureate nursing students. *Nursing Education Perspectives, 36*(1), 8–15.

U. S. Census Bureau. (2011). *2009 American Community Survey.* Retrieved January 2011 from, http://factfinder.census.gov/.

Watson, G., & Glaser, E. M. (1980). *Critical thinking appraisal manual.* San Antonio, TX: Psychological Corp.

Willcoxson, L., & Prosser, M. (1996). Kolb's learning style inventory: Review and further study of validity and reliability. *British Journal of Educational Psychology, 66*, 247–257.

Witkin, H. A., & Goodenough, D. R. (1981). Cognitive styles essence and origins: Field dependence and field independence. *Psychological Issues, 51*, 1–41.

Wolff, A., Ratner, P., Robinson, A., Oliffe, J., & Hall, L. (2010). Beyond multigenerational differences: A literature review of the impact of relational diversity on nurses' attitudes and work. *Journal of Nursing Management, 18*, 948–969.

Wright, J. (2012). Descriptions from accelerated baccalaureate nurses: Determining curriculum and clinical strategies that work best to prepare novice nurses. *International Journal of Nursing Education Scholarship, 9*(1), 1–12.

The Academic Performance of Students: Legal and Ethical Issues*

Linda S. Christensen, EdD, JD, MSN, RN, CNE

3

Nursing faculty have many considerations as they assist students in the learning process. Developing curriculum content, choosing teaching strategies, and developing student evaluation plans can be major areas of focus. However, in carrying out these functions, faculty must also consider the legal and ethical concepts that influence the process and product of nursing education.

Just as nurses in practice have legal and ethical guidelines, nurse educators also have legal and ethical guidelines. Nursing faculty are responsible for understanding the broad legal and ethical principles that apply in all circumstances, as well as those specific to their own setting. Major problems can occur if faculty lack an understanding of these principles and are unable to apply them appropriately.

Many potential problems can be avoided if faculty take a proactive approach to anticipate student concerns. Faculty members who treat students with respect, provide honest and frequent communication about progress toward course goals and objectives, and are fair and considerate in evaluating performance are less likely to encounter student challenges. A learning environment that supports student growth and questioning is likely to reduce the incidence of problems, especially litigation. Suggestions for avoiding such problems are discussed later in this chapter.

The goal of the educational experience remains that students develop knowledge, skills, and values that will enable them to provide safe, effective nursing care. Nursing faculty who are able to apply general legal and ethical principles are much more likely to play their part in effectively meeting that goal.

This chapter provides an overview of the most common legal and ethical issues related to student academic performance that nurse educators face in the classroom and clinical setting. The chapter includes a discussion of the importance of student–faculty interactions and the legal and ethical issues related to academic performance, including the provision of due process, the student appeal process, assisting the failing student, and academic dishonesty.

Student–Faculty Interactions

The student–faculty relationship that is developed during the teaching and learning process is a very important one. Students have often identified student–faculty relationships as the relationships that most often affect learning. The Sullivan Commission Report (2004) identified several factors that "significantly determine the quality of the educational experience" (p. 84) and the student–faculty relationship is among those. There is little doubt that a positive interaction between faculty and students is likely not only to decrease legal issues but also to promote student success.

The National League for Nursing (2005) has asserted that the focus of the faculty should be on establishing a learning environment that is "characterized by collaboration, understanding, mutual trust, respect, equality, and acceptance of differences" (p. 4). Such a learning environment fosters professional growth and development on the part of the nurse.

Effective nurse educators must create interpersonal relationships that promote student development into a competent professional (Halstead, 2007). The National League for Nursing clearly identified the importance of the student–faculty

*The author acknowledges the work of Elizabeth G. Johnson, DSN, RN, and Judith A. Halstead, PhD, RN, ANEF, FAAN, in the previous editions of the chapter.

relationship within the Core Competencies of Nurse Educators (National League for Nursing, 2012). Specifically, in the NLN Competency II, which is focused on facilitating learning development and socialization, the importance of interpersonal interactions on learner outcomes is noted (National League for Nursing, 2012).

Faculty in the classroom and in clinical settings encounter students whose backgrounds and learning needs are extremely diverse. Faculty who are able to address the needs of students from an educational perspective as well as establish positive interpersonal relationships with students of varied backgrounds will make positive contributions in assisting students to meet the desired outcomes. The challenge for faculty in assisting students is to identify ways to address these varied needs. To successfully assist students, faculty must understand and appreciate cultural diversity and be able to use multiple learning strategies to assist students with varying learning styles and needs. The student role in the educational process has changed and must be one of active involvement. When faculty view students as partners or colleagues in an educational experience, they promote the development of a relationship that supports student growth and development and the attainment of educational goals and objectives.

The first step in the process of developing a learning environment that encourages collaborative and positive student–faculty interactions requires faculty to carefully examine and develop an awareness of their own beliefs and values about the teaching–learning process. Working collaboratively with students will require faculty to adopt strategies that involve active student participation and do not place faculty in the role of having sole responsibility for determining learning experiences. Activities such as cooperative group work, debate and discussion, role playing, and problem-solving exercises are examples of interactive teaching strategies that shift the focus from the faculty to the student. Such a pedagogical shift in teaching may also require faculty to leave behind the "safety" and control of the classroom lecture and develop more fully the skills necessary to successfully incorporate interactive teaching strategies into the classroom. Chapter 15 provides further discussion of teaching strategies that promote active learning.

Another important step in the process of developing a positive learning environment is examining attitudes and beliefs that students bring to the learning environment. Students may lack confidence of their abilities in the academic environment, especially those who are first-generation college students and lack role models who have been successful in pursuing higher education. Empowerment of students can occur when faculty demonstrate a sense of caring and commitment to students, and use courtesy and respect in interactions. Having a role in developing their own learning experiences can also prove to be an empowering experience for students.

How can nursing faculty successfully incorporate this concept of empowerment and equity into student–faculty relationships? Educators can assist students in meeting their unique needs by providing various resources (National League for Nursing, 2012). Learning activities can be designed to promote positive faculty–student interactions. For example, the use of computer-mediated communication, such as e-mail and online discussion forums, tends to remove the elements of status and power from communication, thus allowing a freer exchange of information. Integrating content and discussion about empowerment, collaboration, collegiality, and teamwork throughout the curriculum can also help nurture positive student–faculty interactions. Ongoing, open dialogue with students that results in clear communication of mutual expectations and responsibilities is an essential component of all successful student–faculty interactions, as is illustrated in the remaining sections of this chapter.

Legal Considerations of Student Performance

An established responsibility of faculty in nursing education programs is the evaluation of student performance in the classroom (didactic) and clinical setting. This responsibility carries with it accountability because the outcomes of such evaluation have a major effect on the student's progress in the course and even status in the program. In addition, faculty serve as the safeguard for society at large from practitioners who have not demonstrated the ability to practice safely. In a precedent-setting case, the court clearly set the standard that it will not interfere with academic decision making regarding student progress and content (*Board of Curators of the University of Missouri v. Horowitz 1978*). Other courts have followed the Horowitz court by repeatedly affirming faculty members' responsibility for evaluation as long as due process has been provided and there is no finding of arbitrary or capricious facts. However, to ensure due process and avoid being viewed as arbitrary or capricious, the evaluation process must be based on principles that ensure that students' rights are not violated.

Student Rights

Faculty must be aware that students enter the educational experience with rights, just as faculty have rights. A few decades ago it would have been rare to find litigation involving a nursing student and the nursing program, but litigation involving nursing programs has dramatically increased. Many cases involving student litigation within nursing programs have their legal basis in the concepts of due process, fair treatment, and confidentiality and privacy.

Due Process

Due process is a term that is frequently used in education and may be misunderstood. The general concept of *due process* is based in fairness and is intended to ensure that certain rights are respected within the particular situation. There are two types of due process. *Substantive due process* refers to the fairness of the "outcome" in relation to the "infraction." In other words, does the punishment fit the crime? It would most likely be a breach of substantive due process to dismiss a student from a course because he or she arrived to class a few minutes late. The second type of due process is *procedural due process*. Procedural due process ensures that the accused will receive notice and an opportunity to be heard. Providing the student with a clear notice of the potential issue and providing the student the opportunity to present his or her side of the situation is essential to meet the procedural due process requirements.

Student rights in the broadest sense are protected by the Fifth and Fourteenth Amendment of the U.S. Constitution, which limits the restrictions that can be imposed on an individual. These amendments state that no citizen may be deprived of life, liberty, or property without due process of law and require that the federal government provide due process for all citizens (U.S. Const. amend. V & XIV).

Although the Fourteenth Amendment includes language referring to state or government actions (which includes public institutions), the principles of due process are applied by the courts to all educational settings. Within the educational setting, a 1961 case applied the principles of due process to a situation in which students were dismissed without notice and without a hearing (*Dixon v. Alabama State Board of Education*). In *Dixon*, Alabama State College, which was a segregated black college, expelled six students without a hearing for unspecified reasons, although the presumptive cause was that they participated in civil rights demonstrations. The appeals court ruled that a public college could not expel them without a public hearing. The judicial system expanded the holding of the *Dixon* case with *Goss v. Lopez* (1975) when the court clearly noted that the due process protections of *Dixon* applied to all students facing expulsion from a public institution, regardless of whether the institution is a grade school, high school, or college or university. The legal principle of due process has been extended to cases involving private college and university settings, upholding the student's due process rights regardless of attendance at a public or private institution (Kaplin & Lee, 2014).

Student due process rights have their foundation in two types of due process: procedural due process and substantive due process. Procedural due process refers to a step-by-step process including notice and an opportunity to be heard at various levels and appeal options (Christensen, 2010). Procedural due process affords the student an opportunity to be heard—or present the case to parties involved in the decision-making process.

Substantive due process involves the basis for the decision itself (or the substance of the decision) and is based on the principle that a decision should be fair, objective, and nondiscriminatory. Students who might challenge on this principle would seek to prove that a faculty decision was arbitrary or capricious. Substantive due process has often been summarized as asking "Did the punishment fit the crime?"

Other legal concepts that influence student rights come from principles of contract law. Students may also use these concepts in seeking action against an institution. Contract law is applied in this circumstance with the understanding that when students enter a university or college, they actually enter into a contract with the school. If students complete the degree requirements and follow the required procedures, then a degree will be awarded. The implied contract between the student and the school forms the basis for much student rights–oriented precedent law. Courts may view institutional documents as contracts, regardless of whether there may be a written disclaimer on the particular document that the institution does not intend the document to be a contract between the institution and the student. A common example of a document that is often implied to be a contract is a course syllabus. The course syllabus may contain a statement that it is not intended to be a contract between the institution and the student, but is often viewed by the court as being an implied contract. Even in a situation where students agree to a proposed change in the syllabus, the original syllabi terms may govern in a dispute because the students who are voicing agreement may be viewed as unable to object without harassment from other students or teacher reprimand. Additionally, students have successfully won cases against educational institutions based on contract theory when the educational institution was determined to be in breach of implied contract because they did not follow its own policies and procedures (*Boehm v. U. of PA. School of Vet. Med,* 1990; *Schaer v. Brandeis University,* 2000).

There is a difference between student concerns or grievances based on academic performance and those based on disciplinary circumstances. Academic concerns are based solely on grades or clinical performance, whereas disciplinary misconduct is based on violation of rules or policies within the school or department. Academic due process includes the requirement that the student be informed of the academic issue, the requirements necessary to meet academic standards, a time frame for meeting the academic requirements, and notice of the consequences if the academic standards are not met. When disciplinary action is considered, the concept of due process is applied with a higher degree of scrutiny. In this circumstance the individual must receive notice of the specific charge that is being made and the policy and code that has been violated. The student must have an opportunity to present a defense against the charges, usually at a formal hearing, but at least in writing. Because disciplinary dismissals may have more long-lasting effects on the individual, more complicated due process rules apply. Consider the due process rights of the student illustrated in the following scenario:

> Jane Short is a sophomore nursing student who has completed the first nursing course with a barely passing grade. She had difficulty performing the basic nursing skills, stating that having someone watch her made her nervous. She did not come to college with a strong academic background and has struggled in making the adjustment to the required higher-level thinking and need for decision making. However, she was able to complete the course requirements in the basic nursing course, although at a minimal level. As she progresses to the next course, she is having more difficulty. Her study skills need development and she has missed several classes. She is not doing well on tests and has been late for clinical on two occasions in the first 3 weeks of class. Her instructor has asked to meet with her to discuss these concerns. She informs Jane of the issues of concern and relates what needs to be done to address these concerns. She suggests some new study strategies and asks that Jane practice in the lab to become more comfortable with the procedures and skills. She also relates that continued absences and tardiness will negatively affect Jane's classroom performance and her clinical evaluation. She reminds Jane of the School of Nursing Policy that states that students who miss one third of the clinical experiences will be automatically dismissed from the program. The faculty member tells Jane that she needs to demonstrate improvement in these areas within the next 3 weeks. The faculty member asks Jane to add her comments to the documents containing all this information and gives Jane a copy of the document explaining the concerns and including the suggestions for improvement as well as the consequences if no change occurs. The faculty member schedules times to provide regular feedback to Jane about her progress.

What has the faculty done to uphold Jane's due process rights in this circumstance? The faculty member has made Jane aware of the situation and what needs to be done to improve it. She has made suggestions for improvement and provided Jane with a written copy of those suggestions and the consequences if no change occurs. Jane has been informed and duly notified, and her due process rights have been addressed within the student–instructor interactions.

Fair Treatment

Students have the right to expect that they will be treated fairly, consistently, and objectively. Standards of expectations for the course provide the objective guide for evaluation and must be communicated to students early and often. Course requirements should be consistent for all students, including classroom and clinical assignments. Students should receive equivalent assignments, even if they are not identical, that allow them to demonstrate progress toward meeting course objectives. In addition, students must be provided with opportunity and an appropriate time to demonstrate the outcomes required in the course. Students cannot be held accountable for end-of-course outcomes on the first day of class and the same principle applies in the clinical setting. Students must be provided with time to learn before evaluation can take place; students must clearly understand the difference in the learning and the evaluation portion of the clinical experience.

An example of violating fair treatment might occur when a faculty allows one student extra credit in a course, but does not afford the same opportunity to all students to increase their grade. Clinically, holding students to different standards of evaluation will be considered a violation of fair treatment. If the instructor consistently gives a student less challenging assignments and then evaluates the student as not providing a complex case, the issue of fairness is again relevant.

Confidentiality and Privacy

Legislation that has been passed to protect health information and the privacy of patients should remind faculty of their obligation to protect information from and about students. The need for confidentiality in the faculty role is based in the same code of ethics that guides all nurses. Students have a right to expect that information about their progress in the program, their academic and clinical performance, and their personal concerns will be kept confidential.

In the course of the teaching role, faculty are often privy to information about students that is of a personal and private nature. Students often confide in faculty about events that may influence their performance in the classroom or may simply seek advice from persons they feel they can trust. This information, as in a nurse–patient interaction, must be guarded and held in confidence. Morgan (2001) pointed out the conflicts that nursing faculty often feel when deciding whether it is in the student's best interest to divulge information of a personal nature. She suggested that there should be a "compelling professional purpose" (p. 291), such as protection of patients. This conclusion is consistent with the legal precedent set in *Tarasoff v. Regents of the University of California* (1976). In *Tarasoff,* the court held that the patient–provider confidentiality rule did not apply when there was a reasonable belief of impending harm to another individual caused by a patient disclosure. It is easy for caring faculty to disclose private student information based on the belief that it is in the student's best interests. But without the student's consent or the faculty's reasonable belief that harm may come from nondisclosure, the faculty would be violating the student's right to privacy to share confidential information without student consent. Faculty are often anxious to share a student's strengths and weaknesses with other faculty members who will have the student in subsequent semesters. Faculty must seriously consider the implications of such a practice as a standard approach. A student's performance or challenges in one class will not necessarily follow him or her to the next class. Informing other faculty members about an individual student's strengths or weaknesses may provide prejudicial information and could be interpreted as unjust and violate the student's right to privacy. However, alerting faculty to information that may affect patient or student safety may warrant discussion.

In addition to confidentiality, privacy, especially of student records, is essential. Federal Educational Rights and Privacy Act of 1974 (FERPA), often referred to as the *Buckley Amendment,* provides the basis for protection of student records. This law was enacted to ensure that students older than age 18 have access to their educational records and to ensure that they have some input about who can receive information in that record without their consent. The amendment also mandates that a procedure be in place that allows students to contest information in the record that is inaccurate or that they do not agree with. In actual practice, one of the most frequent applications of this law occurs when parents seek information about student progress or grades without student permission. Parents are often dismayed to find that they have no "right" to information about student progress, unless the student provides permission. It is imperative that faculty understand the components of this legislation and follow it implicitly. For example, faculty cannot post grades in any form in public, leave graded materials for students to retrieve in a public place, or circulate a printed class list with student IDs or social security information as an attendance list. All of these constitute violations of FERPA and make faculty and their institutions subject to prosecution. An excellent reference of the requirements of FERPA can be obtained online through the U.S. Department of Education website (http://www2.ed.gov/policy/gen/guid/fpco/ferpa/index.html).

Schools of nursing must follow the guidelines of the institution regarding FERPA, but they must also give particular attention to guarding student health records. These health records are usually kept in a separate file and should follow Health Insurance Portability and Accountability Act, 1996 (HIPAA) guidelines. Student records and evaluation notes maintained by faculty during the process of course evaluation must also be guarded to protect privacy.

Student privacy must be strictly guarded. Whether based in common law privacy standards, FERPA, or HIPAA, students have a legal right to have their information protected within the educational system.

Guidelines for Providing Due Process to Students

Due Process for Academic Issues

The potential for litigation always exists, even in the best of circumstances; therefore it is prudent to take actions and establish policies that decrease the likelihood that litigation will occur as a result of academic failure or dismissal. The following practices help keep students informed of faculty expectations and their progress in coursework, and provide the basis for ensuring that students receive the information they need.

1. *Provide a copy of student and faculty rights and responsibilities in formal documents.* On admission to the program, students should be given a copy of rights, responsibilities, policies, and procedures that apply to students and faculty. Although institutions have the right to establish policies, they also have the responsibility to communicate those policies and guidelines to students and faculty. Policies and procedures that are in effect for all students in the institution, as well as those that are specific to a program, should be available and must be congruent. Policies should address progression, retention, graduation, dismissal, grading, and conduct. Students should also be informed of circumstances that will interfere with progression and those that would result in termination from the program. They should learn the process to follow in filing a grievance. These policies should be readily available and are usually published in faculty and student handbooks. Strategies that ensure that students have read and understand the information contained in these documents should be a part of the orientation process. In every course, faculty should plan to reinforce this information, including providing specific expectations for the course. Written specifics of requirements should be contained in the course syllabus and discussed with students on the first day of class.
2. *Review and update policies in the handbook and catalog periodically.* Published materials given to students and faculty should contain current information about academic policies and procedures. This serves to keep students and faculty informed about the policies and procedures they are subject to, and it is a requirement of institutional and program accreditation agencies. Regular review by faculty of policies and procedures ensures that faculty are aware of current policies and increases the likelihood that they will be consistent in following them.
3. *Course requirements and expectations should be clearly established and communicated at the beginning of the course.* The course syllabus should explain course requirements, critical learning experiences, and faculty expectations of student performance to satisfactorily complete the course. Schools commonly establish guidelines for information to be included in all syllabi developed for nursing courses, and faculty should follow these criteria. A course syllabus should include the following information, at a minimum: description of the course, course objectives, course credit hours, faculty responsible for the course, class schedule, attendance policies, teaching strategies used in the course, topical outlines, evaluation tools and methods, due

dates for assignments, late work policy, and standards that must be met for students to pass the course. Many institutions also require that course syllabi include a statement about the need for students to notify faculty about desired accommodations for a disability. The syllabus for a course should be distributed on the first day of class to provide students the opportunity to understand and clarify course requirements.

4. *Retain all tests and written work in a file until the student has successfully completed at least the course requirements, and in some cases the program requirements.* Student assignments, tests, and evaluations are invaluable, especially in cases of academic deficiency that may result in a student challenge. All evidence of a student's performance in a class should be kept at least until that course is completed. Faculty must be aware of institutional policy or standards that govern maintenance of records and should follow those. There are no universal rules for how long student files should be maintained, and the policy may vary from institution to institution. Student clinical evaluations often become a part of the student's permanent file, although in some programs, these are only retained until the student completes the program. The maintenance of files of student work and tests may also serve to decrease the likelihood of plagiarism of other students' work. Knowing that faculty keep a copy of assignments and tests may make students less likely to attempt to claim other students' work as their own. Files of student work may also serve as examples of assignments to share with evaluators during accreditation visits or to assist in outcome assessment efforts. Samples of student work may also be used to provide positive examples to other students. Faculty must obtain a student's permission to share his or her work with others. Some schools choose to have students sign a standard form granting such permission and to keep this on permanent file.
5. *Students should have the opportunity to view all evaluation data that are placed in the student file.* Students have the right to see all documentation that has been used to determine an evaluation of their performance. Students also have the right to disagree with the appraisal of their performance and should be provided with an opportunity to respond to the comments of the evaluation with comments of their own. Faculty should ask students to sign and date the evaluation form to indicate that the evaluation has been discussed with them, while providing an opportunity for them to register their own comments on the form.
6. *When students are not making satisfactory progress toward course objectives and the potential for course failure or dismissal exists, students must receive notification of and information about their academic deficiencies.* Students should receive regular feedback about the progress they have made toward meeting class and clinical objectives throughout the course. If deficiencies occur, students must receive details of what behavior is unsatisfactory, what needs to be done to improve the behavior, and the consequences if improvement does not occur. Faculty should hold formal conferences with students who are in academic jeopardy, identify the deficiencies in writing, and work with the student to determine a plan to address the deficiencies. Both the faculty member and the student should sign the document to indicate mutual involvement in and agreement to the plan. Subsequent follow-up conferences should be held to note progress or lack of progress made toward achieving the agreed-on goals and note revisions or additional strategies employed. All conferences should be documented in writing, and both parties should receive a copy of the documentation. An example of how this might occur was presented in the earlier example relating to Jane Short.

Faculty who fail to evaluate a student's unsatisfactory performance accurately, through either a reluctance to expose the student to the experience of failure or a fear of potential litigation, are guilty of misleading the student, potentially jeopardizing patient care, placing faculty peers in a difficult situation, and potentially being subject to a claim of educational malpractice. Nursing faculty and even the university are responsible for preparing safe and competent practitioners. When the faculty does not fulfill their responsibilities, they can be held liable for educational malpractice, because they are breaching their duty as an educator. Student deficiencies may eventually be identified and dealt with by subsequent faculty. Students might legitimately ask why they were not notified earlier in the educational experience of these deficiencies and accuse the "failing" faculty of prejudicial behavior. It is much fairer to inform students of their unsatisfactory behaviors when such behaviors are first identified. Informing students of deficiencies in a caring, constructive manner allows them the opportunity to improve performance; to not inform them denies them this opportunity and right.

These procedures help ensure that students receive the due process related to academic failure that is their right by law. Maintaining open lines of communication with a student who is not progressing is a key component in resolving such situations satisfactorily and decreasing faculty liability. Students are much less likely to sue if they perceive that they have been treated in a fair and impartial manner and have been given information throughout the process.

Due Process for Disciplinary Issues

Students who are dismissed because of misconduct or disciplinary reasons should receive additional assurances that due process has been followed. A disciplinary action occurs when a student violates a regulation or law or has engaged in activity that is not allowed. Disciplinary actions brought against the student need to include providing the student with a written copy of the accused violation. The information should include details about what policy or rule was violated, and enough information must be provided to ensure that the student can develop a defense against the charges. Processes included within procedural due process include an impartial decision maker, notice of the charges and evidence against the student, an opportunity to appear before the decision maker, an opportunity to suggest witnesses, protection of the imposition of sanctions against the witnesses, and permitting the student to voluntarily accept discipline or the ruling of the decision-maker (*A v. C. College*, 1994). If the student desires, legal counsel can be present to provide the student with advice but not to question or interview other participants in the proceedings. Legal counsel for the institution is usually available as well. No action should be taken by the faculty or university until a formal hearing has occurred. Depending on the institution, a councilor committee usually decides the outcome of the charges. Courts may be more likely to become involved in disciplinary actions because they involve less professional judgment and evaluation.

In the example presented earlier, if Jane Short's absences continue in clinical and she misses enough clinical days that she is dismissed from the program, then the provision for due process as a disciplinary event must include more faculty action. The faculty member must provide written information about the school policy that has been violated (although one hopes she has done that at the earlier conference) and provide an opportunity for Jane to respond to the accusations. The process must provide an opportunity for Jane to present a defense for her actions or an opportunity to explain her actions to those persons who will make the final decision about the outcome of her situation. In this circumstance, because the issue is a disciplinary one, faculty must take additional steps to ensure that due process rights are protected.

Grievances and the Student Appeal Process

Even when a student has been treated in accordance with due process with a clear communication of policies and expected academic standards, it is possible that the student may wish to seek legal recourse in the face of an academic failure or dismissal. In such cases, the student may appeal to the court on the basis that faculty has acted in a capricious or arbitrary manner. Courts have traditionally not overturned academic decisions unless the student can prove that faculty did not follow "accepted academic norms so as to demonstrate the person or committee responsible did not actually exercise professional judgment" (*Regents of University of Michigan v. Ewing*, 1985]). In this case, a student who was dismissed from medical school brought suit against the university, citing that university faculty moved to dismiss him based on circumstances that were not rational and were capricious. The court ruled that the university faculty did have cause to dismiss the student and thus a "substantive due process claim" had not occurred.

There are other reasons that students may choose to bring suit against an institution. Breach of contract, described earlier, may be charged by students who may not be provided with due process protections, particularly in private institutions. The court has generally followed the "well-steeled rule that relations between a student and a private university are a matter of contract" (*Dixon v. Alabama State Board of Education*, 1961]). However, there is inconsistency in court cases that address grievances of contract issues depending on the substance of the case. Students may also make charges of defamation or violation of civil rights, including discrimination. Courts generally have not hesitated to analyze cases in which discrimination based on any parameter (e.g., race, gender, age, or disability) has been charged. Brent (2001) reported that the best way to avoid such litigation is to maintain policies that clearly demonstrate adherence to the institution's and program's guidelines, which must be in compliance with all federal and state laws regulating civil rights.

The Student Appeal Process

Before seeking the assistance of the court system, students must first use all available recourse within the institution. A well-established principle of educational law is that the courts have generally relied on academic institutions to deal with grade disputes and have intervened only when there is evidence of the violation of student rights. Institutions of higher learning have established policies for hearing student grievances and appeals. The purpose of these guidelines is to establish common procedures to ensure that students are provided due process and that faculty rights are supported.

Institutional and program policies related to student appeals and grievance procedures should be made available in writing to students and faculty. Faculty are usually given this information in the faculty handbook on orientation to the institution and should refer to them periodically as changes are made.

Likewise, students should be informed that a formal grievance process policy exists and that it is their responsibility to initiate the procedure. It is recommended that programs distribute this information to students when they are first admitted to the institution and document that students have received such notification. Students may choose not to initiate the grievance procedure that is their right, but they should always be aware of the option of doing so. Information about the appeal process should be reviewed with an individual student if the situation warrants.

When a grievance occurs and the appeal process is implemented, there are two possible outcomes. It is possible that the appeals board may review the information provided and find that there are insufficient grounds for the student's charge and that the assigned grade or faculty action should stand. The other option is that a recommendation for corrective action may be made based on a review of evidence that indicates that the student's charges have merit. This may mean a change of grade or an opportunity for further evaluation. Implementation of the recommendations may vary depending on the specific charges and circumstances. If, at the conclusion of the institutional appeal process, the student is not satisfied with the outcome, the student has the right to pursue further recourse in the court system.

Faculty Role in the Appeal Process

Being involved in the appeal process can be a stressful experience for both the faculty member involved and the student. When a student indicates dissatisfaction with an assigned grade or evaluation and is considering an appeal, the faculty member should give consideration to reevaluation. If the faculty member finds that the student's evidence is legitimate and that the student truly deserves a higher grade, then the grade should be changed. If the faculty member believes no changes are justified after reviewing the situation and finding that all procedures and standards have been applied consistently and justly, then the faculty member should maintain the assigned grade. However, a faculty member should not act in haste or out of fear in reaction to the threat of a grievance procedure. Changing a grade without justification sets a dangerous precedent and should be avoided. Clear, consistent use of standards for grading that are made known to students will help effectively support grades that are assigned. Planning before the implementation of a course assignment or activity and providing clearly established grading criteria may help decrease student misunderstanding.

Academic Performance in the Clinical and Classroom Settings

One major responsibility of nursing faculty is the evaluation of student academic performance. In many circumstances faculty are charged with evaluating students in both classroom (didactic) and clinical settings. Student evaluation is an expectation of faculty at all levels and requires careful consideration for many reasons.

The outcome of evaluation has a major effect on students, and faculty must always be aware of this. Faculty may have limited preparation in how to evaluate students within the classroom

(Morrison, 2010) or the clinical setting (Suplee, Gardner, & Jerome-D'Emilia, 2014). The outcome of an evaluation usually means that students progress in the program; however, an unsatisfactory evaluation means that students may face having to repeat a course, a delay in their education, or removal from the program. These outcomes have financial, emotional, and other costs for students. In addition, faculty may also experience negative consequences, such as emotional distress, pressure from administration to maintain numbers, and a sense of personal failure when it is necessary to assign a failing grade. In the context of this stressful situation for all involved, faculty must be aware of the legal concepts important to the evaluation process.

Academic Failure in the Clinical Setting

Faculty who teach clinical nursing courses are responsible for guiding students in the development of professional nursing skills and values. Faculty must ensure that the learning experiences chosen provide the student with the opportunity to develop those skills that ensure that they will become safe, competent practitioners. Applying a theoretical knowledge base, developing psychomotor skills, using appropriate communication techniques with patients and staff, exhibiting decision-making and organizational skills, and behaving in a professional manner are examples of the types of competencies that nursing students are expected to achieve through their clinical experiences. Faculty are also expected to make judgments and decisions about the ability of students to satisfactorily meet the objectives of the clinical experience. When students are unable to satisfactorily meet the objectives of the clinical experience, faculty have the legal and ethical responsibility to deny academic progression.

Legal and ethical grounds exist for dismissal of a student who is clinically deficient. Nurse Practice Acts exist in all states to regulate nursing practice and nursing education within a given state. Successful graduation from a nursing program should indicate that the student has achieved the minimum competencies required for safe practice.

When providing clinical care, nursing students will be held accountable for professionally negligent actions, and are required to come to clinical learning situations prepared and to ask for help when needed (Christensen, 2010). Although nursing practice is regulated by state law, which results in variations in practice standards between states, the prevailing view is that students are practicing on their own "fictitious license" and not the license of their instructor (Christensen, 2010). As a result, students will be held to the same standards of practice as a reasonable, prudent nurse with the same education and experience. Patients should expect that the care provided be safe, quality care at the level that is needed. In addition, students and faculty are expected to follow professional standards of practice and codes of ethics that have been developed to guide the profession, even though the students' educational experiences are not completed.

When engaged in clinical learning experiences, the nursing student is under the supervision of the clinical faculty, with input from agency staff. The nursing staff in the facility have ultimate control over patient care that is delivered, so there must be constant and appropriate communication between staff, faculty, and students. The clinical agency contract that allows the school to use the facility for learning experiences may also contain a clause stipulating that the school of nursing will provide supervision of students. It is also common for the agency to retain the right to request removal of students and faculty if the level of performance does not meet the standard of care acceptable to the institution, and could result in the loss of the clinical agency as a site for future clinical experiences. Faculty must accept responsibility for ensuring that students practice with an acceptable level of competence. Each member of the health care team is liable for his or her own potential negligence related to patient care. If the student does not provide care according to applicable standards, the student is liable for any resulting damage. If the nursing faculty does not adequately assign, monitor, and supervise the student, the nursing faculty is liable for resulting damage. And if the clinical staff who retain ultimate responsibility for the patient's care neglect their duties in overseeing the care, they are liable for resulting damage.

Clinical faculty have several responsibilities related to the instruction of students. First, clinical faculty must set clear expectations for student performance and communicate these expectations to students before the onset of any learning experience. These expectations must be reasonable for students to meet and must be consistently and equitably applied to all of the faculty member's assigned students. Second, faculty must determine the amount of supervision to provide to students.

When determining the appropriate level of supervision, faculty should consider the severity and stability of the assigned patient's condition, the types of treatments required by the patient, and the student's competency and ability to adapt to changing situations in the clinical setting. Another responsibility of clinical faculty is to judge the ability of the student to transfer classroom knowledge to the clinical setting.

Application of theory to nursing care is an important component of safe nursing practice, and faculty must engage in data collection to determine the level of student performance in this area. Faculty may collect data in multiple ways. For example, before providing care, students may be asked to develop written care plans and provide the rationale for their proposed nursing interventions. Faculty may also verbally ask students to explain the significance of patient assessment data they have gathered, or students may be asked to keep a weekly journal that provides insight into their clinical decision making. Chapters 17 and 25 provide further discussion of clinical teaching and evaluation. Whatever data collection methods are used by faculty to assess student performance must be consistently applied to all students. Because faculty retain the legal liability for appropriate student assignments and student monitoring to assure applicable standards of care are being followed, the faculty has the responsibility to remove students from providing clinical nursing care when the student is unsafe.

Fearing legal action, faculty may hesitate to fail a student who performs poorly in the clinical setting. However, federal and state courts have frequently upheld the responsibility and right of faculty to evaluate students' clinical performance and dismiss students who have failed to meet the criteria for a satisfactory performance. The courts have long indicated that faculty, as experts in their profession, are best qualified to make decisions about the academic performance of students (Brent, 2001; Christensen, 2014; Guido, 1997; Smith, McKoy, & Richardson, 2001). When teaching a clinical course, faculty must clearly establish and communicate the course and clinical objectives; they must document student performance and effectively communicate with students on an ongoing basis about their progress in the clinical area. These measures are discussed in greater depth in Chapter 17. Key to the success of any of these measures is that there has been clear communication of expectations to students.

As part of this communication, faculty should clearly identify at the beginning of the course, along with the clinical objectives, the level of clinical competence that students will be expected to achieve. These requirements should be stated in the course syllabus, along with information about how the clinical grade will be determined for the course. The clinical syllabus should clearly identify all of the evaluation measures that will be used in determining the clinical grade. Chapter 25 provides more information about the process of clinical evaluation. Students must be informed about how data will be obtained and whether the clinical evaluation will be formative, summative, or a combination. Students must receive continuing input through a formative evaluation process, periodically receiving information about progress and suggestions for improvement. Students must have time to demonstrate the course competency requirements during the clinical experiences and cannot be required to master those competencies until the end of the course. The consequences of not meeting objectives should also be clearly communicated to students.

Written records of all clinical experiences and student–faculty conferences should be kept for each student during the course. Hall (2013) studied the use of anecdotal notes in the clinical setting and suggested that the use of anecdotal notes can promote accurate student clinical evaluations.

Written records of a student's learning experiences document that the student has been provided with adequate opportunity to meet the clinical objectives. If opportunities to meet clinical objectives have not been provided, students cannot be evaluated or failed on unmet objectives.

Anecdotal records should be objectively written, describe both positive and negative aspects of a student's performance, and address the objectives of the course. Faculty should avoid commenting on the personality of the student but instead should reflect on what the student has or has not accomplished in relation to the course objectives. Notes of the student's daily and weekly assignments should be based on fact and should be nonjudgmental. Documenting both aspects of performance indicates that the student's total performance was taken into account when the final clinical grade was assigned.

Throughout the clinical experience, faculty should provide consistent, constructive feedback to students. Identifying positive aspects of a student's clinical performance and areas needing improvement will help that student develop self-esteem and confidence as a practitioner. Feedback is best conveyed in privacy, away from peers, staff, and patients, thus maintaining student confidentiality. Persistent clinical deficiencies should be addressed in conferences with the student, ideally away from the clinical setting. Written records of student–faculty conferences are used to document areas of faculty or student concern that have been discussed, along with the measures that are being taken to correct these deficiencies. Information about the progress the student makes toward correcting clinical deficiencies and any lack of progress should be included in follow-up notes. Both the faculty member and the student should sign these written records.

Communicating effectively with a student who is not performing satisfactorily can be difficult. When feedback is given to a student about deficiencies in performance, it is essential for the faculty member to convey to the student a sense of genuine concern about helping the student to improve his or her performance, as well as to convey the faculty member's responsibility for ensuring patient safety in the clinical setting. McGregor (2007) addressed the importance of the student–faculty relationship in which faculty are supportive when helping students cope with a clinical failure while at the same time retaining a sense of their self-worth and dignity. Students should be allowed the opportunity to clarify and respond to the feedback given by the faculty member. Sometimes an objective third party, such as a department chairperson or course coordinator, can assist by providing an objective perspective of the circumstances and serving as an impartial witness to what was said by both the faculty member and the student.

When notifying a student that course requirements are not being met and failure of the course may result, the faculty member must follow the institutional guidelines that have been established for such situations. Informing a student of unsatisfactory clinical performance can produce a stressful situation for the student. However, it also provides the due process that is the student's right in cases of academic deficiency. It enables the student to understand that his or her performance is unsatisfactory and provides the student with the opportunity to correct deficiencies. It is equally important that the faculty member communicate information about the student's performance to other faculty who are administratively responsible for the course.

Assisting the Failing Student in the Clinical Setting

How do clinical faculty determine when a student's clinical performance is unsatisfactory and warrants failure of the course? How many opportunities should the student be given to learn before being evaluated? These are questions that have been debated in nursing education for decades without resolution. Faculty are responsible for evaluating the cognitive, psychomotor, and affective behaviors of students during clinical learning experiences. Even with reliable and valid evaluation tools, it can be difficult to objectively evaluate the behavior of students, especially in the affective domain.

Clinical evaluation has many inherent challenges for the nurse educator. Clinical evaluation may be subjective, evaluation criteria may be misinterpreted by faculty or students, and clinical nursing practice is very complex (Krautscheid, Moceri, Stragnell, Manthey, & Neal, 2014).

Faculty in the clinical setting need to implement clear clinical evaluation measures and provide the student with frequent feedback as to their progress in meeting the clinical expectations. However, once having determined that a student's performance is unsatisfactory and that failure of the course is likely to occur, faculty must implement actions to protect the student's right to due process and assist the student through what will undoubtedly be a stressful experience.

Faculty may use several guidelines when working with students whose clinical performance is unsatisfactory. For example, as previously mentioned, unsatisfactory clinical behaviors should be identified and discussed with the student as early as possible. Documentation of the student's performance and all conferences with the student should be maintained.

Working in collaboration with the student, faculty should develop a plan or "learning contract" in which the needed areas of improvement are identified, along with appropriate measures to ensure improvement of performance. The student should be made aware that isolated instances of good or inadequate performance will not lead to a passing or failing grade. Instead, it is essential that the student strive to develop a consistency of behavior that portrays continuing improvement in performance and the delivery of safe patient care. The student should also understand that successful completion of any remedial work identified in the plan may not be sufficient to ensure a passing grade for the course; satisfactory completion of the course objectives will be required. After the plan has been detailed in a document, both the student and faculty should sign and date it. The student should be given a copy of the plan for his or her own records and reference.

Frequent feedback sessions are essential during this time, as the student attempts to make an improvement in performance. The number of sessions depends on the situation, but it is often helpful to agree to meet on a regular basis, for example, weekly. The faculty member should maintain objective and factual records of all sessions held with the student, including a description of strategies for intervention that were developed. Student self-appraisal should be a part of the process.

The student should also understand that during this period of evaluation, increased supervision and observation by faculty may be necessary to continue to ensure that patient safety is maintained. The student may report feeling treated unfairly or harassed and indicate that the increased faculty supervision is creating a stressful situation. It may be helpful at this time to refer the student to a counselor or other qualified individual for assistance with stress management. The clinical faculty member should refrain from assuming the role of counselor to the student because a conflict of interest could develop that would interfere with the objective and unbiased judgment of the instructor. Morgan (2001) cautioned that faculty, like counselors and therapists, have a responsibility to avoid assuming dual roles, such as counselor and faculty supervisor, when establishing relationships with students. It is imperative that the nurse educator only act within the boundaries of his or her position and role.

At times, a clinical instructor may experience a sense of concern about a student's performance but have difficulty clearly identifying the unsatisfactory behaviors. The instructor may wish to seek input from another faculty member about the student's performance. Faculty have the right, but no legal responsibility, to obtain an objective evaluation by another faculty member. If this is done, the faculty member must make the student aware of the purpose of this observation and that the results of the objective evaluation may affect the grade awarded.

If the student continues to provide unsafe patient care despite the interventions to improve performance, faculty can withdraw the student from the course before the end of the semester. Students who might qualify for removal from the clinical setting are those who demonstrate a consistent lack of understanding of their limitations, those who clearly and repeatedly cannot anticipate the consequences of their actions or lack of action, and those who consistently fail to maintain appropriate communication with faculty and staff about patient care. If a student is dishonest with faculty and staff about the care provided to a patient, serious, legal and ethical implications occur.

In all of these cases, patient care may be jeopardized and unsafe situations may be created for patients. Clinical faculty can refuse to allow a student to continue to provide care in the clinical setting; however, if the student's performance is safe, the student must be allowed to complete the clinical requirements of the course, even if the student is not meeting course objectives. Students are not required to achieve course objectives until the end of the course.

Following the mentioned procedures helps ensure that a student's right to due process has been upheld. Maintaining effective communication with the student throughout the experience may be difficult but is essential to achieving a satisfactory resolution to the situation for both faculty and student. When students perceive that they have been treated fairly and objectively, most will accept that they were unable to satisfactorily meet the objectives required of the course. Faculty should avoid excessive self-blame for the clinical failure of a student.

Academic Failure in the Classroom Setting

Nursing program curricula are by necessity academically rigorous. Academic classroom failure, with a subsequent attrition from the nursing program, is not uncommon, and retention of nursing students is a familiar concern of nurse educators. However, faculty have a responsibility to uphold academic standards and must at times assign a failing grade in a course.

The reasons for academic failure in the classroom are numerous. First, students may initially underestimate the amount of time that they will need to devote to course study to be successful in the pursuit of a nursing degree. Students may be unprepared and lack the study and time management skills necessary to organize their schedules and study time appropriately. Students can quickly become overwhelmed with the academic demand of a nursing program, and the resulting stress serves to further increase anxiety and the inability to deal with course requirements.

Second, many of today's nursing students are attempting to fulfill numerous roles, simultaneously juggling the responsibilities and demands of work, family, and school. Role overload becomes excessive, and the students' grades are adversely affected. Students are often forced to make difficult decisions and may be ill-equipped to identify appropriate priorities when addressing these issues.

Third, some students have difficulty with the level of cognitive ability required in nursing courses. Although adept at memorizing facts and information, they are not able to apply the concepts and develop the appropriate decision-making abilities. This is usually demonstrated by their inability to perform well on tests that demand application, analysis, and synthesis levels of cognition. Students who have never before been required to think on these levels may become frustrated when they spend much time memorizing information but still do not perform well on tests.

Some students may have learning disabilities that affect their ability to read with comprehension, successfully take tests, memorize information, or maintain concentration. Some students have satisfactory clinical performance but are unable to perform well in the classroom setting. See Chapter 4 for further discussion of students with learning disabilities. Students for whom English is a second language may also experience these difficulties.

Faculty have an ethical responsibility to identify students who are considered to be at high risk for academic failure in the classroom. The same examples of high-risk characteristics Donovan identified in 1989 are still pertinent today, and include low grade point average, low standardized test scores, decreased critical thinking skills, and attendance at several universities without attaining a degree. An additional high-risk characteristic is difficulty achieving satisfactory grades in required science courses (Wolkowitz & Kelley, 2010). When students who have these characteristics are accepted into a nursing program, academic support services must be provided to increase their chances of success. Students who are working more than 16 hours a week and those who have English as a second language have also been documented to be at increased risk for lower academic performance (Salamonson & Andrew, 2006).

Faculty also have the responsibility for developing and providing academic support services that increase students' chances for success and thus increase student retention in the nursing program. There are many services that may be available to assist students academically, such as tutoring programs, individual course study sessions, study skills workshops, faculty–student mentoring programs, test-taking support, peer study sessions, and time and stress management training. Faculty should be aware of resources within other departments in the institution that can offer valuable assistance to students in need. They should also encourage activities that provide a support system for students, such as participation in student clubs and organizations. Peer mentoring can also be an effective educational strategy that benefits both the student serving as the mentor and the student being mentored (Dennison, 2010; Robinson & Niemer, 2010). Developing and providing support services for students with academic difficulties helps ensure that students receive the assistance they need at the earliest possible intervention point.

Assisting the Failing Student in the Classroom Setting

When designing intervention programs that will assist students to be academically successful in a nursing program, faculty must consider the academic experience from the perspective of the student because this may have major implications for student retention and success. Faculty should obtain feedback from students in the program about their areas of concern, both academic and nonacademic. For example, if students believe that large class size is interfering with their ability to learn, strategies that provide students with access to faculty in small groups could be implemented. Student focus groups can provide much feedback, and faculty can use this information to develop interventions.

Faculty also need input about what programs or interventions are working (e.g., tutoring services, orientation programs, peer-to-peer study assistance groups) so that these can be continued or eliminated according to their success. Faculty need to know what concerns students have that can be addressed with appropriate resources. Using this information, faculty would be able to develop a retention intervention program designed to maximize students' positive experiences and enhance academic success.

More specifically, faculty can implement several proactive strategies that support students' academic efforts in the classroom. First, faculty should remain aware of the changing student population and students' different learning styles. Nurse educators need to develop innovative, flexible programs designed to support the academic needs of the increasing numbers of nontraditional adult learners, graduate students, and culturally diverse students.

Flexible class scheduling, the use of technology to provide learning at convenient times for students, campus child care, recognition of students' life experiences, and support for students with English as a second language can all help students achieve their educational goals. The learning expectations and strategies of today's college students are likely to be different than those of students of the past. Much literature has been published that addresses the varying learning styles of the current generation, and information gained from those studies should be used to provide meaningful learning experiences for students.

Students who are successfully integrated academically and socially into the academic environment will more likely be retained in the system. Institutions must realize that students bring diverse needs to the educational process. The role of the faculty adviser is key in assisting students to successfully adjust to their academic responsibilities. Faculty need to be informed about academic policies that affect student advisement so that they are able to provide accurate, timely information.

Academic advising by faculty plays an essential role in the student's academic success as well as in retention in nursing programs (Harrison, 2012). Rosenberg and O'Rourke (2011) suggested that increasing the diversity and cultural competence of the faculty can be used to improve student retention among students from diverse backgrounds. Nursing associations or organizations can be a source of encouragement for students and can serve as a vehicle for socializing students into the nursing profession.

Individually, faculty members can take several steps to assist students who are doing poorly in the classroom. When a student demonstrates evidence of a lack of understanding of content of the course, such as failing a test or not completing an assignment properly, the faculty member should meet with the student to identify the student's perspective of the problem. Students are often able to recognize the problem themselves, such as not enough time spent in preparation, lack of understanding of the material, or personal problems. Each of these reasons for poor performance requires the use of different intervention strategies, and the student should be involved in determining what actions are to be taken. Tests should be reviewed to assess the areas of difficulty and to determine whether the problem is potentially related to, for example, lack of knowledge about content, reading difficulties, anxiety associated with test taking, poor study skills, or personal difficulties. Once the potential causes have been identified, intervention strategies can be designed and implemented to help correct the situation.

Faculty must realize that it is the student's responsibility to learn as well as the student's responsibility to use the resources available to improve academic performance. Students must take responsibility for carrying out the plan of action developed in conjunction with the faculty member. Faculty cannot assume responsibility for ensuring that all students are successful in the course, but they must make certain that students are active participants in identifying concerns, developing strategies to address deficiencies, and improving performance. Faculty should always be willing to listen to student concerns and make referrals to appropriate program resources when appropriate.

If, despite various efforts, a student cannot satisfactorily meet the course requirements, faculty have no alternative but to assign a failing grade. At this point, the student will require guidance and support as the available options are reviewed. If this is the first nursing course that the student has failed, it is commonly program policy to allow one retake of the course. If this is the second nursing course failure for the student, the student may be dismissed from the program. The student should receive appropriate academic advice as he or she plans future educational goals.

Ethical Issues Related to Academic Performance

Many ethical principles that influence student–faculty relationships and interactions are the same ones that guide interactions between nurses and patients. The relationship should be characterized by mutual respect and open communication. Faculty have a responsibility to conduct themselves in a manner that is exemplary, fair, nonjudgmental, and just, and should serve as role models for students in demonstrating honest academic conduct. It is apparent, though, that there is the potential for student–faculty conflict to develop in these interactions. Faculty should consider the ethical implications that exist in relationships developed with students. This section addresses ethical issues that can develop in student–faculty relationships, including academic dishonesty and the nature of interactions occurring between students and faculty. Suggestions for avoiding the development of unethical situations are provided.

Academic Dishonesty

A student copies from another student during a test or uses "crib" notes; another student agrees to help an academically weaker student by providing answers to a test. Lacking the time it takes to write a term paper, a student turns in a paper written by another student, while yet another student plagiarizes portions of a term paper, taking the chance that the professor will not detect the omission of appropriate reference citations. During a clinical experience, a student forgets to administer a medication on time. Fearing the consequences of admitting the error, the student instead documents it as "given." These are all examples of academic dishonesty, or "cheating," representing one of the most difficult situations faculty have to deal with in their interactions with students.

Unfortunately, such incidents are not uncommon and as technology has developed and students have become more proficient, the methods of cheating have become more complicated and complex (DiBartolo & Walsh, 2010; Sifford, 2006). As computer technology has become common-place, students have used more sophisticated high-tech methods of cheating, such as the use of smart phones, cameras, text messages, and inappropriate computer use. Additional cheating methods may include use of tattoos, labels on drinking containers, and papers purchased online. Numerous reports detail alarming statistics that demonstrate an increasing occurrence and acceptance of cheating in schools at every level. Krueger (2014) completed a study of nursing students' engagement in academic dishonesty and identified that more than half of the study participants reported cheating in the classroom and clinical setting. Nursing faculty may be particularly concerned about academic dishonesty because a link between unethical classroom behavior and unethical clinical behavior exists.

McCabe (2009) pointed out that schools and faculty have a major role to play in addressing issues of academic dishonesty. Fontana (2009) noted that the cost to nursing faculty who discover and take action when academic dishonesty occurs is significant. She reported that faculty feel they have significant changes in student relationships, that there is a significant risk associated with confronting students, and that even collegial relationships are altered. However, most faculty are committed to maintaining integrity within nursing education, although they do not always have the knowledge of practices that can assist in deterring cheating (Stonecypher & Willson, 2014).

Many factors may influence a student's decision to cheat. Many authorities note that an alarming number of students do not consider their behavior to be unethical or cheating, but rather see it as acceptable and common. Literature has addressed the concept of academic entitlement, whereby the student feels entitled to the degree because they have paid their tuition, rather than feeling entitled to the opportunity to learn (Karpen, 2014). Dishonesty in the classroom setting is a concern for nursing faculty because of the potential for the student to also demonstrate dishonest behavior within the clinical setting.

Numerous strategies and practices have been identified to deter cheating in nursing education (Stonecypher & Willson, 2014). An initial strategy to address academic honesty should be a careful review of the faculty's own behaviors. For example, do faculty cite sources on materials presented to students in class? Are student contributions to research and publications appropriately acknowledged? Are faculty expectations realistic in terms of time requirements for students? Is there discussion about the importance of values and values development in students, or do these discussions occur only when a crisis situation has occurred? These authors point to the importance of a learning environment that integrates ethics into the entire curriculum and the use of learning strategies that work to develop values and behaviors in students that have lasting consequences. Nursing faculty must role-model a high level of integrity as well as create high-integrity classrooms to promote ethical practices in students (Eby et al., 2013).

Maintaining civility in student–faculty interactions is another important action that faculty can take to serve as positive role models for students (DiBartolo & Walsh, 2010) and to create learning environments that engender respect for all individuals. Bullying occurs at all levels of nursing, including nursing education and nursing practice (Matt, 2012). Faculty are in the power position with respect to the student because faculty hold the power over a student's grade and program progression. Faculty may not think that their actions would be considered bullying, but when the imbalance of power in the teacher–student relationship is considered, actions the faculty perceive as innocent or even helpful may in fact fit the definition of student bullying. It is imperative that faculty not allow an environment of incivility or bullying to occur within the nursing program.

Faculty can take a number of actions to deter cheating in their courses. One of the most common forms of academic dishonesty is cheating on classroom tests. This may be done by copying from another student's test, with or without the cooperation of the other student, concealing and bringing into the classroom potential answers to the test, or obtaining test questions from students who were previously enrolled in the course. Developing alternate test forms that can be used in subsequent semesters can help decrease the likelihood of questions being shared between classes of students. Alternative test forms can also be used among students in the same class, thus decreasing the chance that students can cheat by looking at the test of the student sitting next to them. Requiring students to leave books and other personal items at the front of the classroom or under their desks and rearranging the seating can also make it more difficult for students to cheat. Directing students to look only at their own tests can serve to remind students that their behavior is being observed and that they are responsible for not conveying the appearance of cheating.

Another common method of cheating is plagiarism of written work, through either the use of papers written by other students or the inappropriate citation of references. Students may be unclear about what constitutes plagiarism; therefore faculty should consider clarifying this at the beginning of the course, including how and when citing is to be done and what consequences will take place if plagiarism occurs. The proactive approach has been shown to be more successful, especially when tied to the development of an environment of academic honesty, often linked to an honor code or honor system. This may reduce the number of "I did not know that was wrong" excuses from students. Requesting that copies of the references cited in written work be turned in with the assignment can facilitate faculty review of the materials and reduce the likelihood that students will deliberately plagiarize. Keeping on file copies of past student papers can also decrease the likelihood that students will be able to represent a previous student's work as their own.

Sometimes students are pressured into helping another student cheat on coursework, either through a misguided sense of feeling sorry for and wanting to "help" the student or sometimes through fear. It can be helpful to periodically review the institution's policy on academic dishonesty with students in the class, especially if the faculty member suspects there may be a problem. Many students do not realize that institutional policies commonly state explicitly that a student participating in and enabling another student to cheat is also guilty of academic dishonesty and may be disciplined as well. Also, most institutions have policies that provide guidance for students who feel that they are being verbally and otherwise harassed by another student.

A wide variety of practices are described in the literature to deter cheating (Stonecypher & Willson, 2014). Solomon and DeNatale (2000) described the use of a program-wide convocation to discuss the issue of academic dishonesty, maintaining that drawing the analogy between academic dishonesty and professional ethics is an important first step in socializing students into the nursing profession. Academic honor codes can be used as a proactive stance to discourage dishonesty and to foster the development of a professional value system within an institution. An academic honor code should define what activities constitute academic misconduct, what disciplinary action could result if the student engages in such activity, and the student grievance and appeal procedure. Colleges with honor codes have been reported to have fewer incidences of academic dishonesty (Krueger, 2014). McCabe and Trevino (1996) reported that evidence exists to suggest that the presence of a campus academic honor code creates an environment where cheating is not a socially acceptable behavior and decreases the number of incidences of student dishonesty.

They also point out that student involvement in the outcomes (e.g., student hearings, student courts) may also deter cheating.

It is also helpful if written statements on course syllabi are used to remind students of the institution's policy on academic dishonesty and the academic code of honor, if one exists. The consequences of cheating and violating the honor code should also be clearly delineated in course syllabi. If cheating has occurred, does the student get an F for the assignment or an F for the course? Or are other options a possibility? This information can be included in the evaluation section of the syllabus and lets students know that any incidents of cheating will be taken seriously by the faculty member. It is important that these outcomes be guided by school policy and procedure; all course policies must be congruent with those of the broader school guidelines.

If a faculty member has evidence that a student has engaged in some form of academic dishonesty, it becomes necessary for him or her to confront the student about the incident. Jeffreys and Stier (1995) recommended that the following steps be followed when discussing an incident of academic dishonesty.

Privacy should first be ensured for the student when initiating discussion of the incident. It is appropriate to include an impartial third party, such as the department chairperson or another faculty member, in the discussion. Faculty must clearly communicate to the student the identified dishonest behavior and the potential consequences resulting from this behavior. It is important that faculty convey this information in an objective manner, avoiding blame or anger. The student should be informed of institutional policies and the importance of adhering to professional standards of conduct. The conference should be documented by the faculty member. As mentioned previously in the section regarding disciplinary action and due process, the student's right to due process should be ensured before any action is taken.

Student–Faculty Relationships

As discussed earlier in this chapter, the nature of the relationships that students develop with faculty in the classroom and clinical setting can have a profound influence on the quality of the students' education experiences. The relationship of the student to faculty in nursing may be closer than in other disciplines because of the increased amount of individual contact that occurs between students and faculty. Novice faculty often are uncertain about how to appropriately develop relationships with students. This can have a major effect on the success of faculty in the classroom and their personal satisfaction with their role as an educator. Faculty may indeed be very knowledgeable about the content they teach, but if they cannot relate in a positive manner to students, the students may not listen to the substance of the information being conveyed. Novice faculty should be encouraged to seek guidance on how to develop an effective interpersonal style with students (Halstead, 1996).

Behaviors that help develop effective relationships with students are those that have been described throughout this chapter. Open, ongoing dialogue with students throughout the educational process is essential. Students have the right to expect from faculty respect for their ideas and opinions (although not necessarily agreement); constructive, helpful feedback on their academic performance; a willingness to answer questions and address concerns the student may have; and a respect for student confidentiality. Displaying an appropriate sense of humor and warmth with students is also important and allows students to see the human side of faculty.

Behaviors that are inappropriate and unethical in the teaching situation include using sarcasm or belittling the student, threatening the student with failure, criticizing the student in front of others, acting superior, discussing confidential student issues with other faculty, and displaying inappropriate sexual behavior. Standards and guidelines addressing sexual harassment are part of each institution's policies and procedures. Nursing faculty must be informed about such policies and must follow them explicitly. Faculty may also serve to assist students to access appropriate resources should students have issues with sexual harassment by other members of the university community and need such assistance.

Showing favoritism in the treatment or grading of students, refusing to answer students' questions, behaving rudely, and being authoritarian are other examples of unethical teaching behaviors. Student–faculty interactions that are based on the inappropriate use of power and control cannot result in caring, collegial relationships. In some institutions, policies govern the contact that is appropriate between students and faculty. Those policies must always guide decisions about appropriate student contact and interaction.

Faculty can foster the development of positive student–faculty relationships through the design of learning experiences that promote collaborative, collegial learning exchanges between faculty and students. Faculty need to examine their beliefs about the teaching–learning process and student–faculty relationships to gain an understanding of their own attitudes. The first step in the process of fostering a learning environment that is empowering for both faculty and students is conceptualizing the student–faculty relationship as a collaborative partnership instead of an authoritarian one (Halstead, 1996).

Summary

This chapter provides an overview of the legal and ethical issues that are related to the academic performance of students. The development of positive student–faculty interactions and the faculty role in evaluation of student performance is discussed. The legal and ethical concepts that guide student and faculty interactions and relationships are explained. Academic failure in the classroom and clinical setting is discussed, as are methods of assisting students through this difficult experience while ensuring their rights to due process. The importance of clear, mutual communication of expectations between students and faculty is emphasized.

Nursing students in today's classroom exhibit different characteristics from those of faculty when they were nursing students. Today's diverse students bring a richness of life experiences to the learning experience. Each student is an individual possessing a variety of knowledge, skills, values, beliefs, and needs that will help form the nursing professional that the nursing student wishes to become. It is important for nurse educators to meet the needs of these students by establishing professional relationships that are positive and empowering in nature, ultimately providing students with a learning environment that supports their personal and professional goals.

REFLECTING ON THE EVIDENCE

1. Under what circumstances would it be appropriate to share personal information you have gained from a student with your direct supervisor? With colleagues? Under what circumstances, if any, should it be mandatory that you would do so?
2. What "boundaries" should guide the development of the student–faculty relationship? Are there any activities that are "off limits"?
3. What actions should be considered when a faculty member suspects a student has cheated on an assignment? Is that different than "cheating" in a clinical venue (e.g., altering data, recording data that was not assessed)? Should these situations be treated differently? Why or why not?

REFERENCES

A v. C. College, 863 F. Supp. 156 (S.D.N.Y. 1994).

Board of Curators of the University of Missouri v. Horowitz, 435 U.S. 78 (1978).

Boehm v. U. of PA. School of Vet. Med., 573 A.2d 575 (Pa. Super. Ct. 1990).

Brent, N. (2001). *Nurses and the law: A guide to principles and applications*. Philadelphia, PA: W. B. Saunders.

Christensen, L. (2010). The law and the nurse educator: A look at legal cases. In L. Caputi (Ed.), *Teaching nursing: The art and science* (pp. 83–127). Glen Ellyn, IL: College of DuPage Press.

Christensen, L. (2014, September). *Educational law that all nursing program administrators should know*. In Workshop conducted at the National League for Nursing Education Summit, Phoenix, AZ.

Dennison, S. (2010). Peer mentoring: Untapped potential. *Journal of Nursing Education, 49*(6), 340–342.

DiBartolo, M., & Walsh, C. (2010). Desperate times call for desperate measures: Where are we in addressing academic dishonesty? *Journal of Nursing Education, 49*(10), 543–544.

Dixon v. Alabama State Board of Education, 294 F. 2d 150 (5th Cir. 1961.).

Donovan, M. (1989). The "high-risk" student: An ethical challenge for faculty. *Journal of Professional Nursing, 5*(3), 120.

Eby, R., Hartley, P., Hodges, P., Hoffpauir, R., Newbanks, S., & Kelley, J. (2013). Moral integrity and moral courage: Can you teach it? *Journal of Nursing Education, 52*(4), 229–233.

Federal Educational Rights and Privacy Act (FERPA), 20 U.S.C. § 1232 g; 34 CRF Part 99 (1974).

Fontana, J. (2009). Nursing faculty experiences of students' academic dishonesty. *Journal of Nursing Education, 48*(4), 181–185.

Goss v. Lopez, 419 U.S. 565 (1975).

Guido, G. (1997). *Legal issues in nursing*. Stamford, CT: Appleton & Lange.

Hall, M. (2013). An expanded look at evaluating clinical performance: Faculty use of anecdotal notes in the U.S. and Canada. *Nurse Education in Practice, 13*, 271–276.

Halstead, J. A. (1996). The significance of student-faculty interactions. In K. Stevens (Ed.), *Review of research in nursing education: Vol. VII*. New York: National League for Nursing.

Halstead, J. (2007). *Nurse educator competencies: Creating an evidence-based practice for nurse educators*. New York, NY: National League for Nursing.

Harrison, E. (2012). Development and pilot testing of the faculty advisor evaluation questionnaire. *Journal of Nursing Education, 51*(3), 167–171.

Health Insurance Portability and Accountability Act, Pub.L. 104-191, 110 Stat. 1936 (1996).

Jeffreys, M. R., & Stier, L. A. (1995). Speaking against student academic dishonesty: A communication model for nurse educators. *Journal of Nursing Education, 34*(7), 297–304.

Kaplin, W., & Lee, B. (2014). *The law of higher education* (5th ed., student version). San Francisco, CA: Jossey-Bass.

Karpen, S. (2014). Academic entitlement: A student's perspective. *American Journal of Pharmaceutical Education, 78*(2), Article 44.

Krautscheid, L., Moceri, J., Stragnell, S., Manthey, L., & Neal, T. (2014). A descriptive study of a clinical evaluation tool and process: Student and faculty perspectives. *Journal of Nursing Education, 53*(3), S30–S33.

Krueger, L. (2014). Academic dishonesty among nursing students. *Journal of Nursing Education, 53*(2), 77–87.

Matt, S. (2012). Ethical and legal issues associated with bullying in the nursing profession. *Journal of Nursing Law, 15*(1), 9–13.

McCabe, D. (2009). Academic dishonesty in nursing schools: An empirical investigation. *Journal of Nursing Education, 48*(11), 614–623.

McCabe, D. L., & Trevino, L. K. (1996). What we know about cheating in college: Longitudinal trends and recent developments. *Change, 28*(1), 28–33.

McGregor, A. (2007). Academic success, clinical failure: Struggling practices of a failing student. *Journal of Nursing Education, 46*(11), 504–511.

Morgan, J. E. (2001). Confidential student information in nursing education. *Nurse Educator, 26*(6), 289–292.

Morrison, S. (2010). Test construction and item writing. In L. Caputi (Ed.), *Teaching nursing: The art and science* (pp. 2–44). Glen Ellyn, IL: College of DuPage Press.

National League for Nursing. (2005). *Transforming nursing education*. New York, NY: Author.

National League for Nursing. (2012). *The scope of practice for academic nurse educators*. New York: Author.

Regents of University of Michigan v. Ewing, 474 U.S. 214 (106 S. Ct 507 1985.).

Robinson, E., & Niemer, L. (2010). A peer mentor tutor program for academic success in nursing. *Nursing Education Perspectives, 31*(5), 286–289.

Rosenberg, L., & O'Rourke, M. (2011). The diversity pyramid: An organizational model to structure diversity recruitment and retention in nursing programs. *Journal of Nursing Education, 50*(10), 555–560.

Salamonson, Y., & Andrew, S. (2006). Academic performance in nursing students: Influence of part-time employment, age and ethnicity. *Journal of Advanced Nursing, 55*(3), 342–349. http://dx.doi.org/10.1111/j.1365-2648.2006.03863.x.

Schaer v. Brandeis University, 432 Mass. 474 (2000).

Sifford, K. (2006). Academic integrity and cheating. *Nursing Education Perspectives, 27*(1), 35–36.

Smith, M., McKoy, M., & Richardson, J. (2001). Legal issues related to dismissing students for clinical deficiencies. *Nurse Educator, 26*(1), 33–38.

Solomon, M., & DeNatale, M. (2000). Academic dishonesty and professional practice: A convocation. *Nurse Educator, 25*(6), 270–271.

Stonecypher, K., & Willson, P. (2014). Academic policies and practices to deter cheating in nursing education. *Nursing Education Perspectives, 35*(3), 167–179.

Sullivan Commission Report. (2004). *Missing persons: Minorities in the health professions*. Washington, DC: Report of the Sullivan Commission on Diversity in the Workforce.

Suplee, P., Gardner, M., Jerome-D'Emilia. (2014). Nursing faculty preparedness for clinical teaching. *Journal of Nursing Education, 53*(3), S38–S41.

Tarasoff v. Regents of the University of California, 17 Cal. 3d 425, 551 P.2d 334, 131 Cal. Rptr. 14 (Cal. 1976).

U.S. Const. amend. V & XIV.

Wolkowitz, A., & Kelley, J. (2010). Academic predictors of success in a nursing program. *Journal of Nursing Education, 49*(9), 498–503.

Facilitating Learning for Students with Disabilities

4

Betsy Frank, PhD, RN, ANEF

More than 40 years ago, Congress passed the Rehabilitation Act (1973). This act states that any program or activity that receives federal funding cannot deny access or participation to individuals with disabilities. Section 504 of this act specifically addresses higher education and prohibits public postsecondary institutions that receive federal funds from discriminating against individuals with disabilities. Furthermore, more than 20 years ago Congress enacted the Americans with Disabilities Act (ADA) (1990). This act was further updated in 2008 and is now sometimes referred to as the ADA Amendments Act of 2008 (ADAAA). A summary of key provisions has been published to facilitate use of the Act's provisions (Summary of key provisions, n.d.). Because of these two laws, colleges and universities have experienced an increased number of students with disabilities admitted to their programs, including nursing programs. In the 2008–2009 academic year, more than 640,000 students with disabilities were enrolled across all levels of postsecondary education (National Center for Education Statistics, 2011). Although the numbers of nursing students were not isolated within these data, one can presume that the numbers provided included nursing students enrolled in prelicensure and postlicensure programs.

Dealing with students who have disabilities is not unique to the United States. The Discrimination Act of 1995, with amendments in 2005, and the Nursing and Midwifery Council 2006 standards guide nurse educators in the United Kingdom in educating nursing students with disabilities (Tee et al., 2010).

Nursing students with special needs present a challenge to nursing faculty in both the classroom and clinical settings. Students who have special needs include those who have a physical disability such as a visual, hearing, or mobility impairment; a chronic illness; a learning disability; or a chemical dependency problem. Many nursing programs have had experience in meeting the needs of these students. For example, a recent study by Betz, Smith, and Bui (2012) estimated from a survey of 65 nursing programs in California that approximately 5% of students across associate degree programs, 2% of baccalaureate students, and 0.6% of master's students had some form of disability. Learning disabilities were the most common type of disability reported. Betz et al. (2012, p. 680) also found that the majority of the students did not disclose their disability prior to admission.

Although many students with disabilities are enrolled in nursing programs, faculty often have reservations about their ability to deliver safe patient care. A nationwide survey of baccalaureate programs revealed that nurse educators preferred able-bodied students (Aaberg, 2012). Others, such as Dupler, Allen, Maheady, Fleming, and Allen (2012) have challenged nursing faculty to adopt a more open approach to accommodating students with disabilities. In fact, Griffiths, Worth, Scullard, and Gilbert (2010) suggested that a multifaceted approach to working with students who have disabilities includes holistic, student-centered strategies and encouraged the involvement of practice partners in providing appropriate clinical experiences.

Wood and Marshall's (2010) survey of nurse leaders echoed Griffiths et al. (2010). Wood and Marshall found that nurse managers rated the performance of nurses with disabilities as "exceptional or above average" (p. 182). Furthermore, they discovered that the environment and attitudes of co-workers could hamper work performance despite the fact that accommodations most likely could have been made. As more students with disabilities seek admission to nursing programs, and as those within the profession age, retaining nurses with disabilities in the workforce will be essential. Patient safety concerns notwithstanding, without an open attitude toward students with disabilities, much nursing talent may be lost.

This chapter addresses the issues related to the education of students with disabilities. It specifically focuses on common problems experienced by college students and nursing students: learning disabilities, physical disabilities, mental health problems, and chemical impairment issues. The Rehabilitation Act of 1973, the ADA as amended in 2008 (Summary of key provisions, n.d.), and the significance of these acts to nursing education are also addressed.

Legal Issues Related to Students with Disabilities

Faculty should be aware of the legal issues associated with teaching students with disabilities. The ADA protects the rights of individuals with disabilities in the arenas of education, employment, and environmental accessibility. Higher education institutions must guarantee individuals with disabilities equal access to educational opportunities. Discrimination against individuals with physical and mental disabilities is prohibited by the ADA. However, the ADA does not guarantee that an admitted student will achieve academic success—only that the student has the *opportunity* to achieve academic success. A university or college has the obligation to maintain academic and behavioral standards for all students, disabled or not (Meloy & Gambescia, 2014).

The full effect of the ADA on professional education continues to be determined as more potential students with disabilities seek admission to nursing programs. Focusing on stated program outcomes rather than on specific skills puts faculty in a better position to make decisions about reasonable accommodations for students who are disabled or have other special needs. Aaberg (2012) has recommended that essential functions be more job-related than applied to all nurses or nursing students. For example, not all nurses work in intensive care; therefore not all nurses need to hear a monitor alarm within a prescribed distance. Failure of an institution to make reasonable accommodations for a student who is disabled is considered discrimination (Dupler et al., 2012), and the institution and faculty may be sued for failing to make reasonable accommodations. For example, a Missouri Appeals Court ruled that a nursing program had erred in dismissing a deaf nursing student because she needed accommodations in clinical practice (*Wells v. Lester E. Cox Medical Centers,* 2012).

Implications for Nursing Education

By law, students have the responsibility to notify the institution regarding a disability and the need for accommodation (Dupler et al., 2012). Although disclosure of disabilities is voluntary and not legally required, students who have a disability and require accommodation are encouraged to share this information with the institution's office for students with disabilities. However, many students will not share information regarding their disabilities for fear of rejection.

Barriers to student success may be related more to faculty and practice partners' attitudes rather than to student ability (Aaberg, 2012; Scullion, 2010). Based on faculty interviews, Ashcroft and Lutfiyya (2013) developed a grounded theory about nurse educators' perceptions of working with students with disabilities. Their theory was named "producing competent graduates" (p. 1317). Subthemes within the theory included "let's work with it" (the disability); "it becomes very difficult" (to accommodate); "what would happen if someone died?"(due to unsafe practice); a wary challenge; educator attributes, which included past experience in working with students with disabilities; and perceived student attributes, or kind of disability.

Negative faculty attitudes can change. A study by Tee and Cowen (2012) demonstrated that a variety of strategies can enhance the ability of practice partners to work with students who have disabilities. Such strategies included having students tell their stories and developing a series of DVDs and interactive slide shows that practice partners, called *mentors,* could use to understand the issues faced by students with disabilities and how to appropriately accommodate those students. Education for faculty related to providing accommodations and understanding the possibilities for achievement among students with disabilities is key for students' academic success.

When a student makes known the presence of a disability and gives permission to share this information with faculty, course faculty are notified about the disability that requires accommodation. Course faculty must keep this information confidential and are not to share this information with other faculty, as it is the student's responsibility to decide when and where to disclose the presence of a disability. Students may choose not to disclose a disability in some courses. Even when student consent is given to share information with faculty, the nature of the disability is not disclosed to faculty unless the student decides to disclose it (Meloy & Gambescia, 2014). Box 4-1 is an example of a statement of services provided for students with disabilities. To receive accommodation, the student must disclose the presence of a disability prior to engaging in the learning experience; it is not possible to retroactively claim the need for accommodations after the student has already unsuccessfully engaged in the experience.

Faculty are not allowed to inquire about the nature of the disability. In fact, decisions regarding whether accommodation is possible must be made after the student has been admitted, unless essential abilities are published and *all* students are asked before admission whether they possess the abilities needed for academic success (Aaberg, 2012). However, most lists of essential abilities focus, in part, on physical abilities such as lifting. Recent initiatives call into question such requirements (American Nurses Association, n.d.). Although some schools publish essential abilities that students must achieve, faculty need to consider if they are truly essential to nursing practice. Levey (2014) conducted an integrative literature review on faculty attitudes regarding various aspects of working with nursing students who have disabilities, and concluded that disclosure of disability status prior to admission can be a barrier for students, especially if essential abilities are published. Furthermore, Levey stated that essential functions are more related to employment, not student status. Faculty must remember, however, that students are not required to disclose disabilities prior to admission.

When considering the admission of a student who has a disability, admission committees in schools of nursing must consider the following questions:

- Disregarding the disability, is the individual otherwise qualified to be admitted to the program?
- What reasonable accommodations can the school make to enable the student to be successful in the pursuit of becoming a nurse who can deliver safe patient care?

Although institutions are not expected to lower or alter academic or technical standards to accommodate a student with a disability (Meloy & Gambescia, 2014), they are expected to determine what accommodations would be reasonable for a student who is disabled. Examples of reasonable accommodations include altering the length of test-taking times or methods, providing proctors to read tests or write test answers, allowing additional time to complete the program of study, providing supplemental study aids such as audiotapes of texts, providing note takers, or altering the method of course delivery, such as the use of simulation for some clinical practice (Azzopardi et al., 2014). The same considerations must be given to students who become disabled during their enrollment in a nursing program. Questions to be asked include the following:

- Disregarding the disability, is the student otherwise qualified to continue in the nursing program?
- What reasonable accommodations can be made to allow the student to continue?

Concepts of universal design can accommodate learning styles for all students, not just students with disabilities (Meloy & Gambescia, 2014). Marcyjanik and Zom (2011) have stated that universal design is particularly important for courses offered at a distance. Universal design promotes course design that

BOX 4-1 Services for Persons with Disabilities

Disability Support Services provides reasonable, appropriate, and effective academic accommodations to those with known disabilities. This may include academic adjustments and services such as special testing arrangements. Note-taker services are available to qualified individuals. Services for persons with disabilities are based on individual needs and the University's intent to offer appropriate accommodations according to the student's documentation of need for same. These services are coordinated by the Student Support Services Grant Program. It is recommended that persons with disabilities visit Indiana State University prior to making a decision to enroll.

Courtesy Indiana State University Undergraduate Catalog, 2014–2015.

> ### *BOX 4-2* Universal Design Strategies
>
> 1. Have course materials available in audio and video format.
> 2. Design uncluttered webpages that don't rely on color alone.
> 3. Provide accessible javascript.
> 4. Provide access to webpages that convert text to audio and audio to text.

uses multiple ways of presenting course materials and engaging students in their learning and multiple ways for students to demonstrate course outcomes in the classroom and at a distance (Tobin, 2013). Most learning management systems allow faculty to use universal design in presenting their course materials. (Box 4-2 provides suggested universal design strategies.) Instructional design specialists should be part of the team that designs accessible distance courses.

Faculty should consider that just because a student has a disability, he or she is not necessarily ill, and the type of support needed is not the type needed to cure an illness but to support health (Evans, 2014a). Whether a person's limitations are viewed as a disability is defined by society rather than by the actual abilities of the person involved. Thus the process of deciding what is a reasonable accommodation for a person with a disability is complex and is influenced as much by faculty and practice partner attitudes as by actual student abilities.

As the influence of the ADA, and now ADAAA, on nursing education continues to unfold in the courts and in the workplace, nurse educators must keep current with legal developments that relate to the education of individuals with disabilities who are pursuing degrees in the health professions. Some suggestions for increasing faculty awareness of the needs of students with disabilities include periodic continuing education sessions related to the legal implications of educating such students and the use of consultants who are experts in working with students with disabilities. Most institutions of higher education have an office dedicated to assisting and supporting students with disabilities who are enrolled on campus. This office can provide resources and expert advice to faculty and students. Another source of information may be individuals with disabilities who have successfully developed a career in nursing. These successful nurses can help nursing faculty understand the issues involved in educating students with disabilities and they can serve as mentors to students with disabilities who are pursuing a nursing education. Practicing nurses with disabilities can serve as advocates for students as well as help nursing programs advocate for students who graduate and then seek employment.

Nursing faculty should begin to separate the truly essential components of nursing education from the merely traditional nursing curricula and teaching strategies. Nursing faculty need to consider such philosophical issues as whether nursing education might be extended to those individuals who will never practice bedside nursing in an acute care setting. Such nursing jobs might include staff development, infection control, case management, or a variety of jobs in the community settings where nursing care is delivered. A study of admission and retention practices of California nursing schools (Betz et al., 2012) showed that nursing faculty vary in approaches in dealing with disabilities. In making admission and progression decisions for all students, faculty need to balance student rights, safety, and abilities with issues of patient safety and university responsibility for providing appropriate accommodations according to the ADA. Faculty can use a variety of clinical settings to achieve the prescribed learning outcomes. Working with preceptors in practice not only assists students in their educational process (Tee & Cowen, 2012) but could also demonstrate that disabled students can be successful as graduates by providing evidence of safe practice given by the students.

The Nursing Student with a Learning Disability

Learning disabilities are the most common type of student disability found on college campuses (National Center for Education Statistics, 2011), with approximately 2% of undergraduates having some form of learning disability (Vickers, 2010). A learning disability is an incurable neurologic disorder that interferes with learning in a variety of ways (LD Online, 2015b). Dyslexia, or reading difficulties, is one common form of learning disabilities. Frequently students begin college with undetected learning disabilities. In nursing education learning disabilities are commonly uncovered when faculty notice striking differences between a student's classroom performance and clinical performance. The student may display an adequate knowledge base and competent skills during clinical experiences but be unable to demonstrate the same degree of knowledge when taking tests in the classroom. Such disparities in performance lead to much frustration and stress for the student and, not uncommonly, academic failure. Faculty should have an understanding of the characteristics of learning disabilities so they can refer students to the university or college office that works with students with various disabilities.

Characteristics of Learning Disabilities

Learning disabilities may manifest as a number of characteristics, each necessitating a different treatment and accommodation. Students with learning disabilities may have difficulty following verbal instructions and difficulty organizing ideas in writing, or may be unable to articulate ideas orally but be able to articulate them in writing. Students may also have auditory processing deficits that affect their ability to recite from memory (Kamhi, 2011). Time management may also be a problem for these students (Child & Langford, 2011).

Learning disabilities are highly individualized and each student manifests a different grouping of characteristics. Some students without learning disabilities may experience the same difficulties as those with learning disabilities. In one study, Wray, Aspland, Taghzouit, Pace, and Harrison (2012) screened 242 British preregistration students using the Adult Dyslexia Checklist. Results showed that 28.5% of the sample achieved a score possibly indicative of a learning disability. Of those students who underwent further evaluation, six students were shown not to have a learning disability.

Being accurately diagnosed with a learning disability means students can make adjustments in their study habits and receive support. Using a semistructured questionnaire, Ridley (2011) interviewed seven British students who were diagnosed with dyslexia. Students stated that once diagnosed, they could take action to cope with the diagnosis. They also recognized the need to make sure they didn't make errors and took steps to overcome their limitations and be successful in the clinical environment. Students expressed some anxiety about disclosing their dyslexia to others. Support, which was sometimes difficult to get, was critical to their successfully meeting the academic standards.

In another study, Sanderson-Mann, Wharrad, and McCandless (2012) compared the clinical experiences of students with dyslexia to those without. Students with dyslexia rated reading and writing on patients' charts, using care plans, and following a set of instructions more difficult than those without dyslexia. However, such tasks as change of shift reports, drug calculations, and time management were difficult for all students (Sanderson-Mann et al., 2012).

Evans (2014a) investigated how nursing students with dyslexia construct their identities. Twelve students enrolled in Irish nursing programs were interviewed. Students reported varying feelings regarding their dyslexia, including embracing their identity or having conflicting feelings. Some stated they had experienced being considered stupid by others. Students didn't want their dyslexia to be used as an excuse for poor performance and recognized the need to uphold standards. In another study, Evans (2014b) interviewed 19 nurse educators (lecturers) from two schools in Ireland using vignettes depicting students with various learning disabilities. Themes emerged related to faculty perceptions of students with learning disabilities. Lecturers stated that if students needed support in getting the work done, the students might be viewed as less capable. One lecturer acknowledged that "babysitting" students was problematic and some appeared reluctant to provide accommodations. Evans interpreted these and other similar quotes as indicative of the need for faculty development, to help them understand the need and legal obligation to support students.

Accommodating Learning Disabilities

When faculty believe that a student may have a previously undiagnosed learning disability, the initial action is to refer the student to the campus office that assists students with special needs. After the diagnosis has been made, a plan for accommodation of the disability can be developed. Counseling may also help a student with learning disabilities gain self-confidence in the learning environment. As stated earlier, if the student chooses, the faculty can be made aware of the disability and what accommodations are required. Faculty members who are made aware of a student's disability are not allowed to discuss that information with other faculty members unless the student gives permission.

Depending on the type of learning disability, a variety of accommodations may be appropriate for the student. Once diagnosed, some students may need some accommodation, such as permission to take tests in an alternate setting or more time to complete assignments. The use of color overlays to read text, and written contracts for completing assignments may also be appropriate accommodations (Job Accommodation Network, 2013). McPheat (2014) outlined other strategies that could be useful in both the clinical and classroom settings. For example, printing paperwork on colored paper and using 12- or 14-point Arial font can be easier to read. Audio recordings of lectures also facilitate understanding of complex materials.

Helping students understand their own learning styles helps them discover strategies that promote success. Box 4-2 lists universal design strategies that can guide faculty when teaching students with learning disabilities. The use of simulation is another strategy that can help students to build self-confidence in the ability to develop clinical competence (Azzopardi et al., 2014).

Students may also benefit from the assistance of an in-class note taker, which is a generally accepted accommodation according to ADA. This allows students to concentrate on classroom discussion without the distraction of trying to take notes. Some students have difficulty processing multiple stimuli at once. Students who have difficulty reading, and as a result read slowly, often find this disability to be the greatest barrier to their academic success. Faculty can help students overcome this difficulty by providing an audio recording of textbooks and other readings and providing them with the required reading assignments early in the semester, or helping them identify the key sections of reading assignments. Findings from a research study by Tee et al. (2010) suggested that reading aloud to students and using simple words to describe medical terms may help students to learn better.

Students with learning disabilities may also need accommodations for testing because slow reading skills can affect the student's ability to complete a test within the time allowed. Questions that are grammatically complex or contain double negatives, although difficult for all students, can be particularly challenging for students with learning disabilities and should be avoided. Providing the student with an extended testing time and a quiet room free of distractions may also be necessary accommodations. A test proctor who either reads the test to the student or writes and records the student's dictated answers to the test questions may also be helpful.

An additional strategy that faculty can use to assist students with learning disabilities is to incorporate a multimedia approach, such as computer-assisted instruction. Again, use of universal design principles can help students with learning disabilities, as well as the student body at large. These include providing copies of ancillary learning materials before class and placing visual cues within class notes. The use of smart phones with appropriate applications may also be helpful for all students, but particularly those with learning disabilities. Another strategy that benefits all students, including those with learning disabilities, is to meet with students on a regular basis to ensure that learning goals are being set appropriately and are being achieved.

Accommodation does not mean that academic standards are lowered but that multiple ways to achieve those standards are provided for all students, including those with learning disabilities. All classrooms contain students with multiple learning styles. By structuring classes to account for different learning styles and providing a variety of learning aids, nurse educators also help accommodate those with diagnosed learning disabilities (Tobin, 2013). When faculty consider that students have different ways of learning, they will design learning experiences that accommodate these diverse learning needs.

Campus Support Services

As previously mentioned, most institutions of higher education have established an office responsible for providing support services to students who identify themselves as learning disabled. Use of these services is voluntary, and they are usually available at little or no cost to the student. Services vary among institutions but typically include assessment and diagnosis of learning disabilities, identification of appropriate accommodations for the student, guidance counseling, and development of study and test taking skills. Faculty education about students with learning disabilities is another service commonly provided by these offices. Campus teaching and learning centers can assist faculty with how to design courses in line with universal design principles.

Accommodations for the National Council Licensure Examination

Nurse educators need to be familiar with the accommodations provided students with disabilities in their states when taking the National Council Licensure Examination (NCLEX). Accommodations are offered to individuals with learning and other disabilities in accordance with the ADA (National Council of State Boards of Nursing, 2014). Each state individually determines the degree of accommodation offered to students on a case-by-case basis. Educators should investigate and verify the accommodations offered to students in their respective state and encourage students with disabilities to seek appropriate accommodations. One of the most common accommodations has to do with time allotted for the examination. Regulations do change, and the student and faculty are encouraged to check with the National Council of State Boards of Nursing website (www.ncsbn.org) or the individual state board of nursing for further information. The student must provide documentation as to what accommodations have been made during his or her course of study before arriving at the testing center.

The Student with Physical Disabilities

Thinking of physical disabilities as hindrances as well as providing only environments that favor those without disabilities may limit opportunities for students and nurses with disabilities (Hargreaves & Walker, 2014). Required abilities that schools use to exclude students may include hearing, seeing, and lifting. Essential competencies for basic nursing programs may be different from those required in specialty graduate programs. For example, Helms and Thompson (2005) suggested that nurse anesthetists and nurse anesthetist students must be able to work in a fast-paced environment using complex information that is translated into immediate action. Nurse anesthetists must also be able to work closely with team members, so those who have any impairments that affect their ability to work in groups might not be suited for nurse anesthetist roles.

The United States Supreme Court ruled more than 35 years ago that a prospective nursing student with a hearing impairment could be denied admission because of the potential for lowering educational standards (*Southeastern Community College v. Davis,* 442 U.S. 397 [1979]). However, the ADA and ADAAA have clarified that, with reasonable accommodations, such a student has the potential to succeed. Published reports of students with hearing impairments who have achieved success in nursing programs and in subsequent employment do exist (Manning, 2013; Sharples, 2013). Many aids, such as sophisticated amplified stethoscopes, are now available, and an interpreter could be used for auscultation (Association of Medical Professionals with Hearing Losses, n.d.). Through the use of note takers and tape recorders, many students with hearing impairments have little difficulty participating in the classroom. Pagers and cell phones that vibrate may help students keep in contact with others in the clinical setting.

Much of the evidence regarding physical disabilities is case study evidence. Because some nurses with visual impairments are active in the workforce (American Foundation for the Blind, 2014), faculty could assume that some students with impaired vision may be accommodated. Providing alternative learning environments and enabling students to work with preceptors may be accommodations that can reasonably be made. For example, a student with a visual impairment might need a magnifier to help with reading printed matter, larger font sizes on a computer, or a text-to-voice apparatus.

Students in wheelchairs may also be accommodated and go on to have a successful nursing career (National Organization of Nurses with Disabilities, 2012). Pecci (2013) presented the case of a nurse who has been in a wheelchair and functioned as a staff nurse. Nurses with missing limbs have also functioned as staff nurses, including starting intravenous infusions (Maheady & Fleming, 2012).

Lifting restrictions may not be a barrier because many hospitals and nursing homes are striving for an environment that minimizes lifting. Teaching students how to properly use lifting equipment may help prevent workplace injury and future physical limitations. Students who are in their late teens and early 20s may not be fully physically developed, which makes them susceptible to injury (Kneafsy, 2010). Working with clinical partners to promote role modeling of proper patient handling by teaching students how to safely use lifting equipment may prevent injury on the job (Kneafsy, 2010). However, students often observe poor practice during their program of studies. In a study conducted by Cornish and Jones (2010), students described poor practices by staff for using lifting equipment and using sheets to move patients. Students also shared that they engaged in these practices themselves because of the need to feel a part of the staff and because in some cases the staff may not have been qualified to use the available lifting equipment (Cornish & Jones, 2010).

Students may become disabled during their time in school, and thus reasonable accommodations for students with physical disabilities may include time extensions for assignments and the assignment of an "incomplete" grade for courses that may not have been completed on time. Smith-Stoner, Halquist, and Glaeser (2011) presented a case study of a baccalaureate nursing student who developed cancer. She continued in her classes, but had to delay clinical experiences because of chemotherapy. The student also received extensions on assignment due dates to accommodate treatment. The student did graduate, albeit later than planned. Faculty need to be careful not to assume what a student may or may not be able to do when facing a physical limitation or illness, and should consider ways to provide reasonable accommodations.

Students may have disabilities that are less readily apparent. Dailey (2010) conducted a phenomenological study of 10 students with various chronic illnesses such as multiple sclerosis, diabetes, adrenal hyperplasia, and asthma. Students reported they were determined to finish their programs of study despite feeling ill much of the time. Students expressed a desire to appear normal and they feared being penalized for excessive absences, so they often placed their own health, and perhaps those of their patients, in jeopardy by attending class and clinical experiences when perhaps they should not have done so. Dailey (2010) recommended that faculty accommodate students by providing short rest periods during clinical experiences; promoting group work for learning activities, so that the load for all students was lessened; and incorporating self-care strategies into the curriculum that would benefit all students, not just those with chronic illnesses.

Disabled military veterans are a special population that may require assistance from the veteran support office or the office that handles all students with disabilities. Veterans may have missing limbs or posttraumatic stress disorder (DiRamio & Spires, 2009). The campus support service offices may assist veterans by providing mentors to guide the veterans through the educational process. Learning communities specifically for veterans may also facilitate their academic success (O'Herrin, 2011).

When students with physical disabilities graduate, their successful employment may depend on nurse managers' experience in working with nurses who are disabled. A study by Wood and Marshall (2010) revealed that nurse managers rated disabled nurses' performance as outstanding 22% of the time and rated them as below average only 11% of the time. Most would surmise that disabled nurses' job performance mirrors that of nondisabled nurses.

The Nursing Student with Substance Abuse

Determining the number of nursing students who may be impaired by drug or alcohol use is difficult. However, substance abuse has been found in college students. Results of the 2012 National Survey on Drug Use and Health showed that 22% of college students aged 18 through 22 had used illicit drugs in the past month (Substance Abuse and Mental Health Services Administration, 2013). This same survey showed that among persons aged 18 through 25, 39.5% reported binge drinking at least once in the last month. Binge drinking was defined as consuming five or more drinks at one time.

Other studies have confirmed the extent of college student substance abuse. The college environment does provide students with easy access to alcohol and drugs, including prescription stimulants, such as methylphenidate (Ritalin), and can expose students to situations in which alcohol and drug use is considered an acceptable activity. A study by Garnier-Dykstra, Caldeira, Vincent, O'Grady, and Arria (2012) conducted a longitudinal study of nonmedical use of stimulants such as methylphenidate. The study enrolled 1253 students. Students were followed over a 4-year period. By the fourth year, 61.8% had been offered stimulants and 45.8% had used the stimulants for nonmedical purposes in the year they had been exposed to the drugs. The authors noted that illicit use of drugs was often tied to lower grade point averages.

All college students experience academic pressures, and nursing students have additional stressors. Often nursing programs have retention and dismissal policies that put pressure on students to do well in their studies. Dealing with patients with a variety of complex health problems adds additional stress.

Graduate students also have substance abuse problems. For example, Bozimowski, Groh, Rouen, and Dosch (2014) examined the prevalence of substance abuse in nurse anesthesia students over a 5-year period; 23 out of 111 programs responded to a survey. Of the data reported on 2439 students, 16 students were identified as having a substance abuse problem and opioids were the most commonly abused substance. Of note was the fact that 23 programs had drug testing for cause and 7 conducted random drug screenings throughout the program.

Characteristics of Students with Chemical and Alcohol Impairments

The potential for substance abuse obviously exists among nursing students. Substance abuse, if not dealt with, can affect a student's professional practice after graduation. Monroe, Kenaga, Dietrich, Carter, and Cowan (2013) estimated the number of practicing nurses who had been enrolled in a substance abuse monitoring program during a 1-year period. Using survey data from boards of nursing disciplinary actions, reports of alternatives to discipline programs, and the 2009 National Sample Survey of Registered Nurses, they demonstrated that nationwide 0.51% of employed nurses appeared to have a substance use problem.

To help students deal with potential substance abuse problems that could persist after graduation, faculty need to have an understanding of this issue so they can assist students in receiving the appropriate professional support. Hensel, Middleton, and Engs (2014) investigated the relationship between professional identity, defined as "self-concept," and drinking patterns in undergraduate nursing students. The survey included 333 students across all 4 years of a baccalaureate nursing program. Of these, 33% of the students were classified as heavy drinkers, or more than 7 drinks per week for women and 14 drinks per week for men. Lower grades caused by drinking occurred in 5.1% of the sample. A statistically significant relationship was found between total weekly alcohol consumption and negative general self-concept, but the relationship was weak.

Faculty also have a responsibility to ensure that students deliver safe patient care, which includes protecting clients from the actions of a potentially unsafe student whose clinical performance has been compromised. Faculty should be aware of the characteristics of students who may be chemically dependent, knowledgeable about the policies and procedures within their institution that relate to students who are chemically dependent, and familiar with the support services that are available to students who have a chemical dependency problem. Common signs of substance abuse include slurred speech, smell of alcohol, constricted pupils, sleeping during class, and frequent absences or tardiness. Other signs could include change in dress and convoluted excuses for behavior (Cotter & Glasgow, 2012).

Faculty Responsibilities Related to Students with Impairments

What are the responsibilities of faculty if they suspect that a student is displaying characteristics that are indicative of chemical dependency? Faculty have ethical responsibilities toward the student and the student's patients and therefore should not ignore or make excuses for such behavior. While the ADA considers substance abuse a disability, unsafe clinical practice is not protected under the law (Menendez, 2010).

Mandatory drug testing of nursing students has become more widespread, probably in response to clinical agency requirements. Cotter and Glasgow (2012) discussed the legal and ethical implications of mandatory drug testing. They noted that faculty have the responsibility for seeing that students give safe care. Therefore monitoring for signs of substance abuse is a must. What is not clear is who has the right to know whether a student has tested positive for substance abuse. According to Cotter and Glasgow (2012) policies should be established that protect the rights of all involved, including students, faculty, administrators, and patients. For example, policies need to address whether students can be dismissed from the nursing program for substance abuse.

Before taking any measures, faculty need to clearly understand the policies and procedures for assisting chemically dependent students that are in place within their institution. Behavior must be documented and written policies followed (Cotter & Glasgow, 2012). A faculty member might have to take immediate action if, for example, a student appears impaired in the clinical area, and remove the student from the clinical setting. In cases in which the student does not impose an immediate danger to clients but is suspected of substance abuse, an appointment might be made with the student for the purpose of taking appropriate action. In addition to the faculty, a second person such as an administrator should be present to ensure that the student is dealt with according to policy and due process is not denied.

Written policies about chemical impairment that include the institution's definition of chemical dependency, the nursing faculty's philosophy on chemical dependency, and student and faculty responsibilities related to suspected chemical dependency should be clearly stated in the student handbook. Furthermore, adhering to the institution's established policies helps ensure that the student's right to due process is not denied and protects faculty from possible legal action by the student. The National Student Nurses Association (2009) supports policies that promote treatment and rehabilitation for students with substance abuse problems. In addition, the National Council of State Boards of Nursing (2011) "alternative to discipline policy" model includes student nurses. However, not all states include students in their programs for helping nurses with substance abuse.

Some schools of nursing have formulated their own intervention program for nursing students who are impaired. The following are key considerations: (1) ensuring the confidentiality of students who access the program; (2) clarifying the responsibilities of individuals associated with the program (i.e., faculty, students, administrators, alumni, counselors, and substance abuse professionals); and (3) orienting the student population to the purpose, activities, and responsibilities of the program (Monroe, 2009).

Whether a school should institute a policy for random drug testing is controversial. Although athletes are subject to random testing and most agencies have preemployment drug screening, the extent to which nursing students are required to undergo random screening is unknown. Although schools may not have policies requiring drug testing, students should be made aware that clinical agency policies may require blood or urine testing of individuals, including students, suspected of chemical dependency or as a requirement for engaging in clinical experiences within the agency. Nevertheless, some schools are instituting policies for drug screening prior to admission because of clinical agency requirements, and schools will require a drug screen if chemical impairment is suspected. Much more research is needed to determine the extent and nature of drug screening policies within nursing programs.

Many colleges and universities are attempting to deal with this problem by increasing student awareness of the effects of substance abuse through campus educational programming. Bozimowski et al. (2014) recommended that studies be done to evaluate wellness programs that include drug abuse prevention strategies. One such study was conducted by Cadiz, O'Neill, Butell, Epeneter, and Basin (2012), in which they designed a seminar for students to promote awareness of impaired practice. The seminar included content on the school's substance abuse policy and how confidentiality should be maintained so the stigma of seeking help could be reduced. Pretest and posttest comparisons demonstrated that seminar participants' perceived ability to intervene with students who had substance abuse problems increased. The rating of stigma associated with substance abuse did not increase following the seminar possibly because the seminar was only 2 hours long. Cadiz et al. (2012) suggested that this type of seminar has potential for preventing substance abuse among nursing students and is in line with the recommendations from the National Council of State Boards of Nursing (2011).

Nursing Students with Mental Health Problems

Even though nursing students may be considered to be at risk for developing mental health problems resulting from the high levels of stress that are generally reported among nursing students, little research has been conducted on interventions to alleviate mental health problems in nursing students. What research exists has been primarily descriptive and has focused on behaviors, such as signs of anxiety, stress, and anger. Mental health issues include anxiety, depression, eating disorders, and obsessive compulsive behavior (Storrie, Ahern, & Tuckett, 2010). Some nursing students may have mental health problems before enrolling in nursing school, which may have led them to be attracted to a "helping" profession. Students who experience mental health problems may need assistance in identifying and addressing these problems. Undergraduate and graduate nursing students have many fears and worries about their ability to succeed in their program of studies. Test anxiety is a special form of anxiety often experienced by nursing students. With the advent of high-stakes testing, faculty should be on the alert to signs of extreme test anxiety (Røykenes, Smith, & Larsen, 2014).

Faculty who have close relationships with students may be the first to notice signs of stress and other mental health issues (Chernomas & Shapiro, 2013). Some behavioral indicators, either in the classroom or clinical setting, may include fatigue, poor concentration, change in outward appearance, frequent absenteeism, disruption of logical thought patterns, and a decrease in quality of work (Phimister, 2009). Instituting interventions early can help ameliorate stress and anxiety experienced by nursing students.

It is not necessarily easy to determine the sources of stress for nursing students because of the variety of research instruments used in studies. Pulido-Martos, Augusto-Landa, and Lopez-Zafra (2012) concluded from their systematic review of the literature that, although specific conclusions were difficult to make, some sources of stress in nursing students were problems with studying, workload associated with nursing school, and fear of making mistakes while in the clinical setting. They recommended that faculty examine how assessing students' clinical skills can be conducted in such a way as to decrease stress experienced by students. Alzayyat and Al-Gamel (2014) also commented on how difficult it is to determine the sources of stress in nursing students in the clinical setting, because of lack of consistency with research instruments and inconsistent definitions of *stress*.

Stress and anxiety are prevalent in nursing students globally, especially fear associated with clinical practice, which can lead to depression. Chernomas and Shapiro (2013) measured student levels of depression, anxiety, and stress, and quality of life in 442 Canadian nursing students. Students reported high-normal ranges of depression, anxiety, and stress. Although the majority (84%) rated their quality of life as good or very good, 40% reported sleep disturbances and 41% reported little time for leisure activities. Qualitative comments reinforced that fears related to clinical practice contributed to stress and anxiety. Chernomas and Shapiro recommended that faculty should attend faculty development workshops to learn how to ameliorate students' perceived stress, anxiety, and depression. Moridi, Khaledi, and Valiee (2014) confirmed that clinical practice was a major source of stress for 230 nursing students in Kurdistan. Shaban, Khater, and Akhu-Zaheya (2012) showed that avoidance coping behaviors in Jordanian nursing students in clinical practice increased stress, whereas problem-solving coping behaviors decreased stress.

In their study of depression in nursing students Xu et al. (2014) administered a depression scale to 729 Chinese nursing students. They found a positive relationship between lower depression and better career prospects, academic performance, and quality of interpersonal relationships. Recommendations included developing school- and family-based programs to prevent depression. Cha and Sok (2013) found that anger expression, depression, and self-esteem were related in a sample of 320 Korean students. They recommended that students be taught how to control anger as a way to enhance self-esteem and decrease depression.

A study of 335 graduate and undergraduate Thai nursing students revealed that high stress was correlated with poor health and higher psychological distress (Klainin-Yobus et al., 2014). They found, however, that stress was more related to psychological distress than poor physical health. A study of 123 nursing students in Cyprus showed that strength of religious and spiritual beliefs was related to less depression and stress and more self-esteem (Papazisis, Nicolaou, Tsiga, Christoforou, & Sapountzi-Krepia, 2014).

The aforementioned global studies of factors that contribute to mental health issues in nursing students, certainly confirm the assumption of Papazisis et al. (2012) that nursing faculty cannot draw strong conclusions from this body of descriptive research because few studies were multisite and a variety of data collection instruments were used. Furthermore, these recent studies occurred outside the United States and might not be fully applicable to students in the United States. Nevertheless, the commonality in the findings does lend credence to some generalizability.

Stress in clinical practice has also been shown to be related to organizational characteristics in clinical agencies. Blomberg et al. (2014) examined stress levels in 74 Swedish students from three different universities in their final course of study. As with other studies, a majority of the students experienced stress, especially students who were placed in hospitals for their clinical experiences. Some of the students took a National Clinical Final Examination (NCFE) during the clinical placement. Results demonstrated that students placed in hospitals that were crowded, had multiple supervisors rather than one supervisor or preceptor, and took the NCFE during their placements had higher levels of stress. Such findings could have implications for how clinical experiences are implemented. The investigators recommended that experimental studies be conducted to determine which models of clinical supervision might reduce stress.

Most studies of mental health issues have been descriptive. However, several studies have investigated the effect of interventions on stress and anxiety reduction. Kang, Choi, and Ryu (2009) tested mindfulness meditation as a strategy to decrease stress, anxiety, and depression. Forty-one nursing students were randomly assigned to experimental and control groups. The experimental group participated in 90- to 120-minute sessions for 8 weeks. Before randomization, both groups attended a lecture about stress management. Following the intervention, students in the experimental group had decreased anxiety and stress. However, the amount of depression was not significantly different between the two groups.

Van der Reit, Rossiter, Kirby, Dluzewska, and Harmon (2015) conducted a descriptive, qualitative pilot study with 14 first-year undergraduate and midwifery students designed to evaluate the effects of a 7-week stress management and mindfulness program. From the themes identified, van der Riet and colleagues determined that the program helped students sleep better, have fewer negative thoughts, and promoted better patterns of concentration. However, challenges were encountered during the program, primarily students' inability to attend all sessions because of class commitments.

While specific training can help students learn to control their anxiety, the role of faculty and peer mentoring cannot be overlooked when dealing with anxiety. Appropriate use of humor can also lessen anxiety, help increase self-esteem, and contribute to an overall positive learning environment (Moscaritolo, 2009). A more positive learning environment may lead to better student learning outcomes.

Another strategy that has been tested to decrease stress and increase academic performance is the use of a "home" hospital program (Yucha, Kowalski, & Cross, 2009). The home hospital program involved keeping nursing students, as much as possible, at the same clinical agency throughout their program of study. Nurses in the hospitals served as the clinical instructors. The program was predicated on the fact that familiarity with the clinical agency can decrease stress and, as a side benefit, be used as a recruiting tool for the agencies involved. Students participating in the program reported less anxiety than those students who did not participate in the "home" hospital model.

While some interventions have shown promise in helping students deal with stress and anxiety, students' willingness to participate in interventions may be influenced by their attitudes towards prevalence of stress in themselves and others, and their willingness to seek help. Galbraith, Brown, and Clifton (2014) gathered data from 219 British nursing students regarding willingness to seek help for stress-related conditions. Descriptive analysis of the data demonstrated that 74.9% of the students had experienced stress. Most students (87.2%) would disclose their stress to family and friends. Few would disclose to colleagues or professional institutions because they believed families could best offer advice. Only 11.4% would seek professional help. Students revealed that they would not lose confidence in colleagues who had stress. Another interesting finding was that students had generally recognized existing high levels of stress in the nursing profession. Given these findings, if research-based interventions were offered on a regular basis to nursing students, it's unclear whether students would even avail themselves of the opportunity to engage in stress and anxiety reduction programs.

Faculty Responsibilities Related to Students with Mental Health Problems

Mental health issues range from anxiety, including test anxiety, and stress to severe depression and other mental illnesses. The process used to assist students with suspected mental health problems is similar to the approach used with any student whose academic progress is jeopardized by unsatisfactory performance. First, the ADA/ADAAA prohibits discrimination against individuals who are mentally impaired. Second, all actions taken by faculty must be congruent with existing institutional policies and afford students the due process that is their right. When mental health issues interfere with student behavior, faculty must deal with this behavior in a manner consistent with institutional policy. According to Cleary, Horsfall, Baines, and Happell (2012), policies must include confronting the student with evidence of problematic behavior and the faculty member needs to facilitate reduction of the problematic behavior before action is taken. Students should be made clearly aware of the behavior adversely affecting their academic performance and what they need to do to correct this behavior. A learning contract may be used in this instance to indicate what the student needs to do to improve the behavior and the time frame in which this must be accomplished. Many campuses have student codes of conduct to guide policy development. Policies, according to Cleary et al. (2012), should delineate procedures for assessing, documenting, reporting, intervening, and referring students for treatment. Many university campuses offer this service to students free or for a reduced fee.

If, despite these interventions, the behavior does not improve and the student is unable to perform effectively or patient safety is compromised, administrative withdrawal or dismissal from the program may be necessary. As always, the student who is administratively withdrawn or dismissed has the right to pursue the grievance and appeal process in place within the institution.

Mental health issues may display themselves in the form of student incivility in the classroom and ultimately in anger within the student–faculty relationship and perhaps lead to violent episodes (Clark, 2009). However, mental health issues cannot be used to justify incivility. Behaviors indicative of incivility in students include making sarcastic remarks, sleeping in class, distracting others with side conversations, using cell phones in class, arriving late and leaving early, and making demands of faculty (Clark, Farnsworth, & Landrum, 2009). Clark (2009) has suggested that to deal with incivility, faculty should recognize the risk factors such as competitive academic environments and clinical placements. Faculty can then design strategies to ameliorate the stress and anxiety that results from these factors. Clark (2009) also recommended that faculty test the strategies to determine their efficacy. See Chapter 14 for a more in-depth discussion of student and faculty incivility.

Criminal Background Checks

In addition to mental health issues, which can compromise patient safety, the student who has a record of criminal activity can also compromise patient safety. Patient safety is a major concern for state boards of nursing and health care accreditation agencies. The Joint Commission (2008) states, "Staff, students and volunteers who work in the same capacity as staff who provide care, treatment, and services, would be expected to have criminal background checks verified when required by law and regulation and organization policy" (para 1). Therefore nursing programs often require criminal background checks. Many states, including Louisiana, Ohio, Maryland, and Texas, for example, require applicants applying for a license to practice to have a criminal background check. A search of individual state boards of nursing websites will provide students with information regarding background checks prior to licensure.

The number of nursing programs requiring background checks has increased, although recent data on the number of programs is not readily available. Whether or not a school requires a criminal background check before admission, faculty have a duty to warn students that, although they may have successfully completed the nursing program, licensure could be denied if a student has a criminal background. Additionally, clinical agencies, as noted previously, may have requirements for background checks and may refuse clinical placements based on the results of the criminal background check. An example of a criminal background check policy is found in Box 4-3.

Denying admission based on the results of a criminal background check requires careful consideration. Decisions need to be made in line with

BOX 4-3 Example of Criminal History Background Check Policy

At the time of your application, you were required to submit a current national level criminal background check, which was part of the criteria used to determine your eligibility.

Criminal background information will be maintained in your student nursing file, is considered confidential, and no results will be released.

The student is responsible for notifying the Department Chairperson of any new charges or additions to one's criminal history promptly.

Failure to report new charges may result in dismissal from the program.

Used with permission from Indiana State University Nursing Program Department of Baccalaureate Nursing.

state law and clinical agency policy. Guidelines for making decisions need to be readily available to all faculty and students. When admission decisions are made, faculty need to consider the nature of the criminal conviction and how long ago the offense occurred, and afford due process for those denied admission. Philipsen et al. (2012) question the value of criminal background checks for students, as students are under close supervision of faculty. Nevertheless, they acknowledge that faculty must follow the policy in place for the clinical agency. They also note that the results of the criminal background checks must be evaluated on a case-by-case basis.

Evidence does support that criminal background checks prior to admission may help to identify students who may commit crimes while enrolled as a student (Smith, Corvers, Wilson, Douglas, & Bienemy, 2013). Of the more than 3000 applicants for registered nurse licensure during the year 2006 in the state of Louisiana, 14.7% had a criminal history. One should note that the Louisiana Board also required a criminal background check prior to enrollment in clinical courses. Because of a large difference in sample size, a matched pair cohort was constructed for analytic purposes. Among the findings was the fact that 10% of those who had a criminal record prior to enrollment had subsequent criminal activity, whereas, only 2.3% of those without a prior criminal record did.

The areas of criminal background checks and drug testing continue to evolve and nursing faculty will need to keep apprised of changes in health care agency policies and state laws. The National Council of State Boards of Nursing has published a position paper and a resource packet, including model statutory language for state boards of nursing to use in crafting laws regarding criminal background checks (National Council of State Boards of Nursing, 2006a, 2006b). The National Council of State Boards of Nursing continues to update its policy recommendations.

Summary

This chapter has provided information about the legal and educational issues related to teaching students with disabilities and other special needs. The needs of students with learning disabilities, chemical dependency, and mental health problems are presented, along with faculty responsibilities associated with teaching these students. Interventions are identified for assisting students to cope with a disability or impairment that can be used for all students to promote academic success.

Nursing faculty are responsible for creating a learning environment that supports the teaching–learning process for all students. By creating a caring environment, students may be more willing to disclose their disabilities (Ridley, 2011). Working with students who have disabilities or impairments brings special challenges to the student–faculty relationship. No specific rules say what level of disability or impairment prevents admission to a nursing program. However, faculty who are knowledgeable about the legal issues related to students with disabilities or impairments, their institution's and school's policies and procedures related to students with these special needs, and the interventions designed to help students maintain their self-esteem and be successful will find themselves capable of meeting these challenges in a caring, facilitative manner. Viewing disabilities not as hindrances but as differences may help faculty to better make appropriate accommodations for students while still maintaining academic standards.

Furthermore, if faculty are open to working with students who have disabilities, students might be more inclined to disclose, without fear of adverse consequences, that they have a need for accommodations. Developing strong partnerships with clinical agencies may also be a key to successfully integrating those students with disabilities into the nursing program (Kneafsy, 2010). Educating faculty, nurses in practice, and students to view persons with disabilities not as persons who are ill will go a long way to encouraging those with disabilities to enter the nursing profession. Conducting large-scale studies of nursing students admitted with disabilities and their subsequent success in the program and in practice following graduation will help provide more evidence regarding what accommodations can be made that will foster integration into practice following graduation.

Those with disabilities will continue to seek enrollment in nursing programs. Faculty may need to consult resources that give guidance on how to accommodate those with disabilities.

CASE STUDIES FOR FURTHER DISCUSSION

Case Study 1

Charlie was a 49-year-old construction worker who fell while building an addition to a hospital. He sustained a severe head injury and was in a coma and suffered hemiplegia. With aggressive rehabilitation, Charlie regained full movement of all extremities and was able to pursue a new career. He enrolled in an associate degree nursing program because he believed he needed to redirect his work life. He was able to successfully complete the program in 4 years and pass the NCLEX. Accommodations made during his program of study that contributed to his achievement included allowing his testing to take place in isolation from other students, having tests read to him if needed to promote understanding of what was asked, and permitting additional time to complete tests. As well, he was permitted, as were all students, to pursue part-time study. Support from faculty was crucial to his success. One faculty member in particular had experienced a head injury and was able to help Charlie improve his reading comprehension skills by teaching him to place transparent colored film over and a line above the text he was reading.

Case Study 2

Ann was a nursing faculty member who developed a hearing loss, possibly due to an autoimmune disease while she was in her prelicensure program, although she did not realize it at the time. About a year following graduation, one of her colleagues suggested that she might have a hearing loss and that she should get her hearing tested. Ann acknowledged that she had ringing in her ears for a while that had gotten progressively worse. As she progressed in her career, and following the birth of her first child, she realized the ringing became louder and the sound she heard was different, but she adapted. Finally, after the birth of her second child, her hearing loss became profound to the point that it interfered with her life. A friend connected her with a social worker who worked with individuals with hearing loss. Through the social worker, Ann got connected to the Department of Vocational Rehabilitation. Ann was fitted with appropriate hearing aids, received an amplified stethoscope, and eventually was given a service dog through a philanthropic organization. Throughout her career she has worked in pediatrics, community health, ambulatory care, long-term care, and even intensive care. When in intensive care she has made sure the monitors face her so she doesn't have to rely on alarms to notify her of a potential patient problem. Ann went back to school to get her master's and doctoral degrees. As a faculty member she has taught in classroom and clinical settings. When she had students in community health and long-term care, her service dog accompanied her. The Department of Vocational Rehabilitation installed a surround sound system in a large classroom for her. She placed students in a circle and moved about so she could lip read and hear what students were saying. Ann stated that she views environments as disabled, not people. The service dog accompanied her in the classroom as well. Ann's story can serve as a role model for faculty and students who may question how persons with disabilities can function as a nurse in practice and as a member of a nursing faculty.

("Ann," personal communication, September 22, 2014.)

REFLECTING ON THE EVIDENCE

1. Case studies indicate that nursing students with various disabilities can succeed academically and get jobs. What types of jobs do these graduates get and how successful are they on the job? How do these nurses handle issues of patient safety?
2. There is evidence that some schools of nursing require drug testing of students. How many schools require drug testing? What happens if a student tests positive on a random drug test?
3. Student incivility is an important issue when faculty try to maintain a positive learning environment. What kinds of support do faculty need to deal effectively with aggressive students?
4. What accommodations should faculty make in the learning spaces to maximize learning for all students, both nondisabled and disabled?

REFERENCES

Aaberg, V. (2012). A path to greater inclusivity through understanding implicit attitudes toward disability. *Journal of Nursing Education, 51*(9), 505–510. http://dx.doi.org/10.3928/01484834-20120706-02.

ADA Amendments Act of 2008, 42 USC 12101. Retrieved from, http://www.gpo.gov/fdsys/pkg/PLAW-110publ325/html/PLAW-110publ325.htm

Alzayyat, A., & Al-Gamel, E. (2014). A review of the literature regarding stress among nursing students during their clinical education. *International Nursing Review, 61*(3), 406–415.

American Foundation for the Blind. (2014). *Profile of Leora Heifetz, labor and delivery nurse.* Retrieved from, http://www.afb.org/info/living-with-vision-loss/for-job-seekers/our-stories/mentors/labor-and-delivery-nurse-profile/12345.

American Nurses Association. (n.d.). *Safe patient handling and mobility.* Retrieved from, http://nursingworld.org/Safe-Patient-Handling-and-Mobility.

Americans with Disabilities Act, 42 U.S.C. § 12111 et seq. (1990). Retrieved from, http://www.ada.gov/pubs/ada.htm.

Americans with Disabilities Act, 42 U.S.C.A. § 12101 note. (2008). Retrieved from, http://www.eeoc.gov/laws/statutes/adaaa.cfm.

Ashcroft, T. J., & Lutfiyya, Z. M. (2013). Nursing educators' perspectives of students with disabilities: A grounded theory study. *Nurse Education Today, 33*(11), 1316–1321. http://dx.doi.org/10.1016/j.nedt.2013.02.018.

Association of Medical Professionals with Hearing Losses. (n.d.). *Stethoscope information* (Online forum). Retrieved from, http://www.amphl.org/stethoscopes.php.

Azzopardi, T., Johnson, A., Philips, K., Dickson, C., Hengstberger-Sims, C., Goldsmith, M., et al. (2014). Simulation as a learning strategy: Supporting undergraduate students with disabilities. *Journal of Clinical Nursing, 23*(3/4), 402–409. http://dx.doi.org/10.1111/jocn.12049.

Betz, C. L., Smith, K. A., & Bui, K. (2012). A survey of California nursing programs: Admission and accommodation policies for students with disabilities. *Journal of Nursing Education, 51*(12), 676–684. http://dx.doi.org/10.3928/01484834-20121112-01.

Blomberg, K., Bisholt, B., Engström, A. K., Ohlsson, U., Johansson, A. S., & Gustafsson, M. (2014). Swedish nursing students' experience of stress during clinical practice in relation to clinical setting characteristics and the organisation of the clinical education. *Journal of Clinical Nursing, 23*(15/16), 2264–2271. http://dx.doi.org/10.1111/jocn.12506.

Bozimowski, G., Groh, C., Rouen, P., & Dosch, M. (2014). The prevalence and patterns of substance abuse among nurse anesthesia students. *AANA Journal, 82*(4), 277–283.

Cadiz, D. M., O'Neill, C., Butell, S. S., Epeneter, B. J., & Basin, B. (2012). Quasi-experimental evaluation of a substance abuse awareness educational intervention for nursing students. *Journal of Nursing Education, 51*(7), 411–415. http://dx.doi.org/10.3928/01484834-20120515-02.

Cha, N. H., & Sok, S. R. (2013). Depression, self-esteem and anger expression patterns of Korean nursing students. *International Nursing Review, 61*(1), 109–115.

Chernomas, W. M., & Shapiro, C. (2013). Stress, depression, and anxiety among undergraduate nursing students. *International Journal of Nursing Education Scholarship, 10*(1), 255–266. http://dx.doi.org/10.1515/ijnes-2012-0032.

Child, J., & Langford, E. (2011). Exploring the learning experiences of nursing students with dyslexia. *Nursing Standard, 11*(13), 39–46.

Clark, C. M. (2009). Faculty guide for promoting civility in the classroom. *Nurse Educator, 34*(5), 194–197.

Clark, C. M., Farnsworth, J., & Landrum, R. E. (2009). Development and description of the incivility survey in nursing education (INE) survey. *The Journal of Theory Construction and Testing, 13*(1), 7–15.

Cleary, M., Horsfall, J., Baines, J., & Happell, B. (2012). Mental health behaviours among undergraduate nursing students: Issues for consideration. *Nurse Education Today, 32*(8), 951–955. http://dx.doi.org/10.1016/j.nedt.2011.11.016.

Cornish, J., & Jones, A. (2010). Factors affecting compliance with moving and handling policy: Student nurses' views and experiences. *Nurse Education Today, 10*(2), 96–100.

Cotter, V. T., & Glasgow, M. E. S. (2012). Student drug testing in nursing education. *Journal of Professional Nursing, 28*(3), 186–189. http://dx.doi.org/10.1016/j.profnurs.2011.11.017.

Dailey, M. A. (2010). Needing to be normal: The lived experience of chronically ill nursing students. *International Journal of Nursing Education Scholarship, 7*(1), 1–23. http://dx.doi.org/10.2202/1548-923X.1798.

DiRamio, D., & Spires, M. (Summer 2009). Partnering to assist disabled veterans in transition. *New Directions for Student Services, 2009*(126), 81–88. http://dx.doi.org/10.1002/ss.319.

Disability Discrimination Act 1995. Retrieved from, http://www.legislation.gov.uk/ukpga/1995/50/contents.

Disability Discrimination Act 2005. Retrieved from, http://www.legislation.gov.uk/ukpga/2005/13/contents.

Dupler, A. E., Allen, C., Maheady, D. C., Fleming, S. E., & Allen, M. (2012). Leveling the playing field for nursing students with disabilities: Implications of the Amendments to the American's with Disabilities Act. *Journal of Nursing Education, 51*(3), 140–144. http://dx.doi.org/10.3928/01484834-20120127-05.

Evans, W. (2014a). "I am not a dyslexic person I'm a person with dyslexia": Identity constructions of dyslexia among students in nurse education. *Journal of Advanced Nursing, 70*(2), 360–372. http://dx.doi.org/10.1111/jan.12199.

Evans, W. (2014b). "If they can't tell the difference between duphalac and digoxin you've got patient safety issues": Nurse lecturers' constructions of students' dyslexic identities in nurse education. *Nurse Education Today, 34*(6), e41–e46. http://dx.doi.org/10.1016/j.nedt.2013.11.004.

Galbraith, N. D., Brown, K. E., & Clifton, E. (2014). A survey of student nurses' attitudes toward help seeking for stress. *Nursing Forum, 49*(3), 171–181.

Garnier-Dykstra, L. M., Caldeira, K. M., Vincent, K. B., O'Grady, K. E., & Arria, A. M. (2012). Nonmedical use of prescription stimulants during college: Four-year trends in exposure, opportunity, use, motives, and sources. *Journal of American College Health, 60*(3), 226–234.

Griffiths, L., Worth, P., Scullard, C., & Gilbert, D. (2010). Supporting disabled students in practice: A tripartite approach. *Nurse Education in Practice, 10*(3), 132–137. http://dx.doi.org/10.1016/j.nepr.2009.05.001.

Hargreaves, J., & Walker, L. (2014). Preparing disabled students for professional practice: Managing risk through a principles-based approach. *Journal of Advanced Nursing, 70*(8), 1748–1757. http://dx.doi.org/10.1111/jan.12368.

Helms, L. B., & Thompson, E. S. (2005). Nurse anesthesia students with disabilities: A legal and academic review of potential professional standards. *AANA Journal, 73*(4), 265–269.

Hensel, D., Middleton, M. J., & Engs, R. C. (2014). A cross-sectional study of drinking patterns, prelicensure nursing education, and professional identity formation. *Nurse Education Today, 34*(5), 719–723. http://dx.doi.org/10.1016/j.nedt.2013.08.018.

Job Accommodation Network. (2013). *Accommodation and compliance series: Employees with learning disabilities.* Retrieved from, http://askjan.org/media/downloads/LDA&CSeries.pdf.

Joint Commission. (2008). *Requirements for criminal background checks.* Retrieved from, http://www.jointcommission.org/.

Kamhi, A. G. (2011). What speech-language pathologists need to know about auditory processing disorders. *Language, Speech, and Hearing Services in the Schools, 42*(3), 265–272.

Kang, Y. S., Choi, S. Y., & Ryu, E. (2009). The effectiveness of a stress coping program based on mindfulness meditation on the stress, anxiety, and depression experienced by nursing students in Korea. *Nurse Education Today, 29*(5), 538–543. http://dx.doi.org/10.1016/j.nedt.2008.12.003.

Klainin-Yobus, P., Keawkerd, O., Pumpuang, W., Thunyadee, W. T., Thanoi, W., & He, H. (2014). The mediating effects of coping on the stress and health relationships among nursing students: A structural equation modelling approach. *Journal of Advanced Nursing, 70*(6), 1287–1298. http://dx.doi.org/10.1111/jan.12283.

Kneafsy, R. (2010). Editorial: Musculo-skeletal injury—Are universities doing enough to protect students? *Nurse Education Today, 30*(5), 383–385. http://dx.doi.org/10.1016/j.nedt.2009.10.010.

LD Online. (2015b). *LD basics: What is a learning disability?* Retrieved from, http://www.ldonline.org/ldbasics/whatisld.

Levey, J. (2014). Attitudes of nursing faculty towards nursing students with disabilities. *Journal of Post-Secondary Education and Disability, 27*(3), 321–332.

Maheady, D. C., & Fleming, S. E. (2012). Missing a limb, but not a heart. *Reflections on Nursing Leadership, 38*(1). Retrieved from, http://www.reflectionsonnursingleadership.org/Pages/Vol38_1_Maheady_Fleming.aspx.

Manning, L. (2013). Listen to my story. *Nursing Standard, 28*(12), 66.

Marcyjanik, D., & Zom, C. (2011). Accessibility in online education for persons with disabilities. *Nurse Educator, 36*(6), 241–245. http://dx.doi.org/10.1097/NNE.0b013e3182333f9d.

McPheat, C. (2014). Experience of nursing students with dyslexia on clinical placement. *Nursing Standard, 28*(41), 44–49.

Meloy, F., & Gambescia, S. F. (2014). Guidelines for response to student requests for academic considerations: Support versus enabling. *Nurse Educator, 39*(1), 138–142. http://dx.doi.org/10.1097/NNE.0000000000000037.

Menendez, J. B. (2010). Americans with Disabilities Act—Related considerations: When an alcoholic nurse is your employee: When is a nurse legally considered a "direct threat" to patient safety. *JONA'S Healthcare Law, Ethics and Regulation, 12*(1), 21–24.

Monroe, T. (2009). Addressing substance abuse among nursing students: Development of a prototype alternative-to-dismissal policy. *Journal of Nursing Education, 48*(5), 272–278. http://dx.doi.org/10.9999/01484834-20090416-06.

Monroe, T. B., Kenaga, H., Dietrich, M. S., Carter, M. A., & Cowan, R. L. (2013). The prevalence of employed nurses identified or enrolled in substance use monitoring programs. *Nursing Research, 62*(1), 10–15. http://dx.doi.org/10.1097/NNR.0b013e31826ba3ca.

Moridi, G., Khaledi, S., & Valiee, S. (2014). Clinical training stress-inducing factors from the students' viewpoint: A questionnaire-based study. *Nurse Education in Practice, 14*(2), 160–163. http://dx.doi.org/10.1016/j.nepr.2013.08.001.

Moscaritolo, L. M. (2009). Interventional strategies to decrease nursing student anxiety in the clinical learning environment. *Journal of Nursing Education, 48*(1), 17–23.

National Center for Education Statistics. (2011). *Students with disabilities at degree-granting postsecondary institutions: First look.* Retrieved from, http://nces.ed.gov/pubs2011/2011018.pdf.

National Council of State Boards of Nursing. (2006a). NCSBN 2006 annual meeting: Section 2. In *The threshold of regulatory excellence: Taking up the challenge* (pp. 107–135). Retrieved from, http://www.ncsbn.org/pdfs/II_BB_2006_Section_2a_Recom.pdf.

National Council of State Boards of Nursing. (2006b). *Using criminal background checks to inform licensure decision making.* Retrieved from, http://www.ncsbn.org/pdfs/Criminal_Background_Checks.pdf.

National Council of State Boards of Nursing. (2011). *Substance abuse disorder in nursing: A resource manual for guidelines for alternative and disciplinary monitoring programs.* Retrieved from, https://www.ncsbn.org/SUDN_1v

National Council of State Boards of Nursing. (2014). *2014 NCLEX examination bulletin.* Retrieved from, https://www.ncsbn.org/2014_NCLEX_Candidate_Bulletin.pdf.

National Organization of Nurses with Disabilities. (2012). *As a nurse or nursing student with a wheelchair, how can I perform a head-to-toe physical exam?* Retrieved from, http://www.nond.org/NOND-FAQs/files/e8f98c88835440309b-f66aaaaa48bf49-40.html.

National Student Nurses Association. (2009). *Code of ethics part II: Code of academic and clinical conduct and interpretive statements.* Retrieved from, http://www.nsna.org/Portals/0/Skins/NSNA/pdf/NSNA_CoC_Academic_Clinical_Interp_Statements.pdf.

Nursing and Midwifery Council. (2006). *Guidelines to support learning assessment in practice.* Retrieved from, http://www.nmc-uk.org/Documents/NMC-Publications/NMC-Standards-to-support-learning-assessment.pdf.

O'Herrin, E. (2011). Enhancing veteran success in higher education. *Peer Review [AAC&U], 13*(1), 15–18.

Papazisis, G., Nicolaou, P., Tsiga, E., Christoforou, T., & Sapountzi-Krepia, D. (2014). Religious and spiritual beliefs, self-esteem, anxiety, and depression among nursing students. *Nursing and Health Sciences, 16*(2), 232–238. http://dx.doi.org/10.1111/nhs.12093.

Pecci, A. W. (December 10, 2013). *Give nurses in wheelchairs a chance. Health Leaders Media.* Retrieved from, http://www.healthleadersmedia.com/page-1/NRS-299106/Give-Nurses-in-Wheelchairs-a-Chance.

Philipsen, N., Murray, T. L., Belgrave, L., Bell-Hawkins, A., Robinson, V., & Watties-Daniels, D. (2012). Criminal background checks in nursing: Safeguarding the public? *The Journal for Nurse Practitioners, 8*(9), 707–711.

Phimister, D. (2009). Pressure too much? *Nursing Standard, 22*(33), 61.

Pulido-Martos, J. M., Augusto-Landa, J. M., & Lopez-Zafra, E. (2012). Sources of stress in nursing students: A systematic review of quantitative studies. *International Nursing Review, 59*(1), 15–25.

Rehabilitation Act, 29 U.S.C. 794 § 504 et seq. (1973). Retrieved from, http://uscode.house.gov/download/pls/29C16.txt.

Ridley, C. (2011). The experiences of student nurses with dyslexia. *Nursing Standard, 25*(24), 35–42.

Røykenes, K., Smith, K., & Larsen, T. M. B. (2014). It is the situation that makes it difficult. Experiences of nursing students faced with a high-stakes drug calculation test. *Nurse Education in Practice, 14*(4), 350–356. http://dx.doi.org/10.1016/j.nepr.2014.01.004.

Sanderson-Mann, J., Wharrad, H. J., & McCandless, F. (2012). An empirical exploration of the impact of dyslexia on placement-based learning, a comparison with non-dyslexic students. *Diversity and Equality in Healthcare, 12*(2), 89–99.

Scullion, P. A. (2010). Models of disability: Their influence in nursing and potential role in challenging discrimination. *Journal of Advanced Nursing, 66*(3), 697–707. http://dx.doi.org/10.1111/j.1365-2648.2009.05211.x.

Shaban, I. A., Khater, W., & Akhu-Zaheya, L. M. (2012). Undergraduate nursing students' stress sources and coping behaviours during their initial period of clinical training: A Jordanian perspective. *Nurse Education in Practice, 12*(4), 204–209. http://dx.doi.org/10.1016/j.nepr.2012.01.005.

Sharples, N. (2013). An exploration of deaf woman's access to mental health nurse education in the United Kingdom. *Nurse Education Today, 33*(9), 76–980. http://dx.doi.org/10.1016/j.nedt.2012.10.017.

Smith, D., Corvers, S., Wilson, W. J., Douglas, D., & Bienemy, C. (2013). Prelicensure RN students with and without criminal histories: A comparative analysis. *Journal of Nursing Regulation, 4*(1), 34–38.

Smith-Stoner, M., Halquist, K., & Glaeser, B. C. (2011). Nursing education challenge: A student with cancer. *Teaching and Learning in Nursing, 6*(1), 14–18.

Southeastern Community College v. Davis, 442 U.S. 397 (1979).

Storrie, K., Ahern, K., & Tuckett, A. (2010). A systematic review: Students with mental health problems—A growing problem. *International Journal of Nursing Practice, 16*(1), 1–6. http://dx.doi.org/10.1111/j.1440-172X.01813.x/full.

Substance Abuse and Mental Health Services Administration. (2013). *Results from the 2012 national survey on drug use and health: Summary of national findings.* Retrieved from, http://www.samhsa.gov/data/NSDUH/2012SummNatFindDetTables/NationalFindings/NSDUHresults2012.pdf.

Summary of key provisions: EEOC's notice of proposed rule-making (NPRM) to implement the ADA Amendments Act of 2008 (ADAAA). (n.d.). Retrieved from, http://www.EEOC.gov/laws/regulations/upload/adaaa-summary.pdf

Tee, S., & Cowen, C. (2012). Supporting students with disabilities—Promoting understanding amongst mentors in practice. *Nurse Education in Practice, 12*(1), 6–10. http://dx.doi.org/10.1016/j.nepr.2011.03.020.

Tee, S. R., Owens, K., Plowright, S., Ramnath, P., Rourke, S., James, C., et al. (2010). Being reasonable: Supporting disabled nursing students in practice. *Nurse Education in Practice, 10*, 216–221. http://dx.doi.org/10.1016/j. nepr.2009.11.006.

Tobin, T. J. (2013). Universal design in online courses: Beyond disabilities. *Online Cl@ssroom, 13*(12), 1–3.

Van der Reit, P., Rossiter, R., Kirby, D., Dluzewska, T., & Harmon, C. (2015). Piloting a stress management and mindfulness program for undergraduate nursing students: Student feedback and lessons learned. *Nurse Education Today, 35*(1), 44–49. http://dx.doi.org/10.1016/j.nedt.2014.05.003.

Vickers, M. Z. (2010, March). *Accommodating college students with learning disabilities: ADD, ADHD, and dyslexia.* Raleigh, NC: John W. Pope Center for Higher Education Policy. Retrieved from, http://www.popecenter.org/.

Wells v. Lester E. Cox Medical Centers, 379 S.W.3d 919, (Mo.App. S.D.,2012).

Wood, D., & Marshall, E. S. (2010). Nurses with disabilities working in hospital settings: Attitudes, concerns, and experiences of nurse leaders. *Journal of Professional Nursing, 26*(3), 182–187. http://dx.doi.org/10.1016/j.profnurs.2009.12.001.

Wray, J., Aspland, J., Taghzouit, J., Pace, K., & Harrison, P. (2012). Screening for specific learning difficulties (SpLD): The impact upon the progression or pre-registration nursing students. *Nurse Education Today, 32*(1), 96–100. http://dx.doi.org/10.1177/1744629509355725.

Xu, Y., Chi, X., Chen, S., Qi, J., Zhang, P., & Yang, Y. (2014). Prevalence and correlates of depression among college nursing students in China. *Nurse Education Today, 34*(6), e7–e12. http://dx.doi.org/10.1016/j.nedt.2013.10.017.

Yucha, C. B., Kowalski, S., & Cross, C. (2009). Student stress and academic performance: Home hospital program. *Journal of Nursing Education, 48*(11), 631–637. http://dx.doi.org/10.3928/01484834-20090828-05.

Forces and Issues Influencing Curriculum Development*

5

Linda M. Veltri, PhD, RN
Halina Barber, PhD, MS, RN

Leaders in the nursing profession must remain vigilant to the forces and issues influencing the direction of professional education. In any dynamic organization, curriculum change is not a choice but a requirement. The magnitude, pace, and intensity of change within the health care arena affects providers, consumers, educators, and financers of health care. As a result, nurse educators must continually work to develop and implement relevant curricula congruent with global trends, national events, advancements in science and technology, professional priorities, academic forces, the school's mission, and faculty values. Doing so ensures practitioners entering the workforce are prepared and equipped with relevant knowledge and competencies necessary to provide patient-centered care; effectively intervene in contemporary health care challenges; and advocate for delivery of safe, quality health care.

The ability to deliver meaningful curricula within the dynamic health care environment requires a close understanding of internal and external forces directing change. This chapter describes the current social context for curriculum development, including issues and forces in the environment external to the nursing profession, the higher education environment, and the profession's internal environment. In addition, several strategies are presented that can assist faculty to identify forces and issues that influence the nursing profession and curriculum. Faculty with intimate and current knowledge of the forces and issues influencing nursing curricula are better positioned to navigate the political processes of building consensus and obtaining approval by all significant stakeholders.

*The author acknowledges the contributions of Joanne Rains Warner, PhD, RN, FAAN, in previous editions of this chapter.

Social Context for Curriculum Development Issues External to the Nursing Profession

Understanding issues external to the nursing profession form an essential piece of the foundation necessary to guide contemporary curriculum development. External issues like health care reform, global disasters and globalization, changing demographics, technology, and the environment provide the context for the world in which nurses learn and practice. Collectively these same issues encompass risk factors for health and disease, contribute to the complex web of causation, and describe the current states of humanity and health.

Health issues are increasingly related to the sociopolitical and economic characteristics of the communities where people live, work, and play. Curriculum must acknowledge the broad determinants of health to prepare practicing nurses to effectively intervene in complex problems such as bioterrorism and other mass disasters, climate change, global and domestic violence, economic recession, homelessness, teen pregnancy, emerging infectious diseases, and increasing drug-resistant organisms.

The following six trends, which capture significant developments and concerns for society, are presented as the broad sociopolitical and economic context of nursing practice and education. Although these trends are discussed separately, their interconnectedness is undeniable.

Health Care Reform

The passage and signing of the federal statue known as the Patient Protection and Affordable Care Act (PPACA) in 2010 has become a major force driving health care reform and ultimately curriculum development. Under this act and for the first time in America's history all citizens have access to affordable health care insurance. In conjunction with access to care, a national strategy known as the "Triple Aim" has been implemented with the purpose of improving the quality and access to health care while controlling costs (Institute for Healthcare Improvement, 2009).

Nursing practice and education greatly benefited from the passage of the PPACA through amendments to Title VIII of the Public Health Service Act. As a result, funding priorities of the Nurse Education, Practice, Quality and Retention (NEPQR) program, administered by the Health Resources and Services Administration (HRSA) were shifted to support nursing education, practice, and retention. For example, financial support for pursuit of advanced degrees by nursing students who have a desire to teach increased, as did the amount nursing students from disadvantaged background or with limited financial resources could borrow to pay for their education. In addition, more than $1 billion in new grants were authorized to increase home visits to mothers in high-risk communities and to establish a new grant that will fund nurse-managed health centers (U.S. Department of Human and Health Services, 2011; Wakefield, 2010). In response to this anticipated reformed health care arena, nurse educators must ensure that prelicensure and graduate program nursing curricula prepare nurses to care for patients in ambulatory or community settings, possess skills to coordinate patient care, work as members of interprofessional teams, provide quality as well as value-based care, and develop leadership skills. Nursing program curricula needs to increasingly focus on wellness, prevention, and palliative care versus management of acute patients in acute care settings (Institute of Medicine [IOM], 2010: Sherman, 2012). Nursing curricula should also seek to provide students with the opportunity to envision, create, or actively participate in the redesign of new or revolutionary models of health care delivery systems (Table 5-1).

Global Violence, Threat of Violence, and Other Disasters

It has been more than a decade since hijacked airplanes hit the World Trade Center towers in New York City and the Pentagon near Washington, DC, with a fourth plane crashing in rural Pennsylvania. The tragic September 11, 2001, events along with the emergence of new infectious diseases

TABLE 5-1 New Models of Patient Care Delivery

Accountable Care Organizations	• A group of health care providers (physicians, hospitals; may include specialists, APRNs, and other nurses) providing coordinated care and chronic disease management at a fixed rate of reimbursement. • Goal is to improve quality of patient care and increase care coordination while containing growth. • Achievement of health care quality goals and outcomes resulting in cost savings are tied to the organization's payment.
Patient-Centered Medical Homes	• A team-based primary care practice that includes several different health care professionals, social workers, nutritionists, and educators who coordinate and provide comprehensive care. • Coordinates additional care patients need (specialists; hospital-, home-, and community-based care). • Partners with patients and families, engages in shared decision making and guides self-care management.
Nurse Managed Health Centers	• Nurse-run centers often associated with nursing schools or community-based nonprofit organizations. • Provides comprehensive primary care and other services often serving the medical underinsured. • Many registered nurses provide majority of care. • May employ physicians and other health care workers.

APRN, Advanced practice registered nurse.

Data from: American Nurses Association. (2012, June 29). The Supreme Court decision matters for registered nurses, their families and patients. Retrieved September 20, 2014, from http://www.emergingrnleader.com/wp-content/uploads/2012/07/SupremeCourtDecision-Analysis.pdf

Institute of Medicine. (2010). *The future of nursing: Leading change, advancing health.* Washington, DC: National Academics Press and Sherman, R. (2012). 5 ways the Affordable Care Act could change nursing. Retrieved September 20, 2014, from http://www.emergingrnleader.com/5-ways-the-affordable-care-act-could-change-nursing/

like Ebola and the aftermath of natural disasters like Hurricane Katrina in 2005, the Haiti earthquake in 2010, the tsunami that struck Japan in 2011, and the 2013 Oklahoma tornado have changed our nation and the world. In response to these events and others, the health care system has focused resources on disaster and mass trauma preparedness, bioterrorism responses, and a multitude of strategies to prepare for unpredictable and diverse catastrophic events (Lewis, 2009). Nurses worldwide, regardless of their experience or educational preparation, must have basic knowledge and skills to respond appropriately to mass casualty incidents (International Nursing Coalition for Mass Casualty Education, 2003). To achieve this goal, nursing curricula must prepare practitioners with leadership skills and the ability to work interprofessionally and function as a team member so that nurses can fully participate in the creation of emergency response systems, work within the public health infrastructures characterized by communitywide collaboration and communication, and take their rightful place at the public policy table. Nurses also need clinical knowledge related to biological agents and skills to manage and support surviving individuals, families, and communities experiencing the psychosocial effects in the aftermath of disaster events (Norman & Weiner, 2011; Warsini, West, Mills, & Usher, 2014). Therefore new and redesigned nursing curricula should consider the educational competencies for professional nurses responding to mass casualty incidents developed through the collaborative work of the International Nursing Coalition for Mass Casualty Education (2003). These educational competencies are available at http://www.aacn.nche.edu/leading-initiatives/education-resources/INCMCECompetencies.pdf.

Additionally, the Center for Disease Control and Prevention website (www.bt.cdc.gov) is another useful resource for information and resources related to public health emergency preparation and response.

The Demographic Revolution

The United States is getting more populous, older, and racially and ethnically diverse (Institute of Medicine, IOM, 2010). By 2030 it is estimated people age 65 and older will represent almost 20% of the total U.S. population. The age 85 and older population is also increasing, with a significant trend in "the increase in the proportion of men age 85 and older who are veterans" (Federal Interagency Forum on Aging-Related Statistics [FIFARS], 2012, p. xv). These demographic changes increase the likelihood that nurses and other health care providers will encounter increasing numbers of older and diverse adults who are better educated than prior generations, suffer from a variety of chronic health conditions, and face increased health care costs (Federal Interagency Forum on Aging-Related Statistics, FIFARS, 2012; Institute of Medicine, IOM, 2010). Aging "boomers," including veterans, will enter assisted living or long-term care facilities or be cared for by their families and communities. Initiatives such as those of the Hartford Institute for Geriatric Nursing (http://hartfordign.org/) provide nurse educators with excellent examples of how to incorporate best practices, and other resources to improve the quality of health care of older adults.

End-of-life issues also loom large for the geriatric population and nursing profession. In 2009 the percentage of older Americans dying in hospitals declined while use of hospice services and dying at home increased (Federal Interagency Forum on Aging-Related Statistics, FIFARS, 2012). In 2000 the Robert Wood Johnson Foundation began funding the End-of-Life Nursing Education Consortium (ELNEC) administered by the American Association of Colleges of Nursing (AACN) and the City of Hope National Medical Center. This consortium project is a national education initiative dedicated to educating nurses in excellent palliative care. To date more than 19,300 nurses and other health care professionals, from all 50 U.S. states and 85 countries, have received ELNEC training and are using this innovative strategy to equip the nursing workforce with needed palliative care–related skills and knowledge. More recently, in an effort to improve palliative care for American veterans, the ELNEC-for-Veterans curriculum has been developed to meet the unique needs of nurses caring for those with life-limiting illness (American Association of Colleges of Nursing, AACN, 2014b).

Another important demographic phenomenon affecting nursing curricula is diversification of the U.S. population. Data from the 2010 census revealed the majority of growth in the *total* U.S. population over a 10-year period came from those reporting their races as non-White, Hispanic, or Latino. Although the population of all major race groups increased during this same time frame, the Asian population experienced the fastest rate of growth and the White-alone population the slowest rate of growth (Humes, Jones, & Ramirez, 2011). By 2050 minority groups are anticipated to compose more than half of the total U.S. population (U.S. Census Bureau, 2008).

The changing composition of America has turned this country into a microcosm of the world's peoples. In response, the nursing profession has long recognized the challenges this increasing diversity creates to the provision of high-quality nursing care. Therefore cultural sensitivity has been an essential curricular component of baccalaureate and graduate nursing education (American Association of Colleges of Nursing, AACN, 2008, 2011; Sanner, Baldwin, Cannella, Charles, & Parker, 2010). Although curricular efforts to ensure cultural sensitivity and awareness have been designed and implemented, the fact remains that most nurses, nursing students, and faculty are of White descent (American Association of Colleges of Nursing, AACN, 2014c; Sanner, et al., 2010). It is incumbent on schools of nursing to create and initiate mechanisms to attract, recruit, and retain higher numbers of minority students and faculty from diverse backgrounds (Sanner, et al., 2010). Doing so infuses nursing curriculum with alternative perspectives and helps to establish a nursing workforce that is diverse and equipped to serve a cultural and racially diverse patient population, which is essential to meet the nation's health care needs and reduce health care disparities and feelings of exclusion from the health care system (American Association of Colleges of Nursing, AACN, 2014c).

Whether the demographic shifts include age, diversity, or other population features, there are implications for health and the resources needed to promote health. Future nurses need "the skills to influence policy formulation and the development of creative solutions to respond to changing demographics and the aging chronically ill" (Hegarty, Walsh, Condon, & Sweeney, 2009, p. 5). Preparation of tomorrow's nursing practitioners requires attention to all demographic revolutions of both developed and developing areas of the globe, including patterns of growth, migration, and ethnic or racial composition.

Regardless of the venue in which a culturally diverse and aging population receives care, issues surrounding diversity and geriatric health require educators to equip nurses to promote culturally sensitive health and self-care, prevent disease and disability in an aging population, and provide opportunities to develop political advocacy skills needed to influence public policy decisions related to the allocation of resources toward health and human needs. The responsibility to prepare future nurses in this manner is in keeping with a vision for quality health care explicated by the IOM's 2010 report, *The Future of Nursing: Leading Change, Advancing Health,* which includes discussion of accessible health care for diverse populations, disease prevention, promotion of wellness, and provision of compassionate care across the lifespan.

Technological Explosion

America's transition from a resource-based, industrial economy characterized by semiskilled factory workers and raw materials to a knowledge-based, information-age economy has been reshaping society for decades. Today technology continues to transform nursing practice and education. Most recently, nationwide adoption and use of electronic health record (EHR) systems has required nurses, educators, and students to "use, navigate, and accurately document in the EHR" (Winstanley, 2014, p. 62). The American Recovery and Reinvestment Act of 2009 helped to accelerate the development of standardized EHRs as a means to capture clinical information that could be used to improve health outcomes and lower health care costs. To ensure meaningful use of this new technology and to function in the increasingly complex health care environments, all nurses are expected to "have basic computer competencies, be information literate, and have information management skills" (Tellez, 2012, p. 230).

High-tech, digitalized nursing practice requires educators to incorporate concepts related to information technology into the curriculum and develop teaching strategies requiring students to access, document, collect, and retrieve health care data and other information from electronic sources such as the EHR. Inclusion of informatics education within schools of nursing will assist students to understand data, combine data and knowledge, and make decisions, often through the use of technology (Tellez, 2012). As technology becomes embedded into nursing curricula and health care systems become increasingly automated and digitalized, nurse educators and practitioners must remain mindful of the need to balance the essence of caring and nursing presence at the bedside (Winstanley, 2014).

Technological advancements have also greatly affected nursing education by offering "new opportunities to enhance and broaden learning experiences" (Flynn & Vredevoogd, 2010, p. 7), and by preparing students who are working within complex care environments to be decision makers (Institute of Medicine, IOM, 2010). As technology evolves, increased numbers of nursing programs have found that e-learning, simulation, and mobile devices offer much potential for nursing education (Institute of Medicine, IOM, 2010). Web-enhanced or online learning in particular provides opportunity for practicing nurses to pursue educational programs at times convenient for learners (Institute of Medicine, IOM, 2010; Murray, McCallum, & Petrosino, 2014). As a result, technology allows for educational mobility, provides 24/7 access to education and knowledge, enhances opportunities for teaching and learning or career advancement, and contributes to the availability of a qualified nursing workforce (Institute of Medicine, IOM, 2010).

Technology is also responsible, in part, for how educators have changed their approach to learning in the face-to-face classroom. Educators increasingly are using the "flipped" classroom approach to move select content to an online format. Doing so provides students access to online resources such as voice-over lectures, videos, or links to additional relevant information as a way to learn foundational or knowledge-based content prior to attending a face-to-face class meeting. This instructional strategy allows nurse educators to use class time for applying content learned to new situations, guiding students as they engage in problem solving, as well as engaging students in higher-level thinking (Murray, et al., 2014). Along with the incorporation of the "flipped" classroom, nursing curriculum should take into account how students and educators will engage with and use other available technologies to deliver course content, access information during class and clinical rotations, complete assignments, and communicate with each other.

Simulation is another instructional strategy widely incorporated into nursing curriculum that has come a long way thanks to technological advances (Hayden, 2010; Sanford, 2010). The advent and use of medium- or high-fidelity manikins as well as digital recording capabilities has turned simulation centers into learning environments demanding high levels of technical expertise and the ability to authentically simulate real-work nursing practice; they allow students to learn and practice in a safe environment. Simulation, along with the use of mobile devices such as smart phones or tablets, teaches students real-life skills and prepares them for nursing practice in authentic settings (Institute of Medicine, IOM, 2010; Wolters Kluwer Health, 2014).

Globalization and Global Health

Globalization refers to "a process of interaction and integration among people, companies, and governments of different nations" (The Levin Institute, 2014, para. 1). This process, driven by international trade, investment, and information technology, affects environment, culture, political systems, economic development, prosperity, health, and the well-being of people around the globe (The Levin Institute, 2014). As a result, national boundaries have become less relevant in an era of instantaneous telecommunications, free trade, and multinational corporations. In contrast, global health focuses on issues affecting health that transcend national boundaries and embrace prevention and health equity for all people around the world (Koplan, et al., 2009).

The consequences of globalization are staggering, depend in part on a country's state or development, and have both a positive and negative effect on global health. In the positive sense, globalization has resulted in trade expansion, which in turn increases living standards and improves social and economic status (The Levin Institute, 2014). It has also created an interconnected workforce, including nursing, which "crosses international boundaries, systems, structures, and processes to provide care to and improve the health outcomes of people around the world' (Jones & Sherwood, 2014, p. 60). Another positive and emerging health outcome of globalization is related to the unprecedented spread of mobile technologies such as mobile phones, patient monitoring devices, personal digital assistants, and other wireless devices that are being used to strengthen health systems and achieve health-related goals. In particular, the smart phone and its corresponding medical applications is one example of how mobile technology has transformed the way health information and services are retrieved, delivered, and managed. All of this is made possible by the infiltration of mobile phone networks into a multitude of low- and middle-income countries, resulting in greater than 85% of the world's population being covered by a commercial wireless signal

(Istepanian, 2014; World Health Organization, 2011). However, advances in globalization have also served to negatively affect health. For example, adoption of unhealthy Western habits and lifestyles has resulted in increased obesity and chronic disease. Additionally, open borders and access allow for rapid transmission of infectious agents and disease (Abbott & Coenen, 2008). Globalization has positively increased the mobility of the nursing workforce within and between states, provinces, or countries. However, increased mobility secondary to poor working or living conditions in a nurse's home country, for example, can decrease the local supply of the nurses and thus health of the country or region (Jones & Sherwood, 2014).

Globalization presents a challenge and ethical responsibility for educators to design and implement curricula that will introduce students to the tenets of a global society and global health as well as prepare competent caregivers within a global society (MacNeil & Ryan, 2013). To this end, didactic and clinical teaching and learning strategies should be aimed at developing knowledge, skills, and attitudes nurses need to "identify and influence social, political, and economic determinates of health for marginalized populations" (Peluso, Hafler, Sipsma, & Cherlin, 2014, p. 371). In addition, nurses must gain understanding about the realities of a market-driven or demand-driven health care system based increasingly on a global economy; that health care is a significant industry whose profit margins, stock prices, and bottom lines influence salaries and employment opportunities; and how globalization influences transmission and treatment of disease. Nurses best prepared for changes resulting from economic forces understand the significance of globalization and the global economy.

Environmental Challenges

Just as currency more readily crosses borders, so can environmental and epidemiologic hazards. Besides health issues across the globe, there are concerns regarding sustainable development, energy availability, pollution-free water, and climate change, to name a few. Environmental health involves understanding how the environment influences human health and disease. It involves an awareness of the effect that environmental conditions have on the health of individuals and populations and of interventions that can improve the effect nurses and others have on the environment and the effect the environment has on the health of the people (National Institute of Environmental Health Sciences, 2005; Shaner-McRae, McRae, & Jas, 2007).

Increasingly, Americans are becoming aware that the threats to public health and life are found in the frailty of our earth and our delicate interdependence. Therefore it is important for nurses to be aware that the environment affects our health and that actions in our professional and personal lives can and do make a difference. Nursing curricula should address the content and competencies related to environmental health as well as environmentally responsible clinical practice. Additionally, curricula should encourage and prepare nurses to factor environmental issues into the web of disease causation and to intervene to improve environmental health. The implications of global warming provide an excellent platform for students to discuss the ethics of protecting the environment as well as ways to conserve resources and make educated choices among products that are environmentally friendly. Excellent environmental health resources are available on the American Nurses Association website (http://nursingworld.org/rnnoharm/) and the Alliance of Nurses for Healthy Environments website (http://www.envirn.org/).

Issues in Higher Education

Institutions of higher education sit at an interesting juncture of at least two global themes: the technological explosion and globalization. As learning, knowledge, and skills become the primary resources of a country, the public and private financing of quality higher education becomes more challenging. Colleges and universities, faced with shrinking resources, technological advances, increased enrollments, and the call for globalization of curricula must strive to find a balance between innovation and tradition if they are to remain relevant and current in an ever-changing and evolving world (Flynn & Vredevoogd, 2010; Hornberger, Eramaa, Helembai, McCartan, & Turtiainen, 2014). Therefore affordability, access, accountability, and internationalization continue to be key issues facing higher education. Each issue affects the other, as affordability determines access and, as public concerns related to these issues mount, there are increasing calls for accountability. These challenges must be met in the face of shrinking public higher education budgets.

Affordability

The concern for affordability, noted as early as 1947, persists today as economic and societal factors promote an increased value of a college degree. Current evidence supports that investment in higher education exceeds the cost of that education in the long run. For example, for most people, higher education is associated with a secure lifestyle, significantly increased likelihood of employment, and stable careers, as well as positive financial earnings. It is also associated with a healthier, more satisfying life as well as active participation in civic activities (Baum, Ma, & Payea, 2013). Today, higher education faces many challenges caused by the current economic situation, increasing student enrollment, and rising expectations for quality and equity (Flynn & Vredevoogd, 2010; Heyneman, 2006). Cuts in federal and state funding have affected publicly funded institutions while fluctuations in the stock market have contributed to the declining value of endowments. In short, higher education "will be asked to do more with less" (Flynn & Vredevoogd, 2010, p. 6).

Because of societal concern for a living wage, the financing of higher education becomes a crucial public policy debate. Within that debate, the academy should prepare persuasive arguments for the merits of education beyond salary, society's obligation to invest in human infrastructure, and the importance of public commitment to higher education. The specific charge for schools of nursing is to articulate the cost-effective contribution that nursing makes to the improvement of the health of the nation.

Access

Another issue with historical roots that persists today is access to higher education. The issue of access is important considering society's transformation from an industrial economy to an information-based, global economy because college graduates have "substantially better prospects in the labor market than peers who stop their formal education after high school" (Brock, 2010, p. 110). While access to higher education has increased substantially for women, Hispanics, Asians, and Pacific Islanders, other racial and ethnic groups, such as American Indians and Alaskan Natives, remain underrepresented (Brock, 2010).

The ability of all Americans to take advantage of the multiple benefits and opportunities that higher education affords requires public policies and political will that support access, as well as higher education institutions that make real those opportunities. As administrators of nursing schools pursue robust enrollments of diverse and talented students, affordability and access are crucial considerations for the profession.

Accountability

Worldwide, governments and the taxpaying public are questioning the allocation of scarce public resources. The concept of high-quality, affordable public education is threatened by the competition for funding of other public needs. This, along with rising fear about the deterioration of the U.S. higher education system, low completion rates, and poor preparation of a workforce ready and able to compete in a global marketplace, led to the formation of the Spelling Commission. The purpose of this commission was to recommend a national strategy for postsecondary education reform, with an emphasis on "how well colleges and universities are preparing students for the 21st century workforce" (Floyd & Vredevoogd, 2010, p. 19).

Several forces prompt this increased accountability for higher education. In times of cost cutting and corporate downsizing, business and private sector management looks to education, and its products, for competitive strategies. Also, drastic state budget cuts have caused policy makers and taxpayers to require justification for higher education funding. Legislatures have tended to disallow tuition hikes and request internal moves toward efficiency. Additionally, "publicly funded institutions must be accountable to their principal stakeholder—the public" (Floyd & Vredevoogd, 2010, p. 10). Each of these forces promotes increased public scrutiny and higher expectations.

Accountability therefore becomes a multidirectional force. Institutions of higher education depend on the government for funding and are therefore highly accountable to the public for academic productivity and fiscal prudence. Governments, in response to their perceived accountability to the public, act to regulate and reform higher education. Schools of nursing are accountable to state legislatures, Congress, and the public regarding the preparation of adequate numbers of competent nurses. This accountability includes incorporation of and adherence to regulations set forth by state boards of nursing, accrediting bodies, and others who set standards for prelicensure and graduate nursing education. Clearly accountability will continue as a significant theme in higher education.

Internationalization

In higher education internationalization has served to intensify the "mobility of ideas and of people" in large part because of the technology explosion that continually shrinks time and space (Egron-Polak, 2012, p. 1). It is anticipated over the course of the next 10 years that educational institutes providing English language–based postsecondary education will experience strong demand from international students who have the desire to study outside of their home countries (Ruby, 2013). In turn, institutes of higher education are increasingly open to attracting more international students as well as able to offer faculty opportunities to engage in international research. As a result, new funding sources become available at a time when academic institutions are struggling financially for reasons explicated in the preceding discussion on affordability (Egron-Polak, 2012).

Issues Specific to the Nursing Profession

This chapter began by looking through the lens of the broad socioeconomic and sociopolitical issues that shape the world and influence contemporary life. This section focuses the lens more specifically on the nursing profession and highlights issues of particular consideration within the profession. Included are the context of nursing care delivery, new and reemerging degrees, and competencies for the twenty-first century.

Context of Nursing Care Delivery

The nursing profession influences and is influenced by the health care delivery system, which provides a context for nursing services. The 2010 American Hospital Association Environmental Scan provided insight into several trends affecting the health care field, five of which have great implications for nursing practice and education: science and technology, rising costs, health policy, quality of care and patient safety, and human resources (O'Dell, Aspy, & Jarousse, 2011). These trends inform educators as they determine what and how to teach the next generation of nurses.

Science and Technology

Science and technology continues to revolutionize the health care possibilities at the point of care and within the academic community. For example, from a science perspective the Human Genome Project presents a multitude of individualized genetic therapies, as well as ethical quandaries. As a result, nursing curriculum should incorporate strategies aimed at helping nurses identify, understand, and support patients facing genetic decisions (Forbes & Hickey, 2009). The American Nurses Association's (2008) *Essentials of Genetic and Genomic Nursing: Competencies, Curricula Guidelines, and Outcome Indicators* details basic competencies nurses should possess to "deliver competent genetic and genomic focused nursing care" (Forbes & Hickey, 2009, p. 9) and thus is an excellent resource for those charged with curriculum development and redesign.

A national survey from the Pew Research Center's Internet & American Life Project (2013) indicates just how pervasive technology is in our world. Findings from the Pew survey revealed that one in three American adults have gone online to figure out a medical condition, and 72% of internet users say they looked online for health information within the past year (2013). Through the Internet, consumers have become armed with and have access to information previously available only to clinicians. Today's health care consumers know what they should expect from their health care providers and expect to participate in decisions affecting their health care (Hegarty et al., 2009; Heller, Oros, & Durney-Crowley, 2013). Internet-savvy health care consumers often approach providers with extensive information, requesting treatments or drugs and expecting quality ratings on provider and institution report cards. Therefore nursing needs to appreciate these empowered consumers and "respect, affirm, and share decision-making with increasingly knowledgeable patients" (Hegarty, et al., 2009, p. 6).

The health care industry is following the lead of the aviation industry in providing increased education and assessment using simulation technology, particularly in this era of scarce and complex clinical sites for training. As a result, schools of nursing are challenged to use sophisticated simulations as a way to help students acquire skills and develop critical thinking (O'Dell, et al., 2011). With high-fidelity simulation, nurse educators can replicate many "real-world" patient situations in which students can practice nursing in an environment that does not endanger patients. Findings from a recent randomized control study indicated that substitution of high-quality simulation experiences for up to half of traditional clinical hours produced comparable end-of-program educational outcomes (Hayden, Smiley, Alexander, Kardong-Edgren, & Jefferies, 2014).

Rising Costs

The second trend involves the continued surge in health costs and the need for hospitals and providers to manage care more efficiently within finite budgets. Hospital budgets will be challenged by declining charitable donations and investment income; increasing numbers of Medicare, Medicaid, and self-pay clients; labor shortages; and increased pharmaceutical and supply costs (O'Dell, et al., 2011). Research that documents nursing's contribution to efficient, quality care is needed to advocate in budget negotiations and hospital changes.

Health Policy

Health policy, the third trend, becomes an increasingly significant strategy to shape, finance, and regulate the health care system. With the cost of national health expenditures anticipated to rise from 16% to 20% of the gross domestic product (GDP) by 2017, state and federal policies seek to regulate costs, shift care to less expensive settings, and use market forces to control costs when possible (Henry J. Kaiser Family Foundation, 2009; O'Dell, et al., 2011). Ensuring that everyone in the United States has health insurance is one strategy that would help reduce health care expenditure to only 18.5% of the GDP (O'Dell, et al., 2011). The PPACA represents great progress toward making health care available to and affordable for all Americans. Since its inception, the number of insured Americans has continued to rise. The U.S. Census Bureau (2013) reported that in 2012 both the percentage and number of Americans with health insurance increased to 84.6% and 263.2 million, up from 84.3% and 260.2 million in 2011.

The number of people covered by private health insurance continues to drop while increasing numbers receive coverage by government health insurance. Another feature of the PPACA is the mandate to revitalize primary and public health care infrastructures (U.S. Department of Health and Human Services, 2014). The focus of health care is shifting away from acute and chronic hospital-based care toward community-based care. Nursing will continue to be called on to coordinate collaborative interdisciplinary community-based care and to act as primary care providers, practicing to the full extent of their education and training. The expansion of nursing roles under the PPACA will create a shift in nursing employment statistics and create additional career opportunities for new graduates (Institute of Medicine, IOM, 2010).

The predicted shift from hospital-based to community-based employment has already begun. In 2008, 62.2% of all employed registered nurses (RNs) worked in hospitals. Currently, more than 50% of nurses work outside the hospital setting (Benner, Sutphen, Leonard, & Day, 2010). In 2010 the HRSA estimated a 109% increase in the need for community-based RNs compared with a 36% increased need for hospital-based RNs by 2020.

In response to this shift in where care is delivered, governing agencies are recommending that schools of nursing restructure their curriculums and move away from the traditional primary focus on acute and chronic hospital-based instruction to one that includes more team-focused, community-based practice emphasizing policy technology and leadership development programs (Institute of Medicine, IOM, 2010; U.S. Department of Health and Human Services, 2014). Innovative nurse educators are responding to these recommendations by building collaborative relationships with patient-centered medical homes and nurse-managed health clinics to provide nursing students with clinical experiences that demonstrate the principles of community care, leadership, and client care in community settings (American Association of Colleges of Nursing, AACN, 2013).

Quality of Care and Patient Safety

A need exists to improve patient safety and provide quality care (Forbes & Hickey, 2009). Although the quality of care has improved steadily during the past decade, further improvement continues at a low pace. Not only is health care quality suboptimal, patient safety is also lagging, and there remains a significant geographic variation in quality of care (U.S. Department of Health & Human Services, Agency for Healthcare Research and Quality, 2008; O'Dell, et al., 2011). In 2010 the IOM recommended that patients and their families have access to information regarding a hospital's performance on safety, evidence-based practice, and patient satisfaction (Hinshaw, 2011). This, along with increasing reporting requirements, will challenge health care organizations to collect the most accurate data possible and then improve patient care based on that data. In response to this trend, the Institute for Health Improvement recently developed the Triple Aim framework (2009) as a means to measure health care quality data, interventions in public health, care coordination, universal access to care, and cost control through a financial management system.

Given the loud call from several authorities, including the IOM, the Robert Wood Johnson Foundation, and the Agency for Healthcare Research and Quality, in tandem with the key role nurses play in protecting patient safety and providing quality health care, there exists a need to better prepare today's nurses for professional practice. To this end, the AACN identified the following six essential core competencies for nurses related to ensuring high quality and patient safety: critical thinking, health care systems and policy, communication, illness and disease management, ethics, and information and health care technologies. Teaching strategies and concrete examples of learning activities that nurse educators can use to teach these competencies can be found at the Quality and Safety Education for Nurses website at www.qsen.org. Additionally, educators should assist students to understand the proactive steps that the nursing profession is taking within the changing health care environment to define nursing practice and educate the public on nursing's role in quality care. The Magnet Recognition Program® developed by the American Nurses Credentialing Center (American Nurses Credentialing Center, ANCC, 2008) recognizes health care organizations for quality patient care, nursing excellence and innovations in professional nursing practice. Magnet designation is the ultimate credential for high quality nursing and a powerful example of nursing action that students should understand. Please see the ANCC website for additional information on the Magnet Recognition Program® (http://www.nursecredentialing.org/Magnet/ProgramOverview/New-Magnet-Model.aspx).

Human Resources

Human capital becomes a significant trend with nursing and physician shortages and the unionization of health care providers. In February 2009 three nursing unions merged to form the United American Nurses–National Nurses Organizing Committee. The legislative priorities of this union, which has 150,000 members, include a push for nurse staffing ratios, workplace safety rules, and a national pension for RNs (O'Dell, et al., 2011).

Retention of satisfied employees will be the goal of viable organizations, which is related to the creation and maintenance of healthy and safe work environments. Creation of "workplace cultures that can attract and retain health care workers" will be an important element of hospitals of the future given the "average voluntary turnover rate of new hospital nurses is 27%" during their first year on the job (Joint Commission, 2008, p. 29). In part, respecting human capital means attention to the work environment and relationships as well as sanctions against verbal abuse by physicians, patients, and nurse colleagues; sexual harassment; and workplace violence, including horizontal violence or hostile behaviors within a group of nurse colleagues (Felblinger, 2008; Joint Commission, 2008). In 2005 the American Association of Critical Care Nurses created a document that details six essential standards for establishing and maintaining healthy work environments. Educators would do well to adopt these standards into their curriculum and academic and clinical workplaces. The AACN Standards for Establishing and Sustaining Healthy Work Environments: A Journey to Excellence is available at http://www.aacn.org/wd/hwe/docs/hwestandards.pdf.

In conclusion, future practitioners will need knowledge and abilities to assist informed health care consumers, understand science, use technology, stem rising costs, provide quality health care and protect the safety of patients, advocate for effective health policy, actively participate in the process of health care reform, and work to create a health care system with competent, empowered human capital. In short, "nurses will need to take leadership roles in ensuring quality health care" (Q&A with Kathy Rideout, Associate Dean for Academic Affairs, 2010, p. 11).

Emerging Degrees

Two graduate degrees, the clinical nurse leader (CNL) and the doctor of nursing practice (DNP), have been created and implemented within the profession in the last decade. These two emerging degrees provide one example of efforts within the profession to create roles and curricula to meet changing societal needs for health care.

In 2000, considering declining nursing enrollment among other professional issues, the AACN determined that changes must be made in education, practice, licensure, and credentialing. The AACN recommended a new educational model for a master's entry, the CNL, to improve patient care and maximize patient safety (American Association of Colleges of Nursing, AACN, 2007). To this end, the CNL is intended to be a leader within all health care settings who assumes accountability for patient-care outcomes and provides and manages care to individuals and patient cohorts (American Association of Colleges of Nursing, AACN, 2013). Other fundamental aspects of CNL practices are outlined in Box 5-1. Programs to educate CNLs require ongoing partnerships between practice and education so that both arenas shape the learning and graduates enter practice environments designed to use their skill set.

In 2004 the AACN voted to move the current level of preparation necessary for advanced practice nursing from the master's degree to the doctorate level by 2015, creating the clinical doctorate, the DNP. The drive to create the DNP was the complexity of current health care and curriculum creep that results in some advanced practice degree programs far exceeding the credit hours of a usual master's degree. Since the AACN's membership vote that education for all advanced practice nurses will transition to the DNP, approximately 250 new doctoral programs consistent with the DNP essentials and standards from the particular specialty focus of the program have been created (American Association of Colleges of Nursing, AACN, 2014a). However, other schools perceive budgetary, regulatory, or philosophical barriers to transitioning their MSN degree programs to the DNP degree and will likely continue to offer master's degree advanced practice education as the nursing profession further addresses graduate-level education issues related to advanced practice nursing. Chapter 9 discusses graduate nursing programs in more depth.

BOX 5-1 Fundamental Aspects of CNL Practice

Clinical leadership for patient care practices and delivery, including the design, coordination, and evaluation of care for individuals, families, groups, and populations
Participation in identification and collection of care outcomes.
Accountability for evaluation and improvement of point-of-care outcomes, including the synthesis of data and other evidence to evaluate and achieve optimal outcomes.
Risk anticipation for individuals and cohorts of patients.
Lateral integration of care for individuals and cohorts of patients.
Design and implementation of evidence-based practices.
Team leadership, management, and collaboration with other health professional team members.
Information management or the use of information systems and technologies to improve health care outcomes.
Stewardship and leveraging of human, environmental, and material resources.
Advocacy for patients, communities, and the health profession.

CNL, Clinical nurse leader.
Source: AACN. (2013).Competencies and curricular expectations for clinical nurse leader education and practice. Retrieved September 22, 2014, from http://www.aacn.nche.edu/cnl/CNL-Competencies-October-2013.pdf

Competencies for the Twenty-First Century

The nursing profession needs not only robust workforce numbers, but also practitioners with requisite knowledge, abilities, and work behaviors to meet the health demands of the population as well as nurses who possess leadership skills. Educators are challenged to prepare individuals who, on graduation, can lead; deliver competent, safe, quality, patient-centered, compassionate care; have the ability to navigate future changes in the system; and acquire future abilities associated with evolving roles (Institute of Medicine, IOM, 2010).

Recently, the American Organization of Nurse Executives (2011) released an updated document outlining the competencies common to nurse leaders regardless of educational level or title. These competencies are clustered into five broad categories: (1) communication and relationship building, (2) knowledge of the health care environment, (3) leadership skills, (4) professionalism, and (5) business skills. Box 5-2 presents detailed information about each of these five competency categories, which are pertinent to many issues explicated in the chapter including career planning, performance evaluation, and curriculum development.

BOX 5-2 AONE Nurse Leader Competencies

1. Communication and relationship-building competencies
   a. Effective communication
   b. Relationship management
   c. Influencing behaviors
   d. Diversity
   e. Shared decision-making
   f. Community involvement
   g. Medical, staff relationships
   h. Academic relationships
2. Knowledge of the health care environment
   a. Clinical practice knowledge
   b. Delivery models, work design
   c. Health care economics
   d. Health care policy
   e. Governance
   f. Evidence-based practice, outcome measurement
   g. Patient safety
   h. Utilization, case management
   i. Quality improvement, metrics
   j. Risk management
3. Leadership
   a. Foundational thinking skills
   b. Personal journey disciplines
   c. Systems thinking
   d. Succession planning
   e. Change management
4. Professionalism
   a. Personal and professional accountability
   b. Career planning
   c. Ethics
   d. Evidence-based clinical management practice
   e. Advocacy
   f. Active membership in professional organizations
5. Business skills
   a. Financial management
   b. Human resource management
   c. Strategic management
   d. Marketing
   e. Information management and technology

AONE, American Organization of Nurse Executives.
Adapted from Nurse Executive Competencies, copyright 2011, by the American Organization of Nurse Executives (AONE).

More than a decade ago, Bellack and O'Neil (2000) discussed the recommendations from the Pew Health Professions Commission's fourth and final report, which represented a continuing effort to support the health professions' education reform and align educational programs more fully with the health needs of the population. They presented five recommendations for all health professions schools, including nursing: (1) update professional training to meet new health care demands, (2) ensure diversity in the health professions workforce, (3) require interdisciplinary competence, (4) continue to move health care education into the ambulatory care setting, and (5) encourage health care students to engage in public service. Despite being issued more than 10 years ago, these recommendations continue to provide excellent guideposts for nurse educators as they pursue the preferred future via the current reality.

In many respects, nursing education is still grappling with developing educational models that successfully address the Pew Commission's recommendations from 2000. Most recently, the IOM's (2010) report offers a new set of recommendations that call for significant changes in how nurses are educated and prepared for practice in an era of health care reform. The four key messages delivered in the *Future of Nursing* report are that nurses should: (1) be able to practice to the full scope of their educational preparation; (2) seek higher levels of educational preparation, and be able to do so in seamless academic progression systems; (3) function as full partners in interdisciplinary teams to redesign health care delivery; and (4) benefit from improved data collection and information infrastructures. The IOM report promises to be influential in focusing attention on solutions to the barriers that have kept nurses from being as influential as they can be in leading and advocating for changes in health care.

Strategies to Identify Influential Forces and Issues

The forces and issues that influence the nursing profession and curriculum originate in the external, higher education, and internal environments. This section presents strategies that may be useful to nurse leaders in identifying these influences.

Environmental Scanning

"Strategic planning is critical to the survival of health care organizations in today's turbulent environment" (Layman & Bamberg, 2005, p. 200). Environmental scanning, a component of strategic planning, involves various activities that monitor and evaluate information from the external environment (Layman & Bamberg, 2005). The goal of environmental scanning is for leaders and managers to become aware of general trends and events affecting health care and higher education generally and nursing specifically. Information from the environment can be acquired in various ways, including careful review of scientific and professional journals as well as lay literature and newspapers and attendance and networking at professional meetings. Information gathered from these activities becomes "the basis of future initiatives" (Layman & Bamberg, 2005, p. 200).

Environmental scanning continues to be successfully used by colleges and universities to determine the context of the forces affecting curriculum development. For example, use of strategic environmental scanning led one southeastern university to develop a non–nurse practitioner program designed to prepare nurses for other types of advanced practice roles. Following review of program evaluations and assessment of graduates and other nursing leaders in the community, the Master of Science in Nursing in Advanced Care Management and Leadership program was developed with the goal of preparing nurse leaders who are "equipped to manage and improve client care outcomes" (Aduddell & Dorman, 2010, p. 171).

In curriculum development, environmental scanning allows faculty to be simultaneously reactive and proactive. Through awareness and acknowledgment of significant trends (reactive), faculty can more actively choose a future direction for nursing education and curriculum (proactive). The use of environmental scanning as a strategy to obtain a broad scope of information and evaluate its relevance to nursing is the foundation of the other strategies that follow.

Strategic Planning

Often educators, leaders, and managers are so preoccupied with the "tyranny of the urgent" that they lose sight of their ultimate goals and objectives. Strategic planning is one strategy educators and organizations can use for quality checks, assessments, planning, or analysis. A strategic plan serves as a framework for decisions, provides a foundation for detailed planning, is used to explain "the business" to others, assists with benchmarking and performance monitoring, and stimulates change (PlanWare, 2014).

The process of strategic planning may include the use of the Strengths, Weaknesses, Opportunities, Threats (SWOT) analysis. Educators charged with curriculum development or redesign can use SWOT to guide development and analysis of curricular objectives and key strategies to meet them. SWOT can also be used as an instructional strategy to assist students with job searching and career planning (Weiss & Tappen, 2015).

Epidemiology

Epidemiology is the study of the distribution and determinants of states of health and illness in human populations. Epidemiology provides nursing faculty with systematic ways to understand patterns of disease, characteristics of people at high risk for disease, environmental factors, and shifts in demographic characteristics of the population. Using epidemiologic data with groups or populations, nurses understand and document the need for programs and policies to reduce risk and promote health. Epidemiology can therefore be seen as a method for planned change.

In the same way, nursing faculty responsible for the development of curriculum can use epidemiological data and methods to understand factors affecting the health of populations and trends occurring in health and illness states. Epidemiologic analysis provides faculty with methods for understanding that part of the context that involves the broad determinants of health and patterns of disease and disability in the population.

Survey Research and Consensus Building

Another tool at the disposal of faculty is survey research. Surveys involve systematically collecting information from individuals and deriving statistical statements, such as some measure of central tendency, or consensus statements from groups of experts or involved individuals. If the design is iterative and involves a series of surveys, feedback, and more surveys, it is considered a form of Delphi technique. Surveys and consensus-building processes provide an opportunity to sample the perspectives of various stakeholders and knowledgeable persons, for example, employers or consumers. They facilitate tapping the rich diversity of group wisdom related to complex issues.

The strategies of environmental scanning, forecasting, epidemiology, and survey research and consensus building have utility in preparing for curriculum development or revision. Using some combination of the four strategies presented here, faculty can be equipped to develop curriculum compatible with the current and projected issues influencing nursing and health care.

Summary

The forces and issues that influence and are influenced by nursing curriculum originate in the external, higher education, and internal environments. Educators sensitive to major sociopolitical and economic trends can develop curriculum that matches global characteristics. Educators aware of prevailing higher education issues can assist schools of nursing to be leaders in the academy. Educators attuned to prevailing and visionary thinking within the profession can shape the future through progressive curriculum and pedagogy. Nursing deserves curriculum that is both compatible with the contemporary health care context and flexible enough to be relevant for emerging circumstances and needs.

REFLECTING ON THE EVIDENCE

1. How does your nursing program curriculum remain relevant to the broad societal changes, issues, or health care reform? In what new ways can it become more relevant to broad societal changes, issues, or health care reform?
2. How does your nursing program curriculum prepare students to be engaged citizens in society whose practice matches current issues and trends?
3. How is your nursing program curriculum compatible with new developments in the discipline?
4. In what ways does the faculty in your nursing program incorporate new input and acknowledge new influences on curriculum development? How do faculty respond to those voices of change?
5. How is your nursing program curriculum preparing students to engage in health care reform and collaborative practice as leaders?

REFERENCES

Abbott, P. A., & Coenen, A. (2008). Globalization and advances in information and communication technologies: The impact on nursing and health. *Nursing Outlook*, *56*(5), 238–246. e2. http://dx.doi.org/10.1016/j.outlook.2008.06.009.

Aduddell, K. A., & Dorman, G. E. (2010). The development of the next generation of nurse leaders. *Journal of Nursing Education*, *49*(3), 168–171. http://dx.doi.org/10.3928/01484834-20090916-08.

American Association of Colleges of Nursing (AACN). (2007). *White paper on the education and role of the clinical nurse leader.* Retrieved from, http://www.aacn.nche.edu/.

American Association of Colleges of Nursing (AACN). (2008). *The essentials of baccalaureate education for professional nursing practice.* Retrieved August 8, 2014, from, http://www.aacn.nche.edu/education-resources/BaccEssentials08.pdf.

American Association of Colleges of Nursing (AACN). (2011). *Tool kit of cultural competence in masters' and doctoral nursing education.* Retrieved October 25, 2014, from, http://www.aacn.nche.edu/education-resources/Cultural_Competency_Toolkit_Grad.pdf.

American Association of Colleges of Nursing (AACN). (2013). *Competencies and curricular expectations for clinical nurse leader education and practice.* Retrieved September 22, 2014, from, http://www.aacn.nche.edu/cnl/CNL-Competencies-October-2013.pdf.

American Association of Colleges of Nursing (AACN). (2014a). *The DNP by 2015: A study of the institutional, political, and professional issues that facilitate or impede establishing a post-baccalaureate doctor of nursing practice program.* Retrieved December 30, 2014, from, www.aacn.nche.edu/DNP/DNP-Study.pdf.

American Association of Colleges of Nursing (AACN). (2014b). *ELNEC fact sheet.* Retrieved November 16, 2014, from, http://www.aacn.nche.edu/elnec/about/fact-sheet.

American Association of Colleges of Nursing (AACN). (2014c). *Fact sheet: enhancing diversity in the nursing workforce.* Retrieved November 16, 2014, from, http://www.aacn.nche.edu/media-relations/fact-sheets/enhancing-diversity.

American Nurses Association. (2008). *Essentials of genetic and genomic nursing: Competencies, curricula guidelines, and outcome indicators.* Retrieved November 26, 2014, from, http://www.annanurse.org/essentials-genetic-and-genomic-nursing-competencies-curricula-guidelines-and-outcome-indicators.

American Nurses Association. (2012, June 29). *The supreme court decision matters for registered nurses, their families and patients.* Retrieved September 20, 2014, from, http://www.emergingrnleader.com/wp-content/uploads/2012/07/SupremeCourtDecision-Analysis.pdf.

American Nurses Credentialing Center (ANCC). (2008). *A new vision for magnet.* Retrieved from, http://www.nursecredentialing.org/Magnet/ProgramOverview/New-Magnet-Model.aspx.

American Organization of Nurse Executives. (2011). *The AONE nurse executive competencies.* Retrieved October 22, 2014, from, http://www.aone.org/resources/leadership%20tools/nursecomp.shtml.

Baum, S., Ma, J., & Payea, K. (2013). *Education pays 2013: The benefits of higher education for individuals and society.* Retrieved September 22, 2014, from, http://trends.collegeboard.org/sites/default/files/education-pays-2013-full-report-022714.pdf.

Bellack, J. P., & O'Neil, E. H. (2000). Recreating nursing practice for a new century: Recommendations and implications of the Pew Health Professions Commission's final report. *Nursing and Health Care Perspectives, 21*(1), 14–21.

Benner, P., Sutphen, M., Leonard, V., & Day, L. (2010). *Educating nurses: A call for radical transformation.* San Francisco, CA: Jossey-Bass.

Brock, T. (2010). Young adults and higher education: Barriers and breakthroughs to success. *The Future of Children, 20*(1), 109–132.

Egron-Polak, E. (2012). *Higher education internationalization: Seeking a new balance of values.* Trends & Insights for International Education Leaders. Retrieved October 25, 2014, from, http://www.nafsa.org/Explore_International_Education/Trends/TI/Higher_Education_Internationalization__Seeking_a_New_Balance:of_Values/.

Federal Interagency Forum on Aging-Related Statistics (FIFARS). (2012). Older americans 2012: Key indicators of well-being. *Federal Interagency Forum on Aging-Related Statistics.* Washington, DC: U.S. Government Printing Office.

Felblinger, D. M. (2008). Incivility and bullying in the workplace and nurses' shame responses. *Journal of Obstetrics, Gynecology, and Neonatal Nurses, 37*(2), 234–242.

Flynn, W. J., & Vredevoogd, J. (2010). The future of learning: 12 views on emerging trends in higher education. *Planning for Higher Education, 38*(2), 5–10.

Forbes, M. O., & Hickey, M. T. (2009). Curriculum reform in baccalaureate nursing education: Review of the literature. *International Journal of Nursing Education Scholarship, 6*(1), 1–16.

Hayden, J. (2010). Use of simulation in nursing education: National survey results. *Journal of Nursing Regulation, 1*(3), 52–57.

Hayden, J. K., Smiley, R. A., Alexander, M., Kardong-Edgren, S., & Jeffries, P. R. (2014). The NCSBN national simulation study: A longitudinal, randomized, controlled study replacing clinical hours with simulation in prelicensure nursing education. *Journal of Nursing Regulation, 5*(2), s3–s64.

Hegarty, J., Walsh, E., Condon, C., & Sweeney, J. (2009). The undergraduate education of nurses: Looking to the future. *International Journal of Nursing Education Scholarship, 6*(1), 1–11.

Heller, B. R., Oros, M. T., & Durney-Crowley, J. (2013). *The future of nursing education: Ten trends to watch.* Retrieved from, http://www.nln.org/nlnjournal/infotrends.htm#4.

Heyneman, S. P. (2006). *Global issues in higher education.* Retrieved from, http://www.america.gov/st/econ-english/2008/June/20080608095226xjyrreP0.6231653.html&distid=.

Hinshaw, P. M. (2011). Understanding the triple aim. *Nursing Management, 42*(2), 18–19.

Hornberger, C., Eramma, S., Helembai, K., McCartan, P., & Turtiainen, T. (2014). Responding to the call for globalization in nursing education. The implementation of the transatlantic double-degree program. *Journal of Professional Nursing, 30*(3), 243–250.

Humes, K., Jones, N., & Ramirez, R. (2011). *Overview of race and hispanic origin: 2010.* Retrieved August 8, 2014 from, http://www.census.gov/prod/cen2010/briefs/c2010br-02.pdf.

Institute for Healthcare Improvement. (2009). Optimizing health, care, and cost. *Healthcare Executive, 24*(1), 64–66.

Institute of Medicine (IOM). (2010). *The future of nursing: Leading change, advancing health.* Washington, DC: National Academics Press.

International Nursing Coalition for Mass Casualty Education. (2003). *Educational competencies for registered nurses responding to mass casualty incidents.* Retrieved from, http://www.aacn.nche.edu/leading-initiatives/education-resources/INCMCECompetencies.pdf.

Istepanian, R. (2014). M-health: A decade of evolution and impact on services and global health. *British Journal of Healthcare Management, 20*(7), 334–337.

Joint Commission, The. (2008). *Health care at the crossroads: Guiding principles for the development of the hospital of the future.* Retrieved from, http://www.jointcommission.org/.

Jones, C., & Sherwood, G. (2014). The globalization of the nursing workforce. Pulling the pieces together. *Nursing Outlook, 62*(1), 59–63.

Henry J. Kaiser Family Foundation. (2009). *Health care costs: Key information on health care costs and their impact.* Menlo Park, CA: Author. Retrieved from, http://www.kff.org/.

Koplan, J., Bond, T., Merson, M., Reddy, K., Rodriguez, M., Sewankambo, N., & Wasserheit, J. (2009). Towards a common definition of global health. *The Lancet, 373,* 1993–1995.

Layman, E. J., & Bamberg, R. (2005). Environmental scanning and the health care manager. *Health Care Manager, 24*(3), 200–208.

Levin Institute, The. (2014). *What is globalization.* Retrieved September 21, 2014, from, http://www.globalization101.org/what-is-globalization/.

Lewis, K. L. (2009). Emergency planning and response. In G. Roux & J. A. Halstead (Eds.), *Issues and trends in nursing: Essential knowledge for today and tomorrow* (pp. 261–285). Sudbury, MA: Jones & Bartlett.

MacNeil, J., & Ryan, M. (2013). Enacting global health in the nursing classroom. *Nurse Education Today, 33,* 1279–1281.

Murray, L., McCallum, C., & Petrosino, C. (2014). Flipping the classroom experience: A comparison of online learning to traditional lecture. *Journal of Physical Therapy Education, 28*(3), 35–41.

National Institute of Environmental Health Sciences. (2005). *What is environmental health?.* Retrieved from, http://www.niehs.nih.gov/.

Norman, L., & Weiner, E. (2011). Emergency preparedness and response for today's world. In B. Cherry & S. Jacob (Eds.), *Contemporary Nursing: Issues, Trends, and Management.* (5th ed.)(pp. 317–332). St. Louis, MO: Elsevier.

O'Dell, G. J., Aspy, D. J., & Jarousse, L. A. (2011). 2012 AHA environmental scan. *Hospitals and Health Networks, 64*(8), 13–24.

Peluso, M., Hafler, J., Sipsma, H., & Cherlin, E. (2014). Global health education programming as a model for inter-institutional collaboration in interprofessional health education. *Journal of Interprofessional Care, 28*(4), 371–373.

Pew Research Center's Internet and American Life Project. (2013). *Health online 2013.* Retrieved from, http://www.pewinternet.org/2013/01/15/health-online-2013/.

PlanWare. (2014). *Business planning papers: Developing a strategic plan.* Retrieved September 22, 2014 from, http://www.planware.org/strategicplan.htm#1.

Q&A with Kathy Rideout, Associate Dean for Academic Affairs. (2010). *Nursing.* Rochester, NY: School of Nursing, University of Rochester Medical Center.

Health Resources and Services Administration. (2010). *The registered nurse population: Initial findings from the 2008 national sample of registered nurses.* Retrieved from, http://bhpr.hrsa.gov/healthworkforce/rnsurveys/rnsurveyfinal.pdf.

Ruby, A. (2013). *International education supply and demand: Forecasting the future.* Retrieved October 25, 2014, from, http://www.nafsa.org/_/File/_/ti_supply_demand.pdf.

Sanford, P. (2010). Simulation in nursing education: A review of the research. *The Qualitative Report, 15*(4), 1001–1006.

Sanner, S., Baldwin, D., Cannella, K., Charles, J., & Parker, L. (2010). The impact of cultural diversity forum on students' openness to diversity. *Journal of Cultural Diversity, 17*(2), 56–61.

Shaner-McRae, H., McRae, G., & Jas, V. (2007). Environmentally safe health care agencies: Nursing's responsibility, Nightingale's legacy. *Online Journal of Issues in Nursing, 12*(2), 1–13. http://dx.doi.org/10.3912/OJIN.Vol12No02Man01. Retrieved November, 17, 2014, from, http://nursingworld.org/MainMenuCategories/ANAMarketplace/ANAPeriodicals/OJIN/TableofContents/Volume122007/No2May07/EnvironmentallySafeHealthCareAgencies.html.

Sherman, R. (2012). *5 ways the Affordable Care Act could change nursing.* Retrieved September 20, 2014 from, http://www.emergingrnleader.com/5-ways-the-affortable-care-act-could-change-nursing/.

Tellez, M. (2012). Nursing Informatics education past, present, and future. *Computers, Informatics, Nursing, 30*(5), 229–233.

U.S. Census Bureau. (2008). *An older and more divers nation by midcentury.* Retrieved November 16, 2014, from, http://renewpartnerships.org/articles/older-and-more-diverse/.

U.S. Census Bureau. (2013). *Income, poverty, and health insurance coverage in the United States: 2012.* Retrieved from, http://www.census.gov.

U.S. Department of Health and Human Services. (2014). *12th annual report to the Secretary of the United States Department of Health and Human Services and the Congress of the United States.* Retrieved from, http://www.hrsa.gov/advisorycommittees/bhpradvisory/nacnep/meetings/12thannualreportpublichealthnursing.pdf.

U.S. Department of Health & Human Services, Agency for Healthcare Research and Quality. (2008). *National health-care quality report.* Retrieved from, http://www.ahrq.gov/.

U.S. Department of Health and Human Services. (2011). *Nursing education, practice, quality and retention program report to congress for fiscal year 2011.* Retrieved October 25, 2014 from, http://bhpr.hrsa.gov/nursing/grants/nepqrfy11report.pdf.

Wakefield, M. K. (2010). Nurses and the Affordable Care Act. *American Journal of Nursing, 110*(9), 11. http://dx.doi.org/10.1097/01.NAJ.0000388242.06365.4f.

Warsini, S., West, C., Mills, J., & Usher, K. (2014). The psychosocial impact of natural disasters among adult survivors: An integrative review. *Issues in Mental Health Nursing, 35,* 420–436.

Weiss, S., & Tappen, R. (2015). *Essential of nursing leadership and management* (6th ed.). Philadelphia, PA: Davis.

Winstanley, H. (2014). How to bring caring to the high-tech bedside. *Nursing, 2014,* 60–63. Retrieved from www.Nursing2014.com.

Wolters Kluwer Health. (Septembers 16, 2014). *Wolters Kluwer Health survey finds nurses and health care institutions accepting professional use of online reference & mobile technology.* Retrieved September 21 from, http://www.fiercemobileit.com/press-releases/wolters-kluwer-health-survey-finds-nurses-and-healthcare-institutions-accep.

World Health Organization. (2011). mHealth: New horizons for health through mobile technologies. *Global observatory for eHealth Series. Volume 3.* Geneva, Switzerland: WHO.

An Introduction to Curriculum Development*

6

Dori Taylor Sullivan, PhD, RN, NE-BC, CPHQ, FAAN

The topic of curriculum development and redesign remains a focal point for educators in nursing and other fields. To achieve desired education outcomes in service to society, a curriculum that optimizes student and faculty performance is required. The collective faculty has responsibility for creating an effective, efficient, and contemporary curriculum that prepares graduates to achieve professional practice standards at each level of education to improve the health and well-being of the populations served. The National League for Nursing (NLN) has outlined expected competencies for nurse faculty that include a strong focus on the role of educators in curriculum development, delivery, and evaluation (National League for Nursing (NLN), 2012).

In today's world multiple factors affect and challenge institutions of higher education to demonstrate effectiveness in preparing graduates for entry into the workplace. At the same time, concerns regarding the cost of postsecondary education and a demonstrated shortage of nurse faculty are among other influencing factors and changes affecting the education of nurses (see Chapter 5).

Creative, innovative models of curriculum delivery are being used in an effort to provide cost-effective, quality programming to an increasingly diverse population of students. Flexible curricula are being developed that allow universities to provide programs that quickly respond to the needs of the local, regional, national, and even international constituencies to which they are accountable. Further, the lack of innovation in higher education has led to serious challenges to higher education effectiveness and achievement of important outcomes. A recent assessment (Kirschner, 2012) noted that in the United States there is $1 trillion dollars in student debt during a time when the job market for college graduates is one of the worst. In 2010 the United States ranked only twelfth of 36 developed countries in the number of college degrees held by individuals aged 25 to 34. As institutions of higher education reevaluate how to best achieve their stated missions and position themselves for the future, it is apparent that sweeping changes in higher education are affecting the development and delivery of curricula. Nurse educators in academia need to be actively involved in creating cost-effective, comprehensive curricula (Broome, 2009; National League for Nursing (NLN), 2012; Valiga & Ironside, 2012).

The increase in student diversity provides opportunities and challenges for curriculum development as well. Curricula must be flexible to accommodate work schedules; offer diversity in courses and programs, including distance education options; emphasize cultural sensitivity, leadership, delegation, and negotiation skills; promote oral and written communication and information technology skills; and enhance decision-making skills (Allen & Seaman, 2010; American Association of Colleges of Nursing (AACN), 2009; Jones & Wolf, 2009; Levitt, 2014; Phillips, Shaw, Sullivan, & Johnson, 2010; Valiga, 2012).

The quality, effectiveness, and efficiency of a curriculum in achieving the desired outcomes for a given program of study is of increasing importance to nursing and other health professions. Curricular quality must be assured across all of the curriculum elements that compose a curriculum as depicted in Chapter 7 (see Figure 7-1). These elements include

*The authors acknowledge the work of J. Laidig, EdD, RN, N. Dillard, DNS, RN, L. Siktberg, PhD, RN and D. Boland PhD, RN in the previous editions of the work represented in this chapter.

the institution's mission, vision, and values and those of the school of nursing; professional values and the beliefs, values, and expertise of the faculty; the school of nursing philosophy and organizing or conceptual framework; end-of-program outcomes and competencies; level competencies; curriculum design; courses, teaching strategies, and learning experiences; and resources needed to implement the curriculum.

This chapter provides an overview of curriculum ideologies, a historical perspective on definitions of *curriculum* and *curriculum development,* and descriptions of the elements that compose a curriculum, including curriculum models. The process of curriculum development within a changing environment along with the role of faculty is described. The influence of selected reports, recent evidence related to education methods, and priority-related topics that require significant changes in approaches to nursing education curricula to ensure that nurses are prepared to meet current and evolving health care needs are addressed.

Curriculum Ideologies

A common understanding of how a discipline and a school and its faculty consider the term *curriculum* is crucial to development of a comprehensive curriculum that is current, consistent, and congruent. Understanding the underlying principles and assumptions on which a curriculum is created enhances the structure, processes, and outcomes of that curriculum plan. Schiro (2013) proposes the term *curriculum ideologies* to describe the underlying beliefs and philosophy of educators, and identifies four major approaches to education. The four ideologies are Scholar Academic, Social Efficiency, Learner Centered, and Social Reconstruction. Each of these ideologies has evolved from rich traditions in the field of education and all have the potential to enhance society; however, the approaches and central values of the various ideologies are quite different. A brief description of the four ideologies reveals some of the frequently reported issues of debate that arise when faculty engage in curriculum development or curriculum revision activities.

The *Scholar Academic* ideology is organized around the concept of academic disciplines. Adherents believe that learning should be centered on a growing knowledge of the discipline by novices and expansion of that knowledge base by those more expert. A discipline's knowledge includes ways of thinking, conceptual frameworks, traditions, and specific content (Schiro, 2013, p. 4). A hierarchical relationship flows from the scholar to the teacher to the student, who is the discoverer, user, and consumer of new knowledge. A Scholar Academic approach focuses on ensuring that the curriculum reflects the essence of the discipline.

Social Efficiency ideology focuses on service to society through preparing students to meet the needs of society through their knowledge-based work contributions and through productive lives that enhance societal functioning (Schiro, 2013, p. 5) A curriculum reflecting the Social Efficiency ideology relies on a stimulus-response model that is characterized by faculty creating terminal objectives, and attending to the type and sequencing of learning experiences and to the extent to which learners are able to meet the identified priority societal needs.

The *Learner-Centered* ideology focuses on individuals rather than society as a whole, with the belief that talents and abilities should develop naturally and in harmony with individuals' unique characteristics and preferences. Within this ideology, individual learning goals become the desired learning outcomes and the role of the educator is to create an environment that stimulates growth through social interactions and learner creation of meaning for themselves (Schiro, 2013, p. 6).

The final curriculum ideology is *Social Reconstruction.* The major driving force of those who embrace social reconstruction thinking is that education is the major factor to addressing and changing societal issues and injustices. The goal of education within the social reconstruction frame is to facilitate creation of a new and more just society that benefits all members. As education is viewed from a social perspective, the focus is on meaning as influenced by cultural and other social experiences, with the goal of creating desired societal values that will improve society overall and thereby benefit individual members of society (Schiro, 2013, p. 6). As a profession, nursing is increasingly focused on contributions that will improve society and health for all, requiring inclusion of skill building for nurses to achieve these goals.

Influence of Curriculum Ideologies on Nursing Education

There are examples of nursing curricula that reflect all of the ideologies, with the potential exception of Learner-Centered ideology because of the required focus on demonstrated competencies as established by the State Boards of Nursing to maximize the success of graduates in passing the licensing examination. However, strong and growing support for the use of learner-centered pedagogy strategies is dramatically influencing nursing education and is described later in this chapter.

Scholar Academic ideology is prominent in many schools of nursing and influences both the curriculum as well as the hierarchy of perceived value of faculty contributions (e.g., tenure track researchers versus practice track or clinical experts as a common exemplar). Curricula within this category tend to be closely tied with medical or clinical specialties and are consistent with current practice patterns and health care organization structures (e.g., service lines). Some of the implications of this ideological stance position faculty as the experts with knowledge who make many of the decisions regarding what is to be learned, when it is to learned, and in what manner. Thus, use of learner-centered strategies and learner engagement might be considerably lower in programs that embrace the Scholar Academic ideology model, as compared with schools of nursing that implement other curricular ideologies. The Scholar Academic ideological foundation is most apparent in research-focused institutions as compared with those whose mission is primarily focused on teaching and service.

In response to the increased expectations for accountability from institutions of higher education along with other factors identified in Chapter 5, the Social Efficiency ideology model has become more evident in many schools of nursing. How are professional curricula, such as that found in nursing and the health professions, being affected and what are the implications from a Social Efficiency ideology for faculty in redesigning a content-laden curriculum? Restructuring and reforms in the health care system are rapidly changing the focus of nursing curricula, as graduates must learn to deliver care within a health care environment that is focusing more and more on transitional care and the primary health care needs of individuals. At the same time, there are calls to restructure basic tenets of various societies through education to address social, financial, and other inequities. Nursing practice must be safe and cost effective across patient-care settings and nursing education must continue to maintain standards and meet the requirements of state boards of nursing and national accrediting agencies while meaningfully addressing these crucial considerations and expectations.

Social Reconstruction ideology has implications for developing student and faculty competencies in participating in and leading health care policy and advocacy. Health care disparities, global health issues, and population health issues are increasingly important issues that nurses can and should address as global leaders. Designing learning experiences for students that foster competency in health policy advocacy is an essential program outcome in contemporary nursing education.

Developing Contemporary Nursing Curricula

Faculty need to consider many concepts when developing contemporary nursing curricula. For example, nursing curricula need to include concepts related to patient safety, coordination of care, self-management, and health literacy, with emphasis on the burden of health problems on patient and family, strategies to decrease the gap between practice and evidence-based practice, and strategies that are generalizable across populations (Finkelman & Kenner, 2009; Shattell et al., 2013). Also important to nursing curricula are leadership and other skills to support achieving the stated goals from Healthy People 2020, including a focus on reducing disparities, preventable diseases, disability, injury, and premature death in improving health care for all (Healthy People 2020, n.d.).

There are innumerable position statements, professional standards, recommendations, and guiding principles from various sources that faculty must be knowledgeable about and consider for inclusion in any curricula they are designing. The recent 2014 global outbreak of Ebola demonstrates how quickly current events in health care can affect a curriculum, thus requiring rapid consideration and action from faculty. It is important for faculty to find ways in which they can perform regular environmental scans with a goal of maintaining a curriculum that is dynamic, fluid, and contemporary. To develop relevant undergraduate and graduate nursing curricula for the future, faculty must consider the following questions:

- Are students prepared to practice in a complex and changing health care environment, understanding that they will be required to engage in lifelong learning to have a sustained, relevant nursing career?
- Are students prepared as professionals to demonstrate the requisite knowledge and skills,

including learning to think and make clinical decisions using principles of evidence-based practice within a culture of patient safety?
- Are students prepared to collaborate intra- and interprofessionally, practice as leaders in health care, and demonstrate integrity in their practice within a legal and ethical framework?
- Are students learning essential multicultural and holistic concepts for culturally sensitive patient care within the context of global health needs and challenges?
- Are faculty working dynamically and productively to design curricula, including the design of innovative clinical models of instruction, that will most effectively prepare graduates for the workforce in a variety of settings?
- Does the curriculum integrate a major focus on evidence-based research and practice, promoting faculty and student collaboration with interprofessional colleagues in inquiry and improvement?
- Are curricula congruent with the goals of national and international health efforts (e.g., *Healthy People 2020,* World Health Organization [WHO] goals, and others) and in meeting the needs of older adults, women, children, and culturally diverse and other vulnerable populations?
- Will graduates be prepared to lead care teams in advocating for improved health care outcomes and services locally, nationally, and internationally?
- Are curricula being delivered using active learning strategies, including narrative pedagogies such as unfolding case studies, scenarios, and reflective thought, and are interactive technologies used that require students to engage with the topics and apply their knowledge?
- Are faculty designing learning experiences that will prepare learners for practice in transitional care settings?
- Does the university or college provide programs that are high quality, accessible, and of good value, as compared to peer institutions?
- Are the curricula meeting the needs of the programs' communities of interest and other relevant stakeholders?
- Do the curricula foster use of current and emerging instructional and patient care technologies, and are faculty adequately prepared to integrate these new technologies into their teaching?

Additionally, the exponential expansion of knowledge, dramatically changing sociodemographics and cultural diversity, an economically and consumer-focused political environment, and increasing acts of global terrorism will continue to challenge nursing faculty to critically review current curricula and methods of instruction with the goal of preparing graduates for the future. Nursing education must address the myriad of issues affecting curriculum design and implementation and transform nursing education to prepare graduates at all levels of education for an increasingly complex workforce that has greater practice expectations and a heavier reliance on the use of advanced technologies across the entire health care continuum (Benner, Sutphen, Leonard, & Day, 2010; Valiga, 2012).

Definition of Curriculum

The term *curriculum* was first used in Scotland as early as 1820 and became a part of the education vernacular in the United States nearly a century later. Over time, *curriculum*—derived from the Latin word *currere,* which means "to run"—has been translated to mean "course of study" (Wiles & Bondi, 1989).

In 1949 Tyler published a handbook on principles of curriculum and instruction that has been used for more than five decades (Tyler, 2013). Among other important concepts, Tyler proposed three major criteria for effective organization of a curriculum: continuity, sequence, and integration. Continuity is achieved through careful attention to "vertical reiteration of major curriculum elements" (Tyler, 2013, p. 84). That is, key concepts and skills must be incorporated throughout the curriculum to support knowledge and skill acquisition. Sequence is related to continuity but incorporates attention to new learning experiences building on prior activities, while expanding breadth or depth of the content. Last, "integration refers to the horizontal relationship of curriculum experiences" (Tyler, 2013, p. 85). Integration considers how students will develop appreciation for and the ability to apply skill sets across a variety of subjects and situations. An oft-cited example in nursing education is how the concept of mathematics is used across many topics and settings (e.g., medication calculations, disease prevalence, etc.).

Doll (2002) originally described curriculum in relation to a shifting paradigm, moving from a formal definition to a focus on one's multiple interactions with others and one's surroundings. He defined curriculum as having five concepts: currere, complexity, cosmology, conversation, and community. *Currere* was defined as the process of "negotiating passages" between teachers, students, and the text (pp. 45–46). The concept of *complexity* referred to curriculum as consisting of dynamic and complex interactions that eventually, through vision and perseverance of faculty, formed interconnections (p. 46). *Cosmology* was the term used to depict the "living" nature of the curriculum, evoking creativity and vitality (p. 48). The concept of *conversation* described the respect that faculty and students demonstrate for each other and how they "understand their own humanness" (p. 49–50), and *community* referred to the "ecological, global, and cosmological issues within which all humans are enmeshed" (pp. 51–52).

In later work, Doll (2012) described an evolution in his thinking, noting the importance of integrating the rational, scientific approach (e.g., Tyler) with the aesthetic, spiritual view of education within the context of complexity science, in essence, "developing a different sense of curriculum and instruction—open, dynamic, relational, creative, and systems oriented" (p. 10).

Because of the amorphous nature of the term *curriculum,* it has had a variety of definitions. Educators prefer particular definitions based on individual philosophical beliefs and the emphasis placed on specific aspects of education. Two more recent conceptualizations of curriculum capture some of the most important evolutionary changes. Parkay, Anctil, and Hass (2010) proposed, "Curriculum is all of the educational experiences that learners have in an educational program, the purpose of which is to achieve broad goals and related specific objectives that have been developed with a framework of theory and research, past and present professional practice, and the changing needs of society" (p. 3). Lunenburg (2011) recommended rethinking how to approach a curriculum to encompass "curriculum as content, as learning experiences, as behavioral objectives, as a plan for instruction, and as a nontechnical approach" (p. 1). The nontechnical approach is described as a rejection of traditional curriculum planning and incorporates philosophical, aesthetic, moral and ethical, and other theories that are relevant to the world today.

Common elements found in many definitions of curriculum include the following:

- Preselected goals and outcomes to be achieved
- Selected content with specific sequencing in a program of study
- Processes and experiences to facilitate learning for traditional and adult learners
- Resources required to support curriculum delivery
- Extent of responsibility for learning assumed by the teacher and the learner
- How and where learning takes place
- Interschool activities, including extracurricular activities, guidance, and interpersonal relationships
- Individual learner's experience as a result of schooling

Types of Curricula

Regardless of the ideological interpretation of curriculum, several types of curricula may occur concurrently. The *official (or legitimate) curriculum* includes the stated curriculum framework with philosophy and mission; recognized lists of outcomes, competencies, and learning objectives for the program and individual courses; course outlines; and syllabi. Bevis (2000) stated that the "legitimate curriculum . . . [is] the one agreed on by the faculty either implicitly or explicitly" (p. 74). These written documents are distributed to faculty, students, health care practice partners, and accrediting agencies to document the planned curriculum, including what is to be taught and expected learning outcomes and competencies at program completion.

The *operational curriculum* consists of "what is actually taught by the teacher and how its importance is communicated to the student" (Posner, 1992, p. 10). This curriculum includes knowledge, skills, and attitudes (KSAs) emphasized by faculty in the classroom and clinical settings.

The *illegitimate curriculum,* according to Bevis (2000), is one known and actively taught by faculty yet not evaluated because descriptors of the behaviors are lacking. Such behaviors include "caring, compassion, power, and its use" (p. 75).

The *hidden curriculum* consists of values and beliefs taught through verbal and nonverbal communication by the faculty. Faculty may be unaware of what is taught through their expressions, priorities, and interactions with students, but students are very aware of the "hidden agendas" of the curriculum, which may have a more lasting influence than the written curriculum. The hidden curriculum includes the way faculty interact with students, the teaching methods used, and the priorities set (Bevis, 2000; Posner, 1992).

The *null curriculum* (Bevis, 2000) represents content and behaviors that are not taught. Faculty need to recognize what is not being taught and focus on the reasons for ignoring those content and behavior areas. Examples include content or skills that faculty think they are teaching but are not, such as clinical reasoning. As faculty review curricula, all components and relationships need to be evaluated.

Curriculum Development in Nursing

From an historical perspective, how nurse educators approached curriculum development was greatly influenced by the work of Bevis. Bevis defined curriculum as "those transactions and interactions that take place between students and teachers and among students with the intent that learning takes place" (2000, p. 72). Bevis challenged nurse educators to move from what she termed the *Tylerian behaviorist technical paradigm of curriculum development* to one that focuses on human interaction and active learning, and incorporates a focus on students' and teachers' interactions. Since Bevis' time, several educational scholars in nursing have extended these concepts, most notably Diekelmann and Diekelmann (2009) and Ironside (2014).

The nursing curriculum is often based on current practice, accreditation standards, regulatory requirements, and faculty interests, which leads to lack of curricula standardization. New opportunities abound to foster collaborative debate and dialogue on a number of issues, including how to accomplish the following:

- Enhance students' delegating, supervising, prioritizing, clinical reasoning, decision-making, and leadership skills to effect change.
- Focus on health promotion, disease prevention, and care transitions to improve outcomes in health care disparities across health care settings.
- Enhance student–faculty–preceptor interactions in the learning process.
- Design clinical models that allow for student immersion in the practice setting.
- Develop learner-centered environments.
- Use evidence-based research and nursing practice to deliver efficient and effective care.
- Integrate culture of safety concepts, including care coordination and transitions, in specifically designed interprofessional education and collaborative practice experiences.
- Focus on patient-centered care within the overarching "triple-aim" goal of improving the patient care experience (including quality and satisfaction); improving the health of the populations; and reducing the per capita cost of health care (Berwick, Nolan, & Whittington, 2008).
- Expand culturally sensitive nursing practice with a focus on reducing health disparities.

As Valiga (2012) summarized: "Nurse educators must be proactive, anticipate the future, and not wait until history tells the story of our times. We must act despite uncertainty, and we must be innovative and scholarly as we shape the future of nursing education. Transformation is not easy but it is desperately needed. . . ." (Valiga, 2012, p. 432). The need to craft a national agenda for nursing education research is believed to be crucial to support the necessary transformation in nursing education (Valiga & Ironside, 2012).

Role of Faculty in Curriculum Development

The development of curricula has historically been the responsibility of faculty, as they are the experts in their respective disciplines and the best authorities in identifying the knowledge and competencies students need to acquire by graduation. The NLN's Scope of Practice for Academic Nurse Educators (National League for Nursing, NLN, 2012) outlines nurse educators' responsibility for "formulating program outcomes and designing curricula that reflect contemporary health care trends and prepare graduates to function effectively in the health care environment" (National League for Nursing, NLN, 2012, p. 18).

As the emphasis for designing contemporary and cost-effective curricula continues to increase, so does the need to involve a broader community of stakeholders in the curriculum development process. Practice disciplines such as nursing are actively engaging a diverse array of stakeholders in curriculum design, development, implementation, and evaluation. The desire to increase engagement can and does add to the complexity of the development process and the ability to alter curricula in a timely manner. To address the need to create curricula that are responsive to workforce expectations requires faculty to develop curricula that are flexible in design, open to broader interpretation as expectations change, and capable of being implemented using a variety of different methodologies.

Traditionally, curriculum development has been built on the concepts of frameworks, objectives, and closely orchestrated learning experiences. This approach envisions curriculum development as a logical, sequential process. Although some of this structure is necessary to plan and develop curricula, the more contemporary approach shifts the emphasis from an epistemological to an ontological orientation (Doane & Brown, 2011; Ironside, 2014). An epistemological orientation to education is focused on knowledge, or the "content to be covered." An ontological orientation to the educational process is more learner-centered and focused on the student's "way of being a nurse" (Doane & Brown, p. 22). In this shift in philosophical orientation, knowledge is applied for the purpose of facilitating the learner's transformation into a nursing professional. The move from epistemology to ontology has a profound effect on how curriculum is designed and the teaching–learning strategies chosen to help students think like a nurse and develop competence in their practice.

Nursing faculty have come to approach curriculum development from an outcomes perspective, rather than the traditional teaching process orientation used in the delivery of nursing curricula. Focusing on learning as the product (outcome), the emphasis is placed on how students can use knowledge to practice competently in changing and often uncertain clinical situations. This approach assumes that both students and faculty have some latitude in individualizing the learning experience and related processes used in creating knowledge.

Traditionally, faculty autonomy has been closely tied to curriculum; in fact, faculty are considered to "own" the curriculum. This means faculty are accountable for assessing, implementing, evaluating, and changing the curriculum to ensure quality and relevance in programs. In today's educational climate the value of education is measured against job marketability. In the discipline of nursing, emphasis has been placed on what knowledge and competencies graduates have on completion of their programs as it relates to the expectations of the settings and roles within which they will practice.

Inevitably, when curriculum development is undertaken, the concepts of academic freedom versus curricular integrity arise. As suggested by the prior statements, faculty are collectively charged with using their significant expertise and diverse talents to construct curricula that will produce successful, high-quality graduates. Curricular integrity is achieved through faculty striving for, but not always arriving at consensus decisions. Communication throughout the curriculum is a key determinant in the quality and consistency of the curriculum and the student experience. A statement from the American Association of Colleges and Universities specifically addressed this topic:

> There is, however, an additional dimension of academic freedom that was not well developed in the original principles, and that has to do with the responsibilities of faculty members for educational programs. Faculty are responsible for establishing goals for student learning, for designing and implementing programs of general education and specialized study that intentionally cultivate the intended learning, and for assessing students' achievement. In these matters faculty must work collaboratively with their colleagues in their departments, schools, and institutions as well as with relevant administrators. Academic freedom is necessary not just so faculty members can conduct individual research and teach their own courses, but so they can enable students—through whole college programs of study—to acquire the learning they need to contribute to society (American Association of Colleges and Universities, 2006, p. 1).

This statement emphasizes that academic freedom does not mean that individual faculty can arbitrarily or unilaterally decide what they will teach in their classroom, but that faculty, through faculty governance processes, must work collaboratively to determine curriculum and then are expected to uphold that collective decision to achieve curricular integrity and effectiveness.

National Reports, Education Trends, and Recommendations of Significance

In recent years, several seminal position statements, reports, and recommendations have been issued by prestigious organizations or groups that require substantive curricular change, and in some cases disruptive innovation. Five of the most significant sources requiring substantive curricular changes are reviewed to contextualize the definitions of and processes related to curriculum in nursing.

Institute of Medicine: Quality and Safety Education in Nursing

In 2001, the Institute of Medicine (IOM) released a seminal report titled *Crossing the Quality Chasm* (Institute of Medicine (IOM), 2001) that called for substantive reform of health professions education to enhance quality and safety practices within health care. Simply stated, the report identified five competencies as essential for health professionals of the twenty-first century: patient-centered care, teamwork and collaboration, informatics, evidence-based practice, and quality improvement (including safety). It was also recommended that the disciplines develop common language in important areas, integrate learning experiences, use evidence-based curricula and teaching strategies, and offer faculty development to model these competencies.

The Quality and Safety Education in Nursing (QSEN) project was launched in 2005 with the overall goal of ensuring that all graduating registered nurse students had developed the relevant quality and safety competencies that would prepare them for practice. From feedback received from nursing faculty and practice leaders of the time, it was clear there was an urgent need for faculty development to ensure that faculty were teaching contemporary and accurate information regarding quality and safety practices, and that quality and safety content be integrated into all prelicensure nursing programs as quickly as possible (Sullivan, Hirst, & Cronenwett, 2009). To provide information to nursing faculty that could be immediately incorporated into courses, the QSEN project developed a KSA curricular framework (Quality and Safety Education for Nurses, QSEN, n.d.) that addressed each of the five competencies (separating quality and safety for a total of six) identified in the Institute of Medicine, IOM, 2001 report (Cronenwett, 2012). A QSEN website (www.qsen.org) was established to assist in the dissemination of the KSA framework and serves as a clearinghouse for teaching and learning resources.

The QSEN project was expanded to include graduate-level nursing competency development, resulting in KSAs for this level of nursing program to advance quality and safety competency development (Cronenwett et al., 2009). A partnership with the AACN and communications with the NLN have resulted in continuing faculty development opportunities related to QSEN. Finally, essential content from the QSEN project has been integrated into nursing education program accreditation standards so that a formal review of the presence and effectiveness of QSEN content in nursing education programs is ensured.

Carnegie Foundation for the Advancement of Teaching: Educating Nurses

The Carnegie Foundation for the Advancement of Teaching launched a multiyear comparative study titled "The Preparation for the Professions" focused on professional education in medicine, nursing, law, engineering, and preparation of the clergy in the United States. The goals of this significant initiative were to better understand how the various professions are prepared to practice through identification of educational approaches and how the outcomes of professional education could be strengthened and improved. The fourth volume of this series of studies on the professions was *Educating Nurses: A Call for Radical Transformation* (Benner et al., 2010). Four major recommendations emerged from the Benner et al. (2010) study, which have many implications for curriculum development and implementation:

1. Emphasize teaching for a sense of salience, situated cognition, and action in particular situations, instead of covering decontextualized knowledge. This recommendation is often expressed as teaching students how to "think like a nurse."
2. Integrate clinical and classroom teaching, instead of maintaining a separation of the two. Given the complexity and breadth of knowledge required for today's nursing practice, it is essential that faculty design strategies to better link classroom and clinical teaching to reflect the actual complexities and pace of nursing practice.

3. Emphasize clinical reasoning and multiple ways of thinking, instead of critical thinking. Examples of the multiple ways of thinking include clinical reasoning, clinical imagination, and scientific reasoning.
4. Focus on the formation of professional identity, rather than socialization and role-taking. Nursing students need experiential learning environments that provide the opportunities to learn about and internalize the elements of being a "professional."

These four recommendations, especially when coalesced into actual teaching practices, require educators to think very differently about how curricula are created and to acquire and effectively use many new teaching and learning strategies within the context of a health care system that is evolving rapidly to achieve the "triple aim" of health care. The triple aim seeks to improve the patient experience of care (including quality and satisfaction), improve the health of populations, and reduce the per capita cost of health care (Institute for Health Care Improvement (IHI), 2007).

Use of Simulation

The use of simulation technology in nursing and health professions education has exploded during the last decade in frequency of use, sophistication of the technology, and the teaching and learning strategies employed, and has introduced a number of implications for curriculum development. Specifically, current students expect that simulation activities, including access to a clinical laboratory environment, will be readily available and resemble actual clinical settings. Simulation can be simply defined as activities or events that mimic real-world practice and include both low- and high-fidelity activities. Designing student learning experiences that clearly integrate simulation, classroom, and clinical activities promotes the necessary synergy and learning required to meet desired competencies. See Chapter 18 for an in-depth discussion about the use of simulations.

Interprofessional Education and Collaborative Practice

The importance of interprofessional education (IPE) and collaborative practice to achieving the quality, safety, and innovation goals of the overall health care system within the United States is supported by numerous major reports and statements, including most notably three Institute of Medicine (IOM) (2001, 2003, 2010) studies. The World Health Organization (WHO) (2010) and several organizations promoting interprofessional education have offered definitions of IPE that are guiding efforts in this area. These definitions state that interprofessional education may be described as students from multiple professions learning with and about the various health professional roles so that the foundation for professional collaboration around care will more easily occur in real-world settings.

In 2009 six national education associations representing different health professions (nursing, allopathic and osteopathic medicine, dentistry, pharmacy, and public health) joined forces to create the Interprofessional Education Collaborative (IPEC) and to develop core competencies related to interprofessional collaborative practice (Interprofessional Education Collaborative Expert Panel, 2011). These organizations have the ability to influence curricular changes across the named disciplines. The goals of IPEC include the advancement of substantive IPE to prepare future clinicians for team-based patient care. Thus, IPE is considered a precursor of promoting effective interprofessional collaborative practice across settings. See Chapter 11 for a discussion of interprofessional education and collaborative practice, and the competencies that need to be incorporated into health professions curricula to prepare graduates for interprofessional practice.

The Interprofessional Education Collaborative Expert Panel (2011) core competencies have been incorporated into virtually all of the involved health disciplines' accreditation standards, leading to more widespread adoption within the various curricula. Many colleges have published examples of how the IPEC core competencies are being addressed with numerous evaluation studies of these activities also provided (Sullivan & Godfrey, 2012). Going forward, nursing and other health professions curricula will include substantive IPE experiences to prepare graduates with the now widely accepted IPEC competencies (Thistlethwaite & Moran, 2010).

Web-based Technology and Online Learning

The number of nursing students studying fully or partly in online learning has exploded over the last five years. The reasons for this surge in demand for online learning include easier access, convenience, adult-friendly education and services, and flexible programming schedules that online learning can provide. Established top-tier universities as well as newer nonprofit and for-profit institutions of higher education have increasingly embraced the trend toward online learning, with many incorporating aspects of web-based technologies into campus-based classes resulting in hybrid (blended) courses.

A systematic review of online learning in undergraduate health professions that focused on student knowledge, skills, satisfaction, and cost-effectiveness yielded positive conclusions. In 12 of 50 studies included, significant positive differences in those studying online were noted. And 27 of 50 studies showed no significant differences in learning, or mixed results, suggesting that incorporating online learning is most likely at least as effective as traditional methods (George & Shocksnider, 2014). Evidence exists that similar positive outcomes with online learning can be achieved in graduate study, including doctoral programs (Broome, Halstead, Pesut, Rawl, & Boland, 2011). A metaanalysis of blended learning and technology use in higher education concludes that in terms of achievement outcomes, blended learning worked better than traditional face-to-face classroom instruction. Additionally, the kind of computer support used and the presence of one or more interactions (student-teacher-content) enhance student achievement (Bernard, Borokhovski, Schmid, Tamim, & Abrami, 2014).

Having an awareness of and planning for predicted changes to web-based learning technologies is critical when developing or redesigning curricula at all levels. One of the most important trend reports is the New Media Consortium's (NMC) Horizon Report (New Media Consortium (NMC), 2015). The annual Horizon Report details key trends, significant characteristics impeding higher education technology adoption, and important developments in educational technology for higher education. Some of the key trends of this recent report with significant implications for nursing education include continued focus on and growth of integrated or hybrid learning and the ubiquity of social media. Characteristics reportedly impeding adoption of education technology in higher education included low digital fluency of faculty, relative lack of rewards for teaching, competition from new models of education, and scaling teaching innovations. Flipped classrooms, learning analytics, three-dimensional printing, games and gamification of education activities were also named as important developments for higher education in the near term. Chapters 19, 20, and 21 discuss technology-based education and related pedagogies, as well as faculty implications in more detail.

Curriculum Designs

A well-conceived curriculum is critical to the preparation of practicing nurses at all levels. Once a program's curriculum is designed, curriculum building becomes an on-going task that is indispensable to, yet separate from, the acts of teaching and learning. Curriculum is a dynamic, evolving entity shaped by learner needs and desired achievement, faculty's beliefs about the science and art of nursing, and emerging needs of the populations served within changing health care services, delivery structures, and organization.

Creating a specific curriculum design for a given program must take into account many factors, including the mission, vision, and goals of the educational entity; the philosophy of the educational entity and that of the school of nursing; and the priorities of major stakeholder groups (e.g., students, faculty, employers, alumni, and others). After deciding on desired program outcomes and competencies, faculty are positioned to design the curriculum. It is important to note, however, that it is helpful to create a working organizing framework to guide the development of program outcomes and competencies, as these two components must become synchronized for curricular integrity.

The topic of curriculum design models is complex because of the numerous and often overlapping nomenclature or differential use of the same terms. This discussion is further complicated because nursing education programs frequently use a combination of design models. Descriptions of two of the most commonly used models for curricular design currently in use in nursing education curricula are presented.

Curricular Design Models

The overall organization of a curriculum may be identified as based primarily on one of three models of design: (1) *blocks* of content (often in nursing education reflecting clinical specialties), (2) *concepts* (that often reflect subjects within nursing and from other disciplines thought to be critical for nursing practice), or (3) *competencies* (that reflect broad areas of expected graduate performance that are sequentially "leveled" throughout the curriculum by semester, year, or other time parameter to enable students to advance in knowledge and skill development and achieve desired learning outcomes). Virtually all nursing education programs incorporate a strong focus on competencies because nursing is a practice profession and because program accreditation and professional licensing requirements incorporate expected results or competencies. Competencies can be imbedded throughout either "blocking" or concept design models. A specific challenge that nursing and other practice disciplines share is how to best plan for clinical or practice experiences. The more traditional model consists of a mostly concurrent plan, wherein didactic courses are paired with clinical experience courses with the goal of matching the two. In reality, this rarely works and the logistical issues can be insurmountable. Many programs use a mixed approach, in which some didactic nursing courses have associated clinical experiences and others do not. Some programs are experimenting with front-loading didactic content and sometimes clinical simulation activities after which a clinical intensive or immersion occurs with the goal of integrating the targeted KSA competencies to be achieved. Faculty should also carefully consider clinical learning sites that will provide students with exposure to clinical experiences across the care continuum and in collaboration with learners from other disciplines.

Blocked Course Content Curricula

Faculty who wish to design a curriculum primarily using *blocks* of content must first carefully enumerate the major blocks or clusters of information that need to be represented within the curriculum. Patterns can be built on the premise of sequencing specific courses and corresponding clinical learning experiences. This approach assumes that there is a logical order to sequencing content that will facilitate learning and requires faculty to consider what evidence exists to help them make evidence-based decisions regarding what the "logical" order might be.

Courses in a blocked curriculum are usually structured around clinical specialty areas, patient population, pathologic conditions, or physical systems. Historically, nursing programs have been organized by type of patient (medical condition, specialty, or age) and sometimes by settings (predominantly acute care hospitals with some ambulatory or skilled nursing focus and clinical experiences as well as within the community). Courses with titles based on medical or clinical specialty areas such as adult medical-surgical, pediatric, maternal-child, and community nursing are examples of a blocked approach to curriculum design. Other important content or concepts are taught in separate courses such as research- and evidence-based practice, foundations of professional nursing, among others. Additionally, some important content or concepts are placed in courses that seemed to be the best match; such examples include quality and safety, leadership, and cultural diversity topics. It is also possible to have a predominately blocked approach to curriculum design, with selective integration of some content areas across the curriculum, such as pharmacology and nutrition, or some concepts such as pain or inflammation.

The idea of blocking content organizes both teaching and learning. It facilitates faculty course assignments and complements faculty expertise, allowing faculty to teach primarily in their areas of expertise in a specific location within the curriculum. It is also relatively easy to trace placement of content in the curriculum.

However, the segregation or blocking of content into specific courses can cause content to become isolated from previous or subsequent coursework and can impede the learner's ability to integrate knowledge and transfer concepts, information, and experiences from one course to another. By and large, this curriculum design model produces a curriculum that is highly structured, with little latitude for deviation and meeting individual learning needs. Faculty who design curriculum with a block design also need to guard against the tendency for a strong sense of course ownership to develop among faculty who consider a course to "be theirs," and thus become resistant to changes within their course that need to occur to maintain curricular integrity. Open, ongoing communication and shared faculty decision-making around curriculum development and revision is essential to maintain curricular integrity.

Blocked curriculum design also has the potential to obscure issues with learner development and growth as a professional. When a student does not pass a course, it is not uncommon to hear faculty say that the student failed "pediatrics" or "intensive care," for example. In reality, although the student was not able to apply the expected knowledge, skills, or behaviors to a given population, it was actually the student's inability to transfer and apply the key *concepts* required to demonstrate safe clinical reasoning skills that led to the failure. Faculty must look beyond the "content" to the "concepts" to gain an understanding of what has led to the failing performance.

Concept-based Curricula

Today there is growing interest in a more conceptual approach to curriculum design and the use of core concepts as a focal point of curriculum construction (Giddens, Wright, & Gray, 2012). Concept-based curricula are designed to better reflect the complexity of nursing and health care while using core ideas or concepts important to nursing practice to help learners grasp the connections and master deeper learning of how these concepts explain a variety of conditions and situations they will encounter in nursing practice. These goals are in contrast to a traditional curriculum organized around medical diagnoses or patient groups that use a less flexible and encompassing schema, such as described when "blocking" curriculum.

In a concept-based curriculum, faculty identify and define concepts considered to be core to nursing practice and integral to achieving the program's established end-of-program outcomes for graduates. The concepts are integrated (threaded) throughout the curriculum in a manner that facilitates acquisition of competencies that are leveled throughout the curriculum, ultimately leading to student achievement of expected end-of-program outcomes. Faculty develop learning experiences that will guide the students' application of the concepts across a variety of patient populations and care settings.

Although there is significant variation in the concepts chosen to organize a nursing curriculum, some concepts have emerged across the majority of undergraduate nursing programs. Some examples of these common concepts include oxygenation, cognition, pain, nutrition, pharmacology, and lifespan development. Additionally, nursing roles, communication and teamwork, quality and safety, and ethics and legal issues are also frequently present. Table 6-1 shows the concepts used by the University of Kansas School of Nursing in designing a new undergraduate curriculum. Graduate curricula may also be organized by concepts relevant to advanced practice roles and settings.

An example of content integration may be seen in the following description of the concept of pain. Early in the curriculum, students first learn about the pathophysiologic causes of pain, causes and cardinal characteristics of pain, factors that shape or affect pain, and how to assess and evaluate the characteristics of pain. As students move through the curriculum, they increase their understanding about the manifestations of and treatments for pain, review research related to the concept of pain, and identify appropriate therapeutic nursing interventions related to the care of a patient with pain, thus progressing from a global understanding of pain to a more specific, in-depth understanding of the concept. Eventually, students learn about pain as it relates to acute and chronic health issues, to physical or nondisease–based causes, or to specific situations such as surgery and childbirth in various clinical populations.

In an example of a curriculum that was developed around four conceptual themes, D'Antonio, Brennan, and Curley (2013) described the process used to develop an undergraduate curriculum framework based on judgment, inquiry, engagement, and voice. Faculty used a shared decision-making model to identify concepts that would be meaningful to faculty and students. Additionally, the QSEN standards provide key concepts related to quality and safety that can be used to create a framework to organize curricula along with other important concepts (Chenot & Daniel, 2010; Pollard et al., 2014).

Historically, accreditation standards and performance expectations have had a significant effect on many organizing frameworks as faculty recognize the need to directly address these expectations that include such concepts as clinical reasoning, problem solving, communication, caring, diversity, and therapeutic nursing interventions (Kumm & Fletcher, 2012; Mailloux, 2011). The concept of clinical reasoning or "thinking like a nurse" is increasingly replacing the more general critical thinking concept to better focus on situated knowledge development that leads to action rather than a general intellectual skill (Benner et al., 2010).

Faculty adopting a concept-based, outcome orientation to curriculum must be able to construct the context and meaning that the outcomes will have in the curriculum structure. An outcomes

TABLE 6-1 Concept-based Curriculum Plan: BSN Program

Concepts in Health & Illness I: Foundations of Nursing	Concepts in Health & Illness II: Nursing Across the Lifespan	Concepts in Health & Illness III: Nursing with Diverse Populations	Concepts Related to Professional Practice (various other courses in order of introduction)
Clinical Reasoning 1	Human Development	Addiction	Caring
Comfort	Family Dynamics	Behavior	Professional Identity
Elimination	Fluid Balance	Cellular Regulation	Scholarly Inquiry
Health Promotion	Electrolyte Balance	Clotting	Advocacy
Infection	Metabolism	Cognition	Team
Inflammation	Oxygenation 1	Oxygenation 2	Collaboration 1, 2
Mobility	Acid-base Balance	Intracranial Regulation	Ethics
Nutrition	Perfusion 1	Perfusion 2	Leadership 1, 2
Self-concept	Sensory-Perception	Genetic Predisposition	Change
Sleep	Mood & Affect	Reproduction	Lifelong Learning
Stress & Coping 1	Stress & Coping 2	Sexuality	Diversity
Thermoregulation	Fatigue	Spirituality	Health Literacy
Tissue Integrity	Grief		Health Informatics
	End of Life		Relationships
			Teaching & Learning
			Health Care Quality 1, 2, 3
			Patient Safety
			Evidence and Research
			Communication
			Health Policy 1, 2
			Clinical Reasoning 2
			Care Coordination
			Healthcare Economics
			Health Systems 1, 2
			Health Equity

Fletcher, K., Kumm, S., Buchanan, L., Gay, J., Laverentz, D., Pierce, L., Tarnow, K., Meyer, M., Nelson-Brantley, H., Martin, D., Belchez, C., Johnson, G., Young, E., Barr, N., Godfrey, N., Phillips, C., Schwartz, L., & Klenke-Borgman, L. (2015). Concepts in the University of Kansas School of Nursing Bachelor of Science in Nursing program. Unpublished manuscript, University of Kansas School of Nursing, Kansas City, KS.
Used with permission.

focus reflects the need to achieve designated competencies that students are expected to demonstrate at the completion of the program to demonstrate expected program outcomes. Faculty must identify and integrate the curriculum concepts that will support the students' achievement of the identified competencies and outcomes.

In a concept-based curriculum design, there are no boundaries to knowledge development and skill acquisition, as noted in the blocking approach. The concepts that form the curriculum must be clearly and visibly explicated for students so that they can see and experience the integration of the concepts across the curriculum. Students use clinical experiences to learn the essence of identified concepts and are encouraged to transfer and expand their knowledge and skills to different settings, populations, and experiences. Active, engaged teaching and learning strategies pair naturally with this conceptual approach to nursing education. Problem-based learning, team-based learning, case studies, and reflection are just a few examples of teaching and learning strategies that can be used to facilitate student understanding of the concepts being studied and help them to become "users" of knowledge. See Chapter 15 for further discussion of active learning strategies.

Disadvantages to a more conceptual approach to curriculum design include difficulty in maintaining the integrity of the curriculum because of the lack of discrete boundaries for content and the potential for inadvertently eliminating from the curriculum key aspects of the concept. Faculty must carefully map the concepts across the curriculum to ensure that the students' knowledge of the concept will grow in depth and breadth, and not become mired in repetition or omission. See the "Guiding Principles to Developing an Organizing Framework" section of this chapter for further suggestions on how to select curricular concepts.

Another potential disadvantage is that student learning styles may favor a more traditional and less conceptual approach to learning, as that is how they have likely become accustomed to learning. Faculty need to consider the various learning styles of students in their classroom and design approaches that will facilitate students adjusting to a more conceptual approach to learning.

Competency-based Education

The term *competency-based education* (CBE) as a curriculum approach has a specific, formal definition and is used to define practices embedded in a given curriculum. According to the formal definition, CBE is a "framework for designing and implementing education that focuses on the desired performance characteristics of health care professions. . . . CBE makes explicit [the implicit goal of competence in more traditional education frameworks] by establishing observable and measurable performance metrics that learners must attain to be deemed competent" (Gruppen, Mangrulkar, & Kolars, 2012, p. 1). In contrast, traditional education programs employ learning objectives with definitions of competence that are less clear and precise and sometimes a weaker or inconsistent approach to actually testing and measuring competency achievement. Supporters of CBE cite its systematic and valid assessment of competencies as well as the opportunity for students to progress at their own pace rather than fit into a planned time for and sequence of learning activities. Additionally, CBE may be more resource effective than traditional education methods. Challenges to fully implementing CBE in health-related roles include identifying the health needs of the community, defining competencies, developing self-regulated and flexible learning options, and assessing learners for competence. A formal CBE approach may also not suit all learners' preferences and abilities.

As noted earlier, virtually all nursing and professional education programs incorporate some aspects of CBE as it is required for accreditation and licensure; however, the amount of and consistency to which CBE principles are employed varies widely across nursing education programs.

Ordering or Constructing Knowledge within the Curriculum

Regardless of the curriculum design model chosen, faculty must still make decisions about how knowledge will be ordered or constructed within the curriculum. Wiles and Bondi (2011) describe five patterns of ordering or constructing knowledge in a curriculum. Similar to the blending of curricular design approaches, many nursing education programs use aspects of the five patterns within the overall curriculum, sometimes within the same semester or course. It is helpful that faculty be clear and guide students through how the curriculum and courses are organized to avoid confusion and provide clear expectations.

In a *building blocks design,* content and learning activities commence with foundational knowledge or skills, followed by more detailed or specialized material and, if appropriate, a higher level of depth or specialized knowledge. A *branching design* is similar to a building blocks design in that foundational knowledge or skills occur first, after which there are varied learning option pathways to achieve the desired KSAs. This pattern is typically strongly represented in the blocked curriculum design model.

In a *spiral design,* selected areas of knowledge appear repeatedly through the curriculum, in greater depth or breadth. In some fields, this area is further differentiated into a spiral versus a strand design. In a spiral curriculum, many different topics are covered at designated points throughout the curriculum. The points may be at regular or intermittent intervals because of concerns that students often forget previously covered information as a result of the brief instructional time devoted to each and because students do not have time to master important foundational knowledge. To minimize these issues, some education experts advocate the use of a strand (sometimes also called a *thread*) design. In a strand design, topics are arranged into meaningful groups that are regularly repeated, building better achievement and retention rates. Spiral or strand designs are prominent in concept-based curricula.

A *tasks or skills design* is characterized by presentation of specific knowledge and experiences that are expected to lead learners to achieve the desired competencies. There may be varying pathways for students as individuals or by groupings that reflect learning preferences or other characteristics. This pattern is usually prominent in CBE programs, although the tasks and skills are grouped into the larger competencies for assessment purposes.

The fifth pattern of ordering knowledge is the *process* design where the focus is on the process of learning with specific information or content-provided examples to illustrate the process. Some educators believe that the enhanced focus on narrative pedagogy and related teaching and learning strategies (e.g., the concept of learning to "think like a nurse") reflect a process design.

Curriculum Elements

Curriculum development is a challenging yet rewarding endeavor that ranks among the top responsibilities of a collective faculty. While much has been written about curriculum and its associated processes, there are multiple approaches and terminologies proposed, leading to confusion and disagreements about what elements compose a curriculum. For purposes of this chapter, the following curricular elements are included and discussed: curriculum design, organizing framework, end-of-program outcomes and competencies, level competencies, course design, teaching strategies and learning experiences, and resources needed to implement the curriculum. The terminology and definitions reflect some of the most commonly used across schools of nursing. The influence of contemporary thinking and newer approaches to teaching and learning are highlighted within each element.

Organizing Frameworks

Organizing frameworks can be a means for creating access to knowledge about the phenomena of interest or importance to the discipline. Organizing frameworks do provide a logical structure for cataloguing and retrieving knowledge. This structure, often depicted as a schematic conceptualization, is essential to the processes of teaching and learning as faculty guide students in the development of cognitive linkages among knowledge. This helps faculty and students understand the abstract nature of nursing. Fawcett's (1989) classic work on conceptual models and frameworks can provide readers with a discussion of theories, models, and concepts that is beyond the scope of this chapter.

Organizing frameworks have been used in curriculum development to delineate the constructs embedded in a traditional philosophy statement that reflects the collective faculty belief. It is important that organizing frameworks not be construed as a permanent feature of a program but rather as a kaleidoscope of complex patterns related to what students need to know and how they will best learn it.

The purpose in constructing frameworks is to systematically design a mental picture that is meaningful to the faculty and students when determining what knowledge is important and has value to nursing today, and how that knowledge should be defined, categorized, and linked with other knowledge. Although the majority of nurses continue to practice in acute care settings, with the increasing emphasis on transitional care there needs to be broader orientation to a continuum of care settings within a global context. This thinking is consistent with the IOM's landmark report recommendation (2010) that tomorrow's nurse be prepared to practice across a broad range of care settings and also reflects evolving changes related to the Patient Protection and Affordable Care Act (2011); thus organizing frameworks need to reflect concepts relevant to populations and settings.

Organizing curriculum frameworks provide a blueprint for determining the scope of knowledge (i.e., which concepts are important to include in the teachers' and learners' mental picture) and a means of structuring that knowledge in a distinctive and meaningful way for faculty and students. As such, organizing curriculum frameworks are the educational road maps to teaching and learning. As with any road map, multiple route options are available for arriving at a given destination or outcome. A number of approaches are used in defining and shaping frameworks. However, an organizing framework must reflect the sphere of nursing practice, the phenomena of concern to nurses, and how nurses relate to others who are dealing with health concerns, often referred to as nursing's *metaparadigm* (Lee & Fawcett, 2013).

BOX 6-1 Penn Nursing Organizing Framework

One University, One School, One Curriculum

Penn's baccalaureate curriculum brings structure to the school's mission, vision, and values by centering on the primacy of nursing practice situated in caring relationships that facilitate health and healing. The baccalaureate curriculum builds on this conceptualization of nursing because it moves students toward increasingly contextualized understandings of individuals, families, communities, and populations living with health and illness. It also moves students into increasingly complex situations and care environments because they experience the dynamic nature of nursing's embeddedness in health care systems, social structures, and society.

The baccalaureate curriculum concentrates on four intersecting core themes that characterize the complex and contextual nature of nursing practice: judgment, inquiry, engagement, and voice.

Reprinted from *Journal of Professional Nursing*, 29(6), D'Antonio, P. O. B., Brennan, A. M. W., & Curley, M. A., Judgment, inquiry, engagement, voice: Reenvisioning an undergraduate nursing curriculum using a shared decision-making model, 407-413, (2013), with permission from Elsevier.

Box 6-1 shows one school's depiction of an organizing framework for the undergraduate program (D'Antonio et al., 2013, p. 410). On review of the organizing framework, one would expect to find the following concepts to be further developed and explicitly interconnected for students within the curriculum: nursing practice situated within a caring relationship; health, illness, and healing; nursing's embeddedness within health care systems, social structures, and society; and judgment, inquiry, engagement, and voice. Using this organizing framework as the structural curriculum guidepost for which it is intended, faculty would be held accountable for designing learning experiences that foster students' application of these concepts in increasingly complex and contextualized clinical experiences with patients, families, communities, and populations.

As faculty embrace adoption of an outcome orientation in curriculum building, organizing frameworks or models will continue to serve the same purposes but will be driven by philosophical views and futuristic mental pictures regarding the evolving practice of nursing. For example, the role of nurses in telehealth and retail-based clinics, in both undergraduate and graduate roles, provide new and expanding career options for nurses, so competencies must reflect a wider perspective on nursing practice essentials. Organizing frameworks directly guide development of educational outcomes and end-of-program competencies that are also leveled for more detailed planning purposes.

The process of selecting or designing an organizing framework that will best serve a program or school is not an easy task; however, this process is an exceptional opportunity for faculty to build teamwork and innovation skills. Two general approaches may be used in determining the kind of organizing framework faculty wish to construct. The first approach is to select a single, specific nursing theory or model on which to build the framework, a traditional approach that is used today in some schools. A second, more commonly used approach is more eclectic and blends concepts from multiple theories or models, a method which has gained in popularity as the complexity of nursing and the health care environment has increased.

Developing a Single-Theory Framework

A traditional approach to constructing an organizing framework is to use a particular nursing theory or model to help shape the visual image that is consistent with the philosophy of the faculty. For example, if faculty believe that caring is at the core of nursing, a theory of caring (Hills & Watson, 2011; Swanson, 1999; Watson, 1997) might serve as the anchoring model when explaining the discipline to students and cataloguing knowledge about the discipline of nursing. The advantage to building an organizing framework on a single theory or model is the ability to use a single image with a defined vocabulary that is shared by both the learner and the teacher. Using a single theory or existing conceptual model has limitations and poses challenges, including that it may not reflect everybody's view of nursing and nursing practice. This becomes problematic when faculty have developed or been educated in curricula that have used a different theory or orientation to the discipline. The use of only one theory in a framework may limit the ability of faculty to pull together all elements of their curriculum, which provides a rationale for moving away from this approach as does recognizing that the practice of nursing is being transformed by a dynamic, evolving health care system. Further, it is clear that nursing educators and practitioners will not agree on a single theory. Students educated in a curriculum driven by a single theory are likely to experience frustration and confusion when they find themselves in clinical practice settings that do not ascribe to the same theory, or to any theory for that matter.

Developing an Eclectic Framework

Given the challenges and limitations of using a single theory as an organizing framework, faculty choice does not have to be constrained by a single theory or model. Those who believe that a combination of many theories or concepts are more reflective of their beliefs about nursing may use an eclectic approach to developing a curricular framework. Figure 6-1 shows an eclectic framework that has been used to guide work in several nursing programs. The Care Quality Commission framework incorporates an updated use of traditional nursing role concepts of care, cure, and coordination with the QSEN and IPE competencies as the major guiding structures. The use of a more eclectic approach when designing an organizing framework is not without its pitfalls. Some view this approach as an impediment to the development of a comprehensive nursing theory and the development of a body of knowledge that is uniquely nursing. The advantage to an eclectic approach is the ability to "borrow" concepts and definitions that best fit the faculty's beliefs and values from nursing and nonnursing theories. The eclectic approach may also promote incorporation of contemporary or evolving conceptualizations of nursing, health, the

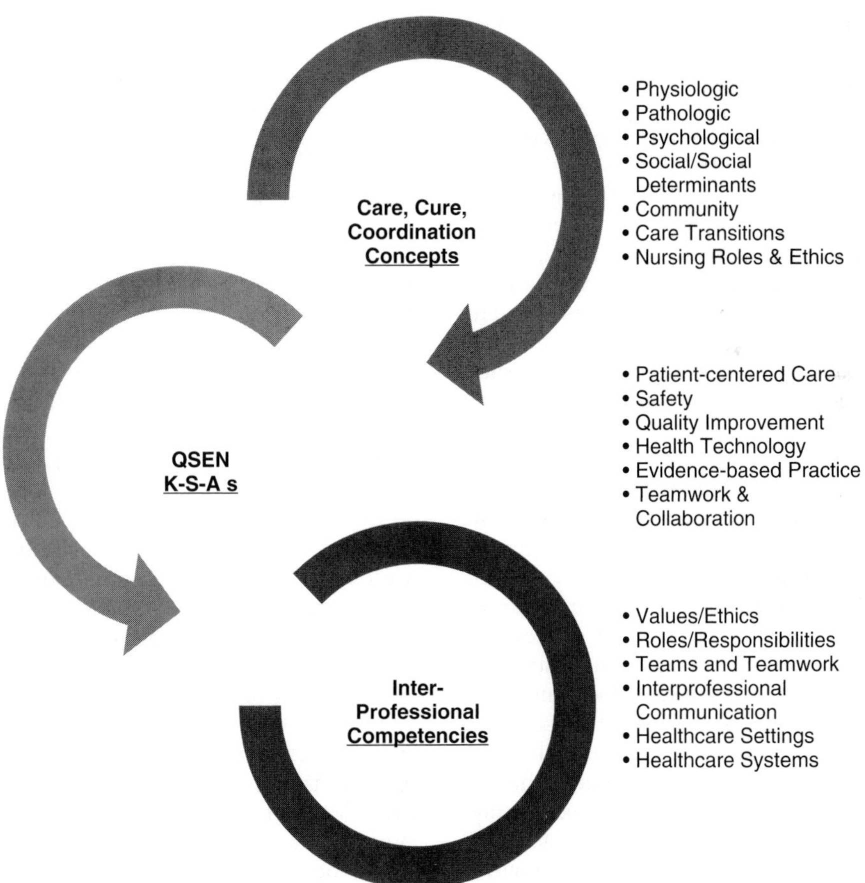

Figure 6-1 Care Quality Commission Organizing Framework for Nursing Education. Courtesy of D.T. Sullivan.

environment, and other key concepts as well as better reflect the practice of nursing across the continuum of settings and patient populations. However, if faculty develop an eclectic framework, where concepts and their definitions are "borrowed" from a number of theories, they need to ensure that in the act of borrowing they have not changed conceptual meaning. It is important to clearly show the relationships among the selected concepts. Therefore it is important to clarify the meaning of concepts that will be used in an organizing framework so that faculty and students are clear about the phenomena being studied.

Guiding Principles for Developing Organizing Frameworks

Although there are no specific steps or "how to's" for developing organizing frameworks for curriculum, there are some guiding principles that faculty can follow. D'Antonio et al. (2013) describe the process used by one school of nursing to identify curricular concepts that illustrates the use of many of these principles.

The first principle is to choose those concepts that most accurately reflect the faculty's beliefs about the practice and discipline of nursing and how students learn. The introduction of contemporary, student-centered approaches to learning, which stem from constructivism theory (see Chapter 13), are becoming more evident in faculty belief statements and are influencing curriculum development. The concepts identified should also reflect or complement the philosophy, mission, and goals of the college or university in which the program is embedded. By creating an organizing framework that reflects concepts valued by both the discipline of nursing and the parent institution, faculty have begun to articulate the contributions their nursing program makes to all stakeholder entities.

The most important aspect of choosing the concepts that tie the curriculum together is relevancy. This means that the concepts chosen need to be relevant and meaningful to the future practicing nurse, consistent with the science and art of nursing, and the needs of the populations served through health care delivery systems. During this phase of the curriculum development, it is important to involve stakeholders in the process. Reading professional standards and recommendations; understanding regulatory and accrediting criteria; and gathering input from practice partners, students, community leaders, and other identified stakeholders can all help faculty with selecting appropriate concepts.

The selected concepts are often organized into a graphic representation to facilitate understanding and recognition of the organizing framework (see Figure 6-1). The concepts included in the organization are further developed through creation of end-of-program outcomes and competencies. The requisite KSAs are then further defined for each of the concepts and integrated throughout the curriculum in course content and learning activities.

The second principle is to clearly define the major concepts underpinning the curriculum framework. Consensus should be established in this process because it will fall to the faculty to articulate these concepts to the students. Consistency in terminology and definitions along with making the organizing framework visible to faculty, students, practice partners, and other program stakeholders will enhance the framework's role in mastery of the desired level of competency at program completion.

The third principle is to explain the linkages between and among the concepts identified. This is critical because the linkages are the basis for how students comprehend, apply, analyze, synthesize, and evaluate knowledge learned throughout the educational process. These principles are analogous to putting together a jigsaw puzzle in which the concepts are the puzzle pieces and the total picture is of high-quality, contemporary nursing practice. Puzzles come in various numbers of pieces. Usually the greater the number of pieces, the greater the challenge in its construction. The outline and coloring of the pieces are the definitions of the concepts. The more clearly the puzzle pieces are defined and the sharper the color delineations, the easier it is to fit the puzzle together. It is critical that faculty and students grasp an understanding of the framework without an intensive investment of time and energy.

Faculty must decide on the major concepts that make up the organizing framework and focus on illustrating the linkages among those concepts. It is not necessary or desirable to identify each and every concept that students will be introduced to. The more faculty focus on minute concepts, the more likely it is that they are defining facts (not concepts) that will quickly become irrelevant. It is important to keep the work of concept identification, definition, and linkage at a broader level involving concepts that will retain salience with safe, quality practice.

However faculty decide to approach the work of developing a framework for their curriculum, the framework eventually constructed must be consistent with the school's mission and philosophy statements, faculty values and beliefs, program goals, professional standards, state and federal regulations, and current and future nursing practice trends. Faculty should have broad-based agreement on the curriculum framework because such agreement is fundamental to the consistent interpretation, implementation, and evaluation of the curriculum in meeting the expected program goals and outcomes. If there is a disconnect among philosophy, values, program expectations, professional practice expectations and outcomes, and the framework, faculty need to raise significant questions as to the utility of the created frameworks.

Once the work has been completed, faculty should share the completed framework with various stakeholders, soliciting feedback on how the organizing framework is interpreted by others. Such an exercise can help faculty determine if they have been successful in publicly articulating their beliefs and values to others.

Outcomes and Competencies

If curriculum frameworks are the road maps to understanding the discipline of nursing, then outcomes can be equated with the trip's destination and competencies with the mileage markers seen along the way. Program outcomes (also referred to as *learning outcomes* or sometimes *expected outcomes*) then take the place of what was traditionally and more generally called *terminal objectives* as the outcomes represent the integrated knowledge, skills, and abilities or competencies students are expected to demonstrate at program completion.

Outcomes, in the simplest of terms, are those characteristics students should display at a designated time, most often at the completion of the curriculum, and reflect a description of the ideal program graduate. Competencies are sometimes described as what students can do with what they know at designated points during and at the end of the educational program. Each broader desired outcome may be linked with multiple competencies to achieve a meaningful level of specificity for student assessment and, in the aggregate, for program evaluation. The chapters in Unit V - Evaluation provide detailed information about assessment of student learning, program evaluation, and related topics.

Identifying Curriculum Outcomes

The movement to an outcomes orientation has developed over time in nursing education as it has in higher education. These resulting changes provide a strong focus on the quality and value of postsecondary education (K–12 has experienced a similar set of changes with a focus on competency testing). Being able to demonstrate achievement of the stated program outcomes is consistent with the Social Efficiency ideology of curricula presented earlier in this chapter. Regional higher education accrediting bodies have fully embraced the idea that educational outcomes should prepare graduates to serve some aspect of societal need or improvement, resulting in strong, and some argue, prescriptive approaches to the assessment of student learning and enhanced review of program evaluation metrics.

An example of this shift in ideology is reflected in a project titled *The Future of Higher Education: Rhetoric, Reality, and the Risks of the Market* by Newman, Couturier, and Scurry (2010). One of the premises growing out of this project was the need for faculty to ask the right questions about educational goals and outcomes when engaged in curriculum development. The questions identified with relevancy to curriculum development include the following:

- What knowledge and skills are needed by all graduates?
- What requisite knowledge needs to be acquired by students to be productive in the workforce?
- What is the gap between current knowledge and skills and those that are needed in the future?
- What is the role of technology in facilitating the acquisition of the requisite knowledge and skills?
- How do we deliver the curriculum in a way that will maximize the outcomes?

Over the past decade, the focus on outcomes in higher education has continued to increase. In response to the provocative questions raised when focusing on program outcomes, the NLN convened an advisory group to explore the outcomes and competencies needed at each educational program level, from licensed practical nurse to the clinical doctorate (National League for Nursing (NLN), 2010). Similar efforts have occurred within the AACN, whose "Essentials" publications contain the expected outcomes and competencies for baccalaureate (2008), master's (2011), and doctor of nursing practice (2006) programs in nursing.

With the need for nursing educators to ensure that the curricula they design keep pace with the ongoing changes in health care and higher education, more emphasis will continue to be placed on the school's ability to demonstrate success. Outcomes assessment has been seen as the key by which school programs can document strengths and weaknesses. A comprehensive assessment program can help faculty determine what works and what does not in achieving academic quality and producing the desired program outcomes (Astin, 2012; McDonald, 2014; Oerrmann & Gaberson, 2014).

This logic is a significant departure from the predominantly process-oriented Tylerian approach to curriculum and evaluation, in which the emphasis was placed on detailed course objectives, the identification of content needed to meet course objectives, and the appropriate pedagogical approaches to complement the type of content needing to be taught. Outcome assessment emphasizes what students have actually learned in their educational experiences, not merely the knowledge and experiences that were designed with the intent of achieving these results (Astin, 2012; McDonald, 2014; Oerrmann & Gaberson, 2014; Wittmann-Price & Fasolka, 2010). These differences, which may seem like nuances to many, are core to the changing focus in curriculum development and student learning assessment and evaluation that continues to evolve in higher education and nursing education.

When moving to a curriculum that is more centered on the development of outcomes relevant to nursing practice, it is often easier to think about curriculum development as starting at a program's end rather than its beginning. Outcomes then become the critical focus of curriculum development. This method of curriculum development places a different emphasis on the need for organizing frameworks as a starting point for curriculum development. Approaching curriculum development beginning with the desired outcome or what the student needs to demonstrate at graduation to be a competent nurse and then working "backward" toward the beginning of the curriculum provides faculty with an opportunity to identify the essential outcomes and competencies that they wish to see their students demonstrate at the completion of the program. It is important to note that development of outcomes should be significantly informed by the mission, vision, values, and philosophy of the program; an environmental scan that includes the perspectives of major external stakeholders; the use of best current evidence in nursing and health professions education; and internal stakeholder preferences from faculty, students, alumni, and appropriate others. See Box 6-2 for an example of BSN program outcomes that are significantly aligned with the mission statement of a religious-affiliated college.

The interrelationship between the organizing framework and the outcomes and competencies becomes clear with the organizing framework being shaped by the theories and concepts embedded in the outcomes and competencies. For example, if faculty believe that students need to possess clinical reasoning, communication, teamwork, and leadership skills, these concepts will be evident in the organizing framework. In an outcomes-focused curriculum, the driver of faculty conversations is not what content must be taught but rather what KSAs (professional values) students need to demonstrate to meet expected curriculum outcomes. Before they can think about curriculum from the outcome, or end stage, faculty first must identify the desired program outcomes using a stakeholder-informed and future-oriented picture of nursing practice (Sroczynski, Gravlin, Route, Hoffart, & Creelman, 2011). Here are some examples of end-of-program competencies that reflect evolving stakeholder priorities with an emphasis on transition care coordination across settings, emerging technologies, and culturally sensitive care.

Upon completion of this BSN program, the graduate will be able to:

- Coordinate care and transitions across providers and settings
- Apply communication and emerging technologies to nursing practice for optimal patient outcomes
- Deliver culturally sensitive care to patients and their families (Thomas Jefferson University College of Nursing, 2015).

As faculty identify outcomes, it is important to embed these outcomes in actions that promote the practice of nursing. Using an outcomes perspective, it is important that faculty not only clarify and define the concepts they wish to use in the development of outcomes but also ensure that they have outcomes that are broad enough to incorporate all of the attributes desired.

A common question is how many program outcomes are needed. There is no evidence-based

BOX 6-2 Aquinas College Mission and Core Principles

The Mission of Aquinas College is a Catholic community of learning in the Dominican Tradition with Christ at its center. The College directs all its efforts to the intellectual, moral, spiritual, and professional formation of the human person in wisdom. Students are formed individually and in a Christian community so that the harmonious integration between faith and reason can permeate every dimension of their lives. Immersed in exploring the relationship between human civilization and the message of salvation, the College community embraces the Dominican imperative to preach the Gospel, serve others, and engage culture in truth and charity.

BSN PROGAM OUTCOMES

Upon the completion of the program the graduate will be able to:

1. Administer evidence-based, clinically relevant holistic care to individuals, families, groups and multi-dimensional populations with diverse demographic and cultural characteristics in a variety of settings.
2. Communicate effectively using oral, written, and electronic methods, to transmit the analysis and integration of data required to provide safe quality care and inform nursing practice.
3. Integrate critical reasoning and problem-solving methods to make effective nursing judgments and help patients make relevant decisions to improve their health and quality of life.
4. Implement interventions that integrate ethical, legal, and Christian principles and behaviors, consistent with the Catholic and Dominican Tradition, in all professional nursing activities in order to advocate for the health, well-being, and the best interests of nurses, patients, families, significant others, and the community.
5. Integrate teaching strategies to assist individuals, families, and communities to achieve the highest level of health and well-being possible.
6. Collaborate in partnership with other healthcare team members to promote, protect, and improve health of patients at any point on the illness/wellness continuum.
7. Engage in leadership and management activities in a multi-disciplinary healthcare environment to plan, implement, delegate, evaluate, and promote safe quality nursing care that is holistic and cost effective.
8. Participate in the ongoing changes in the profession and actions that promote safe quality patient care and engage in ongoing preparation through continued learning and advanced practice education that advance the goals of the profession.

Courtesy of Aquinas College, School of Nursing. Used with permission

answer to this question; however, many programs strive for no more than eight to ten outcomes. Keep in mind that these should be broad-based outcomes that encompass a number of competencies that will evolve with changing practice. If faculty are identifying a large number of program outcomes, it is likely that they have confused program outcomes with the knowledge, skills, or behaviors related to competencies. Program outcomes should not need to be frequently updated; they should stand the test of time. For example, consider the following BSN program outcomes (2 of 9).

As a graduate of the BSN program you will be:

- A culturally sensitive individual who provides holistic, individual, family, community, and population-centered nursing care;
- An effective communicator who collaborates with inter-professional team members, patients, and their support systems for improved health outcomes (Indiana University School of Nursing, 2012).

These outcomes are written broadly and will be contemporary for some time to come. The knowledge, skills, and behaviors (competencies) that the graduate will need to acquire to demonstrate these outcomes will likely change, but the outcomes will remain current. The faculty can review and update the competencies as needed to stay current.

Some of the criteria that will be useful in determining how many outcomes to include are ensuring that the major aspects of the organizing framework are included; that significant professional practice and accreditation standards are appropriately reflected; and that, when considering the outcomes as a collective whole, a clear picture of the major components of a practitioner who is engaged in safe, quality nursing care emerges.

Consideration of a more ontological philosophical approach to defining outcomes adds the perspective of the learner on core characteristics. For example, in the work of Doane and Brown (2011), students are expected to demonstrate "self-initiating, self-correcting and self-evaluating behaviors which they believe are at the core of skillful practitioners" (p. 24). The authors indicate that developing skills of communication is critical and that it is the learners' ability to identify what is not known that shapes the essential content within the curriculum. The importance of reflection and reflective practice is increasingly recognized as a crucial strategy to develop professional identity, emotionally intelligent practitioners, and a commitment to lifelong learning and development (Sherwood & Horton-Deutsch, 2012).

Identifying and Developing Competencies

After the expected program outcomes have been established, the next step in the curriculum development process is to identify the competencies that students need to possess to attain these outcomes. Competency statements identify the knowledge, skills, and professional attitudes and values that students need to develop if they are to achieve the program outcomes. Competency statements are behaviorally anchored and student focused. Nursing faculty must approach curriculum development from the premise that nursing knowledge and skills are built on or interwoven with general education knowledge and skills. Outcomes should include those competencies that are specific to the nursing discipline, as well as those competencies that establish a foundation for lifelong learning. Students achieve the identified competencies, through acquisition of necessary KSAs, leading to the achievement of the expected program outcomes, whether as an undergraduate or graduate student.

Competency statements are important in assessing student learning because they become the foundation that drives evaluation. When identifying competencies, faculty should give attention to determining the right student, the right behavior, the right level of behavior, and the right context of the behavior. Here, *student* refers to the level of student from whom faculty are expecting these behaviors (e.g., prenursing, nursing sophomore, nursing senior, master's or doctoral level, etc.); *level of behavior* refers to the level of learning or performance at which the behavior is to be demonstrated (this is where learning taxonomies are helpful); and *context of the behavior* refers to the environment in which the behavior should occur. For example, if faculty believe that it is essential for students to exhibit a particular skill, knowledge, or attitude across a continuum of health care settings or with a select population of patients, then the competency statement should indicate the parameters in which the behavior should be expressed. It is equally important for faculty to remember not to be so specific as to "paint themselves into a corner" from which there is no escape (e.g., if faculty specify that a certain behavior will be demonstrated with postoperative patients in an outpatient surgical setting, all students must be guaranteed this type of experience for faculty to make an accurate and consistent assessment and evaluation of student performance).

Leveling Competencies

In leveling, or specifying, competencies, faculty must recognize the level at which the KSAs need to be demonstrated to obtain the outcome desired throughout the curriculum. The learning environment will need to be designed to enable the students to acquire knowledge at the level identified. Evaluation measures also need to be consistent with the level of learning identified to ensure consistency in evaluation from the time of input of information through the time of output of the expected competency. Learning occurs at various levels, and the level of learning needs to be explicitly stated in the competencies faculty generate for each level within the curriculum. Table 6-2 provides a sample end-of-program competency related to communication leveled across the last four semesters of a baccalaureate nursing program.

Once competencies have been leveled to a year or semester or academic level, faculty must carefully examine these competencies and determine how courses can be designed to contribute to the ongoing development of these competencies. The behaviors embedded in each competency become the focus for writing course-level competencies. Not all competencies will or should be included in all courses that make up the curriculum. Competencies at the course level are more concrete and detail how the chosen competencies explicitly relate to the course. The faculty will then need to identify what prerequisite and requisite knowledge and skills students will need to possess to demonstrate this behavior.

If, for example, faculty believe that the individualization of a standard care map is critical to a nurse practitioner student learning experience, then a course-level competency resulting in course objectives, learning activities, and evaluation of learning will be included to reflect this behavior.

Because structured learning tends to be grounded in developmental theories, students are expected to

TABLE 6-2 Leveling Competencies Across the Curriculum: Communication

End of Program Competency: Uses appropriate, accurate, and effective communication processes with clients, colleagues, and others

Semester 1	Semester 2	Semester 3	Semester 4
Assess own communication style (verbal, written, and via technology) to evaluate strengths and weaknesses in sending and receiving information accurately.	Access and appraise the quality and appropriateness of information retrieved via information technology sources for professional information and client education uses.	Use principles of effective interpersonal communication theories to enact goal-directed communications with individuals and groups.	Express oneself effectively in a variety of media and contexts to educate, influence, and collaborate with others.

become more accomplished in applying knowledge to increasingly more complex or new situations as they move through the curriculum. Course competencies (course expectations) then should be written to reflect the placement of the course within the curriculum; the expectations of learning for courses that precede, articulate, and follow each course; and how each course can contribute to the development of program competencies. Precision is needed when writing competency statements. The language of the competencies must reflect a continued sense of development. Development may take the form of increasing complexity, differentiation, delineation, or sophistication.

Competency Learning Progression Charts

As noted earlier in this chapter, outcomes are typically measured through more specific competency statements that, in aggregate, provide evidence that the outcome was achieved. To maintain curricula integrity, tracking competencies associated with each program outcome is an important activity; however, tracking the numerous competencies associated with all of the outcomes can become an onerous task. Comprehensive content grids are useful and necessary; however, they can be so voluminous that they lose utility for depicting the building blocks of KSAs desired.

Several methods for documenting learning progression may be used; one exemplar is the competency learning progression chart. A competency learning progression chart (Sullivan, 2014) can succinctly demonstrate the progression of learning (Table 6-3). Each program outcome is measured through multiple derived competencies created to reflect learning achievement. Each of the component competencies is shown in a grid beneath the larger learning outcome, including information regarding the course location, specific learning activities, and evaluation criteria to assess student learning. Once agreed on by faculty and included in the competency learning progression chart, individual faculty may not independently change the key learning activities and evaluation methods. Further, selected assignment products may be used to create student portfolios as an expression of their comprehensive achievement of the desired learning outcomes. Finally, specification of key learning activities is an effective tool to identify content duplication and gaps.

In one recent example within a nursing program, it was discovered that students were asked to perform three community assessments in three different courses using almost identical criteria. Faculty agreed that one community assessment was sufficient and thus freed up precious time for other learning topics. Competency learning progression charts can be reviewed on a regular basis to incorporate new information and concepts, with the designated faculty group making decisions regarding changes. This practice is an exemplar of how curricular integrity can be balanced with the concept of academic freedom discussed earlier.

Course Design

Faculty have now completed the overarching curriculum structure with the identification of the organizing framework, outcomes, and competencies. These competencies now need to be organized, or threaded, through the courses that faculty will develop. To begin this process, faculty must consider the antecedents, or factors, that need to be in place

TABLE 6-3 Competency Learning Progression Chart
Excellence University: BSN Program

Competency Number: 1
Competency Theme/Thread: Nursing/Collaboration
End of Program Competency: Work collaboratively with other health care team members using a process grounded in respect for and knowledge of others' roles.

Competency	Course	Learning Activity	Evaluation
Demonstrate knowledge of other health care team members' contributions to care	N 100	Summarize interviews with 3 nonnursing health care team members regarding their scope of practice and care focus	Assignment Rubric
		Construct a patient education plan that incorporates other disciplines as appropriate to the topic	Peer-rated Group Presentation
Apply knowledge of group behavior and collaboration skills to promote effective team relationships and decisions	N 200	Describe a theory-based approach to effective teamwork	Scholarly Paper with Rubric
		Evaluate two health care team scenarios using teamwork and quality improvement principles	Simulation with Debrief

for the outcomes and competencies to be achieved in each course in the curriculum. *Antecedents* are defined as the prerequisite knowledge needed to develop or foster the identified attributes or characteristics. It is assumed that each course within the curriculum will make a *unique* contribution to the ability of students to meet the identified competencies at each level of the program.

The key is for faculty as curriculum developers to consciously consider and design courses and sequences that will best lead to achieving the desired learning outcomes across the diversity of students within the population. See Chapter 10 for an in depth discussion on designing courses and learning experiences.

Teaching and Learning Trends in Curriculum Design

Seismic shifts have occurred in conceptualizing and designing nursing education programs. Some of these changes have been presented earlier in this chapter. Several additional trends of significance are briefly described here because of their profound and growing influence on nursing education curricula. Among the most important are theories and approaches seeking to promote deeper and more engaged learning while better reflecting the complexity of teaching nursing, especially but not limited to prelicensure students. Four popular trends are overviewed to illustrate the evolution occurring in nursing education: constructivism, narrative pedagogy, problem-based and team-based learning, and flipping the classroom.

Constructivism and Narrative Pedagogy

The influence of constructivism and phenomenological-based approaches to teaching and learning has led to creation of new pedagogies reflecting this shift in foundational beliefs about education. A constructivist perspective embraces elements of cognitive psychology that suggest knowledge is not simply absorbed but must be "created" by and within the learner, with faculty serving as a guide. Hartle, Baviskar, and Smith (2012) published a field guide to constructivism for the college level, noting that there are four essential criteria: prior knowledge assessment, cognitive dissonance creation, application and feedback, and metacognition. *Metacognition* may be simply defined as students reflecting on what they have learned, how they learned it, and why it is important.

With narrative pedagogy, "teachers focus on thinking anew about the experiences they co-create with students, rather than on the activities common in conventional pedagogies . . . and work with students to interpret shared experiences of learning and practicing nursing" (Ironside, 2014, p. 212). Although narrative pedagogy may be interpreted and used as an entirely new paradigm for nursing education, presently it is most often implemented as a strategy and used concurrently with more traditional approaches to curriculum development. Considering Benner et al. (2010) seminal work recommending major changes in nursing education, including contextualizing knowledge, promoting situated clinical reasoning, linking classroom and clinical information, and focusing on professional identity formation, narrative pedagogy provides an evidence-based strategy to revolutionize teaching and learning in nursing. Chapter 13 provides a comprehensive discussion of constructivism, narrative pedagogy, and other learning theories.

Problem-based and Team-based Learning

Although some substantive differences exist between the two, problem-based learning and team-based learning share fundamental characteristics, including the value of peer learning. A systematic review of peer learning in nursing programs revealed improvement in either an objective effect or subjective assessment in 16 of 18 included studies (Stone, Cooper, & Cant, 2013). Additionally, peer learning in nursing education was shown to develop student communication, critical thinking, and self-confidence. Problem-based learning may be defined as a "cognitive endeavor whereby the learner constructs mental models relevant to problems" (Schmidt, Rotgans, & Yew, 2011, p. 792).

Team-based learning is also a learner-centered approach with faculty serving as expert facilitators (Hrynchak & Batty, 2012; Mennenga & Smyer, 2010). As in problem-based learning, cases and scenarios are used to promote problem solving through group interaction and analysis. One major difference is the more structured process generally associated with team-based learning. A benefit of team-based learning is the ability to use the technique with a fairly large group of students; in contrast, problem-based learning is usually conducted in smaller, independent teams. See Chapter 15 for further discussion of problem-based and team-based learning, as well as other active learning strategies.

The "Flipped Classroom"

Last, the concept of "flipping the classroom" has received significant attention in both K–12 and higher education circles. Consistent with much of the prior content, the goal of a flipped classroom is for students to individually prepare for learning with the goal of creating meaningful and engaging learning activities within groups in the classroom. Faculty facilitate the classroom discussions to promote active, engaged learning that results in longer lasting and deeper knowledge gains (Alexandre & Wright, 2013; Dickerson, Lubejko, McGowan, Balmer, & Chappell, 2014). Chapter 19 discusses the concept of interconnectedness in the classroom, including the "flipped classroom."

Clinical Teaching and Learning

As a practice discipline, teaching and learning the role of a nurse in a health care setting is paramount to achieving the desired learning outcomes. The ratio of clinical instructors to prelicensure students is regulated by state boards of nursing to ensure public safety when students are practicing. Clinical teaching is one of the most time- and resource-intensive aspects of nursing education and is of critical importance at all levels of nursing education and any practice discipline. Clinical faculty must develop the teaching skills and strategies to transform their clinical expertise into meaningful experiences for and with students. In numerous clinical placements, especially at the graduate levels, preceptors are used extensively. Thus preceptor identification, development, and evaluation merits the necessary attention and support.

The complexity of health care organizations and competition for clinical sites as schools of nursing increased enrollments to meet health care needs has often suboptimized student clinical experiences through inconsistent scheduling, working 12-hour shifts, and being unable to follow a patient's trajectory of illness and recovery. Students frequently do not care for patients with conditions matching the content being covered in classrooms; may work with different nurses as opposed to an identified preceptor; and struggle to become familiar with the necessary structure, systems, and practices of the several clinical sites they may be assigned to over the course of a semester. The use of concepts to showcase similarities and differences across discrete patient diagnoses is particularly useful given these realities as they help learners to relate information to multiple situations. Last, the underlying pedagogy and role of clinical instructors, who in many cases are not full-time faculty and may not be familiar with the overall curriculum, is often not clear or consistent. Chapter 17 provides a thorough discussion of clinical teaching.

Clinical immersion experiences have waxed and waned in popularity and seem to be experiencing a new wave of popularity. Immersion may be as short as a week or two or as long as one or two semesters, depending on curricular design and clinical site relationships and support. The benefits of immersion include sufficient time to learn the setting and its practices and procedures, opportunities to see the trajectory of patient health and illness patterns over longer periods, and the ability to form work relationships with a variety of health disciplines to master the intra- and interprofessional skills of teamwork and collaboration. Although the increasing support for postlicensure residence programs may bridge some of the gaps related to transition into practice, the importance of clinical practice teaching and learning prior to that time deserves continued attention.

Resources

When designing or revising curricula, it is important to consider the effects of various decisions on the resources that will be required to implement those plans in a manner that will ensure a quality outcome. This assessment and discussion requires collaboration between academic administration and the faculty leading the curriculum efforts. It is most helpful to agree on assumptions regarding resources of faculty (full-time and clinical instructors or others), simulation and related materials, clinical sites, and support services. In some cases, resources will be constrained, requiring that curricula be created with that fact in mind.

Decisions regarding many of the curricular elements have implications for resources with three elements creating the most potential influence on resources: the organizing framework, learning outcomes, and pedagogical strategies. As an example, should a problem-based learning approach be identified as a major teaching strategy, additional faculty facilitators might be desirable for the same number of students. Or, if simulation activities are to be increased in amount and level of complexity, perhaps using simulated patients, the costs of these plans must be considered and approved before the process of curriculum change is completed, not after. Academic administrators and faculty leaders would be well advised to outline the scope of the curriculum development or change project, including an assessment of and future assumptions about resources to avoid disappointment and rework.

Another aspect of resources related to curricular design and change is the amount of faculty time and effort expended to accomplish this important work. Unfortunately, in many cases, curricular change is handled according to existing processes and meetings structures, which may be onerous, time consuming, and sometimes unclear. Viewing the work of curricular change from the lens of project management and quality improvement leads to embracing tested models for data collection, assessment, and decision making within a prescribed timeframe versus an open-ended approach to completing the desired work. More recently, various schools of nursing have reported accomplishing major curricular redesigns within 1 to 2 years; however, it is still common to see curriculum projects expand to 3 or more years. Given that the timeline for receiving various institutional and regulatory approvals can be lengthy and delay curricular implementation even longer, there is the potential for a "new" curriculum to be dated before it has been implemented.

Some potential disadvantages of this more structured approach may include perceptions that faculty decision-making power relationships are shifted and that more time is needed to fully consider all of the issues and topics. Appropriate strategies may be used to proactively address these concerns to accomplish curricular change in an effective manner. Given the central importance of resources in any curriculum, a clear understanding of the assumptions related to and amount and type of available resources will position a curriculum project for success.

Process for Curriculum Development or Revision

Faculty have a responsibility to develop, evaluate, and revise their curriculum. Curriculum evaluation and revision is an ongoing process. Because a significant amount of faculty time is spent in this effort, faculty can consider effective and efficient ways to approach this work.

One of the first steps is to identify the leadership and structure. The leader may be a consultant who is employed to consult or lead the development or revision process, but more often the leader is an appointed or elected faculty member. When undertaking a significant curriculum revision, it may also be helpful to consider using a small group of faculty to serve as co-leaders of the process instead of one individual. In this manner, there is shared responsibility for leading the curricular change, which avoids overwhelming any one individual. Faculty must also determine if the curriculum work will be done by the faculty as a whole, by volunteers, or by faculty who are elected to represent a constituency and serve on the curriculum committee on their behalf. Faculty must also have bylaws in place to define the curriculum process.

Curriculum development or revision is a change process, and some faculty find it helpful to use a change model to guide the process. Several models include Rogers's (2003) *Diffusion of Innovations*; Lewin's (1951) Force Field Analysis; or a Strengths, Weakness, Opportunity, Threat (SWOT) model. Regardless of the model used, if any, faculty will benefit from establishing norms for change, identifying the benefits and risks of change, determining what must change and what can stay the same, and obtaining the needed resources to do the work.

Inevitably there will be barriers and resistance to change. Barriers can include lack of time; large numbers of inexperienced faculty; faculty with a sense of loss of control, lack of trust, or concerns about losing their area of expertise in the curriculum; or uncertainty related to the need to learn new clinical skills, teaching strategies, or content. At the same time, faculty can use strategies to facilitate change. Having key faculty involved in the curriculum development and revision is important, as is having agreed-on goals, a transparent process, and respect for everyone's opinion. Setting a timeline for completion of the work is also important, or the work may stagnate and even become outdated before it is implemented. Recognizing both the barriers and the facilitators improve the curriculum development and revision process.

Summary

Although some traditional concepts of curriculum development continue to provide structure for an important, planned, and sequenced approach to achieving desired educational outcomes, aspects of nursing education are undergoing significant and sometimes disruptive innovations. Although there is often growing support for change, faculty in schools of nursing are challenged to reconceptualize their current curricula while continuing to teach in the current framework and teaching strategies. Major forces influencing curriculum changes provide the context for reenvisioning nursing curricula, using innovative yet evidence-based approaches to achieve the desired learning outcomes and competencies. An approach to designing and documenting curricula was reviewed along with exemplars to support effectiveness of selected elements or strategies.

There are exciting innovations in nursing education today that are expected to result in enhanced outcomes for graduates and in a new excitement about the educator role in this process. Systematic process and outcome evaluation of curriculum development, implementation, and outcomes will be crucial to learning how to best design education curricula to prepare graduates for the ever-expanding and complex role of the nurses across the health care continuum to ensure comprehensive, high-quality care for the populations served.

REFLECTING ON THE EVIDENCE

1. How does a faculty member know if a curriculum framework is providing adequate structure to support the decisions faculty are making regarding curriculum development and implementation?
2. What are some strategies that faculty can adopt to ensure that their program curricula remain fluid and dynamic?
3. What are some of the strategies that faculty may adopt to promote effective and satisfying curriculum change that reflects evidence-based and innovative concepts and practices?

REFERENCES

Alexandre, M. S., & Wright, R. R. (2013). Flipping the classroom for student engagement. *International Journal of Nursing Care, 1*(2), 103–106.

Allen, I. E., & Seaman, J. (2010). *Class differences: Online education in the United States, 2010.* Babson Park, MA: Babson Survey Research Group.

American Association of Colleges and Universities. (2006). *Academic freedom.* Retrieved from, http://www.aacu.org/publications-research/periodicals/academic-freedom-and-educational-responsibility.

American Association of Colleges of Nursing (AACN). (2006). *The essentials of doctoral education for advanced nursing practice.* Washington, D. C: Author.

American Association of Colleges of Nursing (AACN). (2008). *The essentials of baccalaureate education for professional nursing practice.* Washington, D. C: Author.

American Association of Colleges of Nursing (AACN). (2009). *The impact of education on nursing practice.* Washington, D.C: Author.

American Association of Colleges of Nursing (AACN). (2011). *The essentials of master's education in nursing.* Washington, D. C: Author.

Astin, A. W. (2012). *Assessment for excellence: The philosophy and practice of assessment and evaluation in higher education.* Lanham, MD: Rowman & Littlefield.

Benner, P., Sutphen, M., Leonard, V., & Day, L. (2010). *Educating nurses: A call for radical transformation.* San Francisco, CA: Jossey-Bass.

Bernard, R. M., Borokhovski, E., Schmid, R. F., Tamim, R. M., & Abrami, P. C. (2014). A meta-analysis of blended learning and technology use in higher education: From the general to the applied. *Journal of Computing in Higher Education, 26*(1), 87–122.

Berwick, D. M., Nolan, T. W., & Whittington, J. (2008). The triple aim: Care, health, and cost. *Health Affairs, 27*(3), 759–776.

Bevis, E. O. (2000). Nursing curriculum as professional education. In E. O. Bevis & J. Watson (Eds.), *Toward a caring curriculum: A new pedagogy for nursing* (pp. 74–77). New York: National League for Nursing Press.

Broome, M. E. (2009). Building the science for nursing education: Vision or improbable dream. *Nursing Outlook, 57*(4), 177–179.

Broome, M., Halstead, J., Pesut, D., Rawl, S., & Boland, D. (2011). Evaluating the outcomes of a distance accessible PhD program. *Journal of Professional Nursing, 27*(2), 69–77.

Chenot, T. M., & Daniel, L. G. (2010). Frameworks for patient safety in the nursing curriculum. *Journal of Nursing Education, 49*, 559–568.

Cronenwett, L. (2012). A national initiative: Quality and Safety Education for Nurses (QSEN). *Quality and safety in nursing: A competency approach to improving outcomes.* Hoboken, NJ: Wiley-Blackwell.

Cronenwett, L., Sherwood, G., Pohl, J., Barnsteiner, J., Moore, S., Sullivan, D. T., et al. (2009). Quality and safety education for advanced nursing practice. *Nursing Outlook, 57*(6), 338–348.

D'Antonio, P. O. B., Brennan, A. M. W., & Curley, M. A. (2013). Judgment, inquiry, engagement, voice: Reenvisioning an undergraduate nursing curriculum using a shared decision-making model. *Journal of Professional Nursing, 29*(6), 407–413.

Dickerson, P. S., Lubejko, B. G., McGowan, B. S., Balmer, J. T., & Chappell, K. (2014). Flipping the classroom: A data-driven model for nursing education. *Journal of Continuing Education in Nursing, 45*(11), 477–478.

Diekelmann, N., & Diekelmann, J. (2009). *Schooling learning teaching: Toward narrative pedagogy.* Bloomington, IN: iUniverse.

Doane, G. H., & Brown, H. (2011). Recontextualizing learning in nursing education: Taking an ontological turn. *Journal of Nursing Education, 50*(1), 21–26.

Doll, W. E., Jr. (2002). Ghosts and the curriculum. In W. E. Doll Jr., & N. Gough (Eds.), *Curriculum visions* (pp. 23–70). New York: Peter Lang.

Doll, W. E., Jr. (2012). Complexity and the culture of curriculum. *Complicity: An International Journal of Complexity and Education, 9*(1), 10–29.

Fawcett, J. (1989). *Conceptual models of nursing.* Philadelphia: F. A. Davis.

Finkelman, A. W., & Kenner, C. (2009). *Teaching IOM: Implications of the Institute of Medicine reports for nursing education.* Silver Springs, MD: NursesBooks.org.

George, V. M., & Shocksnider, J. (2014). Leaders: Are you ready for change? The clinical nurse as care coordinator in the new health care system. *Nursing Administration Quarterly, 38*(1), 78–85.

Giddens, J. F., Wright, M., & Gray, I. (2012). Selecting concepts for a concept-based curriculum: Application of a benchmark approach. *The Journal of Nursing Education, 51*(9), 511–515.

Gruppen, L. D., Mangrulkar, R. S., & Kolars, J. C. (2012). The promise of competency-based education in the health professions for improving global health. *Human Resources for Health, 2012*(10), 43.

Hartle, R. T., Baviskar, S., & Smith, R. (2012). A field guide to constructivism in the college science classroom: Four essential criteria and a guide to their usage. *Bioscene: Journal of College Biology Teaching, 38*(2), 31–35.

Healthy People 2020. (n.d.) Retrieved from http://healthypeople.gov/2020/TopicsObjectives2020/pdfs/HP2020_brochure.pdf.

Hills, M., & Watson, J. (2011). *Creating a caring science curriculum: An emancipatory pedagogy for nursing.* New York: Springer.

Hrynchak, P., & Batty, H. (2012). The educational theory basis of team-based learning. *Medical Teacher, 34*(10), 796–801.

Indiana University School of Nursing. (2012). *Indiana University Schools of Nursing Baccalaureate Program Outcomes.* Indianapolis: Author.

Institute for Health Care Improvement (IHI). (2007). *The IHI Triple Aim Initiative.*

Institute of Medicine (IOM). (2001). *Crossing the quality chasm: A new health system for the 21st century.* Washington, D.C: The National Academies Press.

Institute of Medicine (IOM). (2003). *Health professions education: A bridge to quality.* Washington, D.C: The National Academies Press.

Institute of Medicine (IOM). (2010). *The future of nursing: Leading change, advancing health.* Washington, D.C: The National Academies Press.

Interprofessional Education Collaborative Expert Panel. (2011). *Core competencies for interprofessional collaborative practice: Report of an expert panel.* Washington, D.C: Interprofessional Education Collaborative.

Ironside, P. M. (2014). Enabling narrative pedagogy: Inviting, waiting, and letting be. *Nursing Education Perspectives, 35*(4), 212–218.

Jones, D. P., & Wolf, D. M. (2009). Shaping the future of nursing education today using distant education and technology. *The ABNF Journal: Official Journal of the Association of Black Nursing Faculty in Higher Education, 21*(2), 44–47.

Kirschner, A. (2012, April 8). *Innovations in higher education? Hah!.* The Chronicle of Higher Education. Retrieved from, http://chronicle.com.

Kumm, S., & Fletcher, K. A. (2012). From daunting task to new beginnings: Bachelor of science in nursing curriculum revision using the new *Essentials. Journal of Professional Nursing, 28*(2), 82–89.

Lee, R. C., & Fawcett, J. (2013). The influence of the metaparadigm of nursing on professional identity development among RN-BSN students. *Nursing Science Quarterly, 26*(1), 96–98.

Levitt, C. G. (2014, July). *Bridging the education-practice gap: Integration of current clinical practice into education on transitions to professional practice.* Paper presented at the 25th international nursing research conference, Hong Kong.

Lewin, K. (1951). *Field theory in Social Science.* New York: Harper and Row.

Lunenburg, F. (2011). Theorizing about curriculum: Conceptions and definitions. *International Journal of Scholarly Academic Intellectual Diversity, 13,* 1–6.

Mailloux, C. G. (2011). Using the essentials of baccalaureate education for professional nursing practice (2008) as a framework for curriculum revision. *Journal of Professional Nursing, 27*(6), 385–389.

McDonald, M. E. (2014). *The nurse educator's guide to assessment of learning outcomes* (3rd ed.). Burlington, MA: Jones & Bartlett.

Mennenga, H. A., & Smyer, T. (2010). A model for easily incorporating team-based learning into nursing education. *International Journal of Nursing Education Scholarship, 7*(1). http://dx.doi.org/10.2202/1548-923X. 1924, January 2010.

National League for Nursing (NLN). (2010). *Outcomes and competencies for graduates of practical/vocational, diploma, baccalaureate, master's, practice doctorate, and research doctorate programs in nursing.* Washington, D.C: Author.

National League for Nursing (NLN). (2012). *The scope of practice for academic nurse educators.* Washington, D.C: Author.

New Media Consortium (NMC). (2015). *Horizon report.* www.nmc.org.

Newman, F., Couturier, L., & Scurry, J. (2010). *The future of higher education: Rhetoric, reality, and the risks of the market.* New York: John Wiley & Sons.

Oerrmann, M. H., & Gaberson, K. B. (2014). *Evaluation and testing in nursing education* (4th ed.). New York: Springer.

Parkay, F. W., Anctil, E. J., & Hass, G. (2010). *Curriculum leadership: Readings for developing quality educational programs.* Boston, MA: Allyn & Bacon.

Phillips, B., Shaw, R. J., Sullivan, D. T., & Johnson, C. (2010). Using virtual environments to enhance nursing distance education. *Creative Nursing, 16*(3), 132–135.

Pollard, M. L., Stapleton, M., Kennelly, L., Bagdan, L., Cannistraci, P., Millenbach, L., et al. (2014). Assessment of quality and safety education in nursing: A New York state perspective. *Nursing Education Perspectives, 35*(4), 224–229.

Posner, G. J. (1992). *Analyzing the curriculum.* New York: McGraw Hill.

Quality and Safety Education for Nurses (QSEN). (n.d.). [Website]. Retrieved from http://www.qsen.org/.

Rogers, E. (2003). *Diffusion of innovations* (5th ed.). New York: Simon and Shuster.

Schiro, M. (2013). *Curriculum theory* (2nd ed.). Los Angeles: Sage.

Schmidt, H. G., Rotgans, J. I., & Yew, E. H. (2011). The process of problem-based learning: What works and why. *Medical Education, 45*(8), 792–806.

Shattell, M. M., Nemitz, E. A., Crosson, N., Zackeru, A. R., Starr, S., Hu, J., et al. (2013). Culturally competent practice in a pre-licensure baccalaureate nursing program in the united states: A mixed-methods study. *Nursing Education Perspectives, 34*(6), 383–389.

Sherwood, G., & Horton-Deutsch, S. (2012). *Reflective practice: Transforming education and improving outcomes.* Indianapolis, IN: Sigma Theta Tau.

Sroczynski, M., Gravlin, G., Route, P. S., Hoffart, N., & Creelman, P. (2011). Creativity and connections: The future of nursing education and practice: The Massachusetts initiative. *Journal of Professional Nursing, 27*(6), e64–e70.

Stone, R., Cooper, S., & Cant, R. (2013). The value of peer learning in undergraduate nursing education: A systematic review. *International Scholarly Research Notices, 2013.* Article ID 930901, 10 pages, http:dx.doi.org/10.1155/2013/930901.

Sullivan, D. T. (2014). *Using competency learning progression charts to enhance assessment of student learning outcomes.* Unpublished manuscript.

Sullivan, D. T., & Godfrey, N. S. (2012). Preparing nursing students to be effective health team partners through interprofessional education. *Creative Nursing, 18*(2), 57–63.

Sullivan, D. T., Hirst, D., & Cronenwett, L. (2009). Assessing quality and safety competencies of graduating prelicensure nursing students. *Nursing Outlook, 57*(6), 323–331.

Swanson, K. M. (1999). What's known about caring in nursing science: A literary meta-analysis. In A. S. Hinshaw, S. Feetham, & J. Shaver (Eds.), *Handbook of clinical nursing research* (pp. 31–60). Thousand Oaks, CA: Sage Publishers.

Thistlethwaite, J., & Moran, M. (2010). Learning outcomes for interprofessional education (IPE): Literature review and synthesis. *Journal of Interprofessional Care, 24*(5), 503–513.

Thomas Jefferson University College of Nursing. (2015). *College of Nursing, BSN curriculum program outcomes.* Philadelphia: Author.

Tyler, R. W. (2013). *Basic principles of curriculum and instruction.* Chicago: University of Chicago Press.

Valiga, T. M. (2012). Nursing education trends: Future implications and predictions. *Nursing Clinics of North America, 47*(4), 423–434.

Valiga, T. M., & Ironside, P. M. (2012). Crafting a national agenda for nursing education research. *The Journal of Nursing Education, 51*(1), 3–6.

Watson, J. (1997). The theory of human caring: Retrospective and prospective. *Nursing Science Quarterly, 10*(1), 49–52 Thousand Oaks, CA: Sage Publishers.

Wiles, J. W., & Bondi, J. C. (1989). *Curriculum development: A guide to practice* (3rd ed.). Columbus, OH: Merrill.

Wiles, J. W., & Bondi, J. C. (2011). *Curriculum development: A guide to practice* (8th ed.). Boston: Pearson Education.

Wittmann-Price, R. A., & Fasolka, B. J. (2010). Objectives and outcomes: The fundamental difference. *Nursing Education Perspectives, 31*(4), 233–236.

World Health Organization (WHO). (2010). *Framework for action on interprofessional education & collaborative practice.* Geneva: World Health Organization. Retrieved from, http://whqlibdoc.who.int/hq/2010/WHO_HRH_HPN_10.3_eng.pdf.

7

Philosophical Foundations of the Curriculum

Theresa M. "Terry" Valiga, EdD, RN, CNE, ANEF, FAAN

Beautiful words. Admirable values. Published prominently on websites and in catalogues, student handbooks and accreditation reports. The philosophical statement of a school of nursing is accepted by faculty as a document that must be crafted to please external reviewers, but for many it remains little more than that. Far too often the school's philosophy remains safely tucked inside a report but is rarely seen as a living document that guides the day-to-day workings of the school.

In reality, the philosophy of a school of nursing should be referenced and reflected upon often. It should be reviewed seriously with candidates for faculty positions and with those individuals who join the community as new members. It should be discussed in a deliberate way with potential students and with students as they progress throughout the program. And it should be a strong guiding force as the school revises or sharpens its goals, outlines action steps to implement its strategic plan, and makes decisions about the allocation of resources.

This chapter explores the significance of reflecting on, articulating, and being guided by a philosophy, examines the essential components of a philosophy for a school of nursing, and points out how philosophical statements guide the design and implementation of the curriculum and the evaluation of its effectiveness. The role of faculty, administrators, and students in crafting and "living" the philosophy is discussed, and the issues and debates surrounding the "doing of philosophy" (Greene, 1973) are examined. Finally, suggestions are offered regarding how faculty might go about writing or revising the school's philosophy.

What Is Philosophy?

The educational philosopher Maxine Greene (1973) challenged educators to "do philosophy." By this she meant that we need to take the risk of thinking about what we do when we teach and what we mean when we talk of enabling others to learn. It also means we need to become progressively more conscious of the choices and commitments we make in our professional lives. Greene also challenged educators to look at our presuppositions, to examine critically the principles underlying what we think and what we say as educators, and to confront the individual within us. She acknowledged that we often have to ask and answer painful questions when we "do philosophy."

In his seminal book, *The Courage to Teach,* Parker Palmer (2007) asserted that "though the academy claims to value multiple modes of knowing, it honors only one—an 'objective' way of knowing that takes us into the 'real' world by taking us 'out of ourselves'" (p. 18). He encouraged educators to challenge this culture by bringing a more human, personal perspective to the teaching–learning experience. Like Greene, Palmer suggested that, to do this, educators must look inside so that we can understand that "we teach who we are" (p. xi) and so that we can appreciate that such insight is critical for "authentic teaching, learning, and living" (p. ix).

Philosophy, then, is a way of framing questions that have to do with what is presupposed, perceived, intuited, believed, and known. It is a way of contemplating, examining, or thinking about what is taken to be significant, valuable, or worthy of commitment. Additionally, it is a way of becoming self-aware and thinking of everyday experiences as opportunities to reflect, contemplate, and exercise our curiosity so that questions are posed about what we do and how we do it, usual practices are challenged and not merely accepted as "the way things are," and positive change can occur. Indeed, each of us—as a fundamental practice of being—must go beyond the reality we confront, refuse to accept it as a given and, instead, view life as a reality to be created.

These perspectives on "doing philosophy" focus primarily on individuals—as human beings in general or as teachers in particular—reflecting seriously on their beliefs and values. There is no question that such reflection is critical and is to be valued and encouraged. However, "doing philosophy" must also be a group activity when one is involved in curriculum work. In crafting a statement of philosophy for a school of nursing, the beliefs and values of all faculty must be considered, addressed, and incorporated as much as possible. In fact, the very process of talking about one's beliefs and values—while it may generate heated debates—leads to a deeper understanding of what a group truly accepts as guiding principles for all it does.

Philosophical Statements

A philosophy is essentially a narrative statement of values or beliefs. It reflects broad principles or fundamental "isms" that guide actions and decision making, and it expresses the assumptions we make about people, situations, or goals. As noted by Bevis in her seminal work (1989, p. 35), the philosophy "provides the value system for ordering priorities and selecting from among various data."

In writing a philosophical statement, we must raise questions, contemplate ideas, examine what it is we truly believe, become self-aware, and probe what might be—and what should be. It calls on us to think critically and deeply, forge ideas and ideals, and become highly conscious of the phenomena and events in the world.

We also must reflect on the mission, vision, and values of our parent institution and of our school itself, as well as on the values of our profession. Figure 7-1 illustrates how a school's statement of philosophy is related to but differs from these other sources. A *mission statement* describes unique purposes for which an institution or nursing unit exists: to improve the health of the surrounding community, to advance scientific understanding or contribute to the development of nursing science, to prepare responsible citizens, or to graduate individuals who will influence public policy to ensure access to quality health care for all. A *vision* is an expression of what an institution or nursing unit wants to be: the institution of choice for highly qualified students wishing to make a positive difference in our world; the leader in integrating innovative technology in the preparation of nurses; or a center of synergy for teaching, research, professional practice, and public service. Institutions and schools of nursing often also articulate a set of *values* that guide their operation: honesty and transparency, serving the public good, excellence, innovation, or constantly being open to change and transformation.

As stated, a *philosophy statement* is the narrative that reflects and integrates concepts expressed in the mission, vision, and values of the institution or profession; it serves to guide the actions and decisions of those involved in the organization. Educational philosophy is a matter of "doing philosophy" with respect to the educational enterprise as it engages the educator. It involves becoming critically conscious of what is involved in the complex teaching–learning relationship and what education truly means. The following statements about education, many by well-known individuals, provide examples of different philosophical perspectives:

> The secret of Education lies in respecting the pupil.
>
> —*Ralph Waldo Emerson*

> If the student is to grow, the teacher must also grow.
>
> —*Confucius*

> I think [education] refines you. I think some of us have rough edges. Education is like sanding down a piece of wood and putting the varnish to it.
>
> —*Suzanne Gordon (1991, p. 131)*

> The whole art of teaching is only the art of awakening the natural curiosity of young minds for the purpose of satisfying it afterwards.
>
> —*Anatole France*

> The teacher learns from the student just as the student learns from the teacher with their encounters as examples of mutual openness to each other's needs.
>
> —*Nili Tabak, Livne Adi, and Mali Eherenfeld (2003, p. 251)*

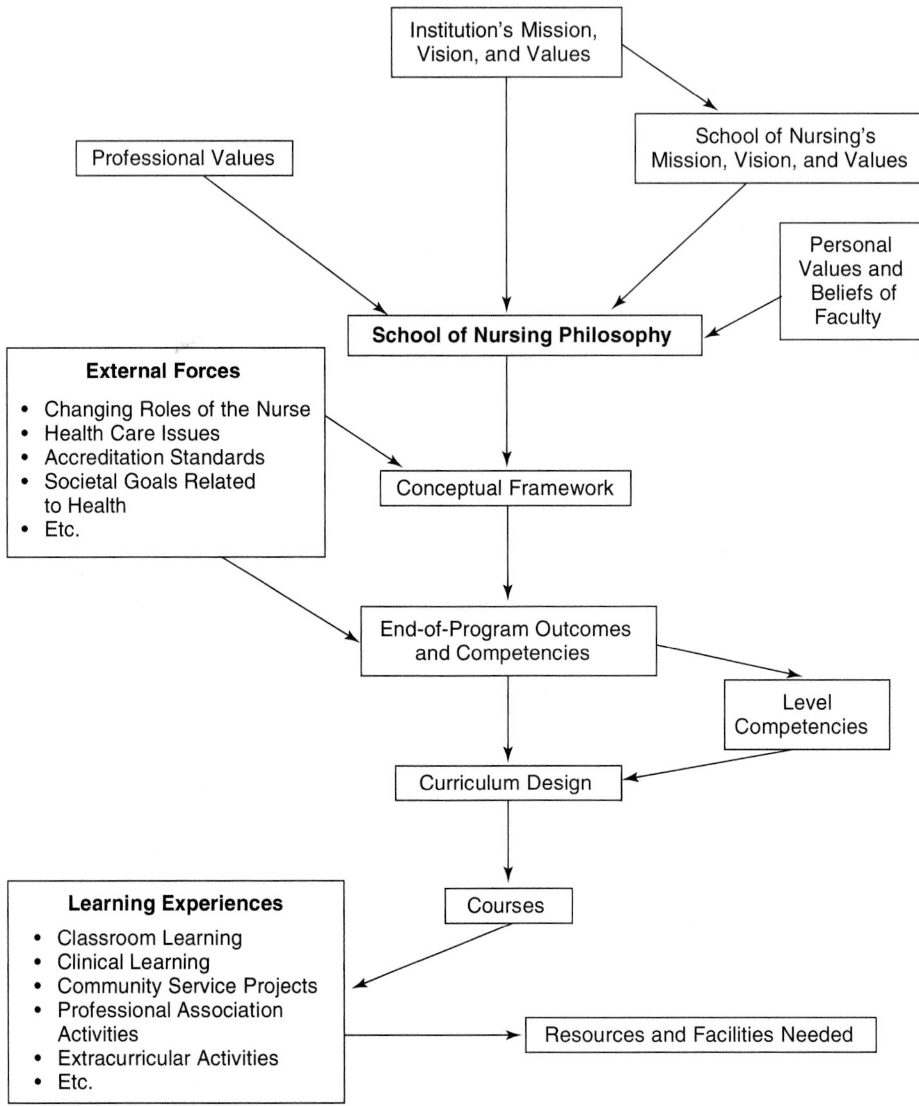

Figure 7-1 Interrelation of curricular elements.

Philosophy as It Relates to Nursing Education

As noted earlier, "doing philosophy" must move from individual work to group work when engaged in curriculum development, implementation, and evaluation. Faculty need to reflect on their own individual beliefs and values, share them with colleagues, affirm points of agreement, and discuss points of disagreement. Table 7-1 summarizes many of the philosophical perspectives expressed through the years, and faculty are encouraged to explore the meaning and implications of each as they engage in developing, reviewing, or refining the philosophical

TABLE 7-1 Summary of Philosophical Perspectives

Philosophical Perspective	Brief Description
Behaviorism	Education focuses on developing mental discipline, particularly through memorization, drill, and recitation. Because learning is systematic, sequential building on previous learning is important.
Essentialism	Because knowledge is key, the goal of education is to transmit and uphold the cultural heritage of the past.
Existentialism	The function of education is to help individuals explore reasons for existence. Personal choice and commitment are crucial.
Hermeneutics	Because individuals are self-interpreting beings, uniquely defined by personal beliefs, concerns, and experiences of life, education must attend to the meaning of experiences for learners.
Humanism	Education must provide for learner autonomy and respect their dignity. It also must help individuals achieve self-actualization by developing their full potential.
Idealism	Individuals desire to live in a perfect world of high ideals, beauty, and art, and they search for ultimate truth. Education assists in this search.
Postmodernism	Education challenges convention, values a high tolerance for ambiguity, emphasizes diversity of culture and thought, and encourages innovation and change.
Pragmatism	Truth is relative to an individual's experience; therefore education must provide for "real-world" experiences.
Progressivism	The role of learners is to make choices about what is important, and the role of teachers is to facilitate their learning.
Realism	Education is designed to help learners understand the natural laws that regulate all of nature.
Reconstructionism	Education embraces the social ideal of a democratic life, and the school is viewed as the major vehicle for social change.

Adapted from Csokasy, J. (2009). Philosophical foundations of the curriculum. In D. M. Billings & J. A. Halstead, *Teaching in nursing: A guide for faculty*. St. Louis, MO: Saunders.

statement that guides their work. A discussion of three basic educational ideologies is presented here to point out how differences might arise if each person on a faculty were to approach education from her or his own belief system only.

One basic educational ideology is that of *romanticism* (Jarvis, 1995). This perspective, which emerged in the 1960s, is highly learner centered and asserts that what comes from within the learner is most important. Within this ideological perspective, one would construct an educational environment that is permissive and freeing; promotes creativity and discovery; allows each student's inner abilities to unfold and grow; and stresses the unique, the novel, and the personal. Bradshaw asserted that "this 'romantic' educational philosophy underpins current nurse education" (1998, p. 104); however, those who acknowledge our current "content-laden curricula" in nursing (Diekelmann, 2002; Diekelmann & Smythe, 2004; Giddens & Brady, 2007; Tanner, 2010) would disagree and posit that, although a "romantic" philosophy is embraced as an ideal, it is not always evident in our day-to-day practices.

A second educational ideology, that of *cultural transmission* (Bernstein, 1975), is more society- or culture-centered. Here the emphasis is on transmitting bodies of information, rules, values, and the culturally given (i.e., the beliefs and practices that are central to our educational environments and our society in general). One would expect an educational environment that is framed within a cultural transmission perspective to be structured, rigid, and controlled, with an emphasis on the common and the already established.

The third major educational ideology has been called *progressivism* (Dewey, 1944; Kohlberg & Mayer, 1972), where the focus is oriented toward the future and the goal of education is to nourish the learner's natural interaction with the world. Here the educational environment is designed to present resolvable but genuine problems or conflicts that "force" learners to think so that they can be effective later in life. The total development of learners—not merely their cognitive or intellectual abilities—is emphasized and enhanced.

Increasingly, education experts agree that development must be an overarching paradigm of education, students must be central to the educational enterprise, and education must be designed to empower learners and help them fulfill their potentials. Beliefs and values such as these surely would influence expectations faculty express regarding students' and their own performance, the relationships between students and teachers, how the curriculum is designed and implemented (see Figure 7-1), and the kind of "evidence" that is gathered to determine whether the curriculum has been successful and effective.

There is no doubt that a statement of philosophy for a school of nursing must address beliefs and values about education, teaching, and learning. However, it also must address other concepts that are critical to the practice of nursing, namely human beings, society and the environment, health, and the roles of nurses themselves. These major concepts have been referred to as the *metaparadigm of nursing,* a concept first introduced by Fawcett in 1984.

Central Concepts in a School of Nursing's Philosophy

Several central concepts are typically contained within a nursing school's statement of philosophy about which faculty communicate their beliefs and values. These concepts include beliefs about human beings, the societal or environmental context in which humans live and act, health, and nursing. Faculty may also add additional concepts about phenomena they hold to be particularly meaningful to the learning environment they are creating within their programs.

In preparing or revising the school of nursing's statement of philosophy, faculty must articulate their beliefs and values about *human beings,* including the individual patients for whom nurses care, patients' families, the communities in which patients live and work, students, and fellow nurses and faculty. It is inconsistent to express a belief that patients and families want to be involved in making decisions that affect them and then never give students an opportunity to make decisions that will affect them. Likewise, it is admirable to talk about respecting others, treating others with dignity, and valuing differences among people, but when faculty then treat one another in disrespectful ways or insist that everyone teach in the same way and do exactly the same thing, the validity of those expressed values must be questioned. Consider the following statements about human beings that might be expressed in a school's philosophy, keeping in mind that *human beings* refers to students, faculty, and administrators, as well as patients:

- Human beings are unique, complex, holistic individuals.
- Human beings have the inherent capacity for rational thinking, self-actualization, and growth throughout the life cycle.
- Human beings engage in deliberate action to achieve goals.
- Human beings want and have the right to be involved in making decisions that affect their lives.
- All human beings have strengths as well as weaknesses, and they often need support and guidance to capitalize on those strengths or to overcome or manage those weaknesses or limitations.
- All human beings are to be respected and valued.

Faculty also need to reflect on their beliefs and values related to *society and environment,* their effect on human beings, and the ways in which individuals and groups can influence their environments and society. The following statements may be ones to consider as faculty write or refine the philosophy of their school of nursing:

- Human beings interact in families, groups, and communities in an interdependent manner.
- Individuals, families, and communities reflect unique and diverse cultural, ethnic, experiential, and socioeconomic backgrounds.
- Human beings determine societal goals, values, and ethical systems.
- Society has responsibility for providing environments conducive to maximizing the health and well being of its members.
- Although human beings often must adapt to their environments, the environment also adapts to them in reciprocal ways.

Because the goal of nursing is to promote *health* and well being, faculty must consider the values and beliefs they hold about health. For example, the following statements express values and beliefs about health that a faculty might consider:

- Health connotes a sense of wholeness or integrity.
- Health is a goal to be attained.

- Health is the energy that sustains life, allows an individual to participate in a variety of human experiences, and supports one's ability to set and meet life goals.
- Health is a dynamic, complex state of being that human beings use as a resource to achieve their life goals; it is therefore a means to an end rather than an end in itself.
- Health can be promoted, maintained, or regained.
- Health is a right more than a privilege.
- All human beings must have access to quality health care.

Finally, it is critical for faculty to discuss their beliefs about *nurses* and *nursing* because this is the essence of our programs. In doing so, it may be important to reflect on the current and evolving roles of the nurse, the purpose of nursing, the ways in which nurses practice in collaboration with other health care professionals, and how one's identity as a nurse evolves. The following statements may stimulate thinking about beliefs and values related to nurses and nursing:

- Nursing is a human interactive process.
- The focus of nursing is to enhance human beings' capacity to take deliberate action for themselves and their dependent others regarding goals for optimal wellness.
- Nursing is a practice discipline that requires the deliberate use of specialized techniques and a broad range of scientific knowledge to design, deliver, coordinate, and manage care for complex individuals, families, groups, communities, and populations.
- Nurses are scholars who practice with scientific competence, intellectual maturity, and humanistic concern for others.
- The formation of one's identity as a nurse requires deep self-reflection, feedback from others, and a commitment to lifelong learning.
- Nurses must be educated at the university level.
- Nurses must be prepared to provide leadership within their practice settings and for the profession as a whole.
- Nurses collaborate with patients and other professionals as equal yet unique members of the health care team.
- Nurses are accountable for their own practice.

Box 7-1 provides examples of actual statements of philosophy regarding these components of the metaparadigm. These examples illustrate the beliefs of various groups of faculty, some of which may express vastly different perspectives and some of which express essentially the same idea but through different words.

BOX 7-1 Examples of Statements of Philosophy from Current Schools of Nursing

CLAYTON STATE UNIVERSITY SCHOOL OF NURSING

We believe that nursing is a dynamic, challenging profession that requires a synthesis of critical thinking skills and theory based practice to provide care for individuals, families, and communities experiencing a variety of developmental and health–illness transitions. Caring, which is at the heart of the nursing profession, involves the development of a committed, nurturing relationship, characterized by attentiveness to others and respect for their dignity, values, and culture. We believe that nursing practice must reflect an understanding of and respect for each individual and for human diversity.

Transitions involve a process of movement and change in fundamental life patterns, which are manifested in all individuals. Transitions cause changes in identities, roles, relationships, abilities, and patterns of behavior. Outcomes of transitional experiences are influenced by environmental factors interacting with the individual's perceptions, resources, and state of well-being. Negotiating successful transitions depends on the development of an effective relationship between the nurse and client. This relationship is a highly reciprocal process that affects both the client and nurse.

Clayton State University, School of Nursing, Morrow, GA. Retrieved from http://www.clayton.edu/health/Nursing/Philosophy

VILLANOVA UNIVERSITY COLLEGE OF NURSING

The Philosophy of the College of Nursing is in accord with the Philosophy of Villanova University as stated in its Mission Statement. While the Philosophy is rooted in the Catholic and Augustinian heritage of the university, the College of Nursing is welcoming and respectful of those from other faith traditions. We recognize human beings as unique and created by God. The faculty believes that human beings are physiological, psychological, social and spiritual beings, endowed with intellect, free will, and inherent dignity. Human beings have the potential to direct, integrate, and/or adapt to their total environment in order to meet their needs.

BOX 7-1 Examples of Statements of Philosophy from Current Schools of Nursing—cont'd

The faculty believes that education provides students with opportunities to develop habits of critical, constructive thought so that they can make discriminating judgments in their search for truth. This type of intellectual development can best be attained in a highly technologic teaching–learning environment that fosters sharing of knowledge, skills, and attitudes as well as scholarship toward the development of new knowledge. The faculty and students comprise a community of learners with the teacher as the facilitator and the students responsible for their own learning.

Villanova University College of Nursing, Villanova, PA. Retrieved from https://www1.villanova.edu/villanova/nursing/about/mission/college_philosophy.html

DUKE UNIVERSITY SCHOOL OF NURSING

Duke University School of Nursing is committed to achieving distinction in research, education, and patient care predicated on our beliefs regarding human beings, society and the environment, health and health care delivery, nursing, and teaching and learning.

Human Beings—We believe that the dignity of each human being is to be respected and nurtured, and embracing our diversity affirms, respects, and celebrates the uniqueness of each person. We believe that each human being is a unique expression of attributes, behaviors, and values which are influenced by his or her environment, social norms, cultural values, physical characteristics, experiences, religious beliefs, and practices. We also believe that human beings exist in relation to one another, including families, communities, and populations

Teaching/Learning—We believe that our purpose is to develop nurse leaders in practice, education, administration, and research by focusing on students' intellectual growth and development as adults committed to high ethical standards and full participation in their communities. We recognize that it is the responsibility of all individuals to assume ownership of and responsibility for ongoing learning and to continually refine the skills that facilitate critical inquiry for lifelong learning.

Duke University School of Nursing promotes an intellectual environment that is built on a commitment to free and open inquiry and is a center of excellence for the promotion of scholarship and advancement of nursing science, practice, and education. We affirm that it is the responsibility of faculty to create and nurture academic initiatives that strengthen our engagement of real world issues by anticipating new models of knowledge formation and applying knowledge to societal issues. This, we believe, equips students with the necessary cognitive skills, clinical reasoning, clinical imagination, professional identity, and commitment to the values of the profession that are necessary to function as effective and ethical nurse leaders in situations that are underdetermined, contingent, and changing over time.

Duke University School of Nursing, Durham, NC. Retrieved from http://nursing.duke.edu/about/academic-philosophy

Purpose of a Statement of Philosophy

Given that "doing philosophy" is hard work, takes time, and may lead to substantial debates among faculty, one may ask, "Why bother?" Perhaps part of the answer to that question lies in a statement made by Alexander Astin, a noted educational scholar whose seminal study (1997) of more than 20,000 students, 25,000 faculty members, and 200 institutions helped educators better understand who our students are; what is important to them; what they value; what they think about teachers; how they change and develop in college; and how academic programs, faculty, student peer groups, and other variables affect students' development and college experiences. Although Astin's original research was completed nearly 20 years ago and focused on traditional-age students enrolled, typically, on a full-time basis—thereby not fully reflecting today's student population—the following comment has relevance for this discussion of why faculty need to "bother" with philosophy: "The problems of strengthening and reforming American higher education are fundamentally problems of *values*" [emphasis added] (Astin, 1997, p. 127).

Engaging in serious discussions about beliefs and values—about human beings, society and environment, health, nurses and nursing, and education—challenges faculty to search for points of congruence, brings to the surface points of incongruence or difference, and highlights what is truly important to the group. In a time when nursing faculty are struggling to minimize content overload and focus more on core concepts, gaining clarity about what is truly important can be helpful in deciding "what to leave in and what to leave out" of the curriculum.

Such exercises also help faculty minimize or avoid what is often referred to as the "hidden curriculum" (Adler et al., 2006; D'eon et al., 2007; Gofton & Regehr, 2006; Smith, 2013) by ensuring that faculty are fully aware of and committed to upholding certain beliefs and values in how they interact with and what they expect of students and one another. Such agreement and consistency is likely to avoid having three components to the curriculum: "what is planned for the students, what is delivered to the students, and what the students experience" (Prideaux, as cited in Ozolins et al., 2008, p. 606). For example, the *plan* may be to help students think of themselves as evolving scholars; what is *delivered* is little more than content about the research process or evidence-based practice; and what is *experienced* by students is minimal discussion by faculty of their own scholarly activities and how they think of themselves as scholars. When what is delivered to and experienced by students does not match what was planned for them, confusion can reign, due process can be challenged, and the relationships between students and teachers can be irreparably damaged. Thus having clear statements of values to which all faculty agree to subscribe can serve a most practical, as well as philosophical, purpose.

Developing or Refining the School of Nursing's Statement of Philosophy

Developing or refining the school's statement of philosophy, while important and valuable, is far from easy. It takes time and effort and is not to be taken lightly. But just how does a group of faculty go about developing a philosophical statement for the school and getting "buy-in" on it? As expected, there are no formulas or step-by-step guidelines on how to go about doing this work, but some examples (Colley, 2012; Snyder, 2014; Thistlethwaite et al., 2014) and suggestions for a process may be helpful.

One approach to engaging in this work may include reflecting on the nursing theories that have been developed to determine if any of them capture the essence of faculty beliefs. For example, if faculty are in agreement that human beings are self-determining individuals who want to take responsibility for their own health and need specific knowledge, skills, and attitudes to do whatever is required to maintain, regain, or improve their health, then Orem's (1971) self-care nursing model may be evident in that school's statement of philosophy. Likewise, Roy's (1980) adaptation model may be reflected in the philosophical statement of a school where the faculty believe that a central challenge to individuals and families is to adapt to their environments and circumstances, and that the role of the nurse is to facilitate that adaptation. Finally, if the concept of caring is essential to a third group of faculty, their philosophy may clearly be congruent with Watson's (2008) theory of human caring.

Whether or not to acknowledge a single nursing theory in a school's statement of philosophy (and then use that theory to develop the school's conceptual framework, end-of-program outcomes or competencies, and other curriculum elements) has been debated in recent years. Those in favor of such an approach argue that it provides students with a way to "think nursing" and approach nursing situations in a way that clearly is nursing-focused, not medical model–focused, and that provides an opportunity to contribute to the ongoing development of the theory and therefore the science of nursing. Those against such an approach argue that it limits students' thinking and engages them with language and perspectives that are not likely to be widely encountered in practice, thereby making it difficult for graduates to communicate effectively with their nursing and health care team colleagues. Obviously, there is no one right answer to this debate. The key question to consider is whether the concepts that are central to a theory—nursing or otherwise—truly are congruent with the beliefs and values of the majority of faculty, because that is what a statement of philosophy must reflect.

The inductive approach can be most useful to faculty when developing or refining their philosophical statement; rather than selecting concepts from existing theories or policy statements or other literature, the faculty themselves generate concepts to include in the philosophy. For example, all faculty may be asked to list no more than five bullet items that express what they believe about each concept in the metaparadigm: human beings, society and environment, health, nurses and nursing, and education and teaching–learning. The responses in each category could then be compiled and faculty—perhaps in small groups—could then engage in an analysis of the items listed for each. These working groups might be asked to note the frequency with which specific ideas were mentioned, thereby identifying those points where there is great agreement and those where only one or a few faculty identified an idea. The fact that only a single faculty member or few faculty identify a particular belief or value, however, does not necessarily mean that it should be discarded. It is possible that other faculty simply did not think of that idea as they were creating their own lists, or it is possible that other faculty did identify the idea but did not include it because they were limited to five bullet items. The compilation from each working group could then be shared with the entire faculty. At this point, a discussion about the meaning and significance of the statements in each category could ensue, or faculty could be asked to review each list, select the three to five statements they believe are most critical to include in the philosophy, and then engage in dialogue about why they selected those statements, what those statements mean to individuals, and so on. A draft statement of philosophy—one that has evolved from an inductive, bottom-up process—could then be written by an individual or small group and circulated to faculty for comment and further discussion.

Another approach that might be used combines deduction—or drawing on existing literature, standards, or policy documents—with induction, or generating ideas "from the ground up" by interviewing faculty. An individual faculty member—one who is viewed as a leader in the group, who is respected and trusted by her or his peers, who has good writing skills, and who is knowledgeable about curriculum development—may be asked to talk to faculty about their beliefs about human beings, society and environment, and so on, and use that input to draft a statement of philosophy that incorporates what faculty expressed. This draft could then be circulated to all faculty for comment, editing, and revision. The original writer would then revise the statement based on feedback from colleagues and present the new statement to the group for discussion and dialogue. This back-and-forth process would continue until there is consensus about what to include in the statement.

In either of these scenarios, or when a philosophical statement already exists but is being reviewed for possible updating and revision, "clickers"—simple online, anonymous surveys—can be used to get a sense of faculty agreement or endorsement. With this approach, each sentence in the draft (or existing) philosophy is listed as a separate item and faculty are asked to indicate the extent to which they agree (e.g., Strongly Agree, Agree, Disagree, or Strongly Disagree). Instead of using the entire sentence as the item to be responded to, it may be more helpful to use phrases or major concepts within each sentence as the item. Regardless of the degree of detail in each item, the anonymous responses can then be compiled, the results shared with the entire faculty, and discussions held to explore the meaning of the data obtained.

Finally, the entire process—whether it involves starting from an existing philosophy or creating a new one—can be prompted or stimulated by the thinking of those outside the school of nursing. For example, faculty may be assigned to review major contemporary documents or reports—for example, the Carnegie study (Benner et al., 2010), the *Future of Nursing* report (Institute of Medicine, 2010), accreditation standards, or published articles about employers' assessment of what new graduates can and cannot do. In reviewing those reports, faculty might identify values that are expressed or implied, beliefs about patients and nurses, or societal expectations related to health, health care, and the role of the nurse. Those values and beliefs could then be compiled and faculty asked to reflect on the extent to which they are aligned with the beliefs of the faculty. Through an iterative process such as one of those described previously, the group could craft its own statement of philosophy, one that has been informed by the larger context in which the educational programs exist.

Regardless of the process used, it is critical that all faculty be involved and that adequate time and safe environments be provided for faculty to disagree, struggle, contemplate, rethink, debate, and "do philosophy." Ending the process prematurely is not likely to be wise. It also is important to remember that this is an iterative process that will continue, to some extent, throughout all of the subsequent steps of curriculum development. For example, the statement of philosophy may have been endorsed and approved-in-concept by faculty, but as various groups work on developing course syllabi, they may generate questions about "what we really meant" by something in the philosophy. Should this occur, it would be worthwhile to revisit the philosophical statement and make revisions to it, if such revisions will lead to greater clarity about its meaning.

The preceding discussion has focused exclusively on the role of faculty in the creation or revision of the school's philosophy. It is assumed that school administrators (e.g., dean, program chair) are faculty who also must be involved in this process. Additionally, consideration should be given to including students in dialogue about beliefs and values; however, in the end, the final document must reflect what faculty believe and are guided by regarding human beings, society and environment, health, nurses and nursing, and education and teaching–learning.

The final statement of philosophy should be clearly written, internally consistent, and easily understood, and should give clear direction for all that follows. It should be long enough to clearly express the significant beliefs and values that guide faculty actions but not excessively detailed, as expressions of detail (rather than fundamental beliefs) often are more congruent with the work that must be done in formulating the conceptual framework, end-of-program outcomes or competencies, and curriculum design. Later chapters explore all of those subsequent curriculum development steps in detail (see Figure 7-1), so only a few examples of how the philosophy gives direction to the development, implementation, and evaluation of the curriculum are offered here.

Implications of the Philosophical Statement for the Curriculum

If the statements included in the school of nursing's philosophy reflect what the faculty truly believe—and are not merely words on a page to "get the task done"—then those values should be evident in how the curriculum is designed, how it is implemented, and how it is evaluated. Examples of this influence are presented in Box 7-2 as if–then statements.

It is hoped that these examples, combined with the detail provided in subsequent chapters, reinforce the importance of the philosophy. Faculty aim to establish positive relationships with students, clinical partners, alumni, administrators, and each other; one way to achieve that goal is to be clear about the values we share and, more importantly, to "live" those values in everything we say and do.

BOX 7-2 Examples of If–Then Statements Regarding Implications of the Philosophical Statement for the Development, Implementation, and Evaluation of the Curriculum

IF *THE PHILOSOPHICAL STATEMENT SAYS . . .*	THEN *ONE WOULD EXPECT TO SEE . . .*
We believe that human beings should have choices regarding what they do . . .	Free, unrestricted elective courses in the curriculum, or choice among several courses to meet a degree requirement (e.g., English)
We believe that human beings engage in deliberate action to achieve goals . . .	Opportunities throughout the curriculum for students to write their own learning goals and collaborate with faculty or clinical staff to design unique learning experiences to achieve those goals
We believe that individuals reflect unique and diverse cultural, ethnic, experiential, and socioeconomic backgrounds . . .	Face-to-face or virtual experiences with a wide variety of patient populations and within communities having a range of resources and challenges
We believe that health can be promoted, maintained, or regained . . .	Equally distributed clinical learning experiences in wellness settings, with patients and families who are managing chronic illnesses, and in acute care settings
We believe that nurses are scholars who practice with scientific competence and intellectual maturity . . .	Courses and learning experiences that expose students to the concept of scholarship, what it means to be a scholar, and how one develops and maintains scientific competence
We believe that nurses must be prepared to provide leadership within their practice settings and for the profession as a whole . . .	Courses and learning experiences that help students appreciate the differences between leadership and management, study nursing leaders, and reflect on their own path toward becoming a leader

BOX 7-2 Examples of If–Then Statements Regarding Implications of the Philosophical Statement for the Development, Implementation, and Evaluation of the Curriculum—cont'd

We believe that nurses collaborate with patients and other professionals as equal yet unique members of the health care team . . .	Face-to-face or virtual experiences where nursing students learn with students preparing for other professional roles, dialogue with or interview members of other health care professions, or undertake projects that call for interprofessional collaboration to meet the health needs of a patient population or community
We believe that the goal of teaching is to awaken the learner's natural curiosity . . .	Problem-based learning experiences where students must identify what it is they need to know to address a problem, seek out that information, judge its quality, ask questions about established practices, and so on
We believe that education involves nurturing students and pulling them forth to a new place . . .	A program evaluation plan that incorporates open forums with students about the extent to which they feel nurtured, supported, and challenged by faculty; dialogue with graduates about how their educational experience changed them as human beings; and surveys of students and alumni regarding the contributions they have made in their practice settings and to the profession

Summary

As noted earlier, "doing philosophy" is hard work. However, it is important and valuable work that has implications for faculty and our practice as teachers, as well as for our students.

"Doing philosophy" may prompt us to attend more deliberately to affective domain learning and identity formation as we design learning experiences and interact with students, a focus that is likely to enhance their educational experience. It may challenge us to ask new questions about our practice as teachers and seek answers to those questions through rigorous pedagogical research efforts, an effort that can contribute to the development of the science of nursing education. It also may direct us to seek out new teaching strategies and evaluation methods that better facilitate student learning, an outcome that may serve to maintain the joy in teaching as we see students become excited about their formation as nurses.

One can conclude that the philosophical foundations of the curriculum extend far beyond mere program designs and course syllabi. Reflections on and clarity regarding those philosophical foundations can help us better understand who we are and how we can best help our students, our colleagues, and ourselves to grow and continue to learn.

REFLECTING ON THE EVIDENCE

1. Although faculty share a commitment to the values of the profession, they are likely to have varied beliefs about the implications of those and other values, particularly in relation to how they "play out" in the educational arena. What effect can such differences have on students? How can such differences be resolved?
2. How can faculty "track" congruence of beliefs, values, and significant concepts from mission, vision, and values to philosophy to framework to end-of-program outcomes and competencies and on through specific learning experiences that are designed for students? How can they assess the congruence of these beliefs and values with their own personal beliefs?
3. What are some signs that a "hidden curriculum" is operating where faculty say one thing but do another, or where beliefs expressed in the philosophy (e.g., nurses must be involved in professional associations) are not evident in what students experience (e.g., faculty never talk about their involvement in professional associations)? What implications might such signals have for reexamining the school's philosophical underpinnings?

REFERENCES

Adler, S. R., Hughes, E. F., & Scott, R. B. (2006). Student "moles": Revealing the hidden curriculum. *Medical Education, 40,* 463–464.

Astin, A. W. (1997). *What matters in college? Four critical years revisited.* San Francisco, CA: Jossey-Bass.

Benner, P., Leonard, V., Day, L., & Sutphen, M. (2010). *Educating nurses: A call for radical transformation.* San Francisco, CA: Jossey-Bass.

Bernstein, B. (1975). *Class, codes and control: Volume III—towards a theory of educational transmission.* New York, NY: Routledge.

Bevis, E. O. (1989). *Curriculum building: A process* (3rd ed.). New York: National League for Nursing.

Bradshaw, A. (1998). Defining "competency" in nursing (part II): An analytic review. *Journal of Clinical Nursing, 7,* 103–111.

Colley, S. L. (2012). Implementing as change to a learner-centered philosophy in a school of nursing: Faculty perspectives. *Nursing Education Perspectives, 33*(4Z), 229–233.

D'eon, M., Lear, N., Turner, M., & Jones, C. (2007). Perils of the hidden curriculum revisited. *Medical Teacher, 29,* 295–296.

Dewey, J. (1944). *Democracy and education: An introduction to the philosophy of education.* New York: The Free Press.

Diekelmann, N. (2002). "Too much content ..." Epistemologies' grasp and nursing education (Teacher Talk). *Journal of Nursing Education, 41*(11), 469–470.

Diekelmann, N., & Smythe, E. (2004). Covering content and the additive curriculum: How can I use my time with students to best help them learn what they need to know? (Teacher Talk). *Journal of Nursing Education, 43*(8), 341–344.

Emerson, E. (1921). *The complete writings of Ralph Waldo Emerson.* In E. Emerson (Ed.), New York: Wm. H. Wise & Co.

Fawcett, J. (1984). The metaparadigm of nursing: Present status and future refinements. *Image: The Journal of Nursing Scholarship, 16*(3), 84–86.

France, A. (1894). *The crime of Sylvestre Bonnard translated by Lafcadio Hearn in The works of Anatole France in an English Translation (1920).* London: J. Lane Publishers.

Giddens, J. F., & Brady, D. P. (2007). Rescuing nursing education from content saturation: The case for a concept-based curriculum. *Journal of Nursing Education, 46*(2), 65–69.

Gofton, W., & Regehr, G. (2006). What we don't know we are teaching: Unveiling the hidden curriculum. *Clinical Orthopaedics and Related Research, 449,* 20–27.

Gordon, S. (1991). *Prisoners of men's dreams: Striking out for a new feminine future.* Boston: Little, Brown.

Greene, M. (1973). *Teacher as stranger: Educational philosophy in a modern age.* Belmont, CA: Wadsworth.

Institute of Medicine. (2010). *The future of nursing: Leading change, advancing health.* Washington, DC: The National Academies Press.

Jarvis, P. (1995). *Adult and continuing education.* London, UK: Routledge.

Kohlberg, L., & Mayer, R. (1972). Development as the aim of education. *Harvard Educational Review, 42*(2), 449–496.

Orem, D. (1971). *Nursing: Concepts of practice.* New York: McGraw-Hill.

Ozolins, I., Hall, H., & Peterson, R. (2008). The student voice: Recognizing the hidden and informal curriculum in medicine. *Medical Teacher, 30,* 606–611.

Palmer, P. (2007). *The courage to teach: Exploring the inner landscape of a teacher's life.* San Francisco, CA: Jossey-Bass.

Roy, C., Sr. (1980). The Roy adaptation model. In J. P. Riehl & C. Roy (Eds.), *Conceptual models for nursing practice* (pp. 179–188). Norwalk, CT: Appleton, Century Crofts.

Smith, B. (2013). *Mentoring at-risk students through the hidden curriculum of higher education.* Lanham, MD: Lexington Books.

Snyder, M. (2014). Emancipatory knowing: Empowering nursing students toward reflection and action. *Journal of Nursing Education, 53*(2), 65–69.

Tabak, N., Adi, I., & Eherenfeld, M. (2003). A philosophy underlying excellence in teaching. *Nursing Philosophy, 4,* 249–254.

Tanner, C. A. (2010). Transforming prelicensure nursing education: Preparing the new nurse to meet emerging health care needs. *Nursing Education Perspectives, 31*(6), 347–353.

Thistlethwaite, J. E., Forman, D., Matthews, L. R., Rogers, G. D., Steketee, C., & Yassine, T. (2014). Competencies and frameworks in interprofessional education: A comparative analysis. *Academic Medicine, 89*(6), 1–7.

Watson, J. (2008). *Nursing: The philosophy and science of caring* (Rev. Ed.). Boulder, CO: University Press of Colorado.

8 Curriculum Models for Undergraduate Programs*

Susan M. Hendricks, EdD, RN, CNE

In this era of unprecedented health care change, opportunities abound for nursing faculty to develop undergraduate curriculum models that respond to emerging challenges and foster innovative thinking. When faculty teaching in an undergraduate nursing program discuss curriculum, they usually are referring to the plan or course of study for a group of students leading to licensure. However, the idea of curriculum considered more broadly should include *what* is taught, *how* it is organized, *how* it is taught (such as delivery method and pedagogy), and *what* student and program outcomes are intended. Dezure (2010) argues that the concept of curriculum should be broad and dynamic, accounting for innovations in methods, sequencing, goals, and content.

A well-conceived curriculum is critical to the preparation of entry-level nurses. Undergraduate curricula in all disciplines have been under increasing scrutiny for the last two decades. There have been a number of reports since the 1980s that have been critical of higher education, suggesting that reform is needed if graduates are to meet the expectations of business and industry (Dezure, 2010). These calls for reform led to a number of initiatives that continue to influence undergraduate curricula today, such as the introduction of learning outcomes in the language of competencies, emphasis on integration of learning experiences, focus on enhancing and streamlining learning, and growth in learning from a more global perspective (Dezure, 2010). Today the priority for learning is not so much on *what* is learned, as much as it is on what graduates can *do* with their learning. For nursing, the curriculum must prepare graduates to function in a dynamic and increasingly complex health care environment.

*The author acknowledges the contributions of Donna Boland, PhD, RN, in previous editions of this chapter.

The challenge facing nurse educators is how to reenvision curriculum to prepare nurses to practice in a changing health care system and proactively create learning that prepares graduates to flourish. Tanner (2010) suggests that the critical questions that curricula designs need to address are what must be taught, how to teach it effectively and efficiently, and where teaching and learning should occur to achieve the best outcomes. Dezure (2010) indicates that the curriculum shifts that shape curricula today are the move to broad learning competencies from a narrower focus on mastery of learning specific content, a shift to more integrative learning experiences from those that emphasize specific skill sets, and an exploration of innovative teaching practices beyond the traditional pedagogical approaches designed to deliver subject matter.

Within the nursing profession, undergraduate curricular design must be flexible. Benner, Sutphen, Leonard, and Day (2010) have called for radical curriculum transformation to best prepare nurses to practice and lead. This transformative process needs to focus on how to design or revise curricula without simply adding onto curricula that are already overloaded with content. Faculty have historically viewed curriculum revisions that meet student learning needs from a content perspective rather than a contextual perspective. As new technologies emerge, new evidence is discovered, and new best practices are identified, they are too often packed into a curriculum structure that is already saturated with content. Instead of simply continuing to add content to the curriculum, the most critical challenge for faculty planning undergraduate curricula is to determine what students need to learn to practice competently and how to design learning experiences that will facilitate acquisition of needed competencies. Mackey, Hatcher, Happell, and Cleary (2013) call for preparation of nurses to practice in new and varied environments, such as the home, community, and through the use of technology. They assert that nurses must be prepared to effectively respond to the social determinants of health, in addition to the physical needs of their patients. This shift will require faculty to redefine what has been identified as traditional competencies critical to nursing practice to more deeply encompass competencies associated with practicing in communities, with populations, and considering the nurse's key role in facilitating transitions in care. Furthermore, as the care environment changes to include new treatment modalities, such as telehealth, consumer devices, and programs that facilitate health, competencies should be modified to reflect these changes. This chapter discusses undergraduate program and curriculum designs. It is important to reflect on the issues that continue to shape nursing curricula as faculty make decisions about the design of curriculum in their programs.

Essential Purposes of Undergraduate Education in Nursing

Undergraduate nursing curricula are primarily designed to prepare students for entry into practice. In addition, some curricula are designed as academic progression models for registered nurses (RNs) to achieve a bachelor of science in nursing (BSN) degree or licensed practical or vocational nurses (LPN/LVN) to pursue an RN degree. Undergraduate curricula also provide a foundation essential to graduate education and advanced nursing practice. In recent years, some health care agencies have been reframing requirements for RN employment with acute care agencies often preferring or requiring applicants to hold a bachelor's degree in nursing. Designing curricula that facilitate the academic progression of the nursing workforce (National League for Nursing [NLN], 2011) will be imperative to achieve the Institute of Medicine (Institute of Medicine [IOM], 2010) recommendations for increasing numbers of baccalaureate and advanced degree–prepared nurses and to meet market demands.

The increased expectation for public accountability has expanded the visibility of nursing education at the national, state, and local levels, which has also increased stakeholder involvement in the education and practice of nurses. As a professional educational degree program, nursing is among the most regulated educational enterprises on higher education campuses. One advantage of regulation for nursing programs is the high level of scrutiny to which they are subjected, and the assurance of minimum standards for most schools of nursing, providing a competent workforce for patient care. Making use of the relative similarities in curriculum plans that exist across nursing programs, in part resulting from regulatory requirements, faculty have adapted plans of study to facilitate articulation and academic progression. A disadvantage to this level of control is the perceived negative effect of prescriptive guidance and rules on innovation; faculty may be discouraged from pursuing new ideas for curriculum organization, content, and teaching methodologies, perceiving too many impediments to innovate.

Compared with curricula in other disciplines, nursing curricula across multiple schools often look quite homogeneous. This does ensure that new graduates have been exposed to knowledge that is commonly accepted to be essential to practice, but on the other hand, having a large body of knowledge that faculty perceive to be essential can potentially stifle innovation. Perhaps this is one reason that examples of innovative curricular responses to the changing environment have been a challenge to initiate. However, innovation is occurring in the area of transforming curricula to meet the needs of more nontraditional students, students pursuing a second degree, and those with unique needs, leading to more creativity and flexibility in curriculum construction and delivery. The expected outcome is to entice, retain, and graduate a diverse population of students.

Historical Influences for Understanding Today's Undergraduate Curricula

Florence Nightingale is considered to be the founder of modern nursing. As a prolific writer who spoke in eloquent tones about the education and practice of nurses, Nightingale envisioned nursing as more than the understanding of disease. She is quoted as having said, "Pathology teaches the harm that disease has done. But it teaches nothing more" (Nightingale, 1969, p. 133). Her nursing orientation focused on health as a broad and encompassing concept that requires an understanding of human nature and the ability of that nature to affect individual health. Nightingale's thinking that nurses need to acquire an understanding of the science and art of human existence has continued to permeate undergraduate education from its original, hospital-based training programs to its current degree-granting educational programs.

Traditionally, nursing philosophy and theory have been crucial to nursing curricula because philosophy and theory state what nursing is and what it should be. Nursing theorists, starting with Nightingale, have provided nursing with the theoretical foundation for educational philosophies, mission statements, curriculum models, and delivery of curriculum content. Despite differing beliefs posited among recognized nursing theorists, they, like the curriculum models that have been predicated on their thinking, have focused on the nature of humans, society, and nursing practice. It appears that the previous emphasis on the roles of nursing philosophy and theory in design of nursing curricula is decreasing as the emphasis has shifted to one that is more outcome-driven. Donohue-Porter, Forbes, and White (2011) point out that as our undergraduate curricula have become saturated with content, the focus on nursing theory has diminished, leading to curriculum structures that are very content-laden, with decreased focus on the theoretical organizing structures of knowledge that allow students to integrate knowledge into practical action. The concept-based movement in curriculum development is one means by which to address the concern about overly content-laden curricula.

The desire to understand human nature and society is still a prevailing factor shaping current undergraduate curricula, especially nursing curricula. Theory that is effectively used in the construction of curricula and teaching–learning methodologies can counter the focus on nurses mainly as "doers" rather than "thinkers" that is often a perception of students in nursing education programs today (Grealish & Smale, 2011). An example of a curriculum structure that effectively uses theory to facilitate integrative thinking is the Popoola holistic praxis model (Popoola, 2012) in which a planned framework of theoretical concepts are organized into a program of study that emphasizes the explicit use of multiple theories throughout the nursing curriculum.

Factors Influencing Undergraduate Program Design

Multiple factors influence the design and development of undergraduate nursing curricula. Nursing curricula should reflect the mission, vision, and values espoused by the university or college, while retaining congruence with the school's philosophy and vision. Further, significant national and international reports create calls to action and change. Along with these influences, schools of nursing design curricula with particular learner characteristics in mind. In planning nursing curricula, schools of nursing must also respond to the expectations of key stakeholders, such as accreditors and boards of nursing. Further, because nursing programs prepare students for licensed practice, attention to licensing requirements is important—successfully licensed students are a publicly recognized marker of program quality. Finally, faculty constructing curricula for nursing programs should consider the present and future trends in health and health care that are likely to affect nurses' practice in the coming years. Although predicting the future issues and needs in health care is an uncertain activity, without such vision, schools of nursing will consistently lag behind the rapidly changing health care environment, to the detriment of the profession.

Faculty designing curricula that meet these extensive design factors require creativity, political savvy, negotiation skills, analytical rigor, psychic energy, and a sense of teamwork. Faculty involved in designing programs and building curricula must possess a clear sense of purpose, a commitment to procuring resources, an understanding of market forces, the ability to anticipate health care trends of the future, and the ability to know when goals have been accomplished. Once programs are designed, curriculum building and revision should continue in a continuous quality improvement process that is related to, but separate from, the acts of teaching and learning. Curriculum is a dynamic, evolving entity shaped by learner needs and faculty beliefs about the science and art of nursing.

Design for Congruence with School and Organizational Forces

Schools of nursing operate in a myriad of different environments, each with a particular world view, set of implicit or explicit values, and encompassing a mission and vision. Faculty working to devise curricula should consider the values, mission, and vision of the parent organization as they develop courses, teaching–learning strategies, and educational outcomes. Mission and vision statements often encompass particular worldviews about the nature and importance of teaching, scholarship, and service; include statements about particular professional values; and also often delineate the scope and focus of areas and populations of interest—such as a focus on the local community, statewide needs, and national and international areas of concern. See Chapter 7 for further discussion of the relationship of mission, vision, and values to curriculum development.

Responding to Major Calls for Reform

One of the ongoing challenges of curriculum development is staying abreast of the many different calls for reform from professional organizations, institutes, and research findings that have the potential to affect nursing practice. When creating nursing curricula for the twenty-first century, Glasgow, Dunphy, and Mainous (2010) recommend that curricula be focused on the integration of science and research and the influences resulting from health care policies. Benner et al. (2010) work on transforming nursing education to some degree complements the recommendations of Glasgow and colleagues. Grown out of her research efforts, Benner and colleagues identified four "shifts" that should guide curriculum design based on the evidence she has collected: a shift toward teaching for a sense of the most important aspects of a situation and related key actions in particular situations; a movement toward integration of didactic and clinical education; a renewed focus on clinical reasoning and many ways of thinking that include critical thinking; and a renewed emphasis on professional formation, much more than simply functioning in a particular role.

The guiding principles that the American Organization of Nurse Executives (AONE), (2010) identified are more prescriptive in nature than those proposed by Benner and colleagues, but also need to be taken into consideration when designing undergraduate curricula, especially those that lead to a baccalaureate degree. The guiding principles are not focused on content, but rather how to access, synthesize, and manage the "knowledge work" of nursing, delivered in the context of a caring, patient-centered environment. The guiding principles also emphasize the importance of interdisciplinary and patient relationships in the delivery of care. Quality and safety are considered to be core concepts to care delivery (American Organization of Nurse Executives, 2010).

In translating some of the expectations of the Institute of Medicine [IOM] (2001, 2010) work into nursing curriculum operating principles, faculty will need to focus on improving the health and functioning of people; preparing students to deliver health care in a safe, effective, patient-centered, timely, efficient, and equitable fashion; and developing competencies to establish care benchmarks and evaluate the outcomes of care according to these benchmarks. The Quality and Safety Education for Nurses (QSEN) competencies have also taken a prominent place in the undergraduate nursing curriculum. Based on the work of Cronenwett et al. (2007) the QSEN Institute has developed competency statements for quality and safety knowledge, skills, and behaviors or attitudes (KSAs) across undergraduate curricula (see www.qsen.org). Many schools of nursing have used either the entire set of KSAs or have mapped their own curricula to this significant body of work.

In another important call for action, the World Health Organization (WHO) published a key report, the *Framework for Action on Interprofessional Education and Collaborative Practice* (2010), issuing a global call for interprofessional health education with the stated goal of improving patient health outcomes worldwide. The WHO asserted there is ample evidence showing that interprofessional education leads to interprofessional collaborative practice. Following this report, the Interprofessional Education Collaborative Expert Panel (2011) published a set of core competencies for interprofessional collaborative practice, including learning outcomes that apply to all health professionals. These two key reports have fostered an international movement toward interprofessional health education that has been endorsed by multiple professional organizations and has relevance for development of undergraduate nursing curricula. See Chapter 11 for a further discussion of interprofessional education and collaborative practice.

Finally, as schools of nursing aim to graduate a workforce that is diverse and representative of the communities served, many have crafted programs aimed to attract and retain a diverse student body. *Diversity* is defined in a myriad of ways, including ethnic and gender diversity, as well as diversity in sexual and gender orientation, socioeconomic status, and even experience. Achieving classes of students who are rich in diverse experience and who mirror the population who will be served by graduates is a focus for many schools of nursing today.

See Chapter 16 for further discussion about achieving inclusivity in the classroom.

Meeting Learner Characteristics through Curriculum Design

With the current emphasis on student learning and student engagement, it is important that curricula be designed to promote the development of individual students. This can be accomplished in part by encouraging interrelationships among the learners, faculty, and what is being learned. Additional factors affecting program design and student development include focusing on health and well-being of society; grounding learning in contemporary evidence; creating a learning environment that is infused with experientially and culturally based learning opportunities; and supporting individual creativity especially as it relates to inquiry, problem solving, and reflection.

For students in undergraduate programs, faculty designing curriculum should consider the particular population of learners that will be served. If there will be a predominance of learners with English as a second language (ESL), strategies for facilitating their success with reading, writing, and testing will be important. If the students in an academic progression program are working in health care and seeking an additional degree (i.e., LPN to associate of science in nursing (ASN) or RN to BSN), learning activities and schedules should be conceived to meet learner needs—being flexible, applicable to "real-world" applications and work experiences, and realistic in terms of pace of the number and type of assignments. Students seeking a second degree appreciate recognition for prior learning, and respond well to a rigorous academic environment. When creating curricula for this population of learners, affording the learners the chance to draw connections between prior degrees and professional work experiences to the field of nursing creates a bridge to exemplary practice that is valued by participants. See Chapter 2 for further discussion about the diverse learning needs of students.

Addressing Stakeholder Expectations

The effect of stakeholder expectations on prelicensure nursing education cannot be overstated: state boards of nursing, nursing accrediting agencies, and the U.S. Department of Education have had tremendous influence on both design and delivery. Today, state boards of nursing are variable in how prescriptive they are relative to nursing curriculum—but they do influence content taught, clinical requirements, and pedagogy. Accreditation criteria are clear influencers regarding criteria to be met in curricular construction, and they are becoming more so as the U.S. Department of Education becomes more explicit in its emphasis on outcome data specified in its standards for recognizing professional accreditation bodies (U.S. Department of Education, 2010).

Furthermore, although it is expected that nursing faculty will use professional standards to shape curricula, sometimes faculty rely on such standards without considering other sources for content and teaching methodology or without considering the unique mission of their own institution. One can look to *The Essentials of Baccalaureate Education for Professional Nursing Practice* (American Association of Colleges of Nursing [AACN], 2013) and the Commission for Collegiate Nursing Education (CCNE) (2009) requirement that programs accredited by CCNE must incorporate them into the curriculum, as an example of how accrediting bodies can influence program development and curricula design.

Professional standards offer critical guidance for nursing programs, but faculty should also attend to other factors relevant in their own institution's mission, their own learners' needs, and the needs of the health care agencies and communities served by the school's graduates. See Chapter 26 for additional information about curriculum evaluation and Chapter 27 for a further discussion of the accreditation process.

Addressing Future Trends in the Design of Prelicensure Curricula

Schools of nursing that are nimble and able to respond to future trends in nursing and health care will be able to maintain a curriculum that prepares learners for their future practice. Faculty who persist in monitoring and responding to identified trends, and who are able to revise curricula in a timely manner, will be rewarded with a curriculum plan that is future oriented and relevant.

Numerous health care trends are predicted to have a major effect on nursing practice at the licensed practical and registered nursing level. Trends that are currently prevalent in health care and well on their way to becoming essential aspects of the nursing role include interprofessional practice competencies, understanding global health challenges, genetics, and genomics. A focus on patient-centered outcomes and further integration of quality and safety concepts into the curriculum will continue. Tella et al. (2014) completed an integrative review of patient safety education practices and their outcomes in schools of nursing and found a wide variety of approaches in this focus area for nursing curriculum.

Other current issues and trends in health care include providing nursing care that is veteran-centric; responding to new care roles to enhance care navigation, health coaching, and telehealth; and use of continuous quality improvement methodologies to enhance the efficiency and reliability of nursing and health care. Kovner, Brewer, Fatehi, and Katigbak (2014) stated the employment patterns of newly licensed RNs is shifting from a heavy focus on acute care more toward care provision in the community; thus nursing curricula need to prepare graduates for this anticipated shift in the care environment. Additionally, building curricula that address workplace readiness and promote healthy work environments (including issues such as civility, bullying, and readiness for practice) has taken on significance in recent years as the cost of high turnover among new nurses is realized—the cost is high in patient safety outcomes, patient satisfaction, nursing job satisfaction, and cost.

Undergraduate Program Models

Various undergraduate nursing program models have been developed to facilitate multiple entry points into the profession and to encourage undergraduate students to pursue graduate study early in their nursing careers. Generally there are many similarities among the program models, with variations occurring within the internal configuration of courses and course content.

Prelicensure nursing programs include those for the LPN, LVN, and RN. For the preparation of RNs, the three most common traditional program models include the 2-year associate degree, the 4-year baccalaureate degree, and the 3-year diploma program. In addition to these three educational models, there are accelerated baccalaureate programs as well as accelerated graduate degree nursing programs for those students who already hold a nonnursing degree. For example, students with previous nonnursing academic degrees may choose to pursue an accelerated bachelor's degree or generic master's degree program, or a clinical nurse leader program. Streamlined academic pathways for undergraduate students that lead to doctoral studies are also available. Diploma, associate, and baccalaureate degree program designs are discussed in further detail in this section, as are LPN and LVN programs. Academic progression models are also addressed.

Licensed Practical and Vocational Programs

LPN programs, also known as LVN programs in some regions of the country, provide an opportunity for many individuals to first enter the nursing workforce. LPN programs are typically 1 year in length and are taught in community colleges and vocational schools. LPNs are employed in structured environments, with approximately 20% employed in hospitals, 29% in long-term care, and 12% in physician's offices, as of 2012 (Bureau of Labor Statistics, U.S. Department of Labor, 2014). It is estimated that the demand for LPNs is expected to grow 25% between 2012 and 2022, mainly because of the expected need for residential care facilities and home health services for the aging baby boomer population. The importance of the growing role for the LPN in the nation's health care system and the importance of developing curricula that adequately prepare LPNs for this role was recently addressed in the NLN's (2014) *Vision for Recognition of the Role of Licensed Practical/Vocational Nurses in Advancing the Nation's Health.* Additionally, a curriculum framework based on the NLN Outcomes and Competencies model (2010) has been developed for LPN/LVN curricula and can be found at www.nln.org under Faculty Development and Resources—LPN Curriculum Resources.

Individuals who are first licensed as LPNs frequently return to school to pursue licensure as RNs, thus increasing their levels of responsibility and accountability within the health care environment. Providing avenues of academic progression for LPNs that recognize their previous learning and experience will continue to be an important component of nursing education academic progression programs.

Diploma Programs

Diploma programs represent the first curriculum model developed for training nurses in the late nineteenth and early to mid-twentieth centuries. Initially affiliated with hospitals, many of today's diploma schools of nursing are also affiliated with institutions of higher education. Diploma programs prepare technical nurses who provide direct patient care in a variety of health care settings. Typically the curriculum is designed to be completed in 3 years and provides an emphasis on clinical practice. General education courses in the biological and social sciences are provided through affiliation with a local college or university. These college course credits can commonly be applied toward a baccalaureate degree in nursing if the student chooses to continue his or her education. With the shift of nursing education into colleges and universities, diploma schools have been gradually closing during the last 30 years, reconfiguring themselves as single-purpose institutions, or merging with existing colleges or universities. Diploma programs compose fewer than 10% of nursing programs educating students in the United States (American Association of Colleges of Nursing [AACN], 2011).

Associate Degree Programs

ASN or associate degree in nursing (ADN) programs were first envisioned in 1952 by Mildred Montag in response to a critical nursing shortage. The intent of the associate degree programs, as originally conceived by Montag, was to prepare in 2 academic years a technical nurse who would provide direct patient care in acute care settings under the supervision of a professional nurse (Dillon, 1997). Despite the persistent call for increasing the level of preparation of the RN, associate degree programs continue to be very popular. According to the Health Resources and Services Administration (HRSA), (2010), in 2008 the percentage was approximately 45.4%. As acute care agencies push for increased numbers of BSN-prepared nurses, the trend is clear that many ASN/ADN nurses are returning to school to pursue baccalaureate or graduate nursing degrees.

Associate degree programs are often situated in community colleges, and have served local community needs for a registered nursing workforce for years. As the demand for registered nurses has increased, associate degree nurses have been an important way workforce needs have been met. As the complexity of the professional nursing role has increased, and the expectations for practice in rapidly changing environments, associate degree nursing programs have responded (Robert Wood Johnson Foundation [RWJF], 2013). One challenge inherent in this response, however, is the difficulty of incorporating a large body of complex information and skills into an associate degree. Some programs have responded by increasing the credits in the program beyond the typical number (60) in a two-year degree, a solution that may extend the program length. As increased attention is placed on the costs of higher education and the amount of student loan debt incurred by students, the number of credits required in associate degree programs is coming under more intense scrutiny. It will be important for faculty who design and revise curriculum plans for ASN/ADN programs to consider the number of credits they are requiring in their programs, and consider ways to ensure that the curricula remain free of excess credit hours.

The curriculum of associate degree programs commonly consists of nursing courses that include concepts and content related to the practice of medical–surgical, pediatric, maternity, and psychiatric–mental health nursing care, focused most intently on what is needed to succeed in the first RN role, consistent with the National Council Licensure Examination test blueprint. Some programs may also include additional topics including management, community health, gerontology, and research. Because the National Council of State Boards of Nursing has responded to changes in the practice environment, most nursing programs leading to licensure as an RN have widened their focus to teach principles and practices related to the management of care, such as prioritization, delegation, and multipatient management.

Students completing the ASN are prepared to practice in structured health care settings.

In response to future workforce needs and employment patterns, faculty teaching in associate degree programs will want to instill in their students a sense of lifelong learning and the expectation of advancing their initial education to at least the bachelor level. The recent Institute of Medicine (IOM) (2010) report on the future of nursing recommended that the profession move to increasing the proportion of practicing nurses with a baccalaureate degree to 80% by 2020. Facilitating the academic progression of associate degree–prepared nurses through innovative curriculum models will become a strategic goal of the profession over the next decade.

Baccalaureate Degree Programs

Baccalaureate degree (BSN, BS, BA) programs are traditionally offered by 4-year colleges and universities. According to the Robert Wood Johnson

Foundation (2013), 19 states now allow community colleges to offer bachelor degrees. The graduate of a baccalaureate nursing program is prepared to deliver care to individuals, families, groups, and communities in institutional, home, and community settings. In addition to content related to specific nursing areas, baccalaureate curricula also include concepts related to management, community health, nursing theory and research, health policy, group and team dynamics, and professional issues. Health promotion, illness prevention, and patient education may also be emphasized.

The baccalaureate curriculum offers a strong foundation of liberal arts and sciences in addition to nursing courses. The program may be designed to require students to take prerequisite courses in the sciences, arts, and humanities before admission to the nursing major, or students may be directly admitted to the nursing program and take these courses concurrently with nursing courses. Faculty must consider the issues related to each program design, their philosophical beliefs about education, the characteristics of the program's student population, and the institution's mission as decisions are made about the design of the curriculum.

It is imperative for the faculty to construct curricula that are flexible enough in adapting to changing practice expectations of baccalaureate-prepared nurses, especially as there is growing evidence and preference for the bachelor degree as entry into nursing practice (Institute of Medicine [IOM], 2010). This growing evidence supports the need for more baccalaureate-prepared nurses in the workforce given the data showing increases in patient safety and patient care outcomes as a result of the practice of baccalaureate-prepared nurses. To develop contemporary curricula and meet the needs of the workforce, and consistent with the IOM's 2010 call for transformational partnerships, there will be a continuing need to stress the creation of academic–practice partnerships (Niederhauser, MacIntyre, Garner, Teel, & Murray, 2010). Faculty must maximize these partnerships as they develop revised program competencies that include but are not limited to such concepts as clinical reasoning, critical inquiry, intra- and interprofessional collaborative practice, leadership, health coaching, complexity thinking, efficient care management and coordination, health policy advocacy, evidence-based decision making, information technology, bioterrorism, genetics and genomics, gerontology, and care redesign. This is certainly not an exhaustive list of competencies but one that will evolve with the dynamics of a changing health care system.

Academic Progression Models

Given the multiple entry points into the nursing profession, and the societal need for nurses who have advanced education and skills, curriculum designs that promote academic progression are an important part of the landscape of nursing education. These programs are designed to provide students a pathway from one educational degree level to another in an expedited fashion. These innovations share three main characteristics: a focus on decreasing the time to move from one academic degree to another; recognition for prior educational and practical or life experience; and the ability to transport educational credit. These programs are critical in partially overcoming the efficiency lost in moving from one degree program to another.

Academic Progression Models for Licensed Practical/Vocational Nurses

Often, students make the choice to begin nursing careers as LPNs or LVNs for a variety of life reasons. For example, students may desire a short time to program completion, early entry into the workforce, and affordability. The most common academic progression models for LPNs are LPN to ASN and LPN to BSN. Porter-Wenzlaff and Froman (2008) described LPN and LVN programs, noting that they offer an entry point into the health professions that is able to draw a greater proportion of ethnic and racial minority students, individuals from disadvantaged personal and academic backgrounds, older students, and students who may have ESL. In nursing, a professional field that has not achieved diversity goals in many areas, this entry point into nursing is a mechanism that could help the profession become more diverse. Successful programs provide supportive services to enhance reading comprehension, to develop writing skills, and to overcome financial obstacles in a supportive environment.

It is expected that nurse educators will continue to design academic progression options that facilitate educational transition for individuals licensed as LPNs and LVNs. One example of an educational model that promotes academic progression is the National League for Nursing (NLN) (2010) Education Competencies Model that identifies outcomes and competencies for all nursing programs from LPN or LVN through doctoral programs, providing a seamless transition across nursing programs.

Academic Progression Models for Registered Nurses with an ASN or Diploma

Many undergraduate nursing program options have been developed to facilitate the academic progression of RNs within the profession. These programs are designed to streamline the articulation of curricula between degree programs. Program designs vary and depend on the philosophy of the nursing faculty and the expectations of the parent institution. The most common include the RN to BSN program and the ASN to MSN programs, which may bypass or grant the BSN during the period in which the MSN is being earned.

Courses in RN to BSN programs typically include additional courses in liberal education to meet general education requirements and to provide graduates with exposure to a broad educational background. Nursing courses in RN to BSN programs usually encompass areas of focus that are not included deeply in associate degree or diploma programs. Most RN to BSN programs include coursework in community health, nursing leadership or management, and research- and evidence-based practice, as well as exposure to topics of concern to professional nurses such as professional communication, health care ethics, and health policy. Many RN to BSN programs include a capstone course, facilitating the integration of learning outcomes. Participation in clinical nursing courses is an expected aspect of this academic progression model, often occurring through the use of precepted coursework.

In recent years, strategies for meeting the needs of diverse learners have led to the proliferation of successful models for structuring curriculum delivery. Some programs schedule educational offerings into a day, evening, or weekend format, allowing the student to continue working while earning credits. Other programs combine online and in person delivery, allowing for the support and collegiality that easily emerges in cohort models of education with the convenience of the online environment. Programs that are fully online have also become common, and allow students to pursue their baccalaureate degree at their own pace and with a great deal of flexibility (Hendricks et al., 2012).

Although nurses entering the profession with an initial BSN are more likely to complete a graduate degree in nursing, there is also a proliferation of academic progression programs facilitating RN (ASN) to MSN degree completion. Some of these programs grant the BSN degree partway through the program and others do not. Such RN to MSN programs provide another streamlined pathway toward advancing the educational level of the nursing workforce.

Second Degree Entry into Practice

Even though the predicted shortage of RNs has not emerged as quickly or acutely as predicted, the need for professional nurses has continued to grow, with projections for nursing shortages well into the future (Auerbach, Buerhaus, & Staiger, 2014). Coupled with this workforce demand, many individuals holding a nonnursing bachelor's degree seek other career opportunities that may be more fulfilling or hold stronger job prospects. Nursing is often an excellent career option to consider. Many schools offering the baccalaureate nursing degree have designed a program track for students seeking a second degree. This BSN degree option is achieved in a short time in a fast-moving, densely packed curriculum, and is sometimes referred to as an *accelerated program.* These second-degree nursing programs may facilitate acquisition of a bachelor's, master's, or even doctoral nursing degree. In light of the nursing shortage that is projected to continue in some regions into the next decade (Buerhaus, Auerbach, Staiger, & Muench, 2013), the proliferation of second-degree programs of study is likely to continue. Students entering the profession through this route are often slightly older than traditional students. Many have experienced a professional work life, and bring a variety of skill sets to the educational experience.

As a result of these multiple program options, those wishing to pursue a nursing career will have many opportunities and choices among educational program offerings. Technology will continue to play a significant role in increasing access to regional and national program offerings. Increasing numbers of online nursing degree programs can be individualized by the student to meet his or her unique learning needs.

The richness in academic progression models has created challenges for nursing faculty and for the public who deal with the products of these educational programs. As noted previously, factors that affect a program choice are related to the type of degree being granted based on workforce needs and compatibility with the mission of the parent institution. This decision then dictates credit hours, program length, required courses, and types of learning experiences that need to be consistent with the degree being awarded. With academic progression models, faculty must make decisions about how to recognize and credit previous learning experiences. This may be accomplished through articulation agreements, advanced placement opportunities, credit transfers, and validation of previous learning through testing and portfolios.

As the nursing profession seeks to increase the number of nurses prepared at the baccalaureate and advanced practice levels, academic progression models will continue to be a quality, cost-effective means of supporting career mobility and accomplishing this goal. Faculty will need to be creative and innovative as they design future programs. They must be willing to engage in experimentation as they find ways to produce and deliver quality, cost-effective programming and consider innovative clinical models of instruction to accompany the classroom experience. Curricula will need to consist of structured and unstructured learning experiences that build on prior knowledge and experiences of the learner. These nursing curricula will also be constructed to maximize the use of the latest technology that will support innovative teaching pedagogies and transformative learning environments.

Collaborative Curricular Models

Gerardi (2014) described the Robert Wood Johnson Foundation's creation and support of the Academic Progression in Nursing (APIN) program, which led to the creation of nine coalitions to support state level initiatives toward seamless academic progression. For example, one model created in New Mexico involved creation of a statewide nursing curriculum. Another model in California, through the APIN initiative at California State University, Los Angeles, created a collaborative model of articulation with eight community colleges. This model incorporated shared faculty, a dual admission process, and an integrated curriculum. Besides creating pathways to achieve the BSN in a timely way, the program also increased diversity in the nursing profession in the area. These collaborative curricular models are becoming increasingly common, and the advantages to students include the clear path toward the BSN, reduction of unnecessary barriers to progression, early introduction to the idea of academic progression as a goal to pursue, and often a community of peers who are engaged in similar progression. For schools of nursing, such models help to ensure a strong and vibrant pipeline, using resources across multiple types of colleges and universities effectively.

Partnerships, Consortia, and Statewide Models

In today's complex social system, nursing practice and education cannot afford to operate in silos. Nursing education programs that engage in partnerships with health care agencies, other schools, state and local government, and community centers situate their practice in a position of strength. Such partnerships can strengthen all involved, align resources to achieve a common goal, and often lead to solutions to problems shared by all stakeholders. For example, Halstead et al. (2012) described an academic and practice consortium between four schools of nursing and an academic health center that resulted in the development of more than 40 nurse educators prepared to effectively use simulation technology. Following a week-long immersion experience in learning how to use the technology, simulation scenarios were collaboratively developed for learning experiences across a wide spectrum of clinical situations that were shared among all of the participating institutions.

Partnerships between communities and schools of nursing also are effective in addressing local health problems, while providing excellent clinical education opportunities. Luque and Castañeda (2013), in a community coalition model, provided mobile clinic services to migrant and seasonal workers in a unique community, resulting in an academic partnership that provided exceptional community health learning experiences for students, while serving a population with significant health service needs. In geographic areas suffering from shortages of nurses, partnerships between service providers and schools may be effective. For example, Murray, Schappe, Kreienkamp, Loyd, and Buck (2010) described a partnership between schools of nursing and the workforce through the state hospital association. The program created pathways for the infusion of nursing faculty, increases in students enrolled, and a sustainable partnership model between schools of nursing and health care agencies. Summarizing these reasons for partnerships, Everett et al. (2012) referred to them as fuel for the future success of each organization.

Designing the Curriculum

Choosing a specific program design, such as an associate or a baccalaureate degree program, does not automatically dictate the design of that program's curriculum. Faculty should develop a curriculum structure that will support the type of program desired and the outcomes envisioned. Chapter 6 provides a discussion of developing program outcomes and competencies. After deciding on desired program outcomes and competencies, faculty are ready to provide additional structure to the curriculum.

There are a number of different ways to think about the construction of a curriculum design. The more traditional approach to designing curricula offers structured courses in a specific sequence. This approach identifies what the student is to learn, when the learning is to occur, and what the outcome of the learning should be. The delineation of nursing and support content, nursing skills, critical learning experiences, and evaluation methods for assessing learning outcomes are emphasized. These pieces are structured into any one of a number of curriculum patterns. Two common curriculum patterns, that of "blocking" course content and that of integrating or "threading" course content or concepts, are described in Chapter 6.

Future Trends in Undergraduate Nursing Curriculum

The more traditional approach to curriculum has focused on the identification of critical content, the sequencing of content, and the efficient delivery of content. The traditional approach has led to an oversaturation of content as faculty have continued to add to the list of critical content needed to practice competently in a rapidly changing health care system. When planning curricular reform, whether on a limited or large scale, an infusion of evidence-based pedagogies that use strategies to engage students in active learning need to be considered. This shifting emphasis requires nothing less than a paradigm shift in how faculty view the education of our future nursing workforce.

Future trends in health care, nursing, and education will have a significant influence on how nursing education programs are designed and implemented during the next decade. Our greatest challenge likely lies in defining how the roles of nurses will transform to meet evolving and changing health care needs and translating these changes into relevant curricula. To meet this challenge, future trends in nursing education will include an increase in the number of collaborative partnerships between nursing practice and education (Everett et al., 2012). Such efforts will focus on maintaining congruence between nursing curricula and contemporary nursing practice, developing initiatives that will help new graduates with the transition into nursing practice, and establishing mechanisms to retain and advance the education of experienced nurses in the workforce. There also will continue to be an increased emphasis placed on collaboration between disciplines.

Barriers to career mobility and articulation will continue to be removed, making articulation between degrees seamless and essentially hassle-free. Past barriers, such as the use of expensive, time-consuming validation examinations; duplication of learning; lack of flexibility; and difficulty with transferring credits, are being addressed. Contemporary articulation models are flexible in design, supported by broad course and credit transferability, and packaged to maximize the use of students' time. Distance learning technologies will continue to play a prominent role in successfully delivering education to geographically dispersed students. These new strategies will play an important role in facilitating the learning of nontraditional students through curricula that will be taught more from an integrated conceptual orientation specially designed for the distance learner.

The ways and means of educating the next generation of nurses must clearly be on the agenda at all nursing schools. Nurse educators must be able to advance innovations in nursing education (Spector & Odom, 2012). Faculty are exploring and will continue to explore the addition of internships and other types of intensive practicum experience either as part of a more formal curriculum design or in partnership with health care partners as part of an orientation program that bridges the gap between graduation and full nurse practice privileges (Tri-Council for Nursing, 2010).

Responding to a health care environment that focuses more on community-based health care between individuals who are well and those who have chronic illnesses has not traditionally been a primary focus in undergraduate nursing education. In the United States, role specialization has historically been reserved for graduate education. However, with the increasing knowledge and technology explosion and the different skills and competencies required for caring for patients with acute illnesses, as opposed to the skills and competencies necessary for teaching health promotion, illness prevention, and caring for patients with chronic illnesses, reconsidering alternative approaches to undergraduate education warrants consideration.

In the world of higher education, the nursing profession has long been the source of much educational innovation. The issues identified here are critical to the future of nursing education, but by no means are they an exhaustive listing of the issues that nursing faculty must consider as they design future nursing programs and curricula. The innovation and creativity that nursing faculty have demonstrated in the past will no doubt continue to identify them as leaders in professional and higher education into the future.

Summary

Nursing leaders have envisioned a future in which nurses play a predominant role in leading the delivery of health care instead of responding to the demands made by others. As nurses take a more active role in leading health care reform, nursing education will need to prepare students, including undergraduate students, with appropriate leadership skills and an understanding of complexity and change. Nursing curricula will need to move away from rigid requirements to flexible learning opportunities to prepare nurses who are capable of managing large amounts of data-rich knowledge in technology-driven health care environments to make patient care decisions.

Designing curriculum provides an opportunity for faculty to use their scientific knowledge base, clinical competence, and creativity. Curriculum development is guided by the need to consistently include in the students' educational experiences opportunities to acquire the knowledge, skills, and competencies that are needed by graduates. Careful attention must also be paid to accreditation requirements and preparation for licensure examinations. Creating innovative curriculum designs that foster the preparation of graduates who are confident in their knowledge and skills and are prepared to meet the challenges of contemporary nursing practice is a challenge that nurse educators must readily embrace.

REFLECTING ON THE EVIDENCE

1. When considering the forces affecting undergraduate nursing education, what do you believe will become most important in the next 5 years? What is the rationale for your projections?
2. What challenges are faced by schools of nursing in managing curricular reform related to rapid changes in the health care and higher education environments?
3. How has the proliferation of various academic progression models influenced the quality of nursing education?

REFERENCES

American Association of Colleges of Nursing (AACN). (2011). *Nursing fact sheet.* Retrieved from http://www.aacn.nche.edu.

American Association of Colleges of Nursing (AACN). (2013). *The essentials of baccalaureate education for professional nursing practice.* Retrieved from, http://www.aacn.nche.edu.

American Organization of Nurse Executives (AONE). (2004a). *AONE guiding principles for the role of the nurse in future patient care delivery toolkit.* Retrieved from, http://www.aone.org/.

American Organization of Nurse Executives (AONE). (2004b). *BSN-level nursing education resources.* Retrieved from, http://www.aone.org/.

American Organization of Nurse Executives (AONE). (2010). *AONE guiding principles for the role of the nurse in future patient care delivery toolkit.* Retrieved from, http://www.aone.org/.

Auerbach, D. I., Buerhaus, P. I., & Staiger, D. O. (2014). Registered nurses are delaying retirement, a shift that has contributed to recent growth in the nurse workforce. *Health Affairs, 33*(8), 1474–1480.

Benner, P., Sutphen, M., Leonard, V., & Day, L. (2010). *Educating nurses: A call for radical transformation*. San Francisco, CA: Jossey-Bass.

Buerhaus, P. I., Auerbach, D. E., & Staiger, D. O. (2009). The recent surge in nurse employment: Cause and implications. *Health Affairs, 28*(2), 124–128.

Buerhaus, P. I., Auerbach, D. I., Staiger, D. O., & Muench, U. (2013). Projections of the long-term growth of the registered nurse workforce: A regional analysis. *Nursing Economic$, 31*(1), 13–17.

Bureau of Labor Statistics, U.S. Department of Labor. (2014). *Occupational outlook handbook, 2014-15 edition, licensed practical and licensed vocational nurses.* on the Internet at http://www.bls.gov/ooh/healthcare/licensed-practical-and-licensed-vocational-nurses.htm (visited July 04, 2015).

Commission for Collegiate Nursing Education (CCNE). (2009). *Standards for accreditation of baccalaureate and graduate degree nursing programs.* Retrieved from, http://www.aacn.nche.edu/Accreditation/pdf/standards09.pdf.

Cronenwett, L., Sherwood, G., Barnsteiner, J., Disch, J., Johnson, J., Mitchell, P., et al. (2007). Quality and safety education for nurses. *Nursing Outlook, 55*(3), 122–131.

Dezure, D. (2010). *Innovations in the undergraduate curriculum.* Retrieved from, http://education.stateuniversity.com/pages/1896/Curriculum-Higher-Education.html.

Dillon, P. (1997). The future of associate degree nursing. *Nursing & Health Care Perspectives, 18*(1), 20–24.

Donohue-Porter, P., Forbes, M. O., & White, J. H. (2011). Nursing theory in curricula today: Challenges for faculty at all levels of education. *International Journal of Nursing Education Scholarship, 8*(1), 1–18. http://dx.doi.org/10.2202/1548-923X.2225.

Everett, L. Q., Bowers, B., Beal, J. A., Alt-White, A., Erickson, J., Gale, S., et al. (2012). Academic-practice partnerships fuel future success. *Journal of Nursing Administration, 42*(12), 554–556. http://dx.doi.org/10.1097/NNA.0b013e318274b4eb.

Gerardi, T. (2014). AONE leadership perspectives. AONE and the Academic Progression in Nursing Initiative. *Journal Of Nursing Administration, 44*(3), 127–128. http://dx.doi.org/10.1097/NNA.0000000000000038.

Glasgow, M., Dunphy, L., & Mainous, R. (2010). Future of nursing. Innovative nursing educational curriculum for the 21st century. *Nursing Education Perspectives, 31*(6), 355–357.

Grealish, L., & Smale, L. (2011). Theory before practice: Implicit assumptions about clinical nursing education in Australia as revealed through a shared critical reflection. *Contemporary Nurse: A Journal for the Australian Nursing Profession, 39*(1), 51–64. http://dx.doi.org/10.5172/conu.2011.39.1.51.

Halstead, J. A., Phillips, J., Koller, A., Hardin, K., Porter, M., & Dwyer, J. (2012). Preparing nurse educators to use simulation technology: A consortium model for practice and education. *Journal of Continuing Education in Nursing, 42*(11), 496–502.

Hendricks, S. M., Phillips, J. M., Narwold, L., Laux, M., Rouse, S., Dulemba, L., et al. (2012). Creating tomorrow's leaders and innovators through RN to Bachelor of Science in Nursing consortium curricular model. *Journal of Professional Nursing, 28*(3), 163–169. http://dx.doi.org/10.1016/j.profnurs.2011.11.009.

Institute of Medicine (IOM). (2001). *Crossing the quality chasm: A new health system for the 21st century.* Washington, DC: The National Academies Press.

Institute of Medicine (IOM). (2010). *The future of nursing: Leading change, advancing health.* Washington, DC: The National Academies Press.

Interprofessional Education Collaborative Expert Panel. (2011). *Core competencies for interprofessional collaborative practice: Report of an expert panel.* Retrieved from, http://www.aacn.nche.edu/education-resources/IPECReport.pdf.

Kovner, C. T., Brewer, C. S., Fatehi, F., & Katigbak, C. (2014). Original research: Changing trends in newly licensed RNs. *American Journal of Nursing, 114*(2), 26–34.

Luque, J., & Castañeda, H. (2013). Delivery of mobile clinic services to migrant and seasonal farmworkers: A review of practice models for community-academic partnerships. *Journal of Community Health, 38*(2), 397–407. http://dx.doi.org/10.1007/s10900-012-9622-4.

Mackey, S., Hatcher, D., Happell, B., & Cleary, M. (2013). Primary health care as a philosophical and practical framework for nursing education: Rhetoric or reality? *Contemporary Nurse: A Journal for the Australian Nursing Profession, 45*(1), 79–84. http://dx.doi.org/10.5172/conu.2013.45.1.79.

Murray, T., Schappe, A., Kreienkamp, D., Loyd, V., & Buck, E. (2010). A community-wide academic-service partnership to expand faculty and student capacity. *Journal of Nursing Education, 49*(5), 295–299. http://dx.doi.org/10.3928/01484834-20100115-03.

National League for Nursing (NLN). (2010). *Outcomes and competencies for graduates of practical/vocational, diploma, associate degree, baccalaureate, master's, practice doctorate, and research doctorate programs in nursing.* New York: Author.

National League for Nursing (NLN). (2011). *Academic progression in nursing education.* New York: Author.

National League for Nursing (NLN). (2014). *Vision for recognition of the role of licensed practical/vocational nurses in advancing the nation's health.* New York: Author.

Niederhauser, V., MacIntyre, R. C., Garner, C., Teel, C., & Murray, T. A. (2010). Transformational partnerships in nursing education. *Nursing Education Perspectives, 31*(6), 353–355.

Nightingale, F. (1969). *Notes on nursing.* New York: Dover.

Popoola, M. (2012). Popoola holistic praxis model—A framework for curriculum development. *West African Journal Of Nursing, 23*(2), 43–56.

Porter-Wenzlaff, L., & Froman, R. (2008). Responding to increasing RN demand: Diversity and retention trends through an accelerated LVN-to-BSN curriculum. *Journal of Nursing Eductation, 47*(5), 231–235.

Robert Wood Johnson Foundation. (2013). The case for academic progression: Why nurses should advance their education and the strategies that make this feasible. *Charting Nursing's Future, 21.* Retrieved from, www.RWJF.org.goto.CNF.

Spector, N., & Odom, S. (2012). The initiative to advance innovations in nursing education: Three years later. *Journal of Nursing Regulation, 3*(2), 40–44.

Tanner, C. A. (2010). 2010—A banner year for nursing education. *Journal of Nursing Education, 49*(6), 303–304.

Tella, S., Liukka, M., Jamookeeah, D., Smith, N., Partanen, P., & Turunen, H. (2014). What do nursing students learn about patient safety? An integrative literature review. *Journal of Nursing Education, 53*(1), 7–13. http://dx.doi.org/10.3928/01484834-20131209-04.

Tri-Council for Nursing. (2010). *Educational advancement of registered nurses: A consensus position.* Retrieved from, http://www.aacn.nche.edu/Education/pdf/Tricouncil EdStatement.pdf.

U.S. Department of Education. (2010). *Accreditation in the United States*. Retrieved from, http://www2.ed.gov.

U.S. Department of Health and Human Services, Health Resources and Services Administration. (2010). *The registered nurse population - initial findings from the 2008 national sample survey of registered nurses*. Retrieved from, http://bhpr.hrsa.gov/healthworkforce/rnsurveys/rnsurveyinitial2008.pdf.

World Health Organization (WHO). (2010). *Framework for action on interprofessional education and collaborative practice*. WHO reference number: WHO/HRH/HPN/10.3. Retrieved from, http://www.who.int/hrh/resources/framework_action/en/.

9 Curriculum Models for Graduate Programs*

Karen Grigsby, PhD, RN

Curriculum Models for Graduate Programs

Graduate nursing education is experiencing a major paradigm shift in response to health care, societal, and professional demands. There is a shortage of nurses prepared with advanced degrees to serve in administrator, educator, nurse scientist, and advanced practice roles. With national calls to increase the number of nurses with advanced practice preparation and doctoral preparation (American Association of Colleges of Nursing [AACN], 2006; Institute of Medicine [IOM], 2010; National League for Nursing [NLN], 2013), much attention is being placed on the curriculum models that nursing has historically used to prepare nurses with graduate degrees. This chapter discusses the evolving nature of U.S. graduate nursing education, curriculum models for master's and doctoral programs, and faculty preparation for teaching in graduate programs, and concludes with future trends that will continue to influence the development of graduate programs in nursing.

Historical Development of Graduate Nursing Education

An understanding of the development of graduate education provides a solid foundation for discussion of the current changes taking place. Graduate education in nursing began to develop early in the twentieth century. Initially, graduate education was reserved for those nurses who worked as supervisors or administrators. Today, graduate education is expected for nurses who want to practice at an advanced level as a nurse practitioner (NP), clinical nurse specialist (CNS), nurse anesthetist, midwife, educator, researcher, or administrator. Curriculum models that facilitate nurses achieving graduate degrees at an earlier stage in their professional careers are emerging to meet the growing demand and maximize their contributions to nursing and health care over the life of their career.

In addition to preparing nurses for advanced clinical care positions, nursing graduate education programs also offer curricula that specifically prepare nurses in areas such as informatics, education, and administration. Although these are not roles that prepare nurses to provide direct care, they are necessary roles to improve systems so that others can deliver safe, quality patient care across settings. These roles increasingly require specialized knowledge and skills beyond a basic nursing education. This preparation can be a focused specialty area in a master's, doctor of philosophy (PhD), or doctor of nursing practice (DNP) program, or can be courses that are added to a specialty area preparing nurses to be advanced practice registered nurses (APRNs).

Master's Programs in Nursing

In 1960 only 14 graduate programs in nursing existed to prepare faculty to teach in schools of nursing (Egenes, 2009). Rutgers University offered the first nursing master's degree, and the focus was a clinical specialist in psychiatric nursing. The demand for master's programs in nursing grew in the areas of research, teaching, administration, and clinical practice areas in response to societal needs for nurses with advanced preparation in theory and research so that they could improve practice and increase the level of competence. As enrollment in master's

*The author acknowledges the contributions of Linda Finke, PhD, RN, in previous editions of this chapter.

programs increased, the focus of master's programs shifted from functional specialization (educator, researcher, and administrator) to an emphasis on clinical areas (CNS). This enabled a growth in application of knowledge to improve care (Egenes, 2009).

The Nurse Training Act of 1964 recommended federal funding to develop graduate programs in nursing. By 1970, graduate nursing programs began to proliferate. Role preparation at this time included the CNS, educator, researcher, and administrator. As the popularity of the CNS increased, fewer nurses selected the role of researcher, educator, or administrator. As this trend grew, programs preparing educators and administrators at the master's level were either eliminated or relegated to supporting courses for programs focused on preparing the CNS (Egenes, 2009).

The NP role developed during this same period as a means to provide primary care to underserved populations at a lower cost. The first program was developed at the University of Colorado in 1965. Initially, NP programs were designed and implemented through continuing education programs and resulted in a certificate. By 1970, NP preparation primarily occurred in graduate nursing programs. A new addition to these programs included developing skill in political activism to influence legislative changes needed to allow NPs to practice to the full scope of their preparation. This effort to influence legislators to make changes in state laws so that NPs can practice to their full scope continues today (Egenes, 2009; Fairman, 2014).

Development of a New Master's Program: The Clinical Nurse Leader

The clinical nurse leader (CNL) role emerged as a master's level generalist prepared to develop methods of improving patient outcomes, coordinating and promoting evidence-based practice, and promote client self-care and decision making. The intended emphasis for this role was for clinicians whose focus was to engage in outcomes-based practice using quality improvement strategies (American Association of Colleges of Nursing [AACN], 2013). CNLs are prepared to deliver care to specific populations and to collaborate with others providing care to a group of patients. The Veterans Administration was one of the first organizations to hire CNLs as a means to provide safe, quality, and cost-effective care to patients (American Association of Colleges of Nursing [AACN], 2013; Keating, 2011b).

The development of the CNL role has not been without controversy. As the CNL role was first introduced, some questioned the need for this new role because CNSs also were prepared to deliver care to populations. However, as the CNL role has become better understood, the differentiation of the two roles has become clearer. The CNS is recognized as an advanced practice nurse who is an expert clinician in a particular specialty or subspecialty of nursing practice. The CNL works at the microsystem level to manage and coordinate client care while the CNS designs, implements, and evaluates patient-specific and population-based programs of care. Ultimately, the CNL works in partnership with the CNS, and both contribute to the delivery of safe, efficient, effective, quality care.

Development of Doctoral Programs in Nursing

Doctoral education for nurses has existed since the 1920s. Originally, doctoral programs prepared nurses for administrative and teaching roles. The first doctoral program for nurses was offered in 1924 at Teachers College, Columbia University; graduates earned an EdD degree (Peplau, 1966). In the 1950s and 1960s, most nurses who wanted doctoral degrees obtained the degree in disciplines other than nursing, such as education, sociology, and psychology.

Although master's programs were growing in the 1970s, nurse leaders were advancing the idea that nursing needed its own theory base to be recognized as a discipline and a profession that could stand alone rather than borrow theory from other disciplines. Doctoral programs in nursing initially developed to stimulate the development of nursing theory and research as well as prepare nurses to teach; development of these programs surged in the later part of the twentieth century (American Association of Colleges of Nursing [AACN], 2012a; Keating, 2011c; Stotts, 2011). These programs resulted in a PhD with a focus in nursing. Today there are currently 131 research-focused doctoral programs (PhD, DNS, EdD) in the United States (American Association of Colleges of Nursing [AACN], 2014a).

As recognition developed that more emphasis was needed for clinical application, the clinical doctorate emerged. The first nursing clinical doctoral program designed to focus on clinical practice opened at Boston University in the 1960s (Carter,

2013). These programs offered a variety of degree titles, such as doctorate of nurse scientist (DNSc). Eventually, it was recognized that these programs were comparable to the PhD but focused on clinical practice improvement rather than research that developed nursing theory. In the 1970s some nurse leaders advocated for the nurse doctorate (ND), which prepared individuals for basic licensure plus application of advanced knowledge in clinical practice areas. The first ND degree was offered at Case Western Reserve University and then was phased out as the DNP degree developed (Carter, 2013).

The idea of the DNP degree was strengthened in response to a recommendation from the National Research Council (2005) that clinical doctorates be offered to prepare faculty to teach. The AACN followed by recommending that a practice-focused doctorate be developed to educate advanced practice nurses and that all APRNs obtain a DNP to enter into advanced practice. The DNP degree focuses on advanced preparation in scientific foundations of nursing practice, leadership, evidence-based practice, health care technologies, health care policies, interprofessional collaboration, clinical prevention and population-based care, and advanced practice in a specialty area (Keating, 2011a). In 2004 the AACN recommended that bachelor of science in nursing (BSN) to DNP programs be developed to shift preparation of the advanced practice nurse from the master's level to the doctoral level. This recommendation and its implementation would increase the number of doctorally prepared nurses, educate nurses to translate research into practice, and improve practice through the application of evidence (American Association of Colleges of Nursing [AACN], 2010a).

The development of DNP programs proliferated early in the twenty-first century, and some nurse leaders began voicing concerns that fewer nurses would enter PhD programs, master's preparation for NPs would be eliminated, and APRNs would not be focused on providing care to people, especially individuals and families living in areas with limited access to health care providers. This belief centered on the understanding that DNP graduates would be focused on leading improvements in health systems rather than providing direct care to populations (Cronenwett et al., 2011). The controversy surrounding the issue of DNP degrees as the entry into advanced nursing practice has economic, societal, and health care delivery implications. The DNP degree is regarded as the highest level of advanced nursing practice that focuses on translating new knowledge into practice and developing evidence-based practice; more than 250 schools currently offer the DNP degree (American Association of Colleges of Nursing [AACN], 2014c).

With AACN's mandate for the DNP degree to be the entry into advanced practice, questions are raised as to how to prepare a nurse for advanced practice while at the same time developing skills in leadership and systems change (Fontaine & Langston, 2011; Malone, 2011). Some leaders argue that engaging young nurses to advance to the DNP degree immediately after completing their BSN degree limits the contributions they can make to the profession, whereas others see an economic benefit for the student as well as a means of improving health care delivery (Potempa, 2011).

The PhD in Nursing Degree

The PhD in nursing degree is designed to prepare nurse scientists who are committed to the generation of new knowledge and can steward the discipline and educate the next generation (American Association of Colleges of Nursing [AACN], 2010a). PhD programs focus on developing researchers who design and implement studies that advance evidence-based practice and inform health policy (Bednash, Breslin, Kirschling, & Rosseter, 2014). These programs mentor students by involving them in a community designed to stimulate students' thinking about their own research agenda and by providing opportunities to prepare grants and manuscripts and initiate a program of research.

PhD programs are designed to accommodate both part-time and full-time students. Delivery of the programs varies from traditional on-campus courses to completely online courses, with most programs using a blended approach to deliver the program. The PhD program prepares a *beginning* nurse scientist. Postdoctoral programs are the next step for nurses who want to continue to develop as a nurse scientist. Postdoctoral programs, often funded by federal grants, give students an opportunity to mature into independent researchers by providing a strong mentoring experience. Postdoctoral programs are not growing at this time, and thus opportunities are limited for students to extend their preparation as nurse scientists before entering the workforce (Bednash et al., 2014).

The Doctor of Nursing Practice (DNP) Degree

The DNP program is designed for those nurses involved in direct practice and those working in areas that support clinical practice, such as administration (Bednash et al., 2014). These programs prepare nurses as advanced practice nurses who are ready to assume leadership roles in clinical organizations, develop and influence health care policy, implement knowledge generated by nurse scientists, advance evidence-based practice, and improve the health care delivery system (Udlis & Mancuso, 2012).

The DNP degree is considered a terminal degree in nursing practice. While not intended to prepare nurses for positions as educators, the DNP degree does provide a terminal degree credential that many institutions accept as qualification for a faculty position and can be instrumental in addressing the profession's shortage of nursing faculty. If DNP graduates are prepared as nurse faculty in addition to advanced practice nurses, these graduates would be well positioned to educate all levels of students and to close the practice-education gap (Danzey et al., 2011).

The Doctor of Education (EdD) Degree

Early in the twentieth century, nurses who wanted to teach selected doctoral programs in schools of education. Schools of education offered PhD and EdD programs ("the practice doctorate" in education). As nursing doctoral programs developed, nurses had more choices about the type of doctoral program they wanted and some chose PhD or DNS programs in schools of nursing while others chose to obtain their degree from schools of education in order to work in schools of nursing and improve programs preparing students to practice nursing. Nurses who want a focus on education still select an EdD program today.

Recently, because of the emphasis on preparing nurse educators at the doctoral level, several schools of nursing are offering an EdD in nursing. These programs may collaborate with the school of education on the campus who can offer foundational courses and major areas of concentration in education. For example, one college of nursing has developed a collaborative doctoral program to prepare nurse scholar teachers; the program results in an EdD degree in instructional leadership and was developed collaboratively by faculty from the college of education and the college of nursing (Graves et al., 2013). This is an innovative way to educate nurses at the doctoral level to become scholars and educators committed to advancing the science of nursing education.

Regulation of the APRN Role

As graduate programs preparing advanced practice nurses continued to grow with expanding enrollments and producing corresponding growth in the APRN workforce, it became apparent that there was a need to achieve some uniformity in the preparation and credentialing of advanced practice nurses. Drawing on collaboration from professional nursing organizations, regulatory agencies, and accrediting bodies, the APRN Consensus Model was developed to describe regulatory requirements in four areas: licensure, accreditation, certification, and education (LACE). Several important outcomes related to APRN education resulted from these collaborations that are still influencing the ongoing development of graduate programs.

National Organization of Nurse Practitioner Faculties

The National Organization of Nurse Practitioner Faculties (NONPF) is an organization formed by NP faculty to promote quality NP education, influence policy to advance NP education, foster diversity, promote scholarship of NP educators, and strengthen resources to sustain NONPF. NONPF has been instrumental, along with the National Council of State Boards of Nursing (NCSBN) and other professional organizations, in leading the development of the APRN Consensus Model.

In 1990 NONPF developed core competencies for NPs. These competencies have been updated (National Organization of Nurse Practitioner Faculty [NONPF], 2012) and now apply to all NPs as they complete either an MSN or DNP program and are ready to enter practice. The competencies are population focused and cover the following areas: scientific foundations, leadership, quality, practice inquiry, technology and information literacy, policy, health delivery system, ethics, and independent practice. NONPF also brings NP educators together to discuss curriculum issues about NP education and develops national recommendations designed to promote excellence and maintain quality in NP programs. Examples of issues that concern NONPF members include faculty/student ratios, number of clinical hours to ensure competencies are met prior to graduation, and use of technology to supervise clinical experiences of students from a distance (National Organization of Nurse Practitioner Faculty, 2012).

The APRN Consensus Model

In 2003 work began to develop the APRN Consensus Model (American Association of Colleges of Nursing, 2008) to regulate the practice of APRNs. Individuals working on this project represented a broad spectrum of stakeholders and included the APRN Consensus Work Group and the NCSBN APRN Advisory Committee. APRNs were defined as certified registered nurse anesthetists, certified nurse midwives, certified CNSs, and certified NPs. The report on the consensus model was published in 2008 and by 2010, 48 organizations had endorsed the report, which recommended alignment of LACE factors of APRNs across states to ensure the safety of patients as well as expand patient access to APRNs. Each state determines the APRN legal scope of practice, roles, criteria for entry into advanced practice, and acceptable certification exams. Because there is no uniform model regulating APRNs across all states, a barrier exists for APRNs to move readily from state to state and may limit access of care to patients. The Consensus Model was designed to diminish this barrier and allow APRNs to move readily from state to state. The goal was to implement this model fully by 2015, a goal which has not yet been achieved.

The LACE mechanism was designed to implement the APRN Consensus Model and operate as a communication mechanism among regulatory organizations. LACE includes the four essential regulatory elements of LACE. The APRN regulatory model has outlined expectations for all four elements of LACE, which will enable the Consensus Model to be implemented. Implementing the LACE mechanism in all states will allow APRNs to more easily move between states, improve the regulation of APRNs, and ultimately improve access to care.

Institute of Medicine

Several landmark reports examining the state of health care in the United States and making recommendations for changes in the health care system and education of professionals working in these systems were published by the IOM beginning in the late 1990s. These reports have stimulated many changes within graduate programs to meet the needs of society (Institute of Medicine [IOM], 2010). *Crossing the Quality Chasm* (2001) identified the need for restructuring the health care system to promote safe, effective, timely, efficient, and equitable health care. In 2003 the IOM recommended that all health professionals be educated to deliver evidence-based, patient-centered care and that all professionals work in interdisciplinary teams using quality improvement strategies and informatics. In 2010 the IOM made recommendations regarding nurses practicing to the full scope of their authority and achieving greater numbers of nurses prepared at the doctoral level.

Curriculum Designs for Graduate Programs

Curriculum design for graduate nursing education has become varied, with a number of program models designed to facilitate academic progression to graduate-level preparation. The quality of graduate nursing education programs is maintained in part through the admission of well-qualified students. This section describes various graduate curriculum models, as well as student qualifications.

Student Qualifications

A variety of factors influence a student's admission to graduate study. Overall, students are evaluated for their potential for success in their chosen program. In research-focused doctoral programs, it is also important that a student's research interest have a match with faculty expertise and scholarship.

Students admitted to a master's program should demonstrate the potential for academic success as indicated by previous academic achievements (grade point average [GPA]), performance on standardized tests such as the Graduate Record Exam (GRE), admission interviews, and professional references. Some master's programs do not require standardized tests for admission. Other common requirements for admission to a master's program as a postlicensure student include graduation from an undergraduate program that is accredited by a national nursing accreditation body and a current, unencumbered licensure as a registered nurse (RN). A number of master's programs have traditionally stipulated a specified amount of work experience prior to admission, but such requirements are increasingly being questioned within the profession as being unduly restrictive to promoting academic progression. In addition, depending on the type of master's program, there may be prerequisite course requirements in selected courses, such as statistics or health assessment.

Admission to doctoral nursing programs tends to be competitive, in part because of the smaller numbers of students admitted and the rigorous qualifications. Requirements vary somewhat depending on the nature of the doctoral program. Successful candidates for admission to either the research-focused doctorate (PhD) or the clinical doctorate (DNP) will demonstrate high levels of academic achievement (GPA) in previous programs and will be expected to submit standardized test scores (GRE). Graduation from an accredited nursing program and a current unencumbered RN license are also common requirements. Graduate level prerequisite course work in selected areas may also be required depending on the focus of the graduate program. Students seeking enrollment in a postmaster's DNP program focused on an advanced practice role will also be asked to provide evidence of the number of clinical hours performed in their master's program.

Interviews and written essays are often key elements to the admission process to doctoral study. It is important for faculty to determine that the student's career goals and research interests are a good fit for the program to which the student is applying. In research-focused doctoral programs, it is important for the research interests of the student to be consistent with the research strengths and interests of the faculty.

Program Designs for Master's Education

Master's degree programs prepare nurses with practice expertise that builds on baccalaureate or entry-level nursing practice. Graduates from master's degree programs have a deeper understanding of the discipline of nursing and are able to engage in higher level practice and leadership in a variety of settings. Graduates of master's degree programs are prepared to enter a research or practice-focused doctoral program (American Association of Colleges of Nursing [AACN], 2011).

The curricular design for a master's degree program builds on a base of sciences and humanities and prepares graduates for practice in a clinical or indirect care nursing specialty. The essentials of the curriculum design include a foundation from the sciences and humanities; organizational systems and leadership; quality improvement and patient safety, translating and integrating scholarship into practice; health policy and advocacy; interprofessional collaboration for improving population health and patient outcomes; clinical prevention and population health for improving health; and an area of master's level nursing practice (American Association of Colleges of Nursing, 2011). Nursing specialty organizations also provide competencies and clinical expectations for a master's degree in their given area of practice.

Master's programs vary in length and focus, and the credit hour allocation for the program may range from 30 credits to 45 depending on the program design and clinical hour requirements. Some areas of focus for master's programs include administration, education, CNL, and informatics. Even with the introduction of the DNP degree, a wide range of master's level advanced practice programs continue to exist.

Most master's programs require 2 years of full-time study, but can range from 12 to 18 months. The length of the program is determined by a variety of factors, including the entry level of the student, curriculum design, credit hours and clinical hours required. Many students do enroll in part-time study, which lengthens their time in the program. Many MSN programs offer their courses fully or partially online, thus making the program accessible to underserved areas of the country and allowing students to remain in their area during the program and upon graduation.

Although many master's programs require an earned baccalaureate in nursing for admission, increasing numbers of academic progression models facilitate student achievement of the master's degree (RN to MSN). There are also entry-level master's programs for nonnurses who have undergraduate degrees in another field. Postmaster's certificates (PMCs) are program options that allow students with a previous master's degree in nursing to obtain credentials in another specialty.

Program Designs for Doctoral Education

There are two types of doctoral programs in nursing, the DNP and the PhD. DNP programs are practice focused and PhD programs are research focused. Doctoral curricula tend to be unique to each institution. Because these two doctoral degrees have different purposes and goals, their program design is significantly different.

PhD Program Design

Doctoral programs that award the PhD are research focused with a program outcome of preparing graduates to engage in knowledge generation and dissemination. Curricula typically consist of coursework related to philosophy and theory construction; statistics and research methodology; state of the science nursing knowledge; social, political, and ethical issues; and teaching and mentoring (American Association of Colleges of Nursing, 2010a, 2010b). Students may also select a minor that complements their major area of study. Although the majority of PhD nursing programs require a master's degree, a growing number of programs admit baccalaureate nursing students, referred to as *BSN to PhD programs.* Students who enter the PhD program with a master's degree will usually engage in full-time study for approximately 3 years and complete a dissertation. Students who enter a PhD program with a baccalaureate nursing degree usually study full time for 5 years and complete a dissertation. These timelines are extended for many students as they choose to pursue part-time study.

On completion of coursework and prior to writing the dissertation, students typically must complete a qualifying examination to demonstrate their ability to conduct research and to be eligible to enter into the final stage of the program. The process used for the qualifying examination varies depending on the institution, but it is common to have a written or oral component, frequently both.

Graduates of PhD programs are required to conduct independent research and prepare a document communicating the process and results of the research. This document historically has been a dissertation. Currently, faculty in PhD programs are reconsidering the value of a lengthy dissertation, and are allowing options for presenting the results of the student's research. These may include writing one or more manuscripts to submit for publication, or even digital products that could include motion, sound, and graphics (Morton, 2015).

DNP Program Design

The DNP program is a practice-focused doctoral program to prepare graduates to provide leadership in the development and application of clinical knowledge in specialized areas of advanced practice (American Association of Colleges of Nursing, 2006). Graduates of this program focus on practice that is innovative and evidence-based, applying research findings to practice, rather than generating the evidence for practice. Curricula for DNP programs can vary significantly, from programs that initially prepare graduates for practice as an advanced practice nurse to programs that focus more on leadership in systems-level indirect care roles, such as administration.

DNP programs have several points of entry (e.g., postbaccalaureate, postmaster's degree, nonnursing degree). Graduates from DNP programs are expected to provide the leadership for implementing evidence-based practice and, with the appropriate preparation to assume a teaching role, could also be prepared as clinical faculty to teach in nursing programs. DNP programs require an additional 35 to 40 credit hours over the master's level, and the length of time to complete the DNP degree depends on the previous academic experiences a student brings to the program. A postmaster's DNP may be completed with 2 years of full-time study, whereas a BSN to DNP program may require 4 or 5 years of full-time study.

The American Association of Colleges of Nursing (2006) has established *The Essentials of Doctoral Education for Advanced Nursing Practice* and these standards can be used by faculty to guide curriculum development. These essentials include scientific underpinnings for practice, organizational and systems leadership for quality improvement and systems thinking, clinical scholarship and analytical methods for evidence-based practice, information systems and technology and patient care technology for the improvement and transformation of health care, health care policy for advocacy in health care, interprofessional collaboration for improving patient and population health outcomes, clinical prevention and population health for improving the nation's health, and advanced practice.

Academic Progression Models for Graduate Education

The Institute of Medicine (IOM) (2010) *Future of Nursing* report set forth recommendations that nurses should achieve higher levels of education through a seamless educational system to achieve quality patient care. Academic progression is a process used to facilitate individuals obtaining higher degrees in a timely manner without duplicating or repeating previous course work. For example, common examples of academic progression models in colleges of nursing are those that facilitate RNs without a BSN degree to achieve a graduate nursing degree. Such programs allow nurses to more rapidly assume an advanced practice role. Academic progression models can help facilitate RNs who are usually working full time while attending school part time to obtain a graduate degree. Part-time graduate program offerings allow the nurse to remain in the workforce while attending school. After graduation the nurses can quickly advance to new positions in the workforce (American Association of Colleges of Nursing, 2014b; American Association of Colleges of Nursing, 2012b; American Association of Colleges of Nursing, 2010b; Pellico, Terrill, White, & Rico, 2012).

Academic progression models can also help facilitate underrepresented minority students achieving a graduate degree, preparing a pipeline of underrepresented student populations qualified to assume faculty roles in schools of nursing. An example of an academic progression program that advances the graduate ethnic underrepresented minorities students to a doctoral degree is a bridge program that partners Winston-Salem State University and Duke University (Brandon, Collins-McNeil, Onsomu, & Powell, 2014).

Articulation Agreements

Another example of an academic model that promotes entry into a graduate program for nurses without a BSN degree is the use of articulation agreements between schools offering graduate nursing programs and community colleges that offer associate degree programs. Sometimes referred to as "bridge programs," the curriculum of the nursing baccalaureate and master's programs are analyzed to identify what content is needed by nurses holding the associate degree to ensure that all BSN and MSN outcomes are met. Using this model means that nurses can enter the workforce as an advanced practice nurse more quickly than if they took the more traditional approach of the RN to BSN program and then applied for entry into a graduate program.

An example of academic progression models that include partnerships and agreements is the Academic Progression in Nursing (APIN) initiative supported by the Robert Wood Johnson Foundation (RWJF) and other similar initiatives. Although many of the partnerships and models emerging from the APIN initiative focus on the RN to BSN pathway, students are also encouraged to consider RN to MSN options, which facilitate a more rapid transition to advanced practice. With approximately 173 RN to MSN programs in existence, many RNs are opting to bypass the BSN degree, instead preferring to focus on obtaining a graduate degree credential (Robert Wood Johnson Foundation [RWJF], 2013). This trend is likely to continue in the future and will increasingly be achieved through the formation of collaborative efforts and partnerships.

Graduate Certificate Programs (Post Master's Certificates)

Graduate certificate programs, also referred to as *post master's certificate (PMC) programs,* are available to advanced practice nurses who already have a master's degree or a DNP degree and want to add another specialty focus to their current practice as an APRN. For example, a nurse prepared as a family NP may return to school to obtain a PMC in psych-mental health. This additional education will allow the nurse to sit for certification as a psych-mental health NP and then to provide services within the scope of practice for both specialties. This approach is especially useful for nurses who practice in rural and community settings such as clinics or emergency rooms.

Graduate certificates may also be available in other specialties besides advanced practice areas. For example, nurses may return to school to obtain a PMC in nursing education, leadership, health care informatics, palliative care, or health care ethics, just to cite a few possibilities, thus enhancing their career options.

Professional standards exist to help faculty design graduate certificate programs for NP programs. Faculty who develop curricula for a PMC program for NPs prepared in a different specialty use the Criteria for Evaluation of Nurse Practitioner Programs (National Task Force on Quality Nurse Practitioner Education [NTF], 2012) to evaluate the knowledge and skills needed for the advanced practice nurse to obtain a PMC in another NP specialty. Typically, this is done using a gap analysis process, which compares the applicant's previous education and work experiences to expected outcomes of another specialty. This process supports the rigor of a program offering while providing the applicant with credit for work already completed.

Academic Progression for Doctoral Programs: BSN to PhD and BSN to DNP

A number of program models are being developed to facilitate acquisition of a doctoral degree earlier in a nurse's career. Typically, in the nursing profession, individuals return to school to seek a doctorate after years in practice. Although this work experience is beneficial to the individual and to nursing, nurses can be more effective at advancing the profession by achieving doctoral degrees earlier in their careers. Thus BSN to PhD and BSN to DNP program models have developed, and nurses who are relatively new to the profession are being encouraged to enter these programs earlier in their careers. Some programs also offer DNP to PhD certificates or degrees for those students who wish to combine their practice skills with a research focus.

The BSN to DNP program model is particularly growing in number. According to the recent American Association of Colleges of Nursing (AACN) (2014c) report outlining progress made in moving to the DNP, approximately 30% of the schools who currently offer APRN programs also offer the BSN to DNP. It is estimated that this figure will grow to greater than 50% over the next few years. Ultimately, it is a possibility that the majority of master's programs may disappear from colleges and universities so that the only degree pathway available for preparing advanced practice nurses will be through clinical doctoral degree (DNP) programs. Some master's programs will remain, such as those preparing the CNL, or in colleges that do not have the resources to offer doctoral-level nursing education.

The American Association of Colleges of Nursing (AACN) (2010a) also has identified some additional academic progression models for PhD programs. In addition to the BSN to PhD, the AACN has proposed two other models, the BSN to DNP/PhD (enrolling in both programs simultaneously) or the BSN to DNP to PhD, for those nurses who wish to receive a degree in an advanced practice role while also receiving the research-focused PhD. These are relatively few in number at this time.

One of the challenges facing nurses who want to apply to a nursing doctoral program is how to select the best program for them. Should they obtain a PhD, which would prepare them as a nurse scientist, or should they obtain a DNP, which would prepare them to translate knowledge into practice? It is important that they consider their career goals and aspirations when selecting doctoral programs. Faculty can develop simple tools to help applicants know whether a PhD program or DNP program is best for the person. An example is the assessment tool used by The University of Nebraska College of Nursing (available at http://www.unmc.edu/nursing/Doctoral_Programs_in_Nursing-DNP_or_PhD.htm).

Curriculum Development for Graduate Programs

Curriculum development for graduate programs follows the same process outlined in Chapter 6. Graduate-level programs build on the mission and philosophy of the school of nursing in which the program resides. Faculty teaching in graduate programs are responsible and accountable for designing, implementing, and evaluating the curriculum.

As graduate programs are developed, faculty must determine which professional standards are appropriate for incorporation into the curriculum as established for a particular specialty. For example, the AACN developed *The Essentials of Master's Education* (American Association of Colleges of Nursing, 2011) and *The Essentials of Doctoral Education for Advanced Practice* (American Association of Colleges of Nursing, 2006) that faculty use when developing graduate programs. The NLN has established Core Competencies for Nurse Educators (2012) that are used to guide graduate curriculum development for nurse educator programs. National Organization of Nurse Practitioner Faculty (NONPF) (2012) has established core competencies for NP curricula and the National Task Force on Quality Nurse Practitioner Education (National Task Force on Quality Nurse Practitioner Education [NTF] (2012) established criteria for the evaluation of nurse practitioner programs. Programs that prepare APRNs are required to provide a stipulated number of clinical hours in the students' program and to maintain student/faculty clinical ratios that follow the national guidelines (National Task Force on Quality Nurse Practitioner Education, 2012). For master's level programs a minimum of 500 clinical hours of supervised direct patient care are required; for clinical doctorate programs, 1000 clinical hours is the current stipulated number. Postmaster's clinical doctorate programs can include the supervised direct patient hours completed in their master's program. National certification is available for all NP specialties as well as CNLs, nurse educators, nurse administrators, and nurse informaticists. National certification is required for all APRNs, and it is an expectation that the curriculum of graduate programs preparing APRNs will design the curriculum in such a way that their graduates will be eligible to take the certification examination for their specialty area.

Additionally when developing curricula, the standards and competencies of nursing accrediting bodies (Accreditation Commission for Nursing Education [ACEN], CCNE, and NLN Commission for Nursing Education Accreditation [CNEA]) must be followed for MSN and DNP programs. PhD programs are not accredited by external accrediting bodies, although the American Association of Colleges of Nursing (AACN) (2001) has published *Indicators of Quality for Research-Focused Doctoral Programs in Nursing* that faculty can use as standards for the PhD program. Instead, PhD programs are usually subject to periodic external and internal academic review procedures, following criteria established by the institution within which they reside.

Curriculum Models for Graduate Programs

Rapid changes in health care demand that traditional models of education that are usually content based be transformed to meet evolving changes in the health care environment. Various curriculum models are emerging in response to this need (Benner, Sutphen, Leonard, & Day, 2010).

Competency or Outcomes Based Models

A key model that needs to be considered in the development of graduate programs is the competency or outcomes-based model (Gibson, 2013; Sroczynski, 2010). This curriculum design focuses on knowledge, skills, and attitudes that encompass professional nursing practice and begins with agreement from stakeholders on the expected outcomes and associated competencies, and ends with implementation and evaluation of the outcomes. Because this model is cyclical, there is no true ending to the process. As the health care environment changes and places new demands on health care practitioners, outcomes and competencies are updated as programs are required to adapt to ensure that new competencies are taught and evaluated. Sroczynski & Dunphy (2012) identified how this model can be used as the foundation for the preparation of primary care NPs. They advocate that using this model will enable nurse educators to quickly adapt curriculum to accommodate the rapid changes in health care so that NPs are prepared to provide quality care for their patients.

Collaborative Models

Collaborative models can be adapted to improve efficiency within schools of nursing that offer multiple specialties at the master's or doctoral level. This is especially critical given the shortage of nurse faculty that exists today. Collaborative curricula are those designed to meet the common needs of learners across specialties. The faculty of each graduate specialty examines their curriculum plans, identifies common outcomes and competencies, and then designs a graduate curriculum that shares content, as appropriate, across specialties. This can increase the efficiency within a school that prepares NPs for several specialties. This type of model calls for core courses such as pharmacology and health assessment to be taught across the specialty programs and then population-focused courses to be taught within the specialty. This model calls for faculty to critically examine the overlaps in content and determine methods of teaching that promote collaboration among nursing faculty while streamlining content that is population-specific.

The Nursing Education Xchange, is another example of a collaborative model that has been established as a national consortium to offer courses for PhD and DNP programs. Schools of nursing participate in the consortium by contributing online courses and faculty to teach them and also by making these courses available to students in participating schools. As a result of the consortium, a greater variety of courses are available than any one school might be able to offer its students (Lobo, Hass, Clark, & McNeil, 2014).

Interprofessional Education Models

A corresponding challenge in today's environment calls for interprofessional education (IPE) that will foster collaborative, patient-centered care (American Association of Colleges of Nursing, 2012a). IPE promotes mutual understanding and respect for what each professional contributes to the care needed by patients and uses multiple strategies such as simulation, collaborative care seminars, and interactive learning experiences (Olenick et al., 2011). IPE programs are being developed regionally as well as within academic medical centers and require collaboration across disciplines to establish a common curriculum core while also maintaining a specialty focus that prepares the student for the role of advanced nursing practice as an NP, educator, administrator, informaticist, or researcher. IPE and collaborative practice promote positive patient outcomes, demonstrate accountability to consumers, and improve efficiency of care delivery systems (Gerard, Kazer, Babington, & Quell, 2014).

Teaching in Graduate Programs

The quality of graduate nursing education programs is maintained through the appointment and selection of well-qualified faculty. Faculty who teach in APRN specialty practice graduate programs at the master's level need to have a master's degree at a minimum with certification in the area in which they teach and remain current in their practice.

To teach in DNP or PhD programs, faculty should have a doctoral degree and have appropriate experience within the field in which they teach. Faculty who teach in PhD programs should have an active research program to mentor PhD students in their development as nurse scientists. There must be a critical mass of faculty in a school of nursing who are active researchers to support a PhD program. Faculty must be excellent teachers as well as scholars to effectively guide and advise students in their development as researchers. As members of the scientific community, faculty disseminate their research findings through publications in peer-reviewed journals and presentations at scientific conferences. PhD students learn by participating with their faculty in their research and dissemination of the findings.

Faculty who are certified as APRNs and teach in DNP programs should have an active clinical practice. In addition to clinical expertise, faculty teaching in a DNP program should have the requisite experience to teach the courses for which they are responsible. Depending on the curriculum, this can include such topics as health policy, epidemiology, complexity science, leadership in complex systems, and health care technology. Given the nature of the curriculum in DNP programs, it is likely that the faculty will be interdisciplinary in nature.

Assessing Graduate Student Readiness for Progression and Graduation

Teaching in graduate programs is both challenging and rewarding. Many issues appear that require faculty to have skillful conversations about what is best for the program and to ensure that students have the knowledge and skills necessary for the career they are planning.

For example, students enrolled in many PhD programs are expected to take a qualifying examination designed to test the student's knowledge of a field as well as the critical and analytical skills needed for success as a researcher and scholar, and complete a dissertation. Although the requirements for both the qualifying examination and dissertation vary with institutions, it is a common expectation that faculty will serve as mentors and advisors to the student. Typically a faculty member is assigned the role of major advisor to a PhD student and has the responsibility to guide the student in course selection, formation of a minor, and in general serving as a resource as the student progresses through the curriculum. Major faculty advisors may chair the qualifying exam committee, bearing primary responsibility for developing the examination according to the school's policies. The major faculty advisor may also chair the dissertation committee and guide the student in the selection of other dissertation committee members. It is the responsibility of the qualifying examination and dissertation committee members to ensure that the student has met the expected competencies and outcomes of the PhD program and is ready to graduate. It is important that the graduate faculty have collectively determined the expected outcomes of the program so that evaluating student outcomes can be accomplished with some measure of objectivity.

Progression and graduation requirements for students enrolled in DNP programs tend to vary based on the expected program outcomes. Some programs follow a format similar to the PhD programs and require a student to take a comprehensive examination before progressing to a scholarly inquiry project. The comprehensive exam process may include a written examination, a self-reflection synthesis demonstrating integration and synthesis of all coursework and practice activities, and an oral examination. Other DNP programs do not require a comprehensive exam. However, all DNP programs require the student to complete a scholarly inquiry project that is most likely designed to improve health care delivery or form health policy. Some schools recognize the scholarly inquiry project as a comprehensive examination that ensures competence of DNP students. To date, there has been tremendous variation across nursing schools as to what the DNP scholarly inquiry project should consist of, even as to what it should be called. It is not intended to be a dissertation similar to the PhD program. National dialogue continues as to the most appropriate model for a culminating scholarly project for DNP graduates.

Similar to the PhD program, most DNP programs assign a faculty as a major advisor and designate a committee of faculty to mentor and guide the student through the program and scholarly inquiry project. Practice partners may also be members of the project committee. The committee will be responsible for determining if the student has met the expected outcomes for the DNP program.

Whatever processes used by faculty to ensure competence of the DNP student, all processes are designed to evaluate the individual student's achievement of the professional standards that faculty have chosen to integrate throughout the curriculum. The professional standard most commonly integrated reflects the *Essentials of Doctoral Education for Advanced Nursing Practice* (American Association of Colleges of Nursing, 2006), and if preparing NPs, the *Criteria for the Evaluation of Nurse Practitioner Programs* (National Organization of Nurse Practitioner Faculty [NONPF], 2012; National Task Force on Quality Nurse Practitioner Education [NTF], 2012).

Preparing Faculty to Teach at the Graduate Level

Preparing faculty to teach at the graduate level is a challenge faced by all schools of nursing. With the current shortage of nursing faculty, it is imperative that nurses who want to teach are prepared for the role. If faculty are hired who do not have educational course preparation in their graduate programs, then the school of nursing must determine how best to assist the new faculty member to gain the necessary skills to teach at the graduate level.

Successful teaching at the doctoral level, in particular, requires a unique skill set. In addition to a solid foundation in nursing science, research, and scholarship, strong writing and oral skills, and a firm grasp on societal, policy, and ethical issues affecting their area of scholarly expertise, faculty need to be able to impart that knowledge and mentor students in the beginning development of their own program of research or clinical practice expertise. Developing such a relationship with students requires a commitment of time and energy to help students conceptualize their research or clinical projects and implement them successfully. It is also important for faculty to be skilled in teamwork and negotiation to help them participate on dissertation and project committees in a manner that is supportive to students and creates an environment for objective evaluation of student outcomes. Faculty who are new to teaching at the graduate level, especially in doctoral education, will require mentoring of their own to help them adjust to the role.

Not all individuals hired into a faculty role have pedagogical course work as part of their graduate preparation. To be effective educators, faculty must be prepared in the science of pedagogy for both classroom and clinical teaching. Some schools deal with this issue by requiring that new faculty take courses to prepare them with the knowledge and skills necessary to teach using a variety of strategies that promote active engagement of students. Effective clinical supervision is another area for faculty skills development. Finally, faculty new to the teaching role in APRN programs must learn how to work effectively with preceptors and understand the responsibilities of the student, preceptor, and faculty in the precepting relationship. If faculty do not take formal course work in nursing education, it is important to establish faculty development programs that provide new faculty with the skills and knowledge needed for success in the teaching role at the graduate level. Mentoring by experienced educators is essential to promote the success of faculty moving into teaching at this level.

Doctoral programs also have an obligation to prepare graduates for faculty positions and the teaching component of the faculty role (National League for Nursing [NLN], 2013). Minnick, Norman, Donaghey, Fisher & McKingan (2010) found that only 20% of PhD programs required a teaching practicum; similarly Udlis & Mancuso (2012) found that only approximately 12% of DNP programs offered any courses that would prepare graduates with educator skills. Strategies that are incorporated in these programs include credit-bearing courses such as Preparing Future Faculty, requirements for students to participate in seminars with content related to the educator role, teaching assistantships, and the use of elective credits for teacher preparation courses (Billings, 2014).

Graduate faculty must balance the roles of teaching, practice, scholarship, and service to advance their own careers in academia. Experienced doctoral faculty are required to mentor and coach younger doctoral faculty on how to be successful in all of these areas. Faculty teaching in PhD programs must be scholars who can mentor and coach younger research scholars in teaching PhD students as well as conducting and disseminating their own research through grant development and implementation, publication in peer-reviewed journals, and presentations at scientific meetings. Faculty teaching in DNP programs must be scholars who can mentor and coach younger DNP-prepared faculty to teach, practice, and develop and implement scholarly projects, as well as disseminate their scholarly projects through publication in peer-reviewed journals and presentations at appropriate meetings. Developing teaching skills and practice skills in faculty who enter academia after completing a BSN to DNP or BSN to PhD program must be considered when developing a program to assist faculty to be successful in academia. Faculty needs to ensure success vary depending on the individual and require individualized plans to help each person be successful.

Future Trends in Graduate Education

Graduate nursing education is in a state of flux striving to respond to changes occurring in the health care environment. Faculty must be willing to make changes in programs to ensure graduates are prepared to meet the health needs of the people they serve. This will involve examining the purpose of all academic programs, determining the viability of the master's degree program, and using the outcomes of successful progression plans and articulation agreements to produce the recommended number of doctorally prepared graduates. Other trends evident at this time include the expansion of IPE, use of social media, use of digital devices in teaching and health care, use of telehealth, integration of technology into programs, and integration of collaboration into programs and across disciplines (Keating, 2011c; Schmitt, Sims-Giddens, & Booth, 2012). Graduate programs will also be affected by national and state legislation regarding professional practice issues, across state licensing, and program requirements. Also of concern are changes in federal legislation regarding financial aid, accreditation of the college or university, and requirements for offering online programs that enroll out-of-state students.

The shift from acute care to community-based settings and ambulatory care will influence what types of nurses and with what level of academic preparation are needed. New roles such as health coach, care manager, transition care coordinator, information specialist, and others still to emerge will require faculty to develop degrees and certificates to prepare nurses to meet these needs of the health care system.

The most significant trend that must be addressed is the need to develop programs that enable nurses to advance to graduate degrees more rapidly. This will require that faculty let go of traditional ways of educating students and explore new ways to prepare nurses who can manage an ever-expanding knowledge base to improve care delivery systems and the care delivered to patients.

The developing workforce shortage in academia requires faculty to determine how new faculty will be developed and prepared to educate graduate students. Graduate faculty need to consider how best to ensure that newer faculty are prepared to teach in the PhD, DNP, or MSN programs as well as continue to develop their careers as researchers, scholars, and practitioners.

With the shortage of doctorally prepared faculty, faculty who work in schools with both PhD and DNP programs advise both PhD and DNP students. This presents a challenge to faculty who may be more grounded in research or practice. It is important that faculty be clear about the differences in expectations for students in each program and support students in meeting outcomes of their particular program.

Summary

This chapter presents an overview of the development of graduate programs. Graduate programs in nursing have grown and morphed into new approaches to educating advanced practice nurses in response to changes in societal, scientific, and professional forces. Today, graduate programs exist to prepare nurses as nurse scientists, advanced practice nurses, administrators, educators, and health policy experts. Graduate curricula are changing from a content focus to a competency or outcomes focus. A driving force influencing change in graduate curricula is the need to collaborate within the discipline and across disciplines. An ongoing challenge is to include preparation to teach as part of graduate education so that graduates of doctoral programs can function as nurse educators in addition to developing the profession's knowledge base or translating knowledge into practice. Graduate programs must continue to change to meet the needs of health care populations and delivery systems.

REFLECTING ON THE EVIDENCE

1. Compare the curriculum of a DNP and PhD program. What are the similarities and differences? Are there areas of overlap? What aspects of the programs could be streamlined to facilitate shortened time from admission to graduation?
2. What end-of-program project, paper, or publication is evidence of attaining DNP program goals? How does this differ from the dissertation in a PhD program?
3. What are the legal and policy implications for advanced practice nurses in providing care via telehealth?
4. What is the future of the MSN degree? Will the programs fold in to DNP degrees? How many BSN to DNP degree programs currently exist? What makes their curriculum design unique? What evidence should be used to guide any decision about discontinuing an MSN program?
5. What evidence is there now about the success of the DNP for preparing nurses for advanced practice?

REFERENCES

American Association of Colleges of Nursing (AACN). (2001). *Indicators of quality in research-focused doctoral programs in nursing*. Retrieved from, http://www.aacn.nche.edu/.

American Association of Colleges of Nursing (AACN). (2006). *The essentials of doctoral education for advanced nursing practice*. Retrieved from, www.aacn.nche.edu/publications/position/dnpessentials.pdf.

American Association of Colleges of Nursing (AACN). (2008). *Consensus model for APRN regulation: Licensure, accreditation, certification & education*. Retrieved from, http://www.aacn.nche.edu/education-resources/APRNReport.pdf.

American Association of Colleges of Nursing (AACN). (2010a). *The research focused doctoral program in nursing: Pathways to excellence*. Retrieved from, www.aacn.nche.edu/education-resources/phdposition.pdf.

American Association of Colleges of Nursing (AACN). (2010b). *Tri-Council for nursing issues new consensus policy statement on the educational advancement of registered nurses*. Retrieved from, http://www.aacn.nche.edu/publications/position/tri-council-sept-2000.

American Association of Colleges of Nursing (AACN). (2011). *The essentials of master's education in nursing*. Retrieved from, www.aacn.nche.edu/education-resources/MastersEssentials11.pdf.

American Association of Colleges of Nursing (AACN). (2012a). *AACN advances nursing's role in interprofessional education*. Retrieved from, www.aacn.nche.edu/news/articles/2012/ipec.

American Association of Colleges of Nursing (AACN). (2012b). *Joint statement on academic progression for nursing students and graduates*. Retrieved from, http://www.aacn.nche.edu/aacn-publications/position/joint-statement-academic-progression.

American Association of Colleges of Nursing (AACN). (2013). *Competencies and curricular expectations for clinical nurse leader education and practice*. Retrieved from, www.aacn.nche.edu/publications/white-papers/cnl.

American Association of Colleges of Nursing (AACN). (2014a). *The doctor of nursing practice: DNP fact sheet*. Retrieved from, http://www.aacn.nche.edu/media-relations/fact-sheets/dnp.

American Association of Colleges of Nursing (AACN). (2014b). *Fact sheet: Creating a more highly qualified nursing workforce*Retrieved from, http://www.aacn.nche.edu/media-relations/NursingWorkforce.pdf.

American Association of Colleges of Nursing (AACN). (2014c). *Progress made in transition to the practice doctorate*. Retrieved from, http://www.aacn.nche.edu/news/articles/2014/dnp-study.

Bednash, G., Breslin, E., Kirschling, J., & Rosseter, R. (2014). PhD or DNP: Planning for doctoral nursing education. *Nursing Science Quarterly*, *27*(4), 296–301.

Benner, P., Sutphen, M., Leonard, V., & Day, L. (2010). *Educating nurses: A call for radical transformation*. San Francisco: Jossey-Bass.

Billings, D. (2014). Preparation for nurse educator and faculty roles in nursing PhD/EdD programs in the United States. In: *Presented at STTI-NLN Research in Nursing Education Conference, April 3, 2014,. Indianapolis, IN*.

Brandon, D., Collins-McNeil, J., Onsomu, E., & Powell, D. (2014). Winston-Salem State University and Duke University's bridge to the doctorate program. *North Carolina Medical Journal*, *75*(1), 68–70.

Carter, M. (2013). The evolution of doctoral education in nursing. In S. DeNisco & A. Barker (Eds.), *Advanced practice nursing: Evolving roles for the transformation of the profession* (pp. 27–36). Burlington, MA: Jones & Bartlett Learning.

Cronenwett, L., Dracup, K., Grey, M., McCauley, L., Meleis, A., & Salmon, M. (2011). The doctor of nursing practice: A national workforce perspective. *Nursing Outlook*, *59*, 9–17.

Danzey, I., Ea, E., Fitzpatrick, J., Garbutt, S., Rafferty, M., & Zychowicz, M. (2011). The doctor of nursing practice and nursing education: Highlights, potential, and promise. *Journal of Professional Nursing, 27*(5), 311–314.

Egenes, K. (2009). History of nursing. In G. Roux & J. Halstead (Eds.), *Issues and trends in nursing: Essential knowledge for today and tomorrow* (pp. 1–26). New York: Jones & Bartlett.

Fairman, J. (2014). *Nurse practitioners: Shaping the future.* Retrieved from, http://www.nursing.upenn.edu/nhhc/Pages/Nurse-Practitioners.aspx.

Fontaine, D., & Langston, N. (2011). The master's is not broken: Commentary on "The doctor of nursing practice: A national workforce perspective." *Nursing Outlook, 59*, 121–122.

Gerard, S., Kazer, M., Babington, L., & Quell, T. (2014). Past, present, and future trends of master's education in nursing. *Journal of Professional Nursing, 30*(4), 326–332.

Gibson, R. (2013). *Competency based learning: Four challenges and impediments.* Retrieved from, www.evolution.com/opinions/competency-based-learning.

Graves, B., Tomlinson, S., Jandley, M., Oliver, J., Carter-Templeton, H., Gaskins, S., et al. (2013). The emerging doctor of education (EdD) in instructional leadership for nurse educators. *International Journal of Nursing Education Scholarship, 10*(1), 1–7.

Institute of Medicine (IOM). (2001). *Crossing the Quality Chasm: A New Health System for the 21st Century.* Washington, DC: The National Academy Press.

Institute of Medicine (IOM). (2003). *Health professions education: A bridge to quality.* Washington, DC: The National Academies Press.

Institute of Medicine (IOM). (2010). *The future of nursing: Leading change, advancing health.* Washington, DC: The National Academy Press.

Keating, S. (2011a). Curriculum planning for master's nursing programs. In S. Keating (Ed.), *Curriculum development and evaluation in nursing* (pp. 241–252). New York: Springer Publishing.

Keating, S. (2011b). The doctor of nursing practice. In S. Keating (Ed.), *Curriculum development and evaluation in nursing* (pp. 253–260). New York: Springer Publishing.

Keating, S. (2011c). Issues and challenges for nurse educators. In S. Keating (Ed.), *Curriculum development and evaluation in nursing* (pp. 353–378). New York: Springer Publishing.

Lobo, M., Haas, B., Clark, M., & McNeil, P. (2014). NEXus: Evaluation of an innovative educational consortium for doctoral education in nursing. *Journal of Professional Nursing.* http://dx.doi.org/10.1016/j.profnurs.2014.07.005.

Malone, B. (2011). Commentary on "The doctor of nursing practice: A national workforce perspective." *Nursing Outlook, 59*, 117–118.

Minnick, A., Norman, L., Donaghey, B., Fisher, L., & McKirgan, I. (2010). Defining and describing capacity issues in US doctoral nursing research programs. *Nursing Outlook, 58*(1), 36–43.

Morton, P. (2015). What is the future of the PhD Dissertation? *Journal of Professional Nursing, 31*(1), 1–2.

National League for Nursing (NLN). (2012). *The scope of practice for academic nurse educators.* Washington, D.C: Author.

National League for Nursing (NLN). (2013). *A vision for doctoral preparation for nurse educators.* Retrieved from, http://www.nln.org/aboutnln/livingdocuments/pdf/nlnvision_6.pdf.

National Organization of Nurse Practitioner Faculty (NONPF). (2012). *Nurse practitioner core competencies.* Retrieved, http://c.ymcdn.com/sites/www.nonpf.org/resource/resmgr/competencies/npcorecompetenciesfinal2012.pdf.

National Research Council of the National Academies. (2005). *Advancing the nation's health needs.* Washington, D. C: The National Academies Press. Retrieved, https://grants.nih.gov/training/nas_report_2005.pdf.

National Task Force on Quality Nurse Practitioner Education (NTF). (2012). *Criteria for evaluation of nurse practitioner programs.* Retrieved from, http://c.ymcdn.com/sites/www.nonpf.org/resource/resmgr/docs/ntfevalcriteria2012final.pdf.

Olenick, M., Foote, E., Vanston, P., Szarek, J., Vaskalis, Z., Dimattio, M., & Smego, R. (2011). A regional model of interprofessional education. *Advanced Medical Education Practice, 2*, 17–23.

Pellico, L., Terrill, E., White, P., & Rico, J. (2012). Integrative review of graduate entry programs in nursing. *Journal of Nursing Education, 51*(1), 29–37.

Peplau, H. (1966). Nursing: Two routes to doctoral degrees. *Nursing Forum, 5*(2), 57–67.

Potempa, K. (2011). The DNP serves the public good. *Nursing Outlook, 59*, 123–125.

Robert Wood Johnson Foundation (RWJF). (2013). *The case for academic progression: Why nurses should advance their education and the strategies that make this feasible.* Retrieved from, http://www.rwjf.org/content/dam/farm/reports/issue_briefs/2013/rwjf407597.

Schmitt, T., Sims-Giddens, S., & Booth, R. (2012). Social media use in nursing education. *Online Journal of Issues in Nursing, 17*(3) Manuscript 2.

Sroczynski, M. (2010). *The competency or outcomes based curriculum model.* Retrieved from, http://campaignforaction.org/sites/default/files/Competency%20%20Model%20Summary.pdf.

Sroczynski, M., & Dunphy, L. (2012). Primary care nurse practitioner clinical education: Challenges and opportunities. *Nursing Clinics of North America, 47*, 463–479.

Stotts, N. (2011). Curriculum planning for doctor of philosophy and other research focused doctoral nursing programs. In S. Keating (Ed.), *Curriculum development and evaluation in nursing* (pp. 261–268). New York: Springer Publishing.

Udlis, K., & Mancuso, J. (2012). Doctor of nursing practice programs across the United States: A benchmark of information. Part 1: Program characteristics. *Journal of Professional Nursing, 28*(5), 265–273.

Designing Courses and Learning Experiences*

10

Martha Scheckel, PhD, RN

The purpose of the curriculum is to create a learning environment that presents students with a cohesive body of knowledge, attitudes, and skills necessary for professional nursing practice. The curriculum is implemented by and for faculty and students through learner-centered courses and learning experiences. This chapter focuses on designing courses and learning experiences for effective implementation of the teaching–learning process, whereby students become educated for self-development and various nursing roles in society. Designing courses and learning experiences cannot be accomplished through a casual, hit-or-miss approach; instead, they must be thoughtfully and cohesively developed to provide students with the opportunities necessary to achieve the intended curriculum outcomes.

Learner-Centered Courses

In recent years, there has been an increased emphasis on learning and learner-centered instruction, shifting the focus in education away from teacher-centered instruction. In teacher-centered instruction, teachers direct the delivery of content, putting great effort into assimilating information, distilling it, and transferring it to students (Stanley & Dougherty, 2010). Freire (2006) most notably names teacher-centered instruction "banking" education where students become receptacles for information. Historically, schools of nursing have adopted banking models of education. This adoption has been largely driven by nurse educators' concerns that students need content to be prepared for nursing practice. Students do need discipline-specific knowledge to provide safe and effective nursing care. However, an over-reliance on providing content through teacher-centered instruction can impede students from integration of the professional apprenticeships: knowledge, skilled know-how, and ethical comportment (Benner et al., 2010, p. 82). Integration requires active rather than passive engagement in learning. Thus courses with learner-centered designs promote "teaching focused on learning" (Weimer, 2013, p. 15). Weimer (2013) conveys that learner-centered foci engage students in learning, empower students by giving them control over learning, encourage collaboration in the classroom, promote reflection on learning, and involve skills in "learning instruction" (p. 15). There are many ways of providing "teaching focused on learning." Most importantly, however, learner-centered course designs require that teachers become familiar with learning theories and instructional strategies that promote four shifts in thinking as outlined by Benner and colleagues (2010, p. 89):

1. Shift from a focus on covering decontextualized knowledge to an emphasis on teaching for a sense of salience, situated cognition, and action in particular clinical situations.
2. Shift from a sharp separation of classroom and clinical teaching to integrative teaching in all settings.
3. Shift from an emphasis on critical thinking to an emphasis on clinical reasoning and multiple ways of thinking that include critical thinking.
4. Shift from an emphasis on socialization and role taking to an emphasis on formation (with formation indicating perceptual abilities, abilities to use knowledge and skilled-know-how, and a way of being and acting in practice [p. 166]).

*The author would like to thank the authors of previous edition Diane Billings, EdD, RN, FAAN, Barbara Norton, MPH, RN and Connie Rowles, DSN, RN.

Course Design Process

Course design follows a sequential process, starting with the broad program outcomes and ending with specific lesson plans (Diamond, 2008; Fink, 2013; Wiggins & McTighe, 2005). Although a sequential process is described here, the process is, in fact, iterative as the course design unfolds. Courses may be designed by a faculty team or an individual with subject matter expertise. Instructional designers, a resource often available at teaching resource centers at many colleges, are an asset to the course development process.

Predesign

Course design begins by understanding the learning background and experience of the students who will enroll in the course, and then identifying how the course fits with overall academic program outcomes and competencies, the curriculum framework, and core concepts and competencies within courses. During the predesign stage, faculty also should review as needed prerequisite, concurrent, or other courses if the course being developed is a part of a sequence. If the course has been taught previously, student course evaluations can provide additional insight for course development.

Prior to writing course outcomes, faculty also should review recommendations from national health care organizations; from influential reports with recommendations for nursing education; and from professional nursing organizations that make recommendations about essential competencies, concepts, and content as they relate to the course being developed. State regulatory and national accrediting agencies may also have prescriptive statements about course content and credit hour allocation.

Course Objectives, Outcomes, and Competencies

Course objectives, outcomes, and competencies are derived from end-of-program (terminal) and program level (year or semester) outcomes and indicate what students should know, be able to do, and value at the end of the course, and how they will be evaluated and graded. Although faculty use terms in different ways, Wittman-Price and Fasolka (2010) suggest that the term *learning outcome* (as opposed to the term *objective)* is less restrictive and more appropriate in a learner-centered environment. Regardless of the term used, these "behavioral indicators" activate the curriculum, direct the choice of learning materials, guide the development of learning activities, and communicate to students what they are expected to learn and how they will be evaluated. Course learning objectives, outcomes, and competencies therefore must be written at appropriate levels or relevance to clinical practice, to be easily understood by students, and to guide evaluation of attainment.

Course Concepts and Content

Once learning outcomes are written, faculty can make decisions about the concepts and content to include in the course. Typically, faculty are selected to develop and teach courses because of their expertise with the content, and may be inclined to include all that is known about the subject. However, they also must design the course to fit within the curriculum and the level of practice for which the student is being prepared.

To prevent having a course burdened by content, Candela et al. (2006) recommend developing a process for making decisions about which content to retain and suggest including only content that is essential to meet program and course outcomes, is required for safe practice, needs to be reinforced and practiced, is included in curriculum recommendations from professional nursing organizations, and cannot be accessed easily when needed. Others (Davis, 2009; Diamond, 2008) recommend distinguishing between essential and optional material, considering core concepts versus details, and including only those topics relevant to practice or common existing problems. If the course is a part of a concept-based curriculum, the course designer must determine which concepts represent contemporary nursing practice, reflect the unique features of a nursing program, and are clear and understandable to students (Giddens et al., 2012).

Organizing the Concepts and Content in Modules

Once core concepts and content are established, the next step is to organize them into modules of related material. Modules can be organized in a variety of ways: using a logical sequence from beginning to end (e.g., across the lifespan); following a sequential process (e.g., the management process); by complexity (from simple to complex or from concrete to abstract); using a body systems approach; or, in the instance of case-based or problem-based learning, by inquiry about a particular problem. Including units within modules breaks material down further to facilitate effective and efficient delivery of material. Regardless of how the concepts and content are organized, the structure should be evident to students and be consistent throughout the course. See Box 10-1 for an example of organizing modules and units for a beginning level undergraduate health promotion and disease and injury prevention course.

Designing Lesson Plans

Once the modules are organized, faculty can design lesson plans within each unit of the modules. The lesson plans should state the name of the module and units included in the module; the unit's purpose; program, level, and course outcomes and competencies related to the lesson; outcomes for the lesson; assignments and learning experiences; and evaluation strategies. Time limits must be considered when determining lesson plan design. The time spent should be in proportion to the relative significance of the concepts and content, the students' ability to learn the material, and time allotted for completion of the course. The following describes general guidelines for each aspect of the example lesson plan displayed in Box 10-2:

- Purpose: Clearly and succinctly describe to students what they will learn and the relevance of the unit.
- Program, level, and course outcomes and competencies: Identify program, level, and course outcomes and competencies that are *most* related to the lesson. This identification allows students to understand the unit's major foci. The identification also allows faculty to determine to what extent course lesson plans collectively address all of the program, level, and course outcomes and competencies, and determine potential gaps in concept and content coverage. Identifying gaps helps faculty balance concepts and content so that students have the best opportunity to obtain a comprehensive understanding of the course material.
- Lesson outcomes: Delineate for students what they will be able to demonstrate at the end of the lesson. When writing lesson outcomes, keep in mind what students will most need to learn for "real-world" nursing practice. This will help faculty narrow content to the most essential elements students need to learn for entry into nursing practice.
- Assignments: Describe assignments so that students clearly understand expectations for learning experiences. Be as specific as possible and elaborate as needed on the assignments in class sessions or in online forums. It is

BOX 10-1 Examples of Modules and Units in a Health Promotion and Disease and Injury Prevention Undergraduate Course

MODULE 1: FOUNDATIONS OF HEALTH PROMOTION AND DISEASE AND INJURY PREVENTION

Units

- Determinants of health
- Health and health care disparities
- Principles of epidemiology

MODULE 2: PRINCIPLES OF HEALTH PROMOTION

Units

- Defining health promotion
- Health promotion theories
- Nursing roles in health promotion

MODULE 3: PRINCIPLES OF HEALTH LITERACY

Units

- Defining health literacy
- Measurements of health literacy
- Nursing roles in health literacy

MODULE 4: DISEASE AND INJURY PREVENTION

Units

- Defining disease and injury prevention
- Levels of prevention
- Epidemiologic principles of injury prevention
- Nursing roles in disease and injury prevention

Courtesy Mary Mundt and Theresa Wehrwein; adapted with permission Michigan State University College of Nursing.

BOX 10-2 Example Lesson Plan in an Undergraduate Health Promotion and Disease and Injury Prevention Course

MODULE 1: FOUNDATIONS OF HEALTH PROMOTION AND DISEASE AND INJURY PREVENTION

- Unit 1: Determinants of Health

PURPOSE: Learn about determinants of health and their influence on health promotion and disease prevention.

Program Outcomes Related to the Lesson:

- Holistic Health Promotion: Empower patients to improve health using a wide range of individual, social, and environmental interventions.
- Cultural Congruence: Apply knowledge, skills, and attitudes to effectively practice within the cultural context of the patient.

Course Outcomes Related to the Lesson:

- Assess health/illness beliefs, values, attitudes, and practices of individuals, communities, and populations.
- Use epidemiology and determinants of health to develop health promotion and disease and injury prevention interventions for individuals, communities, and populations.

Outcomes Related to this Lesson:

- Explain determinants of health.
- Describe *Healthy People 2020*'s focus on determinants of health.
- Demonstrate the nurse's role in influencing determinants of health.
- Discuss how the Centers for Population Health and Health Disparities (CPHHD) are addressing determinants of health.

Assignments Before Class:

- Read Chapter 4 in the textbook.
- Read "About Healthy People" and "Determinants of Health" on the *Healthy People 2020* website.
- Read the introduction to the Centers for Population Health and Health Disparities (CPHHD) on the website.
- Complete the Determinants of Health reading response online journal entry.

Learning Experiences in Class:

- Learning Group #1: Review the textbook case study. Use the principles provided in Chapter 4 to devise a health promotion strategy related to the case. Provide a 5-minute oral report to the class about the health promotion strategy your learning group developed.
- Learning Group #2: Review one of the CPHHDs. Describe a project completed or underway and identify which determinants of health are most affected by the project and why. Complete an illustration of your description to share with the class.

Evaluation Strategies:

- Case Study Discussion Rubric for Oral Reports
- CPHHD Quality Illustration Rubric
- Exam #1: Be prepared to identify health determinants and priority health promotion strategies, which nurses can design and implement.

Courtesy Steve Yelon, Mary Mundt, and Theresa Wehrwein; adapted with permission of Michigan State University College of Nursing.

important to keep in mind that assignments need to be developed in ways that are consistent with course, program, and lesson outcomes. This consistency promotes coherency of the unit and course, and ease of learning for students. Assignments, as much as possible, should involve active learning strategies (see Chapter 15).

- Evaluation strategies: Students need to be informed how faculty will measure learning and what mechanisms they will use to do so. It is important once again to link the evaluation methods to every other aspect of the lesson plan to ensure consistency and coherency of course delivery.

Selecting Learning Materials and Resources

Faculty who are designing courses have a responsibility for choosing the course learning materials. When choosing learning materials, faculty should consider how these materials align with learning outcomes, fit with the course design, and mirror faculty philosophy. They should also ensure the materials support students' learning needs. Ensuring easy access to materials, providing rationale for selected readings, giving directions about how and when to use materials, and explaining how the materials relate to course concepts and methods of evaluation are all ways to use materials to support students' learning needs.

In addition, faculty need to consider the best use of electronic study resources offered by textbook companies and other publishers. E-books are becoming increasingly available. As compared to print copies, e-books offer a number of advantages such as lower costs, availability, accessibility on personal digital assistants in clinical settings, portability, and ability to search quickly for content

(Abell & Garrett-Wright, 2014). Abell and Garrett-Wright (2014) indicate faculty need both education and time to adapt to using e-books; however, the growth of e-books necessitates a need for faculty to prepare for use of these electronic resources.

When making decisions about selecting learning materials and learning resources, it is important for faculty to understand that if prepackaged course materials do not align well with course goals, faculty can develop custom-designed course packs. Faculty may find that course packs with readings that include web-based resources, selected chapters from various textbooks, and journal articles that are pertinent to the course better facilitate learning. Faculty can create course packs for print production or use e-reserve systems at the library.

Faculty can also easily employ learner-centered approaches to select course materials. Weimer (2013), for example, suggests providing students with a selection of various textbooks faculty have determined are appropriate for the course. Students can then use a textbook rating rubric to choose one of the preselected textbooks for use in the course. Another learner-centered approach involves using strategies that avoid assigning excessive amounts of reading that do not respect the principle of effective use of task on time. For instance, Roberts and Roberts (2008) suggest asking students to select an approach that demonstrates their completion and comprehension of assigned readings. Students can choose to create a song or rap about the readings, write a reading response journal, or describe use of a reading study group. Roberts and Roberts (2008) contend that such approaches promote deep learning rather than superficial learning as can be the case when students are provided quizzes as a way to encourage reading compliance.

Principles for Designing Learning Experiences

Successful implementation of course designs requires careful construction of learning experiences within courses. Well-designed learning experiences can provide students with the opportunity to develop higher-order thinking and clinical decision-making skills, and helps them synthesize content and concepts in classroom and clinical practice settings (Benner et al., 2010). Examples of learning experiences include participating in simulations, using case studies, completing writing assignments such as journaling, analyzing narratives of patients' experiences, developing concept maps, engaging in discussions or debates, and using computer-mediated activities and resources such as computer-assisted instruction and the World Wide Web (see Chapter 15 for detailed examples).

Learning experiences can be designed for use by individual students, pairs of students or groups of students. The experiences can be completed as required assignments or as optional, supplemental, or remedial activities, and can take place in class or online, or be assigned as class preparation. The experiences should be reflected in the syllabus and build from course to course, and level to level. The experiences within lesson plans should be congruent with program, level, course, and lesson outcomes and competencies, and provide information about how students will be evaluated. For example, the lesson plan example in Box 10-2 states the purpose of the lesson. The purpose is linked to related program and course outcomes. Lesson outcomes help students specifically understand *what* they will be able to do to achieve the lesson's purpose, and meet course and program outcomes and competencies. The assignments reflect *how* students will achieve the expected competencies and meet the purpose and outcomes. The evaluation strategies describe to students how their learning will be measured. In addition, it is important that faculty plan and organize class time so that students enjoy and benefit from a variety of learning experiences. Variety helps prevent faculty and students from becoming bored and makes it more likely that faculty can accommodate different learning style preferences. Regardless of the learning experiences, faculty should consider the following three major principles when designing learning experiences:

1. Use of structured or unstructured learning experiences
2. Use of active, passive, or both passive and active learning strategies
3. Use of the learning domains (cognitive, affective, and psychomotor)

These principles are outlined in more detail in the following sections.

Structured and Unstructured Learning Experiences

When designing learning experiences, it is important to consider when to use structured or unstructured experiences. Structured learning experiences are frequently used and are important in assisting students to address and pose questions, solve problems, create solutions, and consider alternatives (Pascarella & Terenzini, 2005). Unstructured learning experiences are designed to allow students to acquire knowledge and skill with much less specific direction from faculty. Although unstructured learning experiences may be used at the undergraduate level, they are more likely to be used in honors or honors option courses, independent study courses, and capstone courses. Faculty may also allow students to use unstructured learning experiences for bonus credit.

Structured Learning Experiences

In structured learning experiences, the stimuli for learning are specifically selected. A structured experience consists of a clear, concise description of the purposes, outcomes, and competencies related to the experience and the content and processes to be used while engaged in the experience; specific directions presented in a logical sequence indicating each of the steps to be followed; and the time for the experience and the method to be used to report its completion.

A well-structured experience allows students to function with a great deal of independence and creativity while working to achieve desired outcomes. For example, when assigning students a text, article, or other form of media to study, providing specific suggestions directly related to the desired outcomes assists students in focusing on the essential concepts. Faculty may choose any one of several methods for students to share the results of their learning experiences. For example, students may be asked to do the following:

1. Complete an answer sheet that will be evaluated by peers, faculty or both.
2. Write a general or specific summary report that addresses the concept, content, or processes and submit it to faculty.
3. Present a report to the class.
4. Discuss the experience with another student or small group of students.
5. Initiate a small group or class discussion of the major points, issues, or problems that arise during their work.

These examples can be used separately or in combination with each other. Faculty may also choose to allow the student to select the preferred method of sharing.

Unstructured Learning Experiences

Unstructured learning experiences are derived from Bruner's discovery learning (Bruner, 1977) and, in recent times, have been called *inquiry-based learning* (Levy et al., 2009). Discovery learning is believed to do the following:

1. Promote a disposition toward inquiry.
2. Promote independent thinking and enhanced problem solving.
3. Stimulate student motivation and interest.
4. Improve knowledge retention.
5. Facilitate transfer of learning by stimulating the student to seek and find relationships between information and the situation at hand.

In an unstructured learning experience, students may be given an assignment in which they are asked to apply their previous and current knowledge, skills, and experiences either to a specific faculty-designated situation or to a situation of their choice that fits a general profile described by faculty. The situation may be an actual event in the practice setting or an event that is depicted through a simulation, case study, or form of media. For example, in a community health nursing course, a learning outcome for students may be for them to become familiar with the kinds of activities and interactions that occur during a community meeting. Students would be directed to act as a participant–observer at a community-based meeting of their choosing. The meeting could be a support group for a particular health problem, a meeting of constituents with their legislator, a town board meeting, or a neighborhood association meeting. Students could be given the option of describing their experience verbally in class or at a clinical conference or by writing about it in a journal. A major limitation associated with discovery learning is the need for students to adapt to self-directed learning that is student-centered rather than teacher-centered (Hains & Smith, 2012).

Passive and Active Learning

In designing courses and learning experiences, it is important to take into consideration theories that explain the learning process. Many of these theories are behaviorally, cognitively, or socially based (Andrade, 2013) and include, but are not limited to, constructivism, brain-based learning, experiential learning, and adult learning. Other learning theories are situated in phenomenology and postmodernism, among other philosophical origins (Diekelmann & Diekelmann, 2009). Common to each of these theories is the idea that learning may be a passive or an active process. Students typically experience both types of learning throughout their educational career. See Chapter 13 for an in-depth discussion of learning theories.

Passive Learning

Passive learning occurs when students use their senses to take in information from a lecture, reading assignment, or some form of audiovisual media. Passive learning is used to acquire ideas and information that are internalized through memorization (Michel et al., 2009).

Passive learning provides faculty with the opportunity to present a great deal of information within a short period, and they can select and prepare in advance lecture notes, handouts, and audiovisual media. Faculty usually feel comfortable with these teaching methods because they can present the information that students need to learn in a controlled environment. For a faculty member who is new or one who is teaching new content for the first time, the instructional strategies used in passive learning may enable him or her to feel more comfortable in the teaching situation when presenting the content.

Because many students have been socialized to passive learning, they often prefer this approach to learning. Important concepts and content are identified for students in a concrete manner that helps them organize the material in a meaningful way. With passive learning, students tend to have lower anxiety levels and feel secure in their belief that listening to a lecture, reading the assignments and handouts, taking notes, and copying information from audiovisual media will provide them with all or most of the information they need to be successful in the course.

However, there are disadvantages to passive learning activities. Passive learning activities may leave faculty with little opportunity to understand how well students are learning the content. Unless designed otherwise, the time used for presentation of the content may leave little time for questions, clarification, or discussion. Students may not feel comfortable letting faculty know that they do not understand key points or relationships; furthermore, they may be reluctant to ask questions in class or they may not ask enough questions to clarify their misunderstandings. In addition, students may be unable to articulate what it is they do not know or understand.

Listening to a presentation, taking notes, and copying from printed media require little cognitive effort from students and no consistent use of higher level cognitive skills. Even reading activities, although important, do not provide students with opportunities to apply the concepts about which they are reading. Although many students may prefer passive learning, over time, passive learning experiences tend to become tedious.

Active Learning

Active learning involves helping learners actively process incoming information (Svinicki & McKeachie, 2014). Learning experiences that promote active learning facilitate students' engagement in and response to the learning situation (Price & Nelson, 2011).

The benefits of active learning (Price & Nelson, 2011; Stevenson & Gordon, 2014) include, but are not limited to:

1. Increased attentiveness to learning
2. Greater interest in learning
3. Desire to use multiple ways of learning
4. Increased retention of information
5. Greater assimilation of learning
6. Deeper understandings of course material
7. Increased critical thinking skills
8. Increased problem-solving skills
9. Enhanced teamwork skills
10. Greater sense of accomplishment in learning

It is not always possible to determine whether students are actively involved in learning because their responses during a learning activity may be reticent. Reticence does not necessarily mean students are not learning. However, there are active learning activities that can make it easier for faculty to assess the degree of active learning. For instance, team-based learning, in which small groups of students work together independently within large classes allows teachers to observe the extent of student preparation for class, students' use of materials related to the course, and their level of participation in class sessions (Clark et al., 2008). Peer active learning is an approach in which students make apparent their critical thinking skills through think–pair–share techniques, case-based learning, role playing, interactive presentations, and discussions (Stevens & Brenner, 2009). A "flipped" classroom involves providing students with learning experiences traditionally received in the classroom outside the classroom. For instance, students may listen to lectures through podcasts or take quizzes outside the classroom. When students attend class, integration of learning becomes apparent as students spend time applying what they learned through preclass learning experiences by engaging in activities such as case studies, small-group projects, and deeper discussions (Bergmann & Sams, 2012; Hawks, 2014). Virtual worlds include using computers to mimic actual environments with avatars (an "in-world presence") that interact in social situations (Mastrian et al., 2011, p. 197). For instance, a student may be an avatar providing nursing care in a homeless shelter. The avatar-student nurse is immersed in the shelter environment and is required to actively interact with clients to address health care problems. Fostering active learning in the classroom is a faculty goal, and evidence exists to support the view that active learning is preferred by some students (Lo, 2010; Sisk, 2011).

There can be some disadvantages associated with active learning. Faculty need to be aware of content areas and relationships among concepts that usually pose difficulty for students. Organizing learning experiences so that students are engaged in active learning requires faculty to design teaching strategies that are learner-centered rather than strictly teacher-centered.

Regardless of the active learning strategies employed, the shift to active learning paradigms may be stressful for faculty, particularly when trying these approaches with large groups of students. Furthermore, faculty may have concerns about receiving less favorable evaluations of instruction. Students are often resistant to changes in the way in which they receive instruction because understanding new ways of learning is stressful. They may be impatient with the process and averse to putting forth the effort needed to try new active learning strategies. In fact, White et al. (2010) suggest that, despite recent evidence supporting active learning and teachers' use of it, students may claim to have learned nothing in courses where faculty use active learning strategies. They concluded that students may lack awareness of their own learning in active learning environments. It is important for faculty to receive support from administration and their peers if active learning strategies are to be successfully incorporated into teaching practice.

Domains of Learning and Learning Experiences

Historically, faculty use Bloom's taxonomy (Anderson & Krathwohl, 2001; Bloom, 1956) to address the cognitive, psychomotor, and affective domains of learning and identify the level at which students need to demonstrate competencies that lead to achievement of expected learning outcomes. These domains mirror the knowledge, attitudes, and skills that nursing students need to practice safely and effectively. Figures 10-1, 10-2, and 10-3 illustrate the categories of each domain. Each domain is hierarchical, with learning presented in ascending order of complexity. When designing learning experiences to fit the appropriate domain level, faculty need to use the domains best suited to the learning experiences. However, they should keep in mind that domains are interdependent and

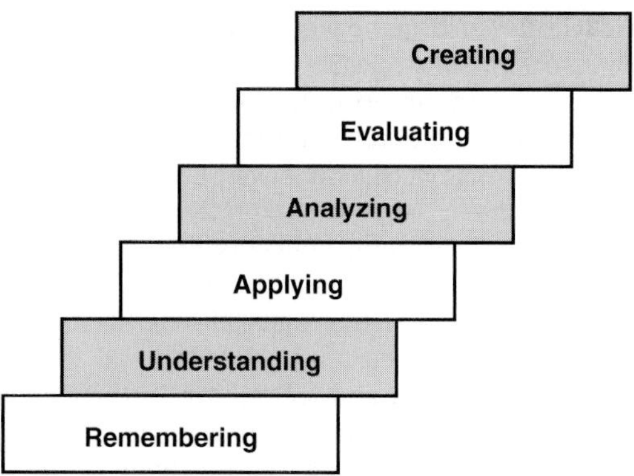

Figure 10-1 Cognitive domain.

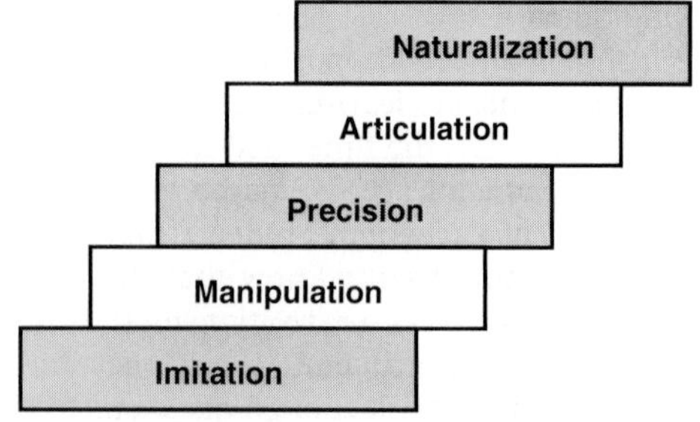

Figure 10-2 Psychomotor domain.

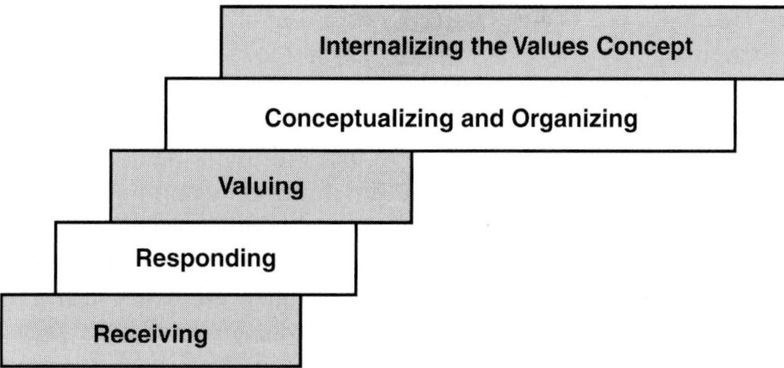

Figure 10-3 Affective domain.

one may be emphasized over another depending on the learning experience and its outcomes. They also need to write learning outcomes expressing the domains using action verbs. Action verbs help faculty level experiences within domains and communicate to students expectations for achievement of outcomes. What follows is a description of each domain with examples of action verbs and an example learning experience within each domain.

Cognitive Domain

The emphasis in the cognitive domain of learning is on knowledge. From a nursing perspective it is important to emphasize the highly complex aspects of this domain. Example action verbs are as follows:

- Remembering: Define, list, label, select, locate, match
- Understanding: Explain, describe, interpret, summarize, predict
- Applying: Solve, apply, use, calculate, relate, change
- Analyzing: Compare, classify, differentiate
- Evaluating: Reframe, critique, support, assess
- Creating: Design, compose, create, formulate, develop

The following example, written for a community health nursing clinical learning experience, illustrates a learning outcome in the cognitive domain with a corresponding learning experience.

> **Learning outcome:** Apply principles of population health to fall prevention in a community-based setting for older adults.
>
> **Learning experience:** Up until this time in your nursing education, your clinical experiences have been in the hospital, and focused on acute care of individual patients. You are preparing to experience your first community-based clinical experience in a respite center for older adults. Before your first clinical experience in the center, read at least two evidence-based articles about fall prevention scales designed to assess fall risk in older adults. Be prepared to discuss clinical settings where fall prevention scales are most applicable for assessing fall risk among older adults. After participating in your first clinical experience, briefly journal about how the respite center setting and the older adults within them changed how you view the use of fall prevention scales in this setting and for this population. Be prepared to share your views with your instructor and your peers in postclinical conference and discuss alterations needed in fall risk assessments based on clinical settings. Discuss the possible meanings of the alterations to respite staff, the older adults, and their families.

This learning experience requires that the students become knowledgeable about fall prevention scales for use in older adults before they enter the respite center. After their first clinical experience, they need to use this knowledge to differentiate use of fall scales in hospitals verses community settings. The experience also requires them to formulate ways to conduct fall risk assessments in various settings. The affective domain is an interdependent domain in this experience because it facilitates valuing what their knowledge of fall risk assessment in a community verses a hospital setting can mean to preventing falls in the non-hospitalized older adult population.

Affective Domain

The affective domain of learning encompasses attitudes, beliefs, values, feelings, and emotions. The aspects of this domain are organized along a continuum of stages of internalization that reflect changes in personal growth, moving from an external to an internal locus of control (Krathwohl et al., 1964). Faculty often find this domain the most difficult to incorporate into learning and the most challenging to assess. Example action verbs are as follows:

- Receiving: Ask, choose, select, locate
- Responding: Discuss, perform, recite, read, help
- Valuing: Differentiate, form, justify, report, share
- Organizing: Alter, arrange, formulate, order, synthesize
- Characterizing: Consistent, revise, judgment, change behavior, reorder priority

The following example, written for a community health nursing course, illustrates a learning outcome in the affective domain with a corresponding learning experience.

> **Learning outcome:** Arranges for patients and families to participate in decisions about self-care practices in the management of chronic illness.
>
> **Learning experience:** Prior to class read the assigned article about a patient newly diagnosed with diabetes. The patient describes the importance of learning to care for his diabetes from family members who also have diabetes. Focus on what the patient values most in learning from his family members about how to manage his self-care. In your small learning groups discuss how you might respond to the knowledge the patient has gained from his family and how you would use this knowledge to design an individualized patient education plan to teach him self-management of his diabetes.

Because this learning experience focuses on what the patient values and the student's responses to these values, it addresses the affective domain of learning. However, the cognitive domain is the interdependent domain because students need to possess clinical knowledge about diabetes management to design a patient education plan that discerns which aspects of the patient's knowledge gained from his family are therapeutic and which aspects indicate that further education is necessary.

Psychomotor Domain

The psychomotor domain of learning deals with the development of manual or physical competencies and is the domain that faculty use most often in developing competencies related to clinical practice. Students initially learn skills through imitation and manipulation, and with repetition eventually internalize the skills. Internalization of skills may not occur until students gain experience as licensed nurses where the repetition eventually requires little conscious thought, like riding a bike or driving a car. Example action verbs are as follows:

- Imitation: Repeat, imitate, follow, show
- Manipulation: Move, manipulate, assemble, display
- Precision: Consistent, precise, demonstrate
- Articulation: Adapt, alter, change, connect, display
- Naturalization: Create, revise, vary, alter

The following example created for a simulated laboratory learning experience in the third semester of a baccalaureate nursing program illustrates a learning outcome in the psychomotor domain with a corresponding learning experience.

> **Learning outcome:** Demonstrate administration of an intravenous (IV) infusion.
>
> **Learning experience:** Prior to demonstrating the administration of IV fluids in a simulated learning scenario, review the steps involved in IV fluid administration. During a simulated patient-care scenario, demonstrate administering a primary maintenance IV solution, including attaching the primary fluid tubing, inserting the IV tubing into the IV pump, setting the appropriate rate of fluid administration, and assessing the IV site. Be prepared to discuss possible complications of IV fluid administration.

Although this learning activity is designed to focus primarily on skill development in the psychomotor domain, the cognitive learning domain is an interdependent domain because students need to use knowledge about proper administration of IV fluids, complications of administration, and an understanding of an IV site assessment. The affective domain is also an interdependent domain because students need to value answering patient questions about an IV infusion.

Evaluating Courses and Learning Experiences

Designing courses and learning experiences requires faculty to determine how they will evaluate student learning, and how they will calculate and assign grades. Where possible, students should be able to choose among several options with regard to how their work will be evaluated and graded. Faculty need to be aware that in education, evaluation of teaching and learning is a continuous process. Two common types of evaluation are *formative* and *summative evaluation.* These types of evaluation are described later in the following sections and are further discussed in Chapter 23. Another type of evaluation, also described later in this chapter, is the prior learning assessment (PLA). This type of evaluation has been increasingly emphasized as an approach to grant credit for prior learning to facilitate postsecondary degree completion.

Formative Evaluation

Formative evaluation is conducted while the teaching–learning process is unfolding. Faculty use formative evaluation to (1) appraise learning experiences while they are developing and using them, (2) assess student learning and ability to apply the content, and (3) identify any difficulties that occur during implementation of the learning experience. Students use formative evaluation to (1) appraise the effectiveness of their learning strategies, (2) determine the extent to which they are grasping the knowledge, skills, and attitudes presented in the course, (3) identify the need for additional clarification of the material, and (4) recognize the need for further study.

Clearly differentiating between learning and evaluation and allocating specific time for each purpose is essential. However, separating learning from evaluation does not mean that frequent formative assessment of student learning can be neglected. Collecting systematic verbal and written feedback from students is an integral and essential component of the teaching–learning process and can easily and effectively occur during class time. These data enable faculty to monitor student progress and design appropriate strategies to improve student achievement.

When students consistently demonstrate problems in achieving the desired outcomes for a specific learning experience, it may be necessary for faculty to select a different learning experience to present and reinforce the content. Faculty can use a variety of other strategies to facilitate student learning, such as giving supplemental assignments, organizing students with different levels of abilities into learning groups, scheduling personal conferences with individuals or groups of students, and referring students to tutors. Students deserve to be informed about when they will be evaluated and the purpose of the evaluation. Because formative evaluation data can provide valuable feedback to students about their performance, faculty should frequently share these data with students in both oral and written form.

Classroom Assessment Techniques

An important approach to formative assessment is classroom assessment technique (CAT). CATs are informal evaluation tools and procedures used to monitor student learning. They involve immediate, continuous interaction between the student and teacher to validate, clarify, and facilitate learning. CATs can be used to assess students' attitudes and knowledge about course concepts, study habits, or even reactions to teaching strategies used in particular courses. Angelo and Cross's (1993) classic work describing various CATs remains a relevant resource for faculty seeking ideas about how to successfully integrate CATs into their teaching practice. Angelo and Cross's three phases of developing and using CATs are planning, implementing, and responding.

Planning Phase

During the planning phase, the teacher selects a particular class in which to implement the CAT. The decision that formative evaluation could improve teaching and learning is based on information the instructor may have about students' progress such as examination scores, student inability to verbalize or implement major course concepts, or frequent questions during class time. The teacher needs to clearly identify the goal of the CAT and the desired information to be gained, and select a CAT that is the best fit for assessing the goal. To effectively use a CAT, the teacher should focus on assessing one specific goal.

Implementation Phase

Implementing the CAT can occur before, during, or after a class period. The class content can be taught, with administration of the CAT following, or the CAT can be administered first to set the stage for the rest of the class period. The timing of the administration of the CAT depends on the goal of the classroom assessment and the particular content of the class session. After implementing the CAT, the teacher must examine and organize the results of the CAT into a meaningful framework that will help inform how the teacher will use the information obtained.

Responding Phase

The responding phase involves reporting the results of the CAT to the students and represents the final step in the administration of a CAT. The feedback is interpreted, organized, and presented in a manner that will enhance student learning. To maximize benefit to students' learning, the teacher should present results of the CAT to the students as soon as they are available. Some CATs involve time-intensive interpretation and analysis. The less time it takes students to receive results, the greater the effect on student learning outcomes. The last activity in the responding phase is reflection (Angelo & Cross, 1993). The teacher evaluates the use of the CAT. Did use of the CAT accomplish the goal established during the first phase? Did implementation of the CAT occur as it was planned? Did the outcome of the CAT enhance student learning? What did the students think about the use of the CAT? What did the teacher think about the use of the CAT? Answering these questions and others posed by the teacher completes the three phases of implementing a CAT. However, this phase usually stimulates further action. Use of another CAT, repeated use of the same CAT at a later date, redesign of a learning experience, and even course revision are some of the future actions that may result from the evaluation. See Box 10-3 and Box 10-4 for two examples of CATs.

Summative Evaluation

Summative evaluation is conducted by faculty to measure student outcome achievement and course and program effectiveness. It is different from formative evaluation. Formative evaluation helps

BOX 10-3 Classroom Assessment Technique Example 1

Title: Minute Paper

Description: An efficient way to collect written information about student learning at the end of a class session. The teacher asks students to write responses to questions such as "What was the most important thing you learned in this class?" or "What important question remains unanswered?"

Purpose: Provides a teacher with a way to assess to what extent students are learning and facilitates any needed adjustments in instruction. The teachers' feedback to students on Minute Papers helps students learn how "experts" discern major points from details.

Goals:

Students can:

- Develop an ability to synthesize and integrate information and ideas.
- Learn to think holistically, seeing the whole rather than just the parts.
- Develop increased abilities to concentrate and listen.
- Improve study skills and habits.
- Learn important concepts and theories.

Exemplar: A faculty just completed instructing students about family theories. She knows that students often struggle to understand the differences between the various theories. To facilitate their learning, she provides students with "real life" deidentified cases. Students work in small groups in the classroom to apply the family theories to the cases. At the end of the class session, she asks students to post on a web discussion forum what questions remain for them following the instruction and the application of the theories to the cases. After reviewing the responses, she identifies the students who remain confused about the differences between some of the theories. To ensure students effectively learn the family theories, she develops a one-page handout describing salient points of each theory, where to review these points in the textbook, and additional examples applying each theory in practice. She reviews the handout with students during the next class. The student response in class to the handout was very favorable, as were exam scores that reflected an average of 92% on content about family theories.

Caution: Although the Minute Paper is a very effective CAT, if this CAT is over or poorly used, students will not take the CAT seriously. Therefore it is important to prepare questions that will effectively obtain adequate information to assess student learning.

CAT, Classroom assessment technique.

Note: A teacher implemented the Exemplar in a nursing classroom. The remaining aspects of this example are derived from Angelo and Cross (1993, p. 148–153).

BOX 10-4 Classroom Assessment Technique Example 2

Title: Course-Related Self-Confidence Surveys

Description: Provides a cursory measure of students' self-confidence regarding a course-specific skill or ability.

Purpose: Helps teachers understand how confident students are in learning skills that correspond with course material. Teachers with an understanding of students' self-confidence can develop assignments that increase confidence while also providing motivation and learning. Students with an awareness of self-confidence can increase their focus on increasing their performance for what Angelo and Cross (1993) describe as a "virtuous" cycle of success (p. 275).

Goals: Students can:

- Develop a desire for lifelong learning.
- Develop self-management skills.
- Develop leadership skills.
- Develop a commitment toward achievement.
- Improve their self-esteem.
- Become committed to personal values.
- Cultivate emotional and physical health and well being.

Exemplar: A faculty teaching a unit about professional communication in a beginning-level leadership in nursing course wants to complete a pre- and post-CAT that assesses students' self-confidence about developing effective communication in clinical settings. Prior to the unit, she surveys the students to obtain the following information:

Circle the most accurate response for how confident you feel about your ability to communicate in the clinical setting.

With other nursing students	**None**	**Low**	**Medium**	**High**
With nursing faculty	**None**	**Low**	**Medium**	**High**
With staff nurses	**None**	**Low**	**Medium**	**High**
With other members of the health care team	**None**	**Low**	**Medium**	**High**

Following instruction about professional communication, the faculty administers the survey again, and engages students in a discussion about their strengths and areas for improvement in learning effective communication in the clinical setting. In collaboration with the students, she selects additional skills the students need to increase their self-confidence to effectively communicate in nursing practice.

Cautions: Although it is important to use this CAT to develop assignments to increase students' self-confidence, a limitation of this CAT is its utility for the overconfident student. Overconfident students may be challenging to teach. In addition it can be discouraging for faculty and students when many students demonstrate low self-confidence in a skill or ability.

CAT, Classroom assessment technique.

Note: The exemplar was contributed by Colleen Thompson, MSN, BSN, Adjunct Faculty Winona State University Department of Nursing, Winona, Minnesota. The remaining aspects of this example are derived from Angelo and Cross (1993, p. 275–279).

teachers regularly (e.g., daily or weekly) understand if students are moving toward achieving learning outcomes (Price & Nelson, 2011). In contrast, faculty use summative evaluation at specified points in time throughout students' course of study for the purpose of determining if students have met expected outcomes. For example, midterm examinations in a course or an end-of-program portfolio of learning are forms of summative evaluation. In general, summative evaluation is aimed primarily at evaluating whether a student has achieved expected student learning outcomes. Summative evaluation data can also be used by faculty to facilitate planning appropriate revisions to the learning experiences of courses within a program of study.

In relation to using summative evaluation to appraise the student's learning outcomes, it is important for faculty to align summative forms of evaluation with program and course outcomes as well as the culmination of lesson outcomes. For example, the lesson plan in Box 10-2 describes program and course outcomes related to the particular lesson. The lesson plan outcomes are also provided. The evaluation strategies for the outcomes are also listed. The last evaluation strategy listed: "Exam #1: Be prepared to identify health determinants and priority health promotion strategies, which nurses can design and implement" informs students how an exam (one form of summative evaluation) will be used to measure their learning. It is important to construct summative evaluation measures so that they describe for students areas of focus in measuring their learning. In the example provided previously, students know to focus their studies on health determinants and the use of clinical judgment in responding to exam questions related to the link between health determinants and the selection of health promotion strategies.

There is great utility in linking program, course, and lesson outcomes to summative evaluation strategies. However, faculty efforts in using summative evaluation to measure learning do not stop there. Faculty need to use the results of summative evaluation methods to determine the effectiveness of learning experiences used during courses. Moss (2013) indicates research about summative evaluation practices conveys that "an accurate and valid description of student achievement is essential to quality and meaningful learning" (p. 251). Moss (2013) further suggests that teachers report high levels of competence in summative evaluation, but they often use "idiosyncratic methods" when interpreting summative evaluation results (p. 252). These methods can lessen the rigor of summative evaluation, leading to lowering standards for achievement. Moss (2013) advocates for a need to have faculty collaborate with one another in the use of summative evaluation methods and their results, and obtain faculty development from those with expertise in summative evaluation. These strategies can help improve faculty competence in summative evaluation methods. Such competence can enhance the accuracy of summative evaluation methods and promote effective use of evaluation results. Once faculty have developed summative evaluation strategies that are aligned with student outcomes, and engaged in a process to ensure rigor of the methods they use, they need to use summative evaluation results to facilitate planning of appropriate revisions to the learning experiences of courses within a program of study. See Box 10-5 for a case study example of how using summative evaluation data can lead to changes in teaching strategies.

Regardless of the summative evaluation strategy faculty use, it is imperative that they work together to examine the results of the evaluation, use an evidence base to adjust learning experiences, and evaluate implementation of new summative evaluation strategies. These efforts can help ensure effective use of summative evaluation methods.

BOX 10-5 Case Study: Using Summative Evaluation Data to Change Teaching Strategies

Faculty in one school of nursing noted that pharmacology scores on exams and National Council Licensure Examination preparation assessments were lower than they desired. They also noticed that students experienced difficulty demonstrating expected competencies in medication administration in the clinical setting. Their evaluation of the results of examination scores along with students' clinical performance indicated that students needed to have a learning experience that facilitated integration of skills, knowledge, and attitudes regarding medication administration. Seeking an evidence-based approach to addressing this issue, faculty reviewed the literature on strategies for teaching pharmacology. This review of literature suggested that objective structured clinical examination (OSCE) in the simulation laboratory could be effective in improving students' pharmacology competencies. OSCEs are an approach to summative evaluation in which students demonstrate competencies through engagement in scenarios often in a simulated setting. They worked together to design and implement a pharmacology OSCE scenario. Initial findings from this experience suggested an increase in pharmacology exam scores and improved performance in medication management in the clinical setting.

Prior Learning Assessment

PLA is "the process of granting college credit, certification, or advanced standing toward further education or training" (Klein-Collins & Werthheim, 2013, p. 51). PLA originated in 1974 through the American Council on Education's College Credit Recommendation Service to help adults obtain college credit for courses and examinations completed outside of traditional degree programs (American Council on Education, 2014). Recently, the need for PLA has increased based on the recognition of historically high college enrollment rates, yet unacceptably low college completion rates (National Commission on Higher Education Attainment, 2013). Subsequently, the PLA has become an important method for assessment of and credit for learning occurring not only in courses and through examinations, but also in the workplace, military, and through self-guided study (Klein-Collins & Werthheim, 2013).

BOX 10-6 Ten Standards for Assessing Learning

1. Credit or its equivalent should be awarded only for learning, and not for experience.
2. Assessment should be based on standards and criteria for the level of acceptable learning that are both agreed upon and made public.
3. Assessment should be treated as an integral part of learning, not separate from it, and should be based on an understanding of learning processes.
4. The determination of credit awards and competence levels must be made by appropriate subject matter and academic or credentialing experts.
5. Credit of other credentialing should be appropriate to the context in which it is awarded and accepted.
6. If awards are for credit, transcript entries should clearly describe what learning is being recognized and should be monitored to avoid credit twice for the same learning.
7. Policies, procedures, and criteria applied to assessment, including provision for appeal, should be fully disclosed and prominently available to all parties involved in the assessment process.
8. Fees charged for assessment should be based on the services performed in the process and not determined by the amount of credit awarded.
9. All personnel involved in the assessment of learning should pursue and receive adequate training and continuing professional development for the functions they perform.
10. Assessment programs should be regularly monitored, reviewed, evaluated, and revised as needed to reflect changes in the needs being served, the purposes being met, and the state of the assessment arts.

Note. Source. "Assessing learning: Standards, principles, and procedures" (2nd ed.) by Fiddler et al., 2006, p. xi. Dubuque, IA: Kendall/Hunt Publishing Company.

There are many approaches to assessing prior learning such as PLA portfolios, challenge and standardized exams, and corporate and military training evaluations (Sherman et al., 2012). These and other approaches are student-centered and facilitate degree completion (Kamenetz, 2011); however, Boilard (2011) critiques PLA for its separation of where teaching actually occurred to the assessment of learning. To ensure appropriate assessment of prior learning, Fiddler et al. (2006, p. xi) provides "Ten Standards for Assessing Learning" (p. xi) that should be used in determining whether to grant credit for prior learning (Box 10-6).

Developing the Course Syllabus

The components of course design and learning experiences should be clearly and succinctly described in the course syllabus. A well-developed syllabus serves as contract between faculty and students and as a student guide to attaining learning outcomes. It is an expectation that students receive the syllabus on or before the first day of class so that they will have a clear understanding of course expectations before the class begins. The syllabus also explains how learning will be assessed, evaluated, and graded. Equally important, the syllabus sets the tone for the course by introducing the faculty and the faculty's philosophy, university, school, and course policies and norms for behavior to be demonstrated during the course; as such it should be written with a learner-centered focus. Harnish and colleagues (2011) describe six characteristics for developing a "warm" or welcoming syllabus (Table 10-1). The syllabus for a learner-centered course also explains the roles of the faculty and students in the teaching–learning process and conveys the attitudes and behaviors that will promote active and effective learning.

A course syllabus is developed for both on-campus and online academic courses. Additional information about using course management systems and course participation from a distance should be included in the syllabus for hybrid (blended) and fully online courses.

A *full* course syllabus includes essential information about the course, information about course implementation, university and school policies, and norms for expected behaviors. The various components of a full course syllabus are described in the following sections (Boxes 10-7 and 10-8).

An *abbreviated* form of the syllabus may be developed as required by the institution or program and contains basic information about course requirements, such as course name, description and outcomes. Some schools publish the abbreviated syllabus on the website and offer full course information in electronic or print format at the beginning of the course.

TABLE 10-1 Six Characteristics of a Warm Syllabus

Characteristic	Description
Positive or Friendly Language	Helps students feel comfortable and welcome. Example: Office Hours Section—"Individual assistance is always available by appointment." "I look forward to seeing you during student hours."
Rationale for Assignments	Motivates students by making clear how assignments relate to course objectives and their learning. Example: Assignment List Section—"Students may believe the worksheets are busy work; however, the questions in the worksheets for this course are designed to help develop your critical thinking about nursing practice."
Self-Disclosure	Provides students with awareness of a teacher's interpersonal style. Example: Learning Resources Section—"We have all needed help at some point in our lives. The learning resources listed are there to support your learning in this course."
Enthusiasm	Increases students' active learning and a teacher's effectiveness. Example: Course Objectives Section—"Think for a moment about how research and evidence-based nursing practice has changed lives and contributed to health and well being."
Compassion	Acknowledges unexpected events and life circumstances. Example: Attendance Section—"Attendance is expected. However, please contact me if you have an unforeseen event such as a death in the family or illness."
Humor	Increases students' active learning and a teacher's effectiveness. Example: Course Objectives Section—Teaching Philosophy Section—"Please beware the use of cartoons is common in this course, and are designed to stimulate your attention to course content."

From Harnish R.J., O'Brien McElwee R., Slattery J.M.,Frantz S., Haney M.R., Shore C.M., and Penley J.,"Creating a foundation for a warm classroom climate: Best practices in syllabus tone" *Observer* Vol. 24, No 1 January, 2011.

BOX 10-7 Example of a Full Syllabus for an Undergraduate Nursing Course

MICHIGAN STATE UNIVERSITY COLLEGE OF NURSING

NUR 324 HEALTH PROMOTION AND DISEASE AND INJURY PREVENTION I

Class Sessions:

Tuesdays, 10:20 am–12:10 pm; Clinical: Mondays or Wednesdays 8 am to 3 pm

Catalog Course Description:

Principles and practices of health education, health promotion/behavior change, and health literacy through understanding epidemiology, determinants of health, and protective and predictive factors of health and well being.

Course Outcomes:

1. Incorporate liberal education principles into application, synthesis, and evaluation of course concepts.
2. Assess health/illness beliefs, values, attitudes, and practices of individuals, communities, and populations.
3. Demonstrate professionalism, including attention to appearance, demeanor, respect for self and others, and professional boundaries with interprofessional team and stakeholders with regard to individuals, communities, and populations.
4. Use epidemiology and determinants of health to develop health promotion and disease and injury prevention interventions for individuals, communities, and populations.
5. Identify interprofessional perspectives needed to ensure health promotion and risk reduction interventions at the individual, community, and population levels.
6. Use creative, evidence-based strategies to help individuals, communities, and populations achieve health promotion and risk reduction behavioral outcomes, considering quality and patient safety initiatives, complex system issues, and stakeholder preferences.
7. Use evidence-based practice to provide health teaching, health counseling, behavioral change techniques, screening, and referral so that care reflects patient age, culture, spirituality, preferences, and health literacy to foster patient engagement leading to health promotion and risk reduction.

(Continued)

BOX 10-7 Example of a Full Syllabus for an Undergraduate Nursing Course—cont'd

8. Demonstrate skills in using health care technologies, information systems, and communication devices that support health promotion and risk reduction interventions at the individual, community, and population levels.
9. Discuss the credibility of sources used for health education and preventive care, including but not limited to databases and Internet resources.
10. Develop a foundational understanding of complementary and alternative modalities and their role in health care.
11. Use an ethical framework to evaluate the impact of social policies on issues of access, equality, affordability, health disparities, and social justice on health care delivery.
12. Uphold ethical standards related to data security, regulatory requirements, confidentiality, and clients' right to privacy.

Prerequisites: HDFS 225 ***Co-requisites:*** NUR 205, NUR 322

Topical Outline:

I. Foundations of Health Promotion and Disease and Injury Prevention
II. Health Promotion
III. Health Education and Health Literacy
IV. Disease and Injury Prevention

Course Faculty:

Names and ranks, contact information, office hours with provision for "arranged" office hours to accommodate student schedules

Faculty Philosophy of Teaching and Learning:

Faculty in this course believe in active learning, and the development of clinical reasoning, clinical judgment, and clinical decision making. They also believe in democratic learning where students and teachers partner in meeting learning outcomes. These beliefs limit the use of passive learning strategies and promote an engaging learning environment.

Teaching and Learning Strategies:

You will learn through assigned readings, lectures, learning groups and learning pairs, case studies, written letters and papers, role-plays and simulations, exams, interviews with nurses, windshield surveys, health screening events, community health education presentations, and teaching holistic health interventions. Detailed instructions for each assignment and assignment due dates are provided in the course pack.

Course Materials and Resources:

Required Texts listed here:

Other readings assigned are in the course pack. All assigned readings need to be completed before class, will be referenced in class, used for class and clinical activities, and to study for examinations.

Evaluation:

Learning Experiences and Corresponding Assessments and Grading:

Classroom Assessments

Infectious Disease Outbreak Computer Game (in class)	5%
Health Insurance Needs Case Study (in class)	5%
Injury Prevention Advocacy Letter (outside of class—1 page)	5%
Review of Literature Paper (outside of class—limit page number to 5 pages)	10%
Exams—Two exams	15%
	40%

Clinical/Lab Assessments

Health Education Presentation	15%
Holistic Health Nursing Intervention	15%
Motivational Interviewing Simulation	15 %
Nurse Advocacy Interview	10%
Windshield Survey and Checklist	5%
	60%

Course Grading Scale:

The standard College of Nursing grading scale will be used.

BOX 10-7 Example of a Full Syllabus for an Undergraduate Nursing Course—cont'd

Assignment and Clinical/Lab Experience Expectations:

Faculty in this course expect students to meet assignment deadlines. In cases such as family emergencies or illnesses, late or missed assignments are accepted per approval of course faculty. Late or missed assignments without just cause can result in a 5% grade reduction/assignment. Faculty also expect attendance at all clinical/lab activities. Students who are absent from clinical/lab experiences for reasons such as family emergencies or illnesses need to arrange with course faculty times to make-up missed clinical/lab assignments.

Professionalism Expectations for this Course:

1. Your clinical experiences in this course will be in community settings. As compared to institutional settings, this setting has a different "look and feel." Sometimes community settings can seem more "casual" than institutional settings. Nonetheless, it is important to use the same professional behavior in this setting as you have in other settings. Your professional behavior sends a positive message to the communities we serve about the MSU CON and the nursing profession.
2. The dress code for this course is your green MSU polo shirt, khaki pants, and your name tag. Please follow all other dress code requirements outlined in the BSN Student Handbook.
3. As with all other clinical settings, please ensure your compliance requirements are all up-to-date by reviewing your record on the University Physicians website at least once a month. You can attend clinical experiences when you are compliant with all compliance requirements.

University and College Policies:

Other specific expectations for professionalism can be found in the appropriate handbook. Please review the information outlined below and act in accordance with the policies and procedures found in the following sources: (source links inserted here)

University Policies:

In addition to being familiar with policies outlined in the sources above, it is important to be familiar with the following University Policies:

Academic Integrity:

Article 2.3.3 of the Academic Freedom Report states that "The student shares with the faculty the responsibility for maintaining the integrity of scholarship, grades, and professional standards." In addition, the College adheres to the policies on academic honesty as specified in General Student Regulations 1.0, Protection of Scholarship and Grades; the all-University Policy on Integrity of Scholarship and Grades; and Ordinance 17.00, Examinations. (See Spartan Life: Student Handbook and Resource Guide http://splife.studentlife.msu.edu/ and/or the MSU Web site: www.msu.edu). Therefore, unless authorized by your instructor, you are expected to complete all course assignments, including homework, lab work, quizzes, tests and exams, without assistance from any source. You are expected to develop original work for this course; therefore you may not submit course work you completed for another course to satisfy the requirements for this course.

Accommodations for Students with Disabilities:

Students with disabilities should contact the Resource Center for Persons with Disabilities to establish reasonable accommodations.

Disruptive Behavior:

Article 2.3.5 of the Academic Freedom Report (AFR) for students at Michigan State University states: "The student's behavior in the classroom shall be conducive to the teaching and learning process for all concerned." Article 2.3.10 of the AFR states that "The student has a right to scholarly relationships with faculty based on mutual trust and civility." General Student Regulation 5.02 states: "No student shall . . . interfere with the functions and services of the University (for example, but not limited to, classes . . .) such that the function or service is obstructed or disrupted. Students whose conduct adversely affects the learning environment in this classroom may be subject to disciplinary action through the Student Faculty Judiciary process."

Attendance:

Students whose names do not appear on the official class list for this course may not attend this class. Students who fail to attend the first four class sessions or class by the fifth day of the semester, whichever occurs first, may be dropped from the course. See the Ombudsman's website for a discussion of student observance of major religious holidays, student-athlete participation in athletic competition, student participation in university-approved field trips, medical excuses and a dean's drop for students who fail to attend class sessions at the beginning of the semester.

Courtesy Steve Yelon, Martha Scheckel, Kathy Forrest, Carol Vermeesch, Judy Strunk, Doug Olsen, Emily Wilson, Theresa Wehrwein, and Mary Mundt; adapted with permission from Michigan State University College of Nursing.

BOX 10-8 Example of a Syllabus for a Graduate-Level Course

WINONA STATE UNIVERSITY DEPARTMENT OF NURSING: GRADUATE NURSING

NURS 608 – ORGANIZATIONAL AND SYSTEMS LEADERSHIP

CREDITS:	**3 Semester credits**
PLACEMENT:	**Fall (Hybrid Online)** **Spring (On Campus-ITV)**
CO- OR PRE-REQUISITES:	**None.**
FACULTY:	**Name, rank, office, office hours, office phone, email**

COURSE DESCRIPTION:

Culturally sensitive organizational and systems leadership skills necessary for improving healthcare outcomes, practice and safety are addressed. Focus is on leadership theories, principles of ethical leadership, and professional communication strategies.

STUDENT LEARNING OUTCOMES:

Upon completion of this course, the student will demonstrate the ability to:

1. Integrate leadership theories and culturally sensitive approaches necessary to lead a diverse workforce to improve patient outcomes.
2. Integrate consultative and leadership skills with intraprofessional and interprofessional teams to create change in health care.
3. Evaluate formal and informal communication processes in nursing care systems that promote quality nursing care.
4. Analyze internal and external factors that influence organizational behaviors, policies, practices, and nursing care systems.
5. Analyze quality improvement methodologies for the promotion of safe, timely, effective, efficient, and equitable patient-centered care.

TOPICAL OUTLINE:

I. Leadership Foundations
II. Leadership Characteristics/Competencies
III. Leading Interdisciplinary Teams
IV. Facilitating Change in Complex Environments
V. Leadership Ethics
VI. Leadership Outcomes
VII. Leadership Challenges
VIII. Power, Influence, and Accountability
IX. Followership
X. Developing Others
XI. Managing Failure/Error
XII. Business Basics for Leaders

TEACHING LEARNING STRATEGIES:

The teaching strategies used in this course reflect a commitment to learning that honors your internal wisdoms and experiences. This course is delivered in hybrid online format and will meet synchronously in a face-to-face or Interactive Television meeting four times per term. Teaching strategies include recorded and live lectures, group discussions, presentations, self-directed study, and written assignments. Active learning is valued and you are expected to participate in course learning activities.

PARTICIPATION AND ATTENDANCE:

As a learning community, your individual participation matters; thus points can be earned through participation and engagement during each face-to-face session. I look forward to your contribution to our learning community and award points for your participation and attendance.

Your experiences are valued and together we will be creating a course learning environment that supports all learners. The University has a Commitment to Inclusive Excellence Statement, which can be found at (insert link here). If you have concerns or wish to speak privately, please connect with me via email or phone. I look forward to answering questions you have.

BOX 10-8 Example of a Syllabus for a Graduate-Level Course—cont'd

COURSE GRADED ASSIGNMENTS:

1. Leadership Development Plan	100 points
2. Analysis of a Global Leader	100 points
3. Business Plan (group assignment)	100 points
4. Participation/Scholarly Contribution to Class	40 points
5. Discussion Café' postings	50 points
	Total: 390 points

GRADING:
Grading scale inserted

Rounding grades will be calculated in accordance with the Graduate Nursing Department policy in the Graduate Nursing Department Student Handbook.

GRADING POLICIES:
All students are responsible and accountable for their own work. Plagiarism will constitute failure of the course. Ethical conduct is described in full in the Graduate Nursing Department Student Handbook. The University academic integrity policy can be found at the following link. (insert link here)

REQUIRED TEXTS:

DISCUSSION EXPECTATIONS:
Discussion Café Participation (10 points maximum/posting): You will be dividing yourselves into discussion groups. Students in the past indicated that the ideal group size for discussions was 4-5 students. Don't worry about knowing who is in your group. You will get to know them as you go along!

All students will self-register into a Discussion Café Group. Please do this by the tenth day of the term. All students will engage in Discussion Cafes the weeks discussions are assigned. The discussion will follow the same period each week that a posting is required.

Discussion Requirements:
Respond to Discussion Questions in a timely manner with evidence of analysis, synthesis and integration

CLASS DISCUSSION EXPECTATIONS (10 POINTS MAXIMUM/CLASS):
Active participation in online and face-to-face seminars is required.

NURS 608: MAJOR ASSIGNMENT DESCRIPTIONS
The Leadership Development Plan, (100 points)
Due XX

This assignment is very personalized to you and your goals for yourself as a leader.

Part I: DUE XX

Complete at least four leadership assessments: Two from the Strengths Based Leadership text, and at least two other assessments OF YOUR CHOICE. I have posted some suggested assessments in the online course system. After completing the assessments, you will evaluate your results and post a reflective summary to the assignment drop box.

Part II: DUE XX

The second part of the plan begins with a concise narrative of your current style and what strengths you bring to your current roles. You will design a plan to improve your leadership skills based on the assessments you completed in Part I, which you see as an opportunity for growth.

Introduction (20 points)
Current Leadership Situation (15 points)
Planned Activities (25 points)
Future Leadership goal and personal mission statement (15 points)
Table of your Leadership Development Plan (15 points)
Writing Form and APA Style (10 points)

(Continued)

BOX 10-8 Example of a Syllabus for a Graduate-Level Course—cont'd

Analysis of a Global Leader (100 points), DUE XX

Reflect on a global leader's accomplishments, context and style, and then apply this leader's attributes to your own strengths and areas of development. This assignment allows you to study a global leader and analyze his or her leadership style. Choose someone you respect, admire, or want to know more about (you will e-mail the name of the leader you choose to faculty by (list date). Using APA format, write a paper summarizing the following points (paper length is usually 6-8 pages):

Introduction (10 points)
Background on the leader (20 points)
Body of the Paper (develop your APA headings as appropriate) (30 points)
Summary (20 points)
APA Format (20 points)

Business Plan (100 points), DUE XX

The purpose of this assignment is to provide you with an opportunity to apply commonly required aspects of a business plan to a service area of your choice within the health care sector. It is a team assignment, and you will choose your team members and project focus.

Business Plan Requirements:

a. Executive Summary: 20 points
b. Problem or Need Identification (Why do it?): 10 points
c. Product Definition: 10 points
d. Market Analysis: 10 points
e. Financial Analysis: 10 points
f. Timeline: 10 points
g. Conclusion and Feasibility Statement: 10 points
h. Presentation: The written business plan will be orally presented as an in-class presentation during our final class time together. Everyone in the group will receive the same grade for this assignment. There will be a separate peer evaluation "quiz" for you to rate one another in the group and this will be added to an individual's grade. The presentation is a total of 20 points.

Courtesy Jane Foote, with permission from Winona State University Department of Nursing. Adapted and condensed for publication.

Course Information

The following essential information should be included in the syllabus: title, description, prerequisites, corequisites, outcomes, teaching–learning strategies, learning experiences, topical outline, policies and procedures, assessment and evaluation strategies, and the grading plan and scale. In addition, faculty should list all dates for course meetings. If the course meets in varied places throughout the semester, such as online at synchronous or asynchronous times, in a learning resources center, or at a clinical agency, it is imperative to indicate this information at the outset. Because the syllabus is an implied contract between the student and faculty, all involved must plan to adhere to the dates posted.

Information about the Faculty's Philosophy of Teaching and Learning

Faculty should include basic information such as name, rank, office hours, general availability, and contact information, with the preferred way of contacting faculty. Faculty should also note their availability inside and outside of class. If providing telephone contact information, it is appropriate for faculty to delineate when students are welcome to contact faculty and for what reasons. In online courses, faculty may include more personal biographical information accompanied by a photograph or a short welcome video. Faculty should also provide a short description of their philosophy of teaching and learning to help students understand their particular point of view.

Course Materials and Resources

In this section faculty can provide information about required and supplemental readings such as textbooks, journal readings, and course pack information. A bibliography and listing of course-relevant websites may also be included.

Course Requirements

A section of the full syllabus should include course requirements, including information about class attendance, clinical assignments, class participation, exams, and written work. Faculty also should specify the consequences of not meeting course requirements and whether there are options for completing late or missed requirements, particularly in courses with clinical practica.

Course Grading Policies

In the full syllabus, faculty can provide detailed information about assignments and how they will be graded; rubrics facilitate clarity. Faculty should provide due dates for assignments and tests, procedures for test makeup, information on the use of optional graded assignments, and procedures for late papers and projects, and should inform students when results from tests and papers will be available.

Study Assistance

If the campus or school provides resources to assist students with study and writing skills, this information can be noted in the syllabus. Faculty can also make suggestions for how students can learn the course material and how students can form their own study groups.

Course, School, and Campus Policies

Each school of nursing and campus has its own set of policies with specified consequences related to codes of conduct, academic honesty, incivility, criminal acts, student privacy, and resources for students with disabilities or special needs. Information about required criminal background checks and substance testing should also be provided as pertinent to the program and course. Information regarding program and campus policies can be provided in the syllabus with links to appropriate campus or school websites.

Course Norms

Course norms are guidelines for behavior in the classroom. Course norms can be written to describe expectations for individual and group participation and active learning within the class, when the use of computers and cell phones is acceptable, how to handle arriving late or leaving early, and how to prevent and manage other annoying or uncivil behavior (see Chapter 14).

At the beginning of each course, faculty should spend time explaining and answering questions, soliciting input from the students, and modifying the syllabus as appropriate. Clark (2009) notes that clarifying expectations at the outset of the course helps to promote desired classroom behavior. Faculty can ask students to commit to the behaviors specified in the syllabus in writing; in online courses, faculty can ask students to send an e-mail or post in the discussion forum indicating their agreement with the document. The syllabus then becomes a learning contract that can be reviewed and referred to throughout the course.

Evaluation of Course Design

Once the course and syllabus are sufficiently developed, and prior to their use with students, faculty can request internal and external review from peers and other curriculum experts. Teaching colleagues can review the syllabus for content accuracy, completeness, and fit with the curriculum. For additional and external review, faculty can consult curriculum and course design experts at the campus teaching center, if available. Ultimately, the course syllabus represents the intended learning outcomes of the course and is the document that is submitted to the course review process of the curriculum committee as designated at the school of nursing and the college.

Constraints to Choosing and Implementing Courses and Learning Experiences

Constraints to designing courses and learning experiences may arise from faculty, students, time, and resources. Although it may not be possible to eliminate all constraints, by making a careful assessment of each source of constraint during the planning phases, faculty will be able to avoid many pitfalls. Faculty gain an appreciation of the benefits and limitations of designing courses and learning experience after implementing them, reflecting on how students responded, and assessing how the experience contributed to learning. Taking time to debrief after course delivery helps faculty decide whether to repeat, revise, or delete the activity. Table 10-2 presents a summary of the sources of constraint in selecting and implementing learning activities.

Faculty Constraints

Some constraints in designing courses and learning experiences arise from faculty. A faculty member's lack of experience in teaching in an academic setting or in teaching students at the course level assigned may present some difficulty when he or she is designing courses and learning experiences. Faculty are more likely to design courses and select appropriate learning experiences when they have a reasonable understanding of the cognitive abilities of their students and some familiarity with the knowledge base and previous school and life experiences that their students bring to the course. Overestimating or underestimating the abilities and experiences of students can undermine the intended value of the learning experience. Another pitfall that faculty may encounter is the failure to adequately appreciate a student's inability to engage in courses and learning experience. This inability may be attributed to an experience that is too sophisticated or complex, or perhaps to a course design and learning experience that is not challenging enough for a student.

TABLE 10-2 Sources of Constraint in Choosing and Implementing Learning Activities

Source	Constraint

Faculty	• Faculty–student ratio
	• Lack of experience
	• Lack of knowledge of course content
	• Lack of understanding of students' knowledge and skills
	• Personal attributes:
	  • Personality
	  • Vocal qualities

Students	• Distractions • Inability to use equipment and technology • Lack of prerequisite knowledge and skills • Resistance to active participation • Stress and anxiety • Student–faculty ratio too large
Time	• Inadequate for activity • Inadequate for debriefing
Resources	• Copyright restrictions • Inadequate clinical or classroom facilities • Inadequate funds • Unavailable audiovisual equipment • Unavailable electronic technology

Novice faculty, and even experienced faculty who are teaching a new course, may not possess a comfortable or adequate command of the content and processes required by the course and learning experiences. In addition, they may not be comfortable in dealing with questions, problems, or issues that may arise during the course. Even under the best of circumstances it is often difficult for faculty to fully appreciate the various perspectives that students may bring to a course. Students may raise questions and issues that faculty may not have considered as being related to the course. Consulting with faculty who have previously taught the course or who have had experience teaching the same level of students before designing the course and learning experiences can provide valuable input that can help reduce the potential for difficulties. Because courses and learning experiences are learner-centered, faculty must not only be prepared to deal with any ambiguity that may arise but also be willing to be flexible, to go with the flow of the course while taking advantage of the opportunity to learn from students how they process the course experience. Feedback from students about the different ways they interpreted the course design and learning experiences, or certain elements of them, can be used as points of discussion and thus expand the course and the learning experiences.

Demands on students outside the classroom can complicate and put constraints on faculty. Retaining standards and rigor, while providing appropriate academic expectations for students with numerous job and family demands, makes teaching a challenge and can have major implications for pedagogy. Learner-centered pedagogies can mitigate challenges teachers face from students who experience demands outside the classroom. Weimer (2013) suggests giving students more control over learning through redistributing the power. Power redistribution can occur in four areas where teachers typically make most of the decisions about student learning: course activities and assignments, course policies, course content, and evaluation of learning (Weimer, 2013, p. 98). Options for power redistribution include providing students with assignment options rather than prescribing assignments, using cooperative learning to establish classroom policies (e.g., rules for participation), providing choices about topics and readings to cover, and involving students in course design through co-constructing syllabi (Weimer, 2013). Redistributing power promotes inclusiveness, responds to students' needs, and accounts for diversity in the classrooms and clinical settings. However, Weimer (2013) emphasizes it does not mean abrogating legitimate instructional responsibility, such as grading and other assessment requirements.

Faculty may have personal attributes that interfere with their ability to establish a climate that engages student interest in courses and learning experiences. Having a soft or a poor-quality voice, talking too fast or too slow, or speaking in a monotone may make it difficult for students to attend to and follow verbal presentations. Faculty with reserved or shy personalities, or those with a matter-of-fact orientation, may be perceived by students as distant, aloof, or uncaring. Personal habits that faculty may be unaware of may also be distracting for students and interfere with their ability to fully focus on the learning experience. Although students may be reluctant to share some of their perceptions about faculty's personal attributes, inviting a colleague to attend a class can provide helpful input that can be used to improve classroom performance. It may also be helpful for faculty to learn the "Concernful Practices of Schooling Learning Teaching." The "Concernful Practices" foster positive learning environments and include being open and welcoming, promoting community, listening, and creating space for questioning and dialogue, among other practices (Diekelmann & Diekelmann, 2009).

Student Constraints

Student constraints may be due to the number of students enrolled in a course. Large numbers of students in a course may affect the faculty's ability to get to know students personally, make it difficult to address various learning styles, and ensure students have a comparable learning experience. The student/faculty ratio may make a particular course or learning experience labor- and time-intensive.

Students may lack some of the prerequisite knowledge and skills required for a course or learning experience, knowledge and skills that faculty reasonably anticipated the students would possess. There are usually some students, regardless of the clarity of the activity and the directions, who do not grasp the course content or the goal of a learning experience. They may be unable to connect course concepts to previously acquired knowledge and experiences. Some students may have difficulty with comprehension and may be unable to follow directions.

Stress or anxiety may interfere with some students' ability to concentrate and participate in coursework and learning experiences. Distractions such as uncomfortable classroom temperature and mechanical noise in the classroom environment may also interfere with learning activities. Students working in groups may also create enough noise to interfere with the learning of students who prefer a quiet environment to concentrate.

Resistance to participation in learning experiences is another constraining force. Students socialized to a passive learning model may be resistant to engaging in learning experiences that require active participation. Students may perceive learning experiences as a form of busywork that has little or no meaning for them and not accept them as meaningful experiences.

Students may not have the skill or experience in using the resources, equipment, or electronic technology required for a learning experience. Although many types of computer equipment are easily and quickly learned, there are students who lack experience, skill, and comfort in using computers for any purpose. Faculty need to be clear about the expectations for use of technology in the course and what competencies are expected of students.

Time Constraints

Time is an all too common constraint in teaching. Faculty must carefully weigh the trade-off between faculty-centered and learner-centered learning experiences when determining how to use class time most effectively. For all courses and learning experiences, faculty must prioritize and then select the outcomes or competencies and the related content and processes. Faculty must also assess the complexity of the course and learning experiences to ensure that they can be accomplished given the ability of the students and the allotted time.

For courses and learning experiences to be meaningful and worthwhile, adequate time needs to be allowed for both students and faculty to actively plan and participate in the course and its learning experiences. Time should also be allowed for debriefing following the completion of the learning experiences within courses. Although the need to debrief depends on the nature of the learning, debriefing is an important part of learning, and it has several benefits for both students and faculty. It extends the learning process because students share what they did with their peers, it enables faculty to gain a more comprehensive perspective of the kinds of thinking processes students use, and it provides a window of opportunity for students to identify issues or problems that came up during the learning experience. Faculty can use this information as the basis for further discussion of issues and problems relevant to the student's immediate learning situation. Information gleaned from students about their difficulties with the directions, elements, or focus of the experience itself is useful to faculty when deciding whether to retain, revise, or delete the experience.

Resource Constraints

Resources may be another source of constraint. The resources used to support courses and learning experiences include clinical facilities, learning resource centers, physical examination rooms, classrooms, supplies and equipment, print materials, audiovisual equipment, computer-assisted instructional programs, and a variety of information technologies. The use of a particular learning experience or type of experience, for example, may not be possible because of a lack of the appropriate resources needed to implement the experience. For instance, a clinical unit may not be able to accommodate the students, the type of clinical facility desired may not be available, classroom size or design may not be adequate, audiovisual equipment may be unavailable for the specific class day and time, or DVDs or computer software may not be accessible because of heavy demand or lack of funds to acquire them. In addition, licensing or copyright restrictions may prohibit or limit faculty use of a particular resource.

Information technology, e-mail, and other electronic messaging and conferencing systems are useful tools that can be used as a vehicle for designing courses and learning experiences. Although faculty may inform students in advance of the course that skill and experience in using electronic technology are required, students often report that they are too busy to allocate the time to acquire the necessary training on their own time. In addition to time, money may also be a barrier. Some academic institutions charge students to learn how to use electronic messaging systems or computer software programs. Faculty who are committed to using some form of computer or electronic technology as a means of implementing one or more learning experiences may find it necessary to schedule training sessions for students during class time.

Summary

Designing courses and learning experiences is an intentional, systematically planned effort. It requires attention to several important issues. Faculty must keep in mind that course designs and the learning experiences within them require students' active engagement in their own learning, which has positive benefits for both students and faculty. Within this context, faculty must use learner-centered approaches to teaching as a mechanism to bridge general curriculum outcomes to specific concepts and content with associated course designs and learning experiences to effectively prepare the student for nursing practice. Faculty must also understand the importance of assessment of student learning through the use of formative and summative assessment techniques and methods. Assembling the syllabus is an equally critical faculty skill that allows them to present the course design and learning experiences to students in welcoming ways and in ways that engage students in learning. How teachers design courses and learning experiences significantly affect learning outcomes. Thus the success of course designs and learning experiences depend on faculty considering and addressing constraints that can threaten the integrity and rigor of the learning experience.

REFLECTING ON THE EVIDENCE

1. Select a teacher-centered learning experience that you want to make learner-centered. What resources would you use to help design a learner-centered experience?
2. Review an existing course. What design elements exist? How were the course concepts and content determined? Is the organizing structure evident?
3. Analyze the learning experiences within a course. Are the experiences active or passive, structured or unstructured? What domains of learning do the experiences address?
4. Compare and contrast formative and summative evaluation. Cite an example of when it is appropriate to use each type of evaluation.
5. How can evidence from summative evaluations lead teachers to use literature to redesign learning experiences that have proven to be ineffective?
6. What are best practices in mitigating constraints to designing courses and learning experiences?

REFERENCES

Abell, C. H., & Garrett-Wright, D. (2014). E-books: Nurse faculty use and concerns. *Nursing Education Perspectives, 35*(2), 112–114.

American Council on Education. (2014). *College credit recommendation services (CREDIT)*. Retrieved from, http://www.acenet.edu/news-room/Pages/College-Credit-Recommendation-Service-CREDIT.aspx.

Anderson, L. W., & Krathwohl, D. R. (2001). *A taxonomy for learning, teaching, and assessing: A revision of Bloom's taxonomy of educational objectives*. New York: Longman.

Andrade, H. L. (2013). Classroom assessment in the context of learning theory and research. In J. H. McMillian (Ed.), *Sage handbook of research on classroom assessment* (pp. 17–34). Los Angeles: Sage.

Angelo, T. A., & Cross, K. A. (1993). *Classroom assessment techniques: A handbook for college teachers*. San Francisco: Jossey-Bass.

Benner, P., Sutphen, M., Leonard, V., & Day, L. (2010). *Educating nurses: A call for radical transformation*. San Francisco: Jossey-Bass.

Bergmann, J., & Sams, A. (2012). *Flip your classroom: Reach every student in your class every day*. Eugene, OR: International Society for Technology in Education and Association for Supervision and Curriculum.

Bloom, B. S. (Ed.), (1956). *Taxonomy of educational objectives. Handbook 1: Cognitive domain*. New York: Longman.

Boilard, S. D. (2011). Prior learning assessment challenges the status quo. *Change, 43*(6), 56–59.

Bruner, J. (1977). *The process of education*. Cambridge, MA: Harvard University Press.

Candela, L., Dalley, K., & Benzel-Lindley, J. (2006). A case for learning-centered curricula. *Journal of Nursing Education, 45*(2), 59–66.

Clark, C. M. (2009). Faculty field guide for promoting student civility in the classroom. *Nurse Educator, 34*(5), 194–197.

Clark, C., Nguyen, H. T., Bray, C., & Levine, R. E. (2008). Team-based learning in an undergraduate nursing course. *Journal of Nursing Education, 47*(3), 111–117.

Davis, B. G. (2009). *Tools for teaching* (2nd ed.). San Francisco: Jossey-Bass.

Diamond, R. M. (2008). *Designing and assessing courses and curricula* (3rd ed.). San Francisco: Jossey-Bass.

Diekelmann, N., & Diekelmann, J. (2009). *Schooling learning teaching: Toward a narrative pedagogy*. New York: iUniverse.

Fiddler, M., Marienau, C., & Whitaker, U. (2006). *Assessing learning: Standards, principles, and procedures* (2nd ed.). Dubuque, IA: Kendall/Hunt Publishing Company.

Fink, L. D. (2013). *Creating significant learning experiences: An integrated approach to designing college course*. San Francisco: Jossey-Bass.

Freire, P. (2006). *Pedagogy of the oppressed: 30th anniversary edition*. New York: Continuum International Publishing Group, Inc.

Giddens, J. F., Wright, M., & Gray, I. (2012). Selecting concepts for a concept-based curriculum: Application of a benchmark approach. *Journal of Nursing Education, 51*(9), 511–515.

Hains, B. J., & Smith, B. (2012). Student-centered course design: Empowering students to become self-directed learners. *Journal of Experiential Education, 35*(2), 357–374.

Harnish, R. J., McElwee, R. O., Slattery, J. M., Frantz, M. R., Haney, C. M., Shore, C. M., & Penley, J. (2011). *Creating a foundation for a warm classroom climate: Best practices in syllabus tone*. Observer. Retrieved from, http://www.psychologicalscience.org/index.php/publications/observer/2011/january-11/creating-the-foundation-for-a-warm-classroom-climate.htmlHoffman.

Hawks, S. J. (2014). The flipped classroom: Now or never? *The Journal of the American Association of Nurse Anesthetists, 82*(4), 264–269.

Kamenetz, A. (2011). The transformation of higher education through prior learning assessment. *Change, 43*(5), 7–13.

Klein-Collins, R., & Wertheim, J. B. (2013). Growing importance of prior learning assessment in the degree completion toolkit. *New Directions for Adult and Continuing Education, 140*, 51–60.

Krathwohl, D., Bloom, B., & Masia, B. (1964). *Taxonomy of educational objectives. Handbook II: Affective domain*. New York: Longman.

Levy, P., Aiyegbayot, O., & Little, S. (2009). Designing for inquiry-based learning with the learning activity management system. *Journal of Computer Assisted Learning, 25*, 238–251.

Lo, C. C. (2010). Student learning and student satisfaction in an interactive classroom. *The Journal of General Education, 59*(4), 238–263.

Mastrian, K. G., McGonigle, D., Mahan, W. L., & Bixler, B. (2011). *Integrating technology in nursing education: Tools for the knowledge era*. Sudbury, MA: Jones and Bartlett.

Michel, N., Cater, J. J., & Varela, O. (2009). Active verses passive teaching: An empirical study of student learning outcomes. *Human Resource Development Quarterly, 20*(4), 397–418.

Moss, C. M. (2013). Research on classroom summative assessment. In J. H. McMillin (Ed.), *Sage handbook of research on classroom assessment* (pp. 235–255). Los Angeles: Sage.

National Commission on Higher Education Attainment. (2013). *An open letter to college and university leaders: College completion must be our priority*. Retrieved from, http://www.acenet.edu/news-room/Documents/An-Open-Letter-to-College-and-University-Leaders.pdf.

Pascarella, E. T., & Terenzini, P. T. (2005). *How college affects students: A third decade of research. (Vol. 2)*. San Francisco: Jossey-Bass.

Price, K. M., & Nelson, K. L. (2011). *Planning effective instruction: Diversity responsive methods and management* (4th ed.). Belmont, CA: Wadsworth.

Roberts, J. C., & Roberts, K. A. (2008). Deep reading, cost/benefit, and the construction of meaning: Enhancing reading comprehension and deep learning in sociology courses. *Teaching Sociology, 36*(2), 125–140.

Sherman, A., Klein-Collins, B., & Palmer, I. (2012). *A resource guide for state leaders: State policy approaches to support prior learning*. Retrieved from, http://www.cael.org/pdfs/college-productivity-resource-guide2012.

Sisk, R. (2011). Team-based learning: Systematic research review. *Journal of Nursing Education, 50*(12), 665–669.

Stanley, M. J. C., & Dougherty, J. P. (2010). A paradigm shift in nursing education: A new model. *Nursing Education Perspectives, 31*(6), 378–380.

Stevens, J., & Brenner, Z. R. (2009). The peer active learning approach for clinical education: A pilot study. *The Journal of Theory Construction & Testing, 13*(2), 51–56.

Stevenson, E. L., & Gordon, H. A. (2014). Students as active learners and teaching partners in the clinical setting. *Nurse Educator, 39*(2), 52–53.

Svinicki, M. D., & McKeachie, W. J. (2014). *McKeachie's teaching tips: Strategies, research, and theory for college and university teachers* (14th ed.). Belmont, CA: Wadsworth.

Weimer, M. (2013). *Learner-centered teaching: Five key changes to practice* (2nd ed.). San Francisco: Jossey-Bass.

White, J., Pinnegar, S., & Esplin, P. (2010). When learning and change collide: Examining student claims to have learned nothing. *The Journal of General Education, 59*(2), 124–140.

Wiggins, G., & McTighe, J. (2005). *Understanding by design*. Columbus, OH: Pearson/Merrill/Prentice Hall.

Wittman-Price, R. A., & Fasolka, B. J. (2010). Objectives and outcomes: The fundamental difference. *Nursing Education Perspectives, 31*(4), 233–236.

11 Interprofessional Education and Collaborative Practice

Elizabeth Speakman, EdD, RN, ANEF, FNAP

In the very near future the system used to deliver health care in the United States and the composition of providers responsible for the delivery of that care will need to be reconfigured and expanded. The need for health care redesign is partly driven by the Patient Protection and Affordable Care Act (PPACA), which was passed by Congress and then signed into law by President Obama in 2010 (U.S. Department of Health and Human Services [HHS], 2012) and promises to provide care by covering millions of additional Americans who have been uninsured and by allowing consumers to be an integral part of their health care decisions. However, the way care is delivered in the future will need to begin to use effective team approaches that are patient centered and person focused. Although some teams exist naturally in certain health care settings, the shift toward team approaches will require retraining of the majority of the current health care workforce and even more urgently will require reconceptualizing health care education to include interprofessional team-based learning opportunities (Interprofessional Education Collaborative [IPEC], 2011).

In recent years, the call for creating more effective health care teams has caused interprofessional education (IPE) and collaborative practice (CP) to receive substantial attention in the health professions. Several reports released from the Institute of Medicine (Institute of Medicine, 2000, 2001, 2003, 2011) and the World Health Organization (World Health Organization, 2010) all describe the value, need for, and effect of interprofessional team work on patient outcomes. But the ability to participate in team approaches to health care delivery depends on clinicians receiving training and education on how to effectively communicate and engage in teamwork. Figures 11-1 and 11-2 illustrates the effect of IPE on creating a CP–ready workforce that affects the quality of health care delivered.

This chapter addresses the implications of IPE and CP on nursing education. Accepting the premise that *IPE* can be defined as occurring when students from two or more professions learn about, from, and with each other (World Health Organization [WHO], 2010), nurse educators must find meaningful and purposeful ways to engage students with other members of the health care team to prepare a practice-ready workforce. The two major tenets of IPE are teamwork and communication. This chapter explores specific ways in which faculty can provide interprofessional and CP experiences in the classroom and in clinical and simulation learning environments.

The Historical Perspective

The call to promote more team-based education in the U.S. health professions is not a new phenomenon. The report of the first Institute of Medicine (1972) conference, *Educating for the Health Team,* described how health care providers from diverse health profession backgrounds were convened to explore ways to teach health care practitioners the art of teamwork. More than two decades later, the Pew Health Professions Commission published a report identifying the need to require interdisciplinary competence in all health professionals (O'Neill, 1998). In 2003 the IOM recommended that educators and accreditation, licensing, and certification organizations ensure that students and working professionals develop and maintain proficiency in five core areas: delivering patient-centered care, working as part of interdisciplinary teams, practicing evidence-based medicine, focusing on quality improvement, and using information technology.

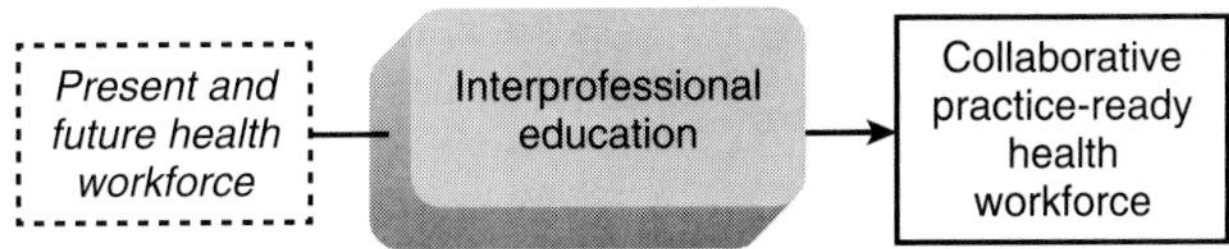

Figure 11-1 Interprofessional education. Reproduced, with permission of the publisher, from Framework for Action on Interprofessional Education and Collaborative Practice, Geneva, World Health Organization, 2010 (Fig. 2, http://www.who.int/hrh/resources/framework_action/en/, accessed 29 October 2014).

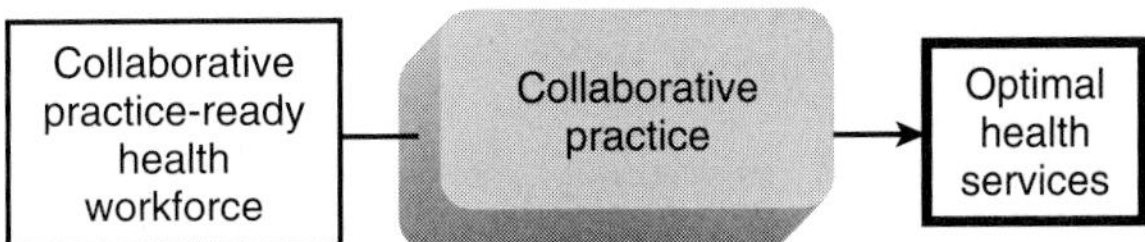

Figure 11-2 Collaborative practice. Reproduced, with permission of the publisher, from Framework for Action on Interprofessional Education and Collaborative Practice, Geneva, World Health Organization, 2010 (Fig. 3, http://www.who.int/hrh/resources/framework_action/en/, accessed 29 October 2014).

It is clear that there have been repeated calls by numerous health care institutes for IPE in the health professions for more than 40 years. But what, if any, academic preparation existed for students to prepare them to function as effective team leaders or members? And more importantly, what, if any, preparation existed for teachers and clinicians who mentor and precept students in teams? The simple truth is that clinicians who had the responsibility for teaching students how to practice in interprofessional teams lacked training themselves in teamwork and effective communication techniques. The World Health Organization (2010) report states, "The health and education systems must work together to coordinate health workforce strategies. If health workforce planning and policymaking are integrated, IPE and CP can be fully supported" (p. 10).

Because students learn from what they experience, a student who is not engaged in a team approach to care as a learner will likely not practice a team approach to care as a practitioner. Chan and colleagues (2009) noted that, as nurses are patients' primary caregivers, nursing students are in a unique position in the care delivery system; it therefore behooves nurse educators to assist students to prepare for the role of team leader and team member. Nursing education programs need to offer a curriculum that has interprofessional classroom, simulation, and clinical experience opportunities.

The "Triple Aim": Connecting Interprofessional Collaborative Practice and Patient Outcomes

The demand for interprofessional CP is related to improving patient care outcomes. The Institute for Healthcare Improvement (IHI) has developed a framework describing the "Triple Aim" with a goal toward optimizing the performance of the U.S. health care delivery system (Institute for Healthcare Improvement [IHI], 2007).

The "Triple Aim" is composed of the three goals of improving the patient's experience of care, improving population health, and reducing per capita costs of health care as represented in Figure 11-3 (Institute for Healthcare Improvement, 2007). The PPACA (2010) promises to provide health care for millions of additional people (U.S. Department of Health and Human Services, 2012) and expanding tele-health modalities such as home-based monitoring gives patients and their family and caregivers an even greater potential to be active members of the health care delivery team. Therefore the manner in which health care is provided will also refocus from episodic acute care to chronic, community-focused

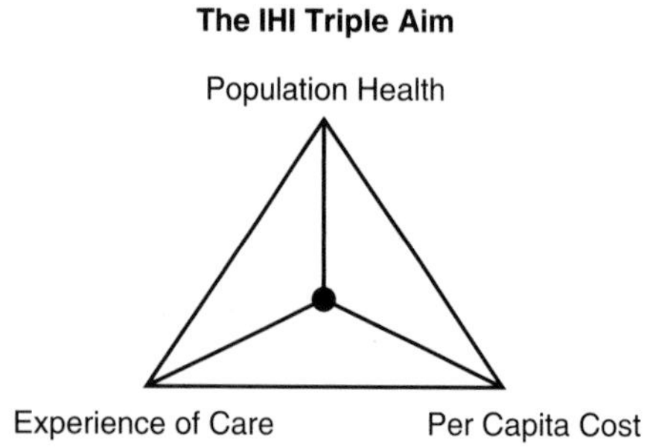

Figure 11-3 The Institute for Healthcare Improvement Triple Aim. The Triple Aim framework was developed by the Institute for Healthcare Improvement in Cambridge, Massachusetts (www.ihi.org). Reprinted with permission.

care (Speakman & Arenson, 2015). Institutions like the Veterans Health Administration have been pioneers in electronic health monitoring at home. In fact, in fiscal year 2013, more than 144,000 high-risk veterans were monitored for chronic conditions including diabetes, high blood pressure, chronic obstructive pulmonary disease, depression, posttraumatic stress disorder, weight management, substance abuse disorder, and spinal cord injuries through tele-health modalities (Conn, 2014).

Using the "Triple Aim" of improving the experience of care, improving the health of populations, and reducing per-capita costs of health care, health care education will need to purposefully prepare students to engage in technology-enriched, patient-centered learning environments. Students will need to become effective collaborators and work in teams that will allow them to learn to function within the fullest scope of their practice. The faculty role in this new paradigm will be to rethink classroom and clinical opportunities so that students have the greatest potential to work in these collaborative environments and learn to be effective members and leaders of the health care team. But the Triple Aim also creates a new dynamic in nursing education that may need to be explored. Berwick et al. (2008) posit that "two additional home outreach nurses might be better for the Triple Aim than another cardiologist" (p. 765). It is equally important that in creating learning opportunities for students, nurse educators need to be cognizant of any changing health care practice patterns in the quest to meet the triple aim of health care and create learning opportunities that support these patterns.

National Standards for Interprofessional Education and Collaborative Practice

Although health care leaders and professional organizations have embraced the concept of IPE as a core strategy to improving the quality of patient care outcomes, widespread integration of IPE in health professions curricula remains limited by perceived and actual barriers at the institutional, program, faculty, and student levels. In addition, questions remain related to the infrastructure required to develop, implement, evaluate, and sustain effective IPE in health professions programs. For example, what faculty competencies and development programs are necessary so that faculty are ready to deliver interprofessional classroom, simulation, and laboratory, and clinical learning experiences? Is teaching productivity and workload affected by faculty participation in IPE? Does engaging in IPE affect faculty satisfaction? To ensure that the promise of IPE education is realized for the benefit of patients, it is important that effective strategies for addressing and overcoming perceived barriers are identified and best practices disseminated.

In 2011 the IPEC established the Core Competencies for Interprofessional Collaborative Practice. The four core competencies are values and ethics, roles and responsibilities, interprofessional communication, and team and teamwork (Table 11-1). It is intended that the core competencies serve as a framework that can be integrated into the curricula of health professions programs. Faculty can design and implement learning experiences to facilitate acquisition of the knowledge, skills, and attitudes represented in the competencies. The core competencies for interprofessional CP are briefly described in this section.

Values and Ethics

> Interprofessional values and related ethics are an important new part of crafting a professional identity, one that is both professional and interprofessional in nature. These values and ethics are patient centered

TABLE 11-1 IPEC Core Competencies for Interprofessional Collaborative Practice

Values and Ethics	Roles and Responsibilities	Interprofessional Communication	Team and Teamwork
Work with individuals of other professions to maintain a climate of mutual respect and shared values.	Use the knowledge of one's own role and those of other professions to appropriately assess and address the health care needs of the patients and populations served.	Communicate with patients, families, communities, and other health professionals in a responsive and responsible manner that supports a team approach to the maintenance of health and the treatment of disease.	Apply relationship-building values and the principles of team dynamics to perform effectively in different team roles to plan and deliver patient population–centered care that is safe, timely, efficient, effective, and equitable.

IPEC, Interprofessional Education Collaborative.
Interprofessional Education Collaborative Expert Panel (IPEC). (2011). Core competencies for interprofessional collaborative practice: Report of an expert panel. Washington, D.C.: Interprofessional Education Collaborative. Retrieved from https://ipecollaborative.org/uploads/IPEC-Core-Competencies.pdf.

> with a community/population orientation, grounded in a sense of shared purpose to support the common good in health care, and reflect a shared commitment to creating safer, more efficient, and more effective systems of care. (Interprofessional Education Collaborative Expert Panel, 2011, p. 17)

Professional values and ethical behavior have always been tenets of nursing practice and major concepts integrated throughout nursing curricula. This is true of all health profession programs. Because values and ethics are so integral to health profession curricula, there are many opportunities in academic programs to create interprofessional learning experiences for students that focus on developing professional values and ethics and exploring the concepts of mutual respect and trust in interprofessional teams. Team-based learning, values clarification, case studies, reflective thought, interprofessional grand rounds with debriefing opportunities, and role play and simulations are examples of teaching and learning strategies that can be effective in facilitating student learning. Chapter 18 discusses the use of simulation as a teaching–learning strategy.

Roles and Responsibilities

> Learning to be interprofessional requires an understanding of how professional roles and responsibilities complement each other in patient-centered and community/population oriented care. (Interprofessional Education Collaborative Expert Panel, 2011, p. 20)

To fully engage in CP, it is important for team members to understand each others' roles and responsibilities; it is also essential for each member of the team to be able to clearly articulate to each other their own roles and responsibilities in patient care (Interprofessional Education Collaborative Expert Panel, 2011). Nurses, by the nature of their profession, are accustomed to working with other health care professionals. However, there is no assurance that a nurse understands the role and responsibilities of other health care providers, or that those other health care providers necessarily understand the nurse's role. Such understandings need to be intentionally cultivated in environments characterized by mutual respect and trust. Developing a reciprocal understanding of the roles and responsibilities of the many members of the health care team should begin in the educational setting. Interprofessional Education Collaborative Expert Panel (2011) states that true "collaborative practice depends on learning, refining and improving the roles and responsibilities of those working together" (p. 20).

Faculty can seek to create opportunities to engage nursing students with other members of the health care team. For example, team debriefings after interdisciplinary rounding in the clinical setting, interprofessional case study presentations in the classroom, and simulated learning activities are just a few strategies that can bring student teams of health care providers together to discuss patient care scenarios, and consciously require them to articulate how their role and responsibilities complement other team members' contributions, forming a collective goal for the patient's care.

Interprofessional Communication

> Communication competencies help professionals prepare for collaborative practice. Communicating a readiness to work together initiates an effective interprofessional collaboration. (Interprofessional Education Collaborative Expert Panel, 2011, p. 22)

Although nursing education prepares students at all levels to strive to be effective communicators, the implementation of interprofessional communication means that all health professionals have equal responsibility to demonstrate leadership and raise concerns with each other within the team. Each team member also has equal value in managing and delivering safe and effective patient care. According to IPEC, "Learning to give and receive timely, sensitive, and instructive feedback with confidence helps health professionals improve their teamwork and team-based care" (2011, p. 22). However, feeling empowered and safe enough within the team to speak and possibly challenge another health professional who either has seniority or is perceived to hold positional authority can be a challenge. Nurse educators must find communication practice opportunities such as the situation, background, assessment, and recommendation technique to help students develop confidence in "speaking up" within the team. The use of simulations can also be an effective strategy in facilitating students becoming more confident in their communication skills. Using clear affirmative communication techniques in practice will have a major effect on safe and effective patient care delivery.

Team and Teamwork

> Working in teams involves sharing one's expertise and relinquishing some professional autonomy to work closely with others. Shared accountability, shared problem-solving, and shared decision are characteristics of collaborative teamwork and working effectively in teams. (Interprofessional Education Collaborative Expert Panel, 2011, p. 24)

The gestalt of IPE and CP is effective teamwork. Nurses must be comfortable with assuming a leadership role on the team as well as being an effective team member. As previously discussed, nurses routinely work in teams, but are these teams always effective at working together to produce quality care outcomes? Interprofessional teams can only be effective if team members understand each others' roles, and everyone is comfortable speaking up and engaging in an open discussion. For many nurses, especially novice nurses, assuming a leadership role on the team can be intimidating. Learning to be an effective team member and patient advocate requires practice. Nursing students can learn to engage in teamwork in a variety of ways. For example experiencing team-based learning in the classroom with peers or group project assignments with students from other disciplines, including those outside the health professions, can help students develop the group dynamic skills necessary to be an effective team leader and member. Interprofessional simulation activities, experiential learning experiences in clinical settings with other health care providers, and community-based interdisciplinary service learning projects are just a few examples of how faculty can intentionally foster the development of teamwork skills in the curriculum.

The literature on interprofessional CP states that teamwork has the potential to positively affect patient outcomes. High-functioning care teams work together, collaborating in collective problem-solving and decision-making processes. As a result, these processes lead to increasing levels of interdependence among those embedded in teams, and in microsystems like hospitals, clinical units, and communities (Interprofessional Education Collaborative Expert Panel, 2011).

Model for Evaluating Learning Effectiveness in IPE

Creating an organizing framework is an essential component to the curriculum of any educational program. Providing faculty with a way of organizing knowledge and skills is critical to achieving the desired educational outcomes. The Kirkpatrick model (Kirkpatrick & Kirkpatrick, 2010), is one framework that is frequently used in IPE to help achieve and evaluate desired learner outcomes (Pardue, 2015).

Smidt et al. (2009) stated that the value of using the Kirkpatrick model is that it provides a framework that educators can use to assess and evaluate whether a training program meets the needs of the organization and learners who are participating in the program. For example, Sheppard and colleagues (2014) used the Kirkpatrick model to evaluate changes in attitudes toward interprofessional teams and older adults in an interprofessional clinical experience in the nursing home setting.

First developed in 1954, the Kirkpatrick model has four components to evaluate educational program effectiveness. Level 1, the reaction level, evaluates how a participant reacts to the training and education programs. Level 2, the learning level, evaluates how much the participant has learned from the actual training. Level 3, the behavior level, evaluates how the participants apply what they learned to their work setting and Level 4, the results level, evaluates the formative outcomes of the training and education programs. Recently the Kirkpatrick model was modified with the addition of a new dimension called return on expectations (ROE). ROE is the practitioner's approach to determining the organizational value of the training and the degree to which the organization's expectations have been satisfied (Kirkpatrick & Kirkpatrick, 2010).

To achieve the desired ROE and effect on patient outcomes, interprofessional learning opportunities should be integrated into the curricula of health professions programs and offered on a continuous basis, using a variety of teaching strategies. Table 11-2 outlines some examples of how the Kirkpatrick model can be used in the evaluation of interprofessional learning activities.

Faculty Development for Interprofessional Education

Incorporating IPE activities and CP initiatives into the curriculum requires faculty development. Although some faculty may already have experience with IPE and can serve as faculty champions for those who have less experience, for many faculty, engaging in IPE and collaborating with faculty from other disciplines will be a change in their practice as educators. There must be a concerted effort to orient faculty on the components of IPE and CP. The following activities can help prepare nursing faculty to engage in IPE:

- Identify a rationale for participating in IPE. The Institute of Medicine (2011) report on the future of nursing can be used to frame faculty discussions and provide context to the importance of integrating IPE and CP into nursing programs. Identify faculty champions for leading the integration of IPE into the curriculum and assign mentors to help less experienced faculty.
- Use up-to-date resources to support the integration of IPE into the curriculum. In 2012 the National Center for Interprofessional Practice and Education was established at the University of Minnesota through federal grant funding. The Center's website (https://nexusipe.org) has a plethora of resources that faculty can use to plan, implement, and evaluate IPE and CP programs. Seeking advice and resources from national IPE champions is another helpful strategy.
- Seek collaborating partners from interdisciplinary colleagues within your own institution and other local and regional colleges, universities, and health care agencies. Although

TABLE 11-2 Application of the Kirkpatrick Model in Interprofessional Education

Reaction	Learning	Behavior	Results
What did the student think and feel about experiencing interprofessional collaboration? How did the student react to the learning activity? Was the response favorable?	How well did the student learn the intended content? Did the student acknowledge an increase in knowledge of interprofessional collaboration?	To what extent was the student able to effectively apply teamwork and communication techniques?	In the health care environment, what were the outcomes resulting from students' learning and practicing in interprofessional collaborative teams?

it is important to explore various types of IPE and CP initiatives that will work in a specific learning environment, it is also important to learn with and from others. Forming local or regional consortiums and partnerships, reviewing the literature for examples of successful IPE programs, and sharing outcomes from such collaborative efforts can be helpful activities. Provide time for faculty to debrief after implementing an IPE initiative to evaluate the experience, acknowledge the lessons learned, and explore new ways to advance IPE in the curriculum.

Implementing IPE and CP Initiatives into the Curriculum

Designing and implementing IPE and CP initiatives into the curriculum can be a daunting task because it requires collaboration and coordination with other professions. Pardue (2015) has proposed a framework that faculty can use to design, implement, and evaluate IPE. She advises starting with the desired learning outcome in mind, prior to designing any specific learning activities. What knowledge, skills, or behaviors (abilities) related to interprofessional practice do faculty expect students to demonstrate as a result of the learning experience? See Box 11-1 for a guide to planning and implementing IPE and CP initiatives.

Cranford and Bates (2015) identified six steps that led to a successful integration of IPE into a nursing curriculum. The six steps included first setting the stage and creating momentum and awareness among the faculty. The next step involved inviting other disciplines to participate in the learning experience and building an interprofessional team that would be responsible for implementing the project. The next steps included identifying objectives for the project and developing the implementation details. The final two steps were evaluating the success of the collaborative effort in terms of student outcomes and then following up as a team to determine next steps to ensure continued expansion of IPE throughout the curriculum (Cranford & Bates, 2015).

The greatest challenge to implementing IPE is usually finding a common time for the learning experiences and resolving competing schedules. It is also important to consider the appropriate level of students from multiple programs to participate in any given learning activity. Depending on the desired learner outcomes, the faculty may decide to partner students of comparable educational levels. For example, students in their first year of clinical experience such as first-year nursing students may be partnered with first- or second-year medical, pharmacy, or physical or occupational therapy graduate students. However, there may also be value to partnering less experienced students with students who are further along in their educational program

BOX 11-1 Guide to Planning IPE and CP Initiatives

- Decide who should participate in planning the experience, ensure representation from each discipline, and find a mutual time to meet.
- Identify key information needed from each discipline to facilitate planning.
- Determine learner level that will be involved in the learning experience, striving for congruency among the various student populations.
- Describe and discuss various program curricula and influence of program accreditation standards.
- Consider placement of clinical learning experiences within the curricula. Use IPEC competencies as a framework for the design of learning activities
- Create a consensus on desired project outcomes using the Core Competencies for Interprofessional Collaboration as a guide.
- Avoid trying to align the entire curriculum of multiple programs. Focus interprofessional efforts where the curricula intersect in some manner (schedule, clinical rotations, common concepts, etc.). Outline the program, deciding who, what, when, where, and how.
- Develop program elements including goals, concepts to be covered, and how the program will be evaluated
- Identify a common time to host the program and a location that ensures easy access by all students.
- Identify needed administrative support and resources to implement the program. Examine and select reliable and valid evaluation tools to measure program outcomes (https://nexusipe.org/measurement-instruments).
- Consider using a systematic plan to facilitate program implementation and evaluation using the core competencies for interprofessional practice.

to foster learning among peers. Subsequently it may be appropriate to partner second-year nursing students with third- or fourth-year medical, pharmacy, or physical or occupational therapy or physician assistant students, as all students are engaged in clinical experiences.

See Table 11-3 for an exemplar of a systematic IPE activities plan used at Thomas Jefferson University that can be used as a guide for implementing IPE and CP initiatives. There may be different challenges to implementing IPE and CP initiatives depending on the type of institution.

Academic Health Centers and Large Universities

Although it is assumed that creating and crafting IPE and CP initiatives in large universities and academic health centers is easy, that may not be the case because of the complexity of the organizations and challenges of competing schedules. There also may not be a preexisting culture of collaboration within the institution. The key to overcoming these challenges is to find an IPE champion in another discipline who will agree to partner in the design and implementation of IPE learning activities. Offering a designated IPE course that addresses the national core competencies and enrolls students from multiple disciplines, either virtually or in a classroom setting, can address some of the scheduling challenges and begin to develop a culture of IPE within the institution.

Nonacademic Health Centers

In addition to logistics, the greatest challenge for faculty in small or large colleges and universities and nonacademic health centers is convening the interested parties, and gaining access to other health care professionals in the community. Designing and planning teamwork and communication opportunities does not require the environment of an academic health center. Smaller institutions can engage in IPE and CP initiatives in several ways. For example, nursing faculty can meet with faculty from another program and identify a common IPEC interprofessional CP core competency on which to focus a collaborative learning activity.

Hall et al. (2014) conducted a pilot study to determine if "humanities can enable learners to meaningfully interact and connect with patients and members of the care team" (p. 519). Using humanities-based learning activities within a clinical placement experience, students were given the opportunity to better understand and experience collaborative teamwork through the lens of the humanities and better understand patients and families as unique and holistic beings (Hall et al., 2014). This pilot study is an exemplar of how students can learn teamwork and communication outside the confines of their own curriculum with an additional benefit of providing nursing students with an opportunity to practice the art of nursing as they engage with students from the humanities.

TABLE 11-3 Systematic Activities Plan

	Classroom Learning—Health Mentors Program					Evaluation Measures
Health Profession Program	**Learner's Level**	**V/E**	**R/R**	**IP Comm**	**TT**	
BSN Nursing	3 & 4	X	X	X	X	• Student Stereotypes Rating Questionnaire (SSRQ)
CFT	1 & 2	X	X	X	X	• Interdisciplinary Education Perception Scale (IEPS)
Medicine	1 & 2	X	X	X	X	• Attitudes Toward Health Care Teams (ATHCT) Scale
Pharmacy	1 & 2	X	X	X	X	• Roles of Health Professions (HP)
PT	1 & 2	X	X	X	X	• Peer and Self Evaluations (P/S Evals)
OT	1 & 2	X	X	X	X	• Team Performance Survey (TPS)

BSN, Bachelor of Science in Nursing; CFT, couple & family therapy; IP Comm, interprofessional communication; OT, occupational therapy; PT, physical therapy; R/R, roles/responsibilities; TT, teams and teamwork; V/E, values/ethics. Thomas Jefferson University. (2014). Jefferson Center for Interprofessional Education Systematic Activities Plan. Philadelphia: Author. Used with permission

Organizing IPE and CP experiences

The individual competencies organized under each of the four core competency domains can be thought of as behavioral learning objectives and can be linked to learning activities and assessments of interprofessional effectiveness (Interprofessional Education Collaborative Expert Panel, 2011). To reiterate, the foundation of IPE and CP is teamwork and communication. Therefore nursing students should be given ample opportunities to interact and engage in teamwork learning experiences with a variety of health care professionals or paraprofessionals to practice collaborative, team-based, patient-centered care. Placing students in a variety of interprofessional and CP experiences will facilitate the student's ability to achieve the four IPEC Core Competencies. Ensuring that each faculty and program has the opportunity to have input into what works for his or her respective college or school has the greatest potential in overcoming any logistical challenges. Changing the culture of non-collaboration can be a challenge, but the addition of IPE in accreditation standards and guidelines of most health education professions has been helpful and will continue to help move organizations toward a culture of collaboration. The following sections contain examples of how faculty can create interprofessional learning opportunities for nursing students.

Natural Interprofessional Relationships

"Natural" interprofessional relationships refers to pairing nursing students with one or more students from medicine, pharmacy, occupational and physical therapy, physician's assistants, diet and nutrition, and social work health care education programs. For the most part, these students are in program plans of study that include didactic and experiential clinical experiences with patients with chronic and episodic health care needs, and therefore are most likely to "naturally" engage with nursing students on the clinical unit. For these partners, interprofessional teamwork can be demonstrated in the classroom and in clinical and simulated learning environments. Some ideas include the following:

- Develop an interdisciplinary case study with partners from other disciplines. Have students work in interprofessional teams to discuss how each profession might manage the care of the patient, creating an interprofessional plan of care.
- Invite an interprofessional team of experts to interact with students, either face-to-face or online, and explain their role in the delivery of patient care. While such a learning experience can be designed and offered to a single student discipline, providing such an experience to students representing multiple disciplines is more powerful.
- Implement a simulated case study regarding a clinical incident or disaster preparedness with an interprofessional team of students. Providing opportunities to practice teamwork, communication skills, and clinical decision-making in a simulated environment is a "low-risk" learning experience and will help students build confidence with implementing these skills in the clinical environment.
- Engage nursing students with other members of the health care team in a rounding experience on the clinical unit. If possible have the students complete a patient assessment together and jointly present findings during a debriefing experience following the rounding activity.

Designed Interprofessional Relationships

"Designed" interprofessional relationships refers to pairing nursing students with one or more of the groups of students enrolled in law, psychology, biological and chemical science, radiologic science, music, art, theater or business programs. For these partners, interprofessional activities that foster teamwork might be limited to the classroom setting with the potential simulation, clinical, or service learning experience. Some ideas include the following:

- Develop a case study with partners from other disciplines. Have students form interprofessional teams to discuss management of the scenario described in the case study. Students should discuss their respective professional roles and responsibilities. As a team, define how their professions intersect in managing the scenario.
- Invite students from multiple professions to attend a common classroom experience to form teams to work on team building skills using such block building exercises as Zoom, Paper Chain building, or Lego. During debriefing have the students describe the techniques they employed during the group process.

- Develop a simulation case study with partners from other disciplines on disaster preparedness, having students practice teamwork and communication skills in interprofessional teams.
- Design a community service learning or joint clinical opportunity. Have students collaborate on an interprofessional care plan or project activity. Confer a joint post conference and discuss the tenets of teamwork and communication.

Teaching Strategies for IPE and CP

Students are not immune to the challenges of organizational culture change. For some students, engaging in IPE is a change from what they previously experienced and for others, it might be contrary to their beliefs and understanding of the role of the nurse in health care. In any event, it is important to create an orientation program for students and include the rationale and expectations for IPE and CP learning experiences. Teaching strategies for IPE are much like general teaching strategies and those principles outlined in Chapter 15.

Summary

The need for safe, quality, patient-centered care remains consistent. Suffice to say that students who are engaged in interprofessional learning experiences and who have ample opportunities to practice effective communication skills in team-based approaches will have the greatest potential to impact patient-centered care. After graduation from interprofessional learning environments, these students can evolve into practitioners who have a repertoire of collaboration and teamwork skills with the greatest hope of avoiding traditional silo approaches to health care delivery. It is important to note that many leaders in IPE are currently examining the correlation between patient outcomes of the "Triple Aim" and interprofessional teamwork (Brandt et al., 2014). The World Health Organization (2010) warns that to ensure future health care workers are qualified for practice, institutions of higher education must create and support a climate of IPE CP. Reeves et al. (2013) noted that, given the complexity of patients, providing IPE opportunities for students is an investment in the future. The very essence of the nurse's role makes him or her central in the delivery of care. It is for these reasons that nurse educators develop IPE and CP learning opportunities as a way to prepare students to practice in a collaborative health care delivery system. Corbridge et al. (2013) concurs that IPE experiences are key in improving communication among team members and provide students the opportunity to collaborate and engage in shared decision making. It is now time to look at the "margins to define the whole" (Guinier et al., 1997).

REFLECTING ON THE EVIDENCE

1. What evidence supports the need to engage nursing students in interprofessional teams?
2. What teaching strategies would you use to create IPE and CP learning opportunities?
3. When designing an IPE or a CP initiative, what key elements should be included from the beginning?
4. What is the value of creating a systematic evaluation plan for IPE or CP activities?

REFERENCES

Berwick, D. M., Nolan, T. W., & Whittington, J. (2008). The triple aim: Care, heath, and cost. *Health Affairs, 27*(3), 759–769.

Brandt, B., Lutfiyya, M. N., Kinga, J. A., & Chioresoa, C. (2014). A scoping review of interprofessional collaborative practice and education using the lens of the triple aim. *Journal of Interprofessional Care, 28*(5), 393–399.

Chan, E. A., Mok, E., Po-ying, A. H., & Man-chun, J. H. (2009). The use of interdisciplinary seminars for the development of caring dispositions in nursing and social work. *Journal of Advanced Nursing, 65*(12), 2658–2667.

Conn, J. (2014). *Staying connected: Providers and patients increasingly relying on home-based monitoring modern healthcare.* Retrieved from, http://www.modernhealthcare.com/article/20140118/MAGAZINE/301189929/staying-connected.

Corbridge, S. J., Tiffen, J., Carlucci, M., & Zar, F. A. (2013). Implementation of an Interprofessional educational model. *Nurse Educator, 38*(6), 261–264.

Cranford, J. S., & Bates, T. (2015). Infusing interprofessional education into the nursing curriculum. *Nurse Educator, 40*(1), 16–20.

Guinier, L., Fine, M., & Balin, J. (1997). *Becoming gentlemen: Women, law school, and institutional change.* Boston: Beacon Press.

Hall, P., Brajtman, S., Weaver, L., Grassau, P. A., & Varpio, L. (2014). Learning collaborative teamwork: An argument for incorporating the humanities. *Journal of Interprofessional Care, 28*(6), 519–525. http://dx.doi.org/10.3109/13561820.2014.915513. Retrieved from, http://informahealthcare.com.proxy1.lib.tju.edu/doi/full/10.3109/13561820.2014.915513.

Institute for Healthcare Improvement (IHI). (2007). *The IHI triple aim initiative.* Retrieved from, http://www.ihi.org/Engage/Initiatives/TripleAim/Pages/default.aspx.

Institute of Medicine. (1972). *Educating a health care team: Report of the Conference.* Washington, DC: National Academies Press.

Institute of Medicine. (2000). *To err is human: Building a safer health system.* Washington, DC: National Academic Press.

Institute of Medicine. (2001). *Crossing the quality chasm: A new health system for the 21st century.* Washington DC: National Academies Press.

Institute of Medicine. (2003). *Health professions education: A bridge to quality.* Washington DC: National Academies Press.

Institute of Medicine. (2011). *The future of nursing: Leading change, advancing health.* Washington, DC: The National Academies Press.

Interprofessional Education Collaborative Expert Panel (IPEC). (2011). *Core competencies for interprofessional collaborative practice: Report of an expert panel.* Washington, D.C.: Interprofessional Education Collaborative. Retrieved from, https://ipecollaborative.org/uploads/IPEC-Core-Competencies.pdf.

Kirkpatrick, J. D., & Kirkpatrick, W. K. (2010, August 15). *ROE's rising star: Why return on expectation is getting so much attention.* T&D: Magazine for the Association of Talent Development.

O'Neil, E. H.(chair) for the Pew Health Professions Commission (1998). *Recreating health: Professional practice for a new century.* San Francisco: Pew Health Professions Committee.

Pardue, K. (2015). A framework for the design, implementation, and evaluation of interprofessional education. *Nurse Educator, 40*(1), 10–15.

Reeves, S., Perrier, L., Goldman, J., Freeth, D., & Zwarenstein, M. (2013). *Interprofessional education: Effects on professional practice and healthcare outcomes (update).* Cochrane Database of Systematic Reviews. Issue 3.

Sheppard, K. D., Channing, R. F., Sawyer, P., Foley, K. T., Harada, C. K., Brown, C. J., et al. (2014, August 20). The interprofessional clinical experience: Interprofessional education in the nursing home. *Journal of Interprofessional Care,* http://dx.doi.org/10.3109/13561820.2014.942776. Retrieved from, http://informahealthcare.com.proxy1.lib.tju.edu/doi/full/10.3109/13561820.2014.942776.

Smidt, A., Balandin, S., Sigafoos, J., & Reed, V. A. (2009). The Kirkpatrick model: A useful tool for evaluating training outcomes. *Journal of Intellectual & Developmental Disability, 34*(3), 266–274.

Speakman, E., & Arenson, C. (2015). Going back to the future: What is all the buzz about interprofessional education and collaborative practice? *Nurse Educator, 40*(1), 3–4.

Thomas Jefferson University. (2014). *Jefferson center for interprofessional education systematic activities plan.* Philadelphia: Author.

U.S. Department of Health and Human Services (HHS). (2012). *The Patient Protection and Affordable Care Act, 42 U.S.C. § 18001 et seq. (2010).* Retrieved from, http://www.hhs.gov/healthcare/rights/law/index.html.

World Health Organization (WHO). (2010). *Framework for action on interprofessional education & collaborative practice.* Geneva: World Health Organization.

12 Service Learning: Developing Values, Cultural Competence, Social Responsibility, and Global Awareness*

Carla Mueller, PhD, RN

For more than two decades, agencies and commissions concerned with higher education and preparation of the professions (American Association of Colleges of Nursing, 2008a; Campus Compact, 2001; National Service-Learning Clearinghouse, 2010; Pew Health Professions Commission, 1998) have recommended that educational programs include experiences that require civic engagement and community involvement. Institutions of higher education and their schools of nursing are therefore seeking opportunities for students to develop moral judgment, civic responsibility, cultural competence, and global awareness, in addition to the basic professional skills set forth in the curriculum. Service learning, a structured component of the curriculum in which students acquire social values through service to individuals, groups, or communities, is one way to provide opportunities for students to develop these values. Service offers opportunities for learning that cannot be obtained any other way. As such, a service experience may be one of the first truly meaningful acts in a student's life. Service learning uses reflective learning to connect learning with students' thoughts and feelings in a deliberate way, creating a context in which students can explore how they feel about what they are thinking, and what they think about how they feel. As it does so, it becomes an integral part of students' education. This chapter explains how service learning can contribute to these outcomes in nursing curricula.

Service Learning

Service learning evolves from a philosophy of education that emphasizes active learning that meets a course objective while also directed toward a goal of social responsibility and civic engagement. Service learning is not merely volunteerism, nor is it a substitute for a field experience or practicum that is a normal part of a course. Service learning is not the same as a nursing clinical experience because the focus of the activity is on meeting both the needs of the host community as well as those of the nursing curriculum. However, student learning is not ignored. Service learning offers a way in which students can meet learning objectives, as well as develop leadership skills, cultural competence, and a sense of civic responsibility congruent with the tenets of social justice and social change (Foli, Braswell, Kirkpatrick, & Lim, 2014; Gillis & MacLellan, 2013). Both the recipient and the student benefit from the experience.

Service learning is an educational experience in which students participate in a service activity that meets the needs of multiple stakeholders in the professional and community environment within the framework of a specific credit-bearing course. Service learning focuses on developing social values rather than providing a discrete type of experiential education. *Service learning* is also defined as a way of connecting academic learning with service; it provides concrete opportunities for students to learn new skills, think critically, and test new roles in situations that encourage risk taking and reward competence.

Service learning is a component of broader educational goals to promote civic engagement). Civic engagement involves individual and collective actions to address areas of societal concern. Civic engagement may include service-learning projects as well as community-focused faculty research. Like service learning, civic engagement involves structured activities that require the student to work with a community to solve a problem, but unlike service

*The author acknowledges the work of Barbara Norton, RN, MPH, in a previous edition of the chapter.

learning, the focus of the activity is to promote civic responsibility and development for citizenship.

Often the terms *service learning* and *experiential learning* are used interchangeably; however, they are distinct entities. Experiential learning includes hands-on work and has the learning of work-related skills as its major goal. Traditional nursing clinical experiences are an example of experiential learning. In contrast, service learning involves work that meets actual community needs, has as one of its goals the fostering of "a sense of caring for others," and includes structured time for reflection (Bailey, Carpenter, & Harrington, 2002). Service learning balances the need of the community and the learning objectives of the students. Community agencies are true partners in design, implementation, and evaluation of the experience.

Service learning expands the learning environment for students and faculty. It is community based and population focused and therefore provides opportunities for students to act locally to solve social problems (Eads, 1994). Although a number of similarities are present, key differences exist between traditional learning and service learning. These differences are summarized in Table 12-1.

TABLE 12-1 Differences between Traditional Learning and Service Learning

	Traditional Learning	Service Learning
Location	Classroom	Classroom, community
Teacher	Professor	Professor, preceptor or facilitator, patients
Learning	Activities Writing	Collaboration with the community Writing
	Examinations	Examinations
	Passive	Active
	Authoritarian	Shared responsibility
	Structured	Reflective
	Compartmentalized	Expansive, integrative
	Cognitive	Cognitive and affective
	Short-term	Short-term and long-term
Reasoning	Deductive	Inductive
Evaluation	Professor	Professor, preceptor or facilitator, community, self-assessment by students

Colleges and universities may engage in service learning differently because of different institutional missions and traditions. Some universities embrace service learning as a philosophy, some as part of their spiritual mission. Others embrace it as part of their commitment to civic responsibility or as a way to foster community partnerships. Regardless of how universities embrace service learning, it must do the following:

1. Be connected to program and course learning outcomes and promote learning
2. Be experiential
3. Allow students to engage in activities that address human and community needs via structured opportunities for student learning and development
4. Provide time for guided reflection in discussion, writing, or media
5. Develop a sense of caring, social responsibility, global awareness, and civic engagement
6. Involve activities that have real meaning for the participants and promote deeper learning
7. Address problems that are identified by the community and require problem solving
8. Promote collaborative learning and teamwork
9. Embrace the concept of reciprocity between the learner and the person, organization, or community being served

Service learning may be a separate course within the college curriculum or integrated as a thread throughout multiple courses. The trend is toward the latter. Faculty members intentionally and strategically plan to incorporate service-learning experiences as part of a course. When it is integrated into existing courses, it is important that it not be added as an "additional" course requirement. Instead, it should be a learning activity that replaces one or more learning activities previously used. Credit should be given for the learning and its relation to the course, not for the service alone. The service activity must match course content and enhance learning by allowing application of the theoretical principles taught in the classroom setting. At some colleges and universities, courses with a service-learning component are identified in the course catalogue as having an opportunity for service learning. At the same time, some colleges allow students to select an alternate learning activity if they do not wish to participate.

Theoretical Foundations of Service Learning

Kolb's (1984) theory of experiential learning has been widely used as a theoretical basis for designing and analyzing service-learning programs. Reflective observation about the experience is essential to the learning process. It links the concrete experience to abstract conceptualizations of that experience. Learning is increased when students are actively engaged in gaining knowledge through experiential problem solving and decision making (Bailey et al., 2002). Use of reflection is built on the work of Kolb (1984) and Dewey (1916, 1933, 1938). In service learning, reflection is both a cognitive process (Mezirow, 1990) and a structured learning activity (Silcox, 1994). Effective reflection fosters moral development and enhances moral decision making. Moral decisions involve an exercise of choice and a corresponding willingness to accept responsibility for that choice (Gilligan, 1981).

Delve, Mintz, and Stewart (1990) developed a service-learning model based on theories of moral decision making and values clarification. Their model includes five phases of development: exploration, clarification, realization, activation, and internalization. It illustrates that service learning is developmental, providing students with an opportunity to move from charity to justice as they become more empathetic. Delve et al. (1990) believe that without that empathy, the student will not come to recognize the members of the patient population as valued individuals in the larger society and as sources for new learning.

The pedagogy of service learning has powerful flexibility. It can be based on subject matter or on learning process; it can connect theory and practice; it integrates several different approaches to knowledge and uses of knowledge; it encourages learning how to learn; and it can focus on a wide range of issues, problems, and interests (Pellietier, 1995). It also lends itself to problem-based learning and case study methodologies.

Outcomes of Service Learning

Service learning in the curriculum provides opportunities for students to attain personal, professional, and curriculum goals. It also contributes to the overall educational experience of the college or university and thus provides benefits to the institution as well. Finally, this benefits the community in which it occurs and the clients it serves.

Benefits to Students

A review of the literature on the outcomes of service learning reveals that students benefit in multiple and integrated ways (Amerson, 2010; Gillis & MacLellan, 2013). Benefits can include personal and professional development as well as mastering course outcomes.

Direct participation in this activity assists with socialization into the profession, introduces new technical or professional skills, increases motivation to learn, encourages self-directed learning, facilitates acquisition of leadership skills, and promotes preparation of nurses who are capable of serving as advocates for social justice (Foli et al., 2014; Gillis & MacLellan, 2013). Several schools of nursing have integrated service-learning components into the freshman experience as a way to introduce nursing students to the role of the nurse (Baumberger, Krouse, & Borucki, 2006). It can also be an opportunity for interprofessional learning and developing collaborative relationships with other professions. Although the majority of service learning occurs in undergraduate programs, graduate programs in nursing are beginning to explore community engagement to further develop students' leadership skills and sense of responsibility, as well as enhancement of their critical thinking skills and learning of academic content (Francis-Baldesari & Williamson, 2008; Sheikh, 2014).

Service learning has been found to provide a more thorough understanding of "self " and provides insight into personal strengths and weaknesses (Batchelder & Root, 1994). It also has been found to contribute to the development of personal vision, moral sensitivity, clarification of values, and spirituality.

Service learning facilitates academic inquiry by connecting theory and practice, enhancing disciplinary understanding and understanding of complex material, bringing greater relevance to course material, and helping students generalize their learning to new situations (Jarosinski & Heinrich, 2010). Service-learning experiences also develop critical thinking, communication, collaboration, leadership, and professional skills. Reising, Allen, and Hall (2006a) found that participating in a blood pressure screening service-learning project in the university community provided skills of blood pressure assessment, history taking, and health counseling.

The social effect includes the development of civic responsibility, increased orientation to volunteerism, increased political and global awareness, development of cultural competence, and improved ethical decision making (Gehrke, 2008; Reising, Allen, & Hall, 2006b). Students also learn the value of community health promotion (Reising et al., 2006a, 2006b).

Benefits to Faculty

Identifying benefits to faculty are key to obtaining buy-in because of the time commitment involved. Even though faculty may not be on-site with students directly supervising the service activities, significant faculty time commitment is required to plan the assignment, obtain community partners, read student journals, and facilitate reflection sessions. Faculty who link service-learning activities in their courses with their research and service interests have increased commitment to continuing its use. Some universities have adopted the Boyer model of scholarship, which enlarged the scholarship perspective to include teaching, service, and practice, in addition to research. By enlarging the scholarship perspective, Boyer (1990) believed that there would be a stronger connection between universities and the communities they served. This scholarship model facilitates integration of service learning into the faculty member's academic role as well as promotion and tenure requirements. The Carnegie Academy for the Scholarship of Teaching and Learning in Higher Education provides an online gallery of interdisciplinary projects, including those that involve service learning that can be used by faculty to transform their teaching. This gallery is available on the Carnegie Foundation for the Advancement of Teaching's website at http://gallery.carnegiefoundation.org/gallery_of_tl/castl_he.html.

Benefits to the Institution

Service learning also has institutional benefits. These include invigoration of the campus educational culture, development of a strong sense of campus community, increased institutional visibility, enhanced appeal to potential donors, and retention of students. It invigorates the campus culture by increasing students' engagement in their own learning, revitalizing faculty, and allowing faculty to mesh service projects with research interests. The interdisciplinary nature of service learning helps the campus regain a strong ethos of community, keeps students and faculty more engaged in the life of the college, and contributes to student retention (Hamner, Wilder, Avery, & Byrd, 2002). By placing service-learning experiences early in the program, for example as a freshman-year experience, the student retention rate can be increased because students develop self-efficacy and an understanding of the field of study. Increased institutional visibility contributes to increased student recruitment by providing a visible link between the community and the institution and by providing a perception of access to higher education to community members who have not believed higher education to be within their reach. Service learning enhances the institution's appeal to potential donors by providing a direct link between the college and the community, and it appeals to donors interested in community service educational reform (Pellietier, 1995).

The mentoring environment that is created between students, faculty, staff, administration, and the broader community becomes a "complex ecology of higher education . . . that can provide knowledge, support, and inspiration" (Daloz, Keen, Keen, & Parks, 1996). Service learning also provides a real-world learning environment in the community that facilitates transfer of knowledge and transition to the practice environment. A smooth transition to practice and increased use of community and public health settings were key recommendations for nursing education in the Institute of Medicine (Institute of Medicine, 2010) report. The new alliances formed between academic institutions and community service agencies and organizations eliminate or minimize the traditional separation between the "gown and the town."

Benefits to the Community

The community also benefits when colleges and universities include service learning and civic engagement outcomes in their academic programs. For example, Reising et al. (2006b) found that as a result of a service-learning project in which nursing students conducted hypertension screening and health counseling, 1 year later the community recipients had made modifications in their health-management behaviors such as diet change and weight loss. In another service-learning course, students in a nursing research course established partnerships with community organizations to develop research proposals, some of which led to submission for grant funding (Rash, 2005). Benefits to the community may also include students' increasing awareness of community health needs and an interest in working in community settings (Ligeikis-Clayton & Denman, 2005).

Benefits to the Health Care System

Although traditional service learning has occurred in community settings, it can also occur within a traditional acute care setting. Service learning benefits the nursing staff because the ideas for projects are initiated by the staff based on their needs and priorities, and implemented in collaboration with the students, resulting in the development of meaningful outcomes such as evidence-based patient care protocols and guidelines and improved patient care outcome measures. Hospitals working toward Magnet status can use these projects to provide support for their application for Magnet recognition.

Integrating Service Learning into the Curriculum

The Pew Health Professions Commission (1998) identified service learning as a key competency for programs educating health professionals. National organizations such as the American Association of Colleges of Nursing (2008b), the National League for Nursing (2005), and the Institute of Medicine (2010) have noted that nursing curricula should prepare nurses to practice in diverse settings that are global in nature. The IOM report (2010) advocated interdisciplinary learning to facilitate a smooth transition to the workplace, where working as part of an interdisciplinary group is a key skill. Service learning lends itself to interdisciplinary endeavors, and the interdisciplinary nature of the endeavor would enrich and change the experience.

Community-based service learning is increasingly being integrated into nursing courses (Gillis & MacLellan, 2013). Some service-learning endeavors are part of a larger consortium. An example is the Community-Campus Partnerships for Health (CCPH), an independent, nonprofit organization that organized the Partners in Caring and Community: Service-Learning in Nursing Education project. The Partners in Caring and Community project works with teams of nursing faculty and students and their community partners to facilitate the integration of service learning into nursing education curricula, increase the understanding and support for it in nursing education, and disseminate new knowledge and information about best practices and models of service learning and nursing education (Campus Community Partners for Health, n.d.). The CCPH website (http://depts.washington.edu/ccph/index.html) provides links to participatory institutions and a wide variety of information.

Support Structures

Faculty support is important to cultivating success. Support begins with campus and school administrators who value service learning and will commit resources to its implementation in the curriculum. Although universities have embraced service learning, they have been slow to implement support systems needed for effective implementation (Schmidt & Brown, 2008). Faculty can organize a faculty service-learning committee or advisory board to provide needed support. This group could be an invaluable advocate of service learning as a teaching tool. The committee can establish faculty handbooks and guidelines for service-learning courses, sponsor lunch-and-learn sessions on service learning for particular departments or the entire college, develop webinars, ensure that faculty receive continuing education units for attending service-learning workshops, and organize faculty development opportunities regarding service learning pedagogy (American Association of Community Colleges [AACC], 2010). This committee also encourages the development of interdisciplinary professional relationships and provides an avenue for sharing ideas, successes, and failures.

The goal of planning is to work for sustainability of service learning throughout the curriculum. Funding can be obtained from the community, from grant funding available locally and nationally, and often from the college or university itself. Although service learning is not expensive, it does require time for planning and course development and the personnel to make the arrangements. A number of colleges and universities have a service-learning office or coordinator. Staff from this office provide assistance in structuring the program, identifying community partners, and placing students according to mutual needs.

Integrating service-learning experiences into the curriculum requires careful planning. The experience must be developed and resources acquired before the course is offered. Identifying enthusiastic faculty champions and faculty development are keys to success (American Association of Community Colleges, 2010).

Challenges

Some of the challenges to implementing service learning result from ordinary budgetary constraints in higher education. Multiple departments and programs compete for limited resources. Those beginning a service-learning initiative may need to search for external funding sources and rely on the goodwill of faculty members willing to spend extra time learning about service learning and then incorporating it into their courses without extra compensation.

Institutions that lack a dedicated service-learning office may struggle with organization and effective evaluation strategies. When funding issues prevent the establishment of a service-learning office, a service-learning council composed of faculty members from each department on campus can provide direction for faculty development, coordinate student learning activities with community agencies, evaluate service-learning experiences, and facilitate the sharing of information.).

Convincing faculty members to adopt service learning as an effective pedagogical device can also be a challenge. This resistance is understandable because of the time and effort involved in incorporating it into courses. Faculty members involved in service learning often serve as the best change agents as they extol the benefits of service learning, including increased student engagement in the learning process and increased sense of collegiality because of their intradisciplinary and interdisciplinary activities.

Challenges encountered by faculty include time constraints; students' commitments to work and family; and students', faculty's, and community partners' heavy workloads. Community partners may struggle with orienting new students each semester and with the lack of students during summer break. There are also challenges when service learning experiences last more than one semester or students taking multiple courses with service-learning components are to remain at the same community agency to increase continuity.

Planning Faculty Development

Planning for a change to service learning begins with faculty development that may be available from the academic institution, workshops, and independent study. These resources will help faculty obtain essential information about how to design and implement service learning. A few of the practical considerations involved in planning include establishing good relationships with community agencies, identifying the types of experiences suitable for the course content, finding agency representative supervisors, structuring the types of activities, and scheduling the activities.

Preparation links the service-learning activities to specific learning outcomes and prepares students to perform the activities. The service needs to be challenging, engaging, and meaningful to the students, and it must focus on meeting an actual community need that students can perceive as important and relevant to their own development.

Preparation also includes finding agencies for student placement. Students involved typically work in voluntary not-for-profit community or public tax-supported service agencies and organizations that provide services that meet people's actual needs. Agencies and programs are selected on the basis of their congruence with the academic program or course and student goals and objectives. Faculty must also assess the agency's capacity for students and determine that the students' abilities are a match for the agency's needs.

Faculty development provides an explanation of a new pedagogy for many and establishes a common definition and a sound knowledge base. Consultants can be an invaluable aid in this early development process, and many campuses have offices of service learning that can provide or assist with faculty development. It is also helpful for faculty to make contact with faculty in other colleges to identify what others have been doing. The Internet can be a means of making contact with other faculty involved in service learning. Electronic mailing lists are available, and many sources of information that list faculty involved in service learning are available on the Internet. The Internet can also be a source of information about starting service-learning programs, sample course descriptions, syllabi, electronic mailing lists, funding resources, and best practices. Some of the most widely recognized Internet resources are:

Campus Compact: www.compact.org
Corporation for National and Community Service: www.cns.gov
Learn and Serve, National Service-Learning Clearinghouse: www.servicelearning.org

Developing Placement Sites

Anstee, Harris, Pruitt, and Sugar (2008) presented a process model for incorporating service learning into an academic class. The six stages of their model were "(a) establishing community collaboration, (b) partnering in the classroom, (c) student training, (d) delivering the service, (e) returning to the classroom, and (f) reporting to the stakeholders" (p. 599). Selecting a placement site and establishing collaboration within the community are important early steps. It is important to match the type of community organization and service with the institutional mission of the college when service-learning experiences are being planned. Before making plans regarding service placements, faculty should conduct a community needs assessment and develop a resource inventory, either informally through personal and telephone contact or formally through surveys or needs assessments. Community agency staff are invaluable in determining where students are needed the most and what the greatest need is. Allowing community partners to control the identification of the service helps ensure that projects meet agency needs. Involvement of agency staff in the planning process also helps educate community agencies about service learning. Community advisory boards often help ensure continual contact between agencies, students, faculty, and staff and ascertain evolving community needs. Student safety is also an issue, and the agency and school have a responsibility to choose sites that are appropriate for the students' safety needs.

Once placement sites have been determined and projects are finalized, preceptors must be identified and dates for student orientation and initial meetings must be planned. Written project descriptions, contact information, and a schedule of initial meetings should be available for students on the first day of class. Organization before the start of the semester ensures that students get started on projects promptly and are likely to complete projects within the semester time limit.

Although careful planning prevents many problems, faculty members should be prepared for the unexpected. Occasionally the needs of community agencies change (e.g., because of funding cuts or receiving a grant), there may be conflicts between agencies' needs for services and students' schedules, or there may be dissatisfaction. Sources of dissatisfaction may include students' perception of inequality of time investment between groups, failure of the reality of the situation to match expectations, and problems in communication. Faculty members may need to intervene to prevent the escalation of problems and to renegotiate expectations.

Planning Learning Activities

Service learning can be used as an experientially based pedagogy to bring excitement and vitality to the classroom, to assist community members in need while at the same time learning from them, and to provide students with information and experiences through which they can engage in critical reflection about society's needs and one's responsibility to the community. Opportunities may be discovered from a number of sources. Faculty may identify appropriate situations for service learning from their own service activities in a wide variety of community agencies. Opportunities may also be suggested by friends, colleagues, agency personnel, or students, or they may be found in the professional or secular literature. When faculty have identified potential service-learning experiences that seem to be appropriate for the course, discussions and negotiations are held with the agency staff.

Legal issues also need to be considered when planning service activities. Any time a student performs service off campus in conjunction with coursework, liability issues can arise. Faculty should seek legal counsel from the college or university regarding activities with potential liability, just as legal counsel is sought when contracts with clinical agencies are established. Institutional Review Board approval should be sought if students are collecting data as a part of their service-learning projects.

Once service-learning experiences have been planned, students must be engaged. Faculty can use groups such as the student nurses association, student government, the student life office, and campus publicity mechanisms (e.g., newspaper, radio station, online learning system bulletin boards) to inform students about service learning. Often courses or service-learning components of courses are open to students from a variety of disciplines, and faculty should distribute the course announcements widely. Service learning's best promoters are its own students, who attract other students by word of mouth.

Student activities are planned so that they relate to the course objectives and content (Phillips, Bolduc, & Gallo, 2013). Types of agencies and programs that could be used for nursing students engaged in service learning include state or county services for persons with different forms of impairment or disability, various types of health and health care facilities, social welfare agencies and day care programs, Meals on Wheels, senior centers, youth services, civic leagues, drug education programs, and groups or committees related to some aspects of government. Community agencies offer many opportunities for students to collaborate with the agency to fulfill unmet needs. Some service experiences will involve assessment, others work in ongoing programs, and still others work on development and implementation of new programs or services. During the final phase of the service experience, students who have developed new programs should work with agency partners to establish plans for sustainability. Students should compile materials to facilitate this continuation. Although the community agency should be an active partner throughout the activity, a summary meeting with the stakeholders should be held to close the service experience.

Implementing Service Learning in the Nursing Curriculum

The nursing literature provides a variety of examples for ways to integrate service learning into the curriculum. In one program students spent the first half of the semester in the classroom learning background material and the second half of that semester and all of the following semester in a service-learning experience. Service-learning courses are also designed to provide students an opportunity to work with underserved and vulnerable populations. For example, at one school, course placement sites include a child care center for homeless children, a senior citizens program, a center serving teenage parents, a mission for homeless individuals, Habitat for Humanity, and Head Start (Hales, 1997). Another course provides opportunities for students to work with an underserved sector of society that has a variety of needs and challenges that are often different from their own. Students provide health and developmental screenings, create handouts for parents, assess the social behavior of children, read safety storybooks to the children, and assist with classroom activities (Kulewicz, 2001). Health promotion activities such as education on tobacco use can help to reduce the prevalence of cigarette smoking (Bassi, Cray, & Caldrello, 2008). In another example, working in partnership with a sheriff's department, students conducted health assessments, participated in case findings, and provided health education (Fuller, Alexander, & Hardeman, 2006).

Service learning can also be integrated into faith-based curricula and faith-based nursing practices (Brown, 2009; Lashley, 2007). In one service-learning project, several Catholic Charities programs were targeted for service experiences, including an emergency shelter for battered women and their children, an addiction recovery treatment center for economically disadvantaged individuals, food pantries, and an inner-city school counseling service. Initially the Department of Nursing focused on students' ability to apply theoretical knowledge during the service experience. However, Herman and Sassatelli (2002) report that as the program evolved, it embraced Brackley's (1988) challenge to have the "courage not to turn away from the eyes of the poor, but to allow them to break our hearts and shatter our world" (p. 38). They also incorporated Dorr's (1993) emphasis on the importance of not only feeling for economically disadvantaged individuals but also discovering what it means to be with them. Faculty and students found that companionship with economically disadvantaged individuals during the service experience encouraged understanding of what it means to be humanly weak and powerless (Herman & Sassatelli, 2002). Brown (2009) reported that a faith-based service-learning experience reduced mental illness stigma in an underserved community and increased students' understanding of mental health problems and substance abuse. Because of the decreased stigma, patients reported greater willingness to seek treatment and use community resources.

Global Awareness through Service Learning

Global service learning programs support global citizenship, provide an understanding of diverse cultural communities, and promote a paradigm shift to global citizenship and global health care (Burgess,

Reimer-Kirkham, & Astle, 2014; McKinnon & Fealy, 2011). Global citizens "identify not primarily or solely with her own nation but also with communities of people and nations beyond the nation-state boundaries" (Abowitz & Harnish, 2006, p. 675). Global citizenship expands the boundaries of social justice concerns beyond one's own city, state, and nation. McKinnon and Fealy (2011) believe that global service learning programs should be built around the Seven Cs of Best Practice: "compassion, competence, curiosity, capacity building, courage, creativity, and collaboration" (p. 95). Collaboration is key to foster partnership and avoid cultural and linguistic misunderstanding.

Despite the increased interest in global health care, fewer than half of U.S. nursing programs offer international service opportunities and faculty identify significant obstacles to developing new programs such as cost, time, interest, and logistics (McKinnon & McNelis, 2013). Help for faculty in overcoming obstacles can be located in the National League for Nursing (2012) resource Faculty Preparation for Global Experiences Toolkit.

The course objectives and needs of the host community must be linked in deliberate ways to meet the needs of both groups. One school set up an experience in Nicaragua for students who conducted a nutritional needs assessment; provided prenatal education for community health workers and lay midwives, with a special emphasis on nutrition; and supported the relief efforts in refugee camps following Hurricane Mitch (Riner & Becklenberg, 2001). Students were provided with information about the Nicaraguan culture before starting the experience. This is critical because the ability to provide culturally responsive health care is important.

In an interdisciplinary global service project, a school brought a mobile medical clinical to Honduras staffed by nurse practitioner students, baccalaureate nursing students, and medical students (Green, Comer, Elliott, & Neubrander, 2011). Another school set up a 2-week immersion experience in Guatemala for senior baccalaureate nursing students who provided nursing assessments and health teaching at prenatal and well-child clinics, an adult day program, and rural health clinics (Curtin, Martins, Schwartz-Barcott, DiMaria, & Ogando, 2013). The faculty provided seminars about the culture and language prior to the trip, and used journals and postexperience seminars to facilitate reflection on the experience. The faculty identified that by linking the reflective process to curricular goals and the nursing program mission, students were able to articulate learning about global engagement, cultural awareness, and building professional competence (Curtin et al., 2013).

International travel involves additional steps and advance planning, including learning about the host country and its culture, getting passports, arranging for a translator if a foreign language is spoken, vaccinations (for some regions), and arranging for safe accommodations. The Center for Global Education provides a variety of helpful information that assists with preparation and the U.S. Department of State Bureau of Consular Affairs has an Overseas Travel Checklist that is also helpful. Travelers may wish to be accompanied by a guide familiar with the area to enhance safety and should travel in groups at all times. The U.S. Department of State Bureau of Consular Affairs is a resource for region-specific travel and health warnings when traveling abroad. Additional vaccinations may be needed. Health concerns vary by region and may include traveler's diarrhea, Ebola, yellow fever, and typhoid. Students should check their medical insurance to identify what it will cover when traveling abroad should they become ill.

When traveling abroad, communication via telephone and Internet may be limited. Contacting cellular providers ahead of time can avoid last-minute problems. Apps are designed for international travel and may be helpful in language translation and for phone and text message service. Internet access may be limited, but some countries have Internet cafés where service is available. Organizations such as the International Service Learning Alliance and the International Partnership for Service Learning and Leadership may be helpful sources of information.

Although international travel takes more time and effort to plan, it helps prepare nurses for the diverse world in which they live by enhancing cultural knowledge, commitment to global social needs, and forming valuable global connections (Crabtree, 2013).

Adapting Service Learning for Distance Education

Service learning has traditionally been structured as a part of an on-ground nursing program. However, as more and more programs move in whole or in part to distance education, consideration must be given to service-learning experiences for this student population.

Service learning for distance learning students can occur in a number of ways. First, the online student can identify a community partner in his or her local community for a service experience and take advantage of online learning technologies. For example, faculty teaching an online RN to BSN leadership course used service learning to enhance the collaborative teaching–learning relationship and provide a venue for a required change project (Anderson & Miller, 2007). An asynchronous forum allowed discussions with opportunities for reflection. Descriptions of agencies and service projects used by on-campus students were posted online to help distance education students find comparable experiences within their own community. Faculty members worked collaboratively with students to finalize arrangements with those agencies.

Second, the students enrolled in an online program could travel to an international site for a service learning experience together with other students enrolled in the course (whether online or on-ground).

Third, the service could become e-service learning. This would overcome the traditional time and geographic boundaries and allow students to conduct their service online. E-service learning provides opportunities for engagement, skill building, and practical experience that might otherwise be limited or lacking in an online course (Waldner, McGorry, & Widener, 2012). E-service learning requires both the student and the community partner to have access to technology (chat rooms, e-mail, videoconferencing, Skype, wikis, or discussion boards), but it removes the traditional geographic boundaries. Best practices for e-service learning include providing training on any technology that will need to be used, creating clear written communication of expectations between students and community partners, scheduling meeting times to enhance communication, and maintaining faculty engagement throughout the e-service learning experience (Waldner et al., 2012). Using these guidelines, service learning opportunities can be expanded to distance education students.

Preparation for Service Learning

Once student placements and focus of the service have been selected, preparation must extend to the classroom setting. Conceiving of service learning as simply a matter of mutually beneficial service ignores the important concept of readiness for the encounter. Radest (1993) introduced the idea of *solidarity*: "the name of my relationship to the stranger who remains unknown—only a person in an abstract sense—but who is, like me, a human being. Solidarity is then a preparation for the future and at the same time a grounding in the present" (p. 183). Sheffield (2005) notes that "Radest's concept of solidarity develops into a disposition toward democratic interaction and service" (p. 49) and that academic preparation for the encounter is essential. Preparation develops a sense of understanding in students that gives increased meaning to the service and a realization that the strangers are much like them, further developing the sense of solidarity.

Preparation should include exploration of social issues as well as an introduction to the service environment and the people who will be encountered. It can take the form of reading materials from the agency, reading text-based materials, exploring material available on the Internet, or viewing films, and should be accompanied by discussions to prepare students for the service experience. Preparatory classroom activities should have an overall goal of enhancing understanding and helping the stranger become familiar. Sheffield (2005) notes that "academic preparation not only undergirds the particular service activity, but also advances solidarity generally for future encounters with future 'strangers' and develops a habit of readiness to interact open-mindedly with others" (p. 52). Preparation also brings participants a greater understanding of diversity, the ability to embrace and celebrate differences, and a realization of their ethical responsibility to connect with others in the community. Sheffield (2005) notes that "without that understanding, service degenerates into volunteerism where act rather than connection is the focus" (p. 52).

Incorporating Reflection

Reflection is a critical and essential aspect of service learning that further differentiates it from volunteerism, community service activities, and nursing students' clinical experiences. Reflection is an active, persistent, thoughtful, and intentional consideration of the service activity. Reflection must include the student's behavior, practice, and achievement. Within the reflective process, students must respond to basic questions such as "What am

I doing?" "Why am I doing it?" and "What am I learning?" As well, they should critically examine their actions, feelings, and thoughts. During this examination and while responding to the questions posed, students contemplate, think, reason, and speculate about their service experiences (Gillis & MacLellan, 2013).

Reflection is a learning tool that serves to maximize students' highly individualized learning experiences by linking the service experiences with the learning objectives established for the course and curriculum. Reflection combines cognitive and affective activities in a way that bridges the gap between the service experience and the course.

Reflection also provides opportunities for students to improve their self-assessment skills and have insights that help build on their strengths. Because reflection and self-assessment are skills that require development, many students new to service learning find faculty facilitation and journaling helpful with the reflective process (Gillis & MacLellan, 2013).

Faculty responsibilities include designing reflection activities, coaching students during reflection, monitoring students' reflections, and providing feedback (Rama, 2001). Faculty will also find a wealth of other information on reflection activities available on the Internet.

Reflection is most effective when it is continuous, connected, contextual, and challenging. Continuous reflection involves reflection before, during, and after the service-learning experience. Connecting service learning with classroom learning assists students to develop a conceptual framework for their service project and to apply concepts and theories learned in class to the experience. Reflection must be appropriate for the context and setting of the experience. Some service-learning experiences lend themselves to formal methods of reflection, such as written papers, whereas others are best suited to informal discussions. Whether formal or informal methods are used, reflection should challenge students to think in new ways, question their assumptions, and formulate new understandings and new ways of problem solving (Rama, 2001).

Including service partners in the reflective dialogue enhances communication and increases the depth and breadth of learning. Without an emphasis on dialogue between individuals and community partners, reflection becomes one sided, focusing on the isolated views and perceptions of the individual student without coming to an understanding of each person's perspective (Rama, 2001). Keen and Hall's (2009) study noted that this dialogue across boundaries of perceived differences that happened during the service experience and in reflection exercises was the core experience, not the service itself.

One common approach to stimulate reflection is to have students keep a journal or engage in directed writing that faculty read and respond to frequently throughout the course. Journals allow students to record thoughts, observations, feelings, activities, questions, and problems encountered and solved during the service-learning experience. If students are working on a service-learning project as a team, a team journal can be used to promote interaction between team members on project-related issues and to introduce students to different perspectives on the project (Rama, 2001). The team concludes its work with a collective reflection on the service learning.

Portfolios can be developed to organize materials related to the service-learning project and document accomplishments and learning outcomes. Other reflective activities include small-group discussions and presentations that relate the service experience to classroom concepts, introduce students to different perspectives, and challenge them to think critically about the service experience. It is helpful for faculty to pose a few questions to guide the discussion, but students should also be allowed to freely discuss and reflect on ideas and issues. In such discussions students often disclose expectations and myths about the service experience. Themes that may emerge during reflections include social analysis of community needs and the importance of civic responsibility (Bailey et al., 2002). A final reflective paper based on the writing done during the semester provides a comprehensive description of students' learning.

Bringle and Hatcher's (1996) guidelines help clarify the nature of effective reflection activities in a service-learning course. Effective reflection activities:

1. Link the service-learning experiences to the learning objectives.
2. Are designed, structured, and guided by faculty.
3. Are planned so that they occur across the span of service-learning experience.

4. Permit faculty feedback and assessment of progress and learning.
5. Foster the clarification and exploration of values.

Debriefing

Following the experience, debriefing is essential to reinforce classroom theory, allow students to share differing experiences, and reinforce the sense of solidarity that was developed. Debriefing adds to the intentional nature of the service experience and facilitates a dialogue between students who may have been placed in different locations throughout the community. Debriefing can be combined with an evaluation of the service experience. Community partners can also be engaged in the debriefing experience and share their views of outcomes of the experience and what effect the service learning had on the agency in which the students served.

Evaluation

After the completion of service learning, the community partner, faculty, and students should evaluate the usefulness of the service project in meeting their needs, the strengths and areas for improvement of the service project, and student performance. Faculty should evaluate student outcomes and the contribution of the experience to overall curriculum goals. Evaluation of students' achievement is based on the students' learning and not merely on their experience or participation in the service activities. Faculty, the agency supervisor, and students' self-assessment provide the evaluation data.

Many faculty administer preservice and post-service surveys that measure students' attitudes toward community service and civic responsibility and toward their coursework. Such instruments not only help faculty evaluate their students and assess the usefulness of service learning, but also help students see how much they have learned and how their attitudes may have changed because of their service-learning experience. In addition to the short-term course evaluation, a systematic long-term follow-up of students helps determine any additional learning that may have occurred after the course is completed.

Summary

The ultimate goal of providing opportunities for civic engagement, development of cultural competence, leadership, advocacy skills, and service learning in institutions of higher education and their schools of nursing is to develop a more caring society, foster advocacy for social justice, and increase the focus on global health care. Students, schools, and the community benefit when service learning is a part of the curriculum. Service-learning experiences have the benefits of increasing retention of academic material and fostering global awareness and a sense of social responsibility within participants. Following service-learning experiences, students are often inspired to continue to work for social justice as engaged citizens in their communities. Although integration of service learning into the curriculum requires faculty development and thoughtful planning, service learning is a win–win–win situation for the college, the students, and the community.

REFLECTING ON THE EVIDENCE

1. In what ways is service learning similar to and different from a clinical practicum experience in a nursing program?
2. Plan a service-learning project for a particular curriculum.
   a. How does service learning fit within the mission of the college or university and school of nursing?
   b. What needs to be considered before initiating service learning in the United States or overseas?
   c. What resources are already available on campus? What barriers and facilitators exist?
   d. Where is (are) the most appropriate place(s) for the experience(s)?
3. What are the best practices for service learning in the curriculum?
   a. What evidence exists?
   b. What additional evidence needs to be established?
   c. Pose a research question and design a study.

REFERENCES

Abowitz, K. K., & Harnish, J. (2006). Contemporary discourses of citizenship. *Review of Educational Research, 76*(4), 653–690.

American Association of Colleges of Nursing. (2008a). *Cultural competency in baccalaureate nursing education.* Retrieved from, http://www.aacn.nche.edu/Education/pdf/competency.pdf.

American Association of Colleges of Nursing. (2008b). *The essentials of baccalaureate education for professional nursing practice.* Retrieved from, http://www.aacn.nche.edu/Education/ pdf/BaccEssentials08.pdf.

American Association of Community Colleges (AACC). (2010). *Creating a climate for service learning success.* Retrieved from, http://www.aacc.nche.edu/Resources/aaccprograms/horizons/Documents/creatingaclimate_082010.pdf.

Amerson, R. (2010). The impact of service-learning on cultural competence. *Nursing Education Perspectives, 31*(1), 1822.

Anderson, S., & Miller, A. (2007). Implementing transformational leadership as a model for service learning activities in an online RN to BSN leadership course. *Online Journal of Nursing Informatics, 11*(1). Retrieved from, http://ojni.org/11_1/Miller.htm.

Anstee, J. L. K., Harris, S. G., Pruitt, K. D., & Sugar, J. A. (2008). Service learning projects in an undergraduate gerontology course: A six-stage model and application. *Educational Gerontology, 34*(7), 595–609.

Bailey, P. A., Carpenter, D. R., & Harrington, P. (2002). Theoretical foundations of service-learning in nursing education. *Journal of Nursing Education, 41*(10), 433–436.

Bassi, S., Cray, J., & Caldrello, L. (2008). A tobacco-free service-learning project. *Journal of Nursing Education, 47*(4), 174–178.

Batchelder, T. H., & Root, S. (1994). Effects of an undergraduate program to integrate academic learning and service: Cognitive, prosocial cognitive, and identity outcomes. *Journal of Adolescence, 1*(4), 341–355.

Baumberger, M. L., Krouse, A. M., & Borucki, L. C. (2006). Giving and receiving: A case study in service learning. *Nurse Educator, 6*, 249–252.

Boyer, E. L. (1990). *Scholarship reconsidered: Priorities of the professoriate.* New York: The Carnegie Foundation for the Advancement of Teaching.

Brackley, D. S. J. (1988). Downward mobility: Social implications of St. Ignatius's two standards in studies of spirituality of Jesuits. *Studies in Spirituality of Jesuits, 20*(1), 38.

Bringle, R. G., & Hatcher, J. A. (1996). Implementing service learning in higher education. *Journal of Higher Education, 67*(2), 221–239.

Brown, J. F. (2009). Faith-based mental health education: A service learning opportunity for nursing students. *Journal of Psychiatric and Mental Health Nursing, 16*(6), 581–588.

Burgess, C. A., Reimer-Kirkham, S., & Astle, B. (2014). Motivation and international clinical placements: Shifting nursing students to a global citizenship perspective. *International Journal of Nursing Education Scholarship, 11*(1), 1–8.

Campus Community Partners for Health. Retrieved from http://depts.washington.edu/ccph/index.html.

Campus Compact. (2001). Retrieved from http://www.compact.org.

Crabtree, R. D. (2013). The intended and unintended consequences of international service learning. *Journal of Higher Education Outreach and Engagement, 17*(2), 43–66.

Curtin, A. J., Martins, D. C., Schwartz-Barcott, D., DiMaria, L., & Ogando, B. M. S. (2013). Development and evaluation of an international service learning program for nursing students. *Public Health Nursing, 30*(6), 548–556.

Daloz, L. A., Keen, C. H., Keen, J. P., & Parks, S. D. (1996). Lives of commitment. *Change, 28*(3), 11–15.

Delve, C. I., Mintz, S. D., & Stewart, G. M. (1990). Promoting values development through community service: A design. *New Directions for Student Services, 50*(2), 7–29.

Dewey, J. (1916). *Democracy and education.* New York: Macmillan.

Dewey, J. (1933). *How we think.* Boston: Heath.

Dewey, J. (1938). *Experience and education.* New York: Macmillan.

Dorr, D. (1993). *Options for the poor: A hundred years of Vatican social teaching.* Maryknoll, NY: Orbis Books.

Eads, S. E. (1994). The value of service learning in higher education. In R. J. Kraft & M. Swadner (Eds.), *Building community: Service learning in the academic disciplines* (pp. 35–40). Denver: Colorado Campus Compact.

Foli, K. J., Braswell, M., Kirkpatrick, J., & Lim, E. (2014). Development of leadership behaviors in undergraduate nursing students: A service learning approach. *Nursing Education Perspectives, 35*(2), 76–82.

Francis-Baldesari, C., & Williamson, D. C. (2008). Integration of nursing education, practice, and research through community partnerships: A case study. *Advances in Nursing Science, 31*(4), E1–E10.

Fuller, S. G., Alexander, J. W., & Hardeman, S. M. (2006). Sheriff's deputies and nursing students service-learning partnership. *Nurse Educator, 31*(1), 31–35.

Gehrke, P. M. (2008). Civic engagement and nursing education. *Advances in Nursing Science, 31*(1), 52–66.

Gilligan, C. (1981). Moral development in the college years. In A. Chickering (Ed.), *The modern American college* (pp. 139–157). San Francisco: Jossey-Bass.

Gillis, A., & MacLellan, M. A. (2013). Critical service learning in community health nursing: Enhancing access to cardiac health screening. *International Journal of Nursing Education Scholarship, 10*(1), 1–9. http://dx.doi.org/10.1515/ijnes-2012-0031.

Green, S. S., Comer, L., Elliott, L., & Neubrander, J. (2011). Exploring the value of an international service-learning experience in Honduras. *Nursing Education Perspectives, 32*(5), 302–307.

Hales, A. (1997). Service-learning within the nursing curriculum. *Nurse Educator, 22*(2), 15–18.

Hamner, J. B., Wilder, B., Avery, G., & Byrd, L. (2002). Community-based service learning in the engaged university. *Nursing Outlook, 50*(2), 67–71.

Herman, C., & Sassatelli, J. (2002). DARING to reach the heartland: a collaborative faith-based partnership in nursing education. *Journal of Nursing Education, 41*(10), 443–445.

Institute of Medicine. (2010). Transforming education. In Institute of Medicine (Eds.), *The future of nursing: Leading change, advancing health.* (pp. 139–186). Retrieved from, http://books.nap.edu/openbook.php?record_id=12956&page=139.

Jarosinski, J. M., & Heinrich, C. (2010). Standing in their shoes: Student immersion in the community using service-learning with at-risk teens. *Issues in Mental Health Nursing, 31*(4), 288–297.

Keen, C., & Hall, K. (2009). Engaging with difference matters: Longitudinal student outcomes of co-curricular service learning programs. *Journal of Higher Education, 80*(1), 59–79.

Kolb, D. A. (1984). *Experiential learning: Experience as the source of learning and development.* Englewood Cliffs, NJ: Prentice Hall.

Kulewicz, S. J. (2001). Service learning: Head Start and a baccalaureate nursing curriculum working together. *Pediatric Nursing, 27*(1), 27–43.

Lashley, M. (2007). Nurses on a mission: A professional service-learning experience with the inner-city homeless. *Nursing Education Perspectives, 28*(1), 24–26.

Ligeikis-Clayton, C., & Denman, J. Z. (2005). Service learning across the curriculum. *Nurse Educator, 30*(5), 191–192.

McKinnon, T. H., & Fealy, G. (2011). Core principles for developing global service learning programs in nursing. *Nursing Education Perspectives, 32*(2), 95–101.

McKinnon, T. H., & McNelis, A. M. (2013). International programs in United States schools of nursing: Driving forces, obstacles, and opportunities. *Nursing Education Perspectives, 34*(5), 323–328.

Mezirow, J. (1990). How critical reflection triggers transformative learning. In J. Mezirow (Ed.), *Fostering critical reflection in adulthood: A guide to transformative and emancipatory learning* (pp. 1–20). San Francisco: Jossey-Bass.

National League for Nursing. (2012). *Faculty preparation for global experiences toolkit.* Retrieved from, http://www.nln.org/facultyprograms/facultyresources/toolkit_facprepglobexp.pdf.

National League for Nursing. (2005). *Transforming nursing education.* Retrieved from, http://www.nln.org/aboutnln/PositionStatements/transforming052005.pdf.

National Service-Learning Clearinghouse. (2010). Retrieved from, http://www.servicelearning.org/.

Pellietier, S. (1995). The quiet power of service learning: Report from the National Institute on Learning and Service. *The Independent, 95*(4), 7–10.

Pew Health Professions Commission. (1998). *Recreating health professional practice for a new century.* San Francisco: The Center for Health Professions.

Phillips, A., Bolduc, S. R., & Gallo, M. (2013). Curricular placement of academic service-learning in higher education. *Journal of Higher Education Outreach and Engagement, 17*(4), 75–96.

Radest, H. (1993). *Community service: Encounter with strangers.* Westport, CT: Praeger.

Rama, D. V. (2001). *Using structured reflection to enhance learning from service.* Retrieved from, http://www.compact.org/disciplines/reflection.

Rash, E. M. (2005). A service learning research methods course. *Journal of Nursing Education, 44*(10), 477–478.

Reising, D. L., Allen, P. N., & Hall, S. G. (2006a). Student and community outcomes in service-learning: Part 1—Student perceptions. *Journal of Nursing Education, 45*(12), 512–515.

Reising, D. L., Allen, P. N., & Hall, S. G. (2006b). Student and community outcomes in service-learning: Part 2—Community outcomes. *Journal of Nursing Education, 45*(12), 516–518.

Riner, M. E., & Becklenberg, A. (2001). Partnering with a sister city organization for an international service-learning experience. *Journal of Transcultural Nursing, 12*(3), 234–240.

Schmidt, N. A., & Brown, J. M. (2008). Girl Scout badge day as a service learning experience. *International Journal of Nursing Education Scholarship, 5*(1), 1–14.

Sheffield, E. C. (2005). Service in service-learning education: The need for philosophical understanding. *The High School Journal, 89*(1), 46–53.

Sheikh, K. R. (2014). Expanding clinical models of nurse practitioner education: Service learning as a curricular strategy. *The Journal for Nurse Practitioners, 10*(5), 352–355.

Silcox, H. C. (1994). *A how to guide to reflection: Adding cognitive learning to community service programs.* Holland, PA: Brighton Press.

Waldner, L. S., McGorry, S. Y., & Widener, M. C. (2012). E-service learning: The evolution of service learning to engage a growing online student population. *Journal of Higher Education Outreach and Engagement, 16*(2), 123–150.

Theoretical Foundations of Teaching and Learning*

13

Lori Candela, EdD, RN, APRN, FNP-BC, CNE

Teaching is a complex undertaking that must always consider the learner, the intended learning outcome, the environment in which it will occur, and how it will be known if learning has indeed occurred. Central to these is the learner. The learners who enter nursing programs are diverse in every way imaginable. They differ from one another in previous education, work, and life experiences and in gender, age, ethnicity, religion, socioeconomic status, social support systems, learning style, language, and technological abilities. Each comes with his or her own motivations and expectations. Some may appear disinterested in the class and may have difficulty achieving the expected learning outcomes. The seven principles of good practice in undergraduate education proposed by Chickering and Gamson (1987) addressed this and articulated concepts for teachers to use in their teaching such as *learner activity, cooperation, interaction,* and *responsibility.*

Adding to the complexity of teaching and learning are changing societal demographics and trends, the constant influx of new information in health care, and the practice of education. Clearly, to teach effectively, the teacher must also continue to learn. This makes the use of educational theories to explain, guide, and even predict teaching practice an imperative.

Theory helps to explain the "whys" of the teaching–learning process, thus allowing for a more direct influence on the learner. Applying a theory in the practice of teaching provides a way of understanding these complex learners and the learning processes within the context of escalating new information and the rapid pace of health care change. This understanding is prerequisite for making decisions regarding what concepts and content to include in the curriculum or course, sequencing of learning experiences, and determining learner involvement and methods for assessment and evaluation. Taking the time to consider various theories and applying them as a regular part of the practice of teaching can result in improved learning outcomes and greater learner engagement. This chapter provides an overview of selected teaching–learning theories, their primary premise, and implications for use.

Learning Theories

Learning theories explain the complex nature of the interaction of students with their faculty, the learning environment, and the subject matter. Learning theories are descriptive in that they focus on and describe the processes used to bring about changes in either the way in which students perform or the way in which they understand or organize elements in their environment.

Learning theories provide the structure that guides the selection of instructional strategies and student-centered learning activities. Faculty's beliefs about learning provide the assumptions that underlie the approaches used in their teaching. Being cognizant of various theories is a prerequisite to effective teaching. When choosing which theories to use, faculty must consider those that support the school philosophy, meet student learning needs, and complement their teaching preferences

Learning theories derive from work in a variety of fields such as philosophy, educational psychology,

*The author would like to thank previous edition writers Melissa Vandevier and Barbara Norton for their contribution to earlier versions of the chapter.

higher education, and, recently, neuroscience. In this chapter the learning theories are categorized by their paradigms. These include behaviorist, cognitivist, and constructivist views of learning, as well as those derived from humanistic approaches, interpretive pedagogies, human development theories, and the emerging field of neuroscience. See Table 13-1.

Behavioral Learning Theories

Ivan Pavlov and Edward Thorndike established the roots for behaviorism in the late nineteenth century with their systematic, scientific investigation of how animals and human beings learn (Hilgard & Bower, 1966). This work provided the basis for what

TABLE 13-1 Learning Theories

Theory	Premise	Theorists
Behaviorism	All behavior is learned and can be shaped and rewarded. Behavior is directed by behavioral objectives and competency statements.	Skinner, Mager, Pavlov
Cognitivism	Conditions of learning influence acquisition and retention of knowledge by modifying cognitive structures and forming "schema" and mental models. Assimilation and accommodation are processes of learning.	Lewin, Ausubel, Bruner Piaget, Gagne
Constructivism	Learning is constructed by the learner; learners build on existing knowledge through personal interpretation of experience. Past learning is connected to new learning.	Bruner
Social learning theory	Learning involves active information processing. Students learn by observing others as models of behavior. Students who believe they can perform well have high self-efficacy and have confidence when taking on complex tasks.	Bandura
Sociocultural learning	Learning occurs in a context of social interaction. Learners have a zone of proximal development (ZPD) in which they can perform some skills independently; to learn other skills they need to have assistance. The assistance provided by a teacher or peer is known as *scaffolding*, and the support is gradually withdrawn as the student attains the skill.	Vygotsky
Situated learning	Learning takes place in the context in which it can be applied.	Lave & Wenger, Benner*
Cognitive Development	Learning occurs in stages, over time.	
Adult education	Adults are self-directed and problem centered. Adults need to learn useful information and are self-directed.	Knowles
Intellectual, moral, and ethical development	Students progress through categories of development in a sequential fashion (dualism, multiplicity, relativism, and commitment) as they acquire intellectual skills and values	Perry
Novice to expert	Nurses develop expertise in 5 stages: novice, advanced beginner, competent, proficient, expert	Benner*
Humanism	Education motivates the development of human potential. Goal is to become self-actualized.	Maslow, Rogers
Caring	Education consists of an integration of humanistic-existential, feminist, and caring ideologies.	Watson*
Interpretive Pedagogies	Learning occurs as experience is explored, deconstructed, and critiqued.	Diekelmann*
Phenomenology	Philosophical approach to understanding human behavior, the lived human experience.	Heidegger, Benner,* Tanner*
Narrative pedagogy	Knowledge is gained through experiences of students, teachers, patients, clinicians.	Dieklemann,* Ironside*
Neuroscience, Brain-based Learning, Deep Learning, Multiple Intelligences	Learning is understood by studying biological changes in the brain as information is processed.	
Deep learning	Taking advantage of the many functional areas of the brain, students integrate previous knowledge to what is being learned. Learning is for application vs. memorization.	Smith & Colby
Brain-based learning	Enhancing the conditions in which the brain learns best: relaxed alertness; active processing of experiences.	Connell; Caine & Caine
Multiple intelligences	Learning involves developing and using multiple intelligences: linguistic, logical-mathematical, spatial, kinesthetic, musical, intrapersonal, interpersonal.	Gardner

*Nurse theorists

became known as *behaviorist psychology.* According to Skinner's (1953) principles of operant conditioning, the focus is on arranging consequences for learner behavior. A behavior is strengthened or weakened in response to positive or negative consequences. Positive consequences are referred to as *reinforcers* because they strengthen or increase the frequency of behaviors, whereas negative consequences weaken the behavior by not reinforcing it (Slavin, 1988). Complex behaviors are acquired by shaping them by providing reinforcement. Reinforcement is an essential condition for learning because reinforced responses are remembered. Building on the evolving science of behaviorism, Mager (1962) developed a model for writing highly prescriptive behavioral objectives that consist of three components: specification of the behavior to be acquired, conditions under which the behavior is to be demonstrated, and the criteria for how well the behavior is to be performed. Prominent nurse educators of the 1970s and 1980s who adopted the behavioristic paradigm into their works included Bevis, deTornyay, and Reilly. During this time, many programs in nursing education made extensive use of the principles of behaviorism.

Premise

The main premise of behavioral learning theories is that all behavior is learned; it can be shaped and rewarded to achieve appropriate and desired ends

Implications for Nursing Education

Principles of behaviorism are used in classrooms, clinical settings, and learning resource centers. The organization of instruction is directed by behavioral objectives and learning outcomes that can be specified, and behavior can be observed and measured. Behaviorist principles are appropriate for structured situations in which the objectives can be clearly established in a step-by-step sequence and the desired behavior can be defined, quickly learned, and observed.

In the behaviorist paradigm, *faculty* facilitate the learning environment by designing the learning experience (e.g., simulations, skills demonstrations) and offer positive reinforcement through ongoing feedback. Faculty's focus is on what the student is doing correctly while making suggestions for improving incorrect behavior. Student attainment of learning goals is monitored by looking for behavior patterns demonstrated over a period.

Students use the behavioral objectives or competency statements as a guide for what is to be learned. Students work to achieve and demonstrate the desired behavior and plan the time needed to practice as much as necessary to attain the desired behavior. Student motivation for achievement is obtained from the tangible rewards that reinforce the desired behavior.

Cognitive Learning Theories

Cognitive learning theories focus on the internal learner environment and the mental structures of thinking. The initial focus on the cognitive aspects of learning is attributed to the work of the Gestalt psychologists during the early 1900s. Gestalt psychologists believe that people respond to whole situations or patterns rather than to parts. Insight is an important concept in Gestalt psychology. Insight, or the "aha" phenomenon, is a matter of perception that is explained as a procedure of mental trial and error that results in a solution. When a person's perceptual field is disorganized, order is imposed by restructuring problems into a better gestalt (pattern); the restructuring may occur through a process of trial and error. Lewin (1951) believed that because human beings have a basic need to bring order to the situation, the motivation to learn is stimulated by the ambiguity or chaos perceived in the situation. Cognitive psychology has several perspectives and approaches that try to explain particular aspects of human behavior (Weinstein & Meyer, 1991). Other theorists associated with cognitive learning theory are Anderson (1980, 1985), Ausubel (1960, 1978), Tulving (1985), and Wittrock (1977, 1986).

Premise

Cognitive theorists focus on and emphasize the mental processes and knowledge structures that can be inferred from behavioral indices. Cognitive learning theorists are concerned with the mental processes and activities that mediate the relationship between stimulus and response; the learner selects from stimuli in the environment according to his or her own internal structures (Grippin & Peters, 1984; Slavin, 1988). Cognitive theorists seek the factors that explain complex learning; they are concerned with meaning rather than behavior. In cognitive systems of learning, behavior is not automatically strengthened by reinforcers; the reinforcers provide affective and instructional information. The specific focus is on mental processes that include perception, thinking, knowledge representation, and memory, with emphasis on understanding and acquisition of knowledge and not merely on acquiring a new behavior or learning how to perform a task.

Information processing is an important aspect of cognitive learning. In this theory, memory is viewed as a complex organized system in which information is processed through three components of the memory system: sensory register, short-term memory, and long-term memory. The goal of learning is to practice information for retention in short-term memory so that the information will move to long-term memory for later recall and use.

Cognitive theories define *learning* as an active, cumulative, constructive process that is goal oriented and dependent on the learner's mental activities. Learning is an internal event in which modification of the existing internal representations of knowledge occurs. Learning is processing information; it is experiential and formed by a person's experience of the consequences.

Implications for Nursing Education

In a cognitivist approach to learning, students have active rather than passive roles in the instruction and a new responsibility for learning. Faculty emphasis is on developing students in how to think (Torre, Daley, Sebastian, & Elnicki, 2006). It is not the transfer of information that results in learning; rather, students must discover meaning by using information processing strategies, memories, and attentional and motivational mechanisms to organize and understand it (Wittrock, 1992).

Constructivist Learning Theories

Constructivism as a learning theory is based on the work of Piaget (1970a, 1970b, 1973), Vygotsky (1986/1962), and Bandura (1977). Constructivism holds that learning is development (Fosnot, 1996) and that assimilation, accommodation, and construction of knowledge are the basic operating processes in learning. A learner constructs new knowledge by building on an internal representation of existing knowledge through a personal interpretation of experience; faculty coach and facilitate (Brandon & All, 2010). Constructivists believe that learners build knowledge in an attempt to make sense of their experiences and that those learners are active in seeking meaning. Learners form, elaborate, and test their mental structures until they get one that is satisfactory. In the constructivist paradigm, knowledge representation is open to change as new knowledge structures are added to the existing foundational structure and connections.

Constructivism is also helpful in understanding how interactive social situations foster learning. Social constructivist views involve both individual cognition and social interactions in the learning process.

From this perspective, also known as *social interactivist,* construction of knowledge is enhanced because of interactions with others (Frank, 2005; Hean, Craddock & O'Halloran, 2009: Vianna & Stetsenko, 2006). Packer and Goicechea (2000) described this as learning via communities of practice. According to the authors, learning is constructed in those social types of settings. Learner participation and relating is indicative of a social constructivist learning environment, which includes learning from others, and drawing on context from the topic of the lessons being studied (Adams, 2006). The learning environment is one that engages students with one another and promotes comfort and safety for expression of creative ideas and novel thought (Powell & Kalina, 2009). Social learning theory, sociocultural learning, and situated (authentic) learning are discussed as examples of constructivist theories that are of interest to nurse educators.

Social Learning Theory

In social learning theory as proposed by Bandura (1977), learning involves active information processing. Students learn by observing others as models of behavior. A key component of this theory is that students who believe they can perform well have high self-efficacy and will be able to take on complex tasks with confidence. The goal of learning is to develop self-efficacy. The environment, cognition, and behavior all interact through a series of processes that consist of attention (such as complexity and value), retention (remembering, coding, mental images), reproduction (trying it and observing how it went), and motivation (compelling reason) to affect learning and performance (Bahn, 2001).

Premise

The basic premise of social learning theory is that people can learn through observation (such as role modeling) and that individual mental state (such as value perceived) affects all learning.

Implications for Nursing Education

Social learning theory with its emphasis on self-efficacy is used in nursing education to guide teaching–learning strategies such as role-play, simulation, and clinical learning experiences to develop students' self-efficacy. Bandura's theory is also used as a framework for nursing education research (Lasater, Mood, Buchwach, & Dieckelmann, 2015).

Sociocultural Learning

Sociocultural learning theory (SCT) is attributed to Lev Vygotsky. Although acknowledging a biological base to the human development potential and recognizing cognitive learning theory such as that suggested by Piaget, Vygotsky (1986/1962) believes that learning involves (1) cognitive self-instruction, (2) assisted learning, and (3) the zone of proximal development (ZPD). Assisted learning requires that a senior learner (adult, teacher) provide the learner with the necessary support to allow the learner to eventually solve the problem. The senior learner gradually withdraws instruction and coaching as the student gains independence. Support includes clues, affirmation, reducing the problem to steps, role modeling, and giving examples. Real learning occurs in the ZPD, the point at which the learner cannot solve the problem alone but has the potential to succeed and can do so with assistance. The teacher or facilitator must understand what the learner has mastered and what comes next.

Premise

The main tenet of SCT is that learning is interactive and occurs in a social context. Students interact with an expert (faculty, clinician) to assume increasing responsibility for mastering the knowledge, skill, or attitude. The faculty work with the student in the ZPD and provide "scaffolding" or necessary support while the student is learning, and then withdraw the support as the student demonstrates mastery.

Implications for Nursing Education

SCT can be used in the classroom, online, and in the clinical or laboratory setting. To facilitate further learning, faculty recognize learners' zones of proximal development and provide assistance through encouragement, affirmation, role modeling, and the breakdown of steps. They support students and motivate then to learn through the use of innovative teaching strategies (Phillips & Vinton, 2010). Sanders and Sugg (2005) discussed the actions of faculty as assisted performance that includes feedback and cognitive structuring. The focus is on student development through participation with others. Faculty must be comfortable in letting learning emerge and trust the student when "scaffolding" is withdrawn.

Faculty can encourage student identification of the sociocultural nature of their previous learning through personal reflection, storytelling, and comparisons between textbook or clinical examples and their own experience. Encouraging students to communicate in their own voice in both written and oral presentations can serve to both illuminate and enrich individual and peer learning. Sanders and Welk (2005) developed strategies to scaffold student leaning, applying Vygotsky's ZPD (1986). Scaffolding techniques to be constructed or gradually diminished based on student needs include modeling, feedback, instruction, questioning, and cognitive structuring.

Group interactions in activities such as examination of issues from an actual clinical day promote sociocultural learning. Debriefings following simulation activities provide rich opportunities for feedback and learning. Authentic case studies can be used to foster questioning, dialogue, and even debate among student groups. This may be enhanced if cases are given that are complex and contain less than all of the information needed. Peer and McClendon (2002) noted that teachers need to focus on connection-making activities, such as peer and reciprocal questioning techniques and cooperative learning. Sociocultural learning aimed at constructing new knowledge can also be used in interprofessional education (Hean et al., 2009; Sthapornnanon, Sakulbumrungsil, Theeraroungchaisri, & Watcharadamrongkun, 2009).

Students are responsible for their learning by communicating and collaborating with others. This includes reflection, sharing, and questioning as ways to learn from others. Students participate in the design and evaluation of learning. Students may discover the meaning by presenting analogies, using and describing prior knowledge and experiences, and having dialogues with faculty and peers about real-life situations that require application of the content. With faculty and peer support and scaffolding, students can acquire an increased self-awareness about what is known and become aware of how the new knowledge fits into their existing knowledge structure. Student reflection on the meaning of the content and the learning experiences is a process they can use to enhance and extend their learning.

Situated (Authentic) Learning and Situated Cognition

Situated learning occurs in the context of the actual nursing practice setting. The goal is to bring the "real" world into the academic setting so that students are better prepared to navigate the complex and often ill-defined environments in which they will ultimately be employed. Rule (2006) notes that these situations are typically open-ended and require investigation through multiple sources, collaboration with others, and individual and group reflection. An important aspect of situated learning is situated cognition, or thinking embedded in the context in which it occurs (Elsbach, Barr, & Hargadon, 2005). Benner, Sutphen, Leonard, and Day (2010) note that situated learning is the hallmark of nursing education, and in their call for transformation of nursing education, recommend a shift from teaching decontextualized knowledge to teaching for a sense of salience and situated cognition through a closer integration of classroom and clinical experiences.

Premise

Focusing on real-world situations provides opportunities for students to develop skills important to practice, including collaboration, clinical decision making, communication, and creativity.

Implications for Nursing Education

Faculty design learning experiences such as case studies, unfolding case studies, role play, simulation, and learning in clinical settings to immerse students in situations they will experience in actual nursing practice. Students focus on learning for application in clinical practice. There is less emphasis on memorization, with increased learning and practice for synthesizing information for safe and quality patient care.

Cognitive Development Theories

Cognitive development theories focus on the sequential development of learning over time. These theorists believe that learning depends on student's maturation, experiences in the real world, and time. Three cognitive development theories of interest to nurse educators are Knowles' (1980) adult learning theory, Perry's (1970) theory of intellectual and moral development and Benner's (1984) theory of learning from novice to expert.

Adult Learning Theory

According to Malcom Knowles (1980), adults learn in ways that are different from children. He used the term *andragogy* to refer to the education of adults, in contrast to *pedagogy*, the term used for the education of children. Knowles described adult learners as persons who do best when asked to use their experience and apply new knowledge to solve real-life problems. Adult learners' motivation to learn is more pragmatic and problem centered than that of younger learners. Adults are more likely to learn if they view the information as personally relevant and important (Mitchell & Courtney, 2005; Peterson, 2005). The basic assumptions about adult learners are that they are increasingly self-directed and have experiences that serve as a rich resource for their own and others' learning. Their readiness to learn develops from life tasks and problems, and their orientation to learning is task centered or problem centered.

The following five additional characteristics of adult learners have been described by Jackson and Caffarella (1994):

1. Adults have more and different types of life experiences that are organized differently from those of children.
2. Adults have preferred differences in personal learning style.
3. Adults are more likely to prefer being actively involved in the learning process.
4. Adults desire to be connected to and supportive of each other in the learning process.
5. Adults have individual responsibilities and life situations that provide a social context that affects their learning.

The learning behaviors of adults are shaped by past experiences; their maturity and life experiences provide them with insights and the ability to see relationships. Adults are not content centered; adults are self-directed and motivation to learn is internal (Goddu, 2012). They are problem centered, and need and want to learn useful information that can be readily adapted. Adults need a climate that enables them to assume responsibility for their learning.

Premise

The basic assumptions about adult learners are that they are increasingly self-directed and have experiences that serve as a rich resource for their own and others' learning. Their readiness to learn develops from life tasks and problems, and their orientation to learning is task centered or problem centered.

Implications for Nurse Educators

Because adults fear failure, faculty must create a relaxed, psychologically safe environment, while developing a climate of trust and mutual respect that will facilitate student empowerment. Faculty facilitate, guide, or coach adult learners. Although faculty assume responsibility for being the content expert, a collaborative relationship and use of the democratic process are essential with adult learners. Faculty can design meaningful learning activities so that learning transfer becomes a reality. Learning activities should stimulate and encourage reflection on past and current experiences and be sequenced according to the learners' needs. Faculty attend to adult learners' needs and concerns as legitimate and important components of the learning process; this helps ensure that their learning experiences are maximized.

Course materials and learning experiences are sequenced according to learner readiness. Learning plans are actually learning contracts established with learners. Learning contracts are often used with adult learners in formal academic classrooms and staff development. Contracts are developed collaboratively and should specify the knowledge, skills, and attitudes that students will acquire; the means by which students will attain the objectives; the criteria and evidence by which they will be judged; and the date for completion of the work (Knowles, 1980).

Learning activities should include independent study and inquiry projects that focus on inquiry and experiential techniques (Caffarella & Barnett, 1994). Field-based experiences such as internships and practicum assignments provide experiential learning. Reflective journals, critical incidents, and portfolios are other types of activities that allow adult learners to introduce their past and current experiences into the content of the learning events. These activities also help learners make sense of their life experiences, providing added incentive to learn (Caffarella & Barnett, 1994). Evaluation is shared with the students and peers; students should have some options for selecting the methods of evaluation.

The use of adult learning principles actively involves students and stimulates the use of a broader variety of resources as students work collaboratively with others to achieve their personal learning objectives. Box 13-1 identifies the teaching and learning principles associated with Knowles' adult learning model (Knowles, Holton, & Swanson, 2005). Students must be able, with support from faculty and peers, to determine their own learning needs and work collaboratively in negotiating

BOX 13-1 Adult Teaching and Learning Principles Based on Knowles' Model of Adult Learning

1. Faculty
   a. Relate to learners with value and respect for their feelings and ideas.
   b. Create a comfortable psychological and physical environment that facilitates learning.
   c. Involve learners in assessing and determining their learning needs.
   d. Collaborate with learners in planning the course content and the instructional strategies.
   e. Help learners to make maximum use of their own experiences within the learning process.
   f. Assist learners in developing their learning contracts.
   g. Assist learners in developing strategies to meet their learning objectives.
   h. Assist learners in identifying the resources to help meet their learning objectives.
   i. Assist learners in developing their learning activities.
   j. Assist learners in implementing their learning strategies.
   k. Encourage participation in cooperative activities with other learners.
   l. Introduce learners to new opportunities for self-fulfillment.
   m. Assist learners in developing their plan for self, peer, and faculty evaluation.
2. Learners
   a. Accept responsibility for collaborating in the planning of their experiences.
   b. Adopt learning experiences as their goals.
   c. Actively participate in the learning experience.
   d. Pace their own learning.
   e. Participate in monitoring their own progress.

their learning experiences. Self-directedness and the ability to pace learning and monitor progress toward completion of goals are essential attributes of adult learners.

Theory of Intellectual and Moral Development

The theory of intellectual and moral development features an understanding of how college students come to understand knowledge and the ways in which they develop the cognitive processes of thinking and reasoning. Perry (1970) proposed that college students pass through a predictable, developmental sequence of positions from simple to complex thinking. Learners move from viewing truth in absolute terms of right-and-wrong, dualist thinking to a more elaborate set of viewpoints. At any point in time, however, further development may be halted or suspended. Growth is usually not linear and usually occurs in fluctuating surges. Students develop the ability to abstract and weigh information to problem solve in specific situations. In the end, students understand that making a commitment is necessary to become oriented to a world of relativism.

Premise

According to Perry (1970), students progress through stages of intellectual and moral development. Student growth begins with a narrow, dualistic view of the world; develops to the point in which knowledge and values are perceived as contextual and relative; and finally commits to establishing a personal identity in a pluralistic world.

Implications for Nursing Education

Findings from studies in which Perry's model was used in nursing have particular relevance because of the responsibility faculty have for preparing graduates with highly developed moral and intellectual skills and the ability to deal with uncertainty when they provide care in an increasingly complex society and health care system. Valiga (1988) summarized several variables identified through research with Perry's (1970) model that relate to cognitive development. Variables that pertain to the student include age, sex, socioeconomic status, verbal fluency, student's hometown population, educational motivation, and learning style preference. Variables related to the development and implementation of the curriculum and courses include the subject matter discipline of the curriculum, the amount of structure and flexibility, the degree of challenge and support given, the types of course assignments, the nature of student–peer interactions, the openness of student–faculty relationships, and the degree of fit between the students' positions in the Perry model and the learning environment.

Frisch (1990), in a study of junior baccalaureate nursing students, revealed that most students operated at the end of the dualistic stage, whereas only one had attained multiplicity which occurs at the beginning of the relativism state. Valiga (1988) found in her study that at the beginning and at the end of the academic year, most of the students were at the dualistic stage. Although some showed no change, a few gained almost two positions, moving them into the relativism stage.

Faculty using Perry's model are attentive to developing not only intellectual capacity, but also the ethical and moral capacity of the students. Faculty develop an open, honest, and supportive partnership with students while facilitating intellectual growth. Valiga (1988) recommended that faculty design curricula that require students to have organized experiences with other students who have alternative ways of thinking, reasoning, and viewing the world. These experiences should be introduced during the freshman year. Requiring courses in different disciplines that provide gradual degrees of complexity should be part of the curricular design. Interprofessional courses can provide the situated learning that blends complexity and uncertainty with the collaboration necessary for successful clinical practice (Sargeant, 2009).

When using Perry's theory, students must be willing to be socialized to the college experience and risk entering into new experiences with others whose backgrounds and views are different than their own. Having an open and receptive attitude and a disposition to become comfortable in revealing aspects of the self is important. Students' being aware of the importance of their active participation in new and challenging experiences that will stretch their cognitive abilities is beneficial for their development. Students can also expect that progression through school will bring increased intellectual demands, challenging faculty expectations, and some disruptions in their sense of certainty about their world.

Students who developmentally focus on certainty or absolute answers may be stressed to develop answers to contextual situations that exist in nursing practice. These students may adopt a negative attitude about the amount of time and effort required to meet the program and course objectives. Thus the context of their learning becomes a negative experience in and of itself.

Novice to Expert

As patient acuities continued to increase during the past several decades, it was becoming clear that new nurse graduates would require ongoing development and guidance throughout their early practice and beyond. Benner (1984) used the Dreyfuss model of skill acquisition, to explain the differences of proficiencies of nurses at various levels. Benner described these levels as novice (more concrete level of knowledge; needs close supervision), advanced beginner (developing more working knowledge of practice, more use of judgment; needs overall supervision), competent (increasing working knowledge of practice, mostly able to use own judgment), proficient (growing depth of understanding of practice and of nursing, responsible for self and some others), and expert (authoritative knowledge of practice and discipline, responsible for self and others, creates new interpretations beyond standards).

Premise

The premise of this theory is that nursing expertise develops over time. Nurses pass through five stages as they fully develop their expertise as nurses. Student nurses begin as novices and may progress to advanced beginner stages, but it is the experience of real-world nursing practice that provides opportunities for progressive development of expertise.

Implications for Nursing Education

Although the novice-to-expert model was developed with practicing nurses in mind, it is relevant to nursing students who progress in levels of knowledge and experience throughout their nursing program. The educator must first understand what level of students they are working with, such as those in the first semester versus the final semester of the program as well as what learning and experiences they have previously had. Ways to gather more information include reviewing the sequence of the curriculum and course descriptions, discussions with other nurse faculty who have taught previous courses, and querying the students. Throughout the learning process, the skills of student self-reflection on what is known, what needs to be learned, and how it can be learned should be fostered. Continual assessment of student performance in didactic and clinical settings is necessary to make adjustments to teaching. These adjustments could involve reinforcing previous concepts, breaking down abstract concepts, or increasing the depth and scope of what is being learned and related assignments. The novice to expert theory is used to guide the development of capstone experiences, internships as well as orientation programs, internships, and residency programs.

Humanism

Humanism, sometimes referred to as the *human potential movement,* became an important force during the 1970s as a strong reaction to the excessive use of behaviorism and focus on skills development. Humanistic psychologists are primarily concerned with motivating students for growth toward becoming self-actualized. Individual behavior is described according to the person rather than the observer. Humanistic education has been defined as an educational practice in which the teaching–learning process emphasizes the value, worth, dignity, and integrity of all individuals. Two humanistic learning theories are relevant for nursing education: humanism and caring.

The humanistic approach supports and promotes the dignity of the individual, values students' feelings, and promotes the development of a humanistic perspective toward others. Learning is defined as a process of developing one's own potential with the goal of becoming a self-actualized person. Proponents of the humanistic movement in education include theorists such as Combs, Glasser, Kohlberg, Learn, Leininger, Maslow, and Rogers.

Premise

Education motivates students to develop their human potential so that they can progress toward self-actualization.

Implications for Nursing Education

Educators adopting this approach use learning experiences that emphasize the affective aspects of development, promoting the students' sense of responsibility, cooperation, and mutual respect. Honesty and caring are considered equally important as the learning goals that focus on the cognitive and psychomotor domains. Humanistic education involves a climate in which there is recognition and valuing of individual freedom and worth. It may be used in academic courses, continuing education courses, staff development programs, and personal development seminars and courses.

Faculty create a learning environment that fosters and promotes self-development by establishing an informal and relaxed climate. This can be accomplished by taking a few minutes at the beginning of the first few classes to use "icebreaker" strategies that invite students to mingle and become acquainted with each other and the teacher. One way to help students learn the behaviors consistent with the humanistic movement is through modeling. Faculty can model the desired behaviors and attitudes that are integral components of humanistic education: being a caring, empathetic person and demonstrating genuineness while being consistently respectful of self and others. Faculty's recognition of themselves as a co-learner in educational transactions encourages more egalitarian student–teacher relationships. Faculty help students recognize and develop their own unique potential by facilitating their growth process. This may be facilitated by praising students' positive behaviors, asking students to draw on and share their own experiences, asking questions that enable students to contribute to discussions, and elaborating on students' responses and questions.

Students are responsible for their own learning; determine their own needs, goals, and objectives; and conduct self-evaluations. Students become actively engaged in the learning process, assume responsibility, are open to discussion, and are able to use reflection and introspection. In addition, students adopt the respectful and caring behaviors modeled by faculty.

Caring

The caring theory, as proposed by Watson (1989), integrates within a human science orientation concepts and principles drawn from the humanistic-existentialist perspective and feminist philosophy, as well as from phenomenology. The primary concepts of the theory are:

- Practice of loving-kindness and equanimity
- Authentic presence: enabling deep belief of other (patient, colleague, family, etc.)
- Cultivation of one's own spiritual practice toward wholeness of mind/body/spirit—beyond ego
- "Being" the caring-healing environment
- Allowing miracles (openness to the unexpected and inexplicable life events)

Premise

The main premise of this theory is caring for self and others based on a moral, ethical, philosophical foundation of love and values. Essential to the theory is the use of 10 carative factors which are vital in caring for another. The 10 factors include promotion of transpersonal teaching–learning; assisting with gratification of human needs; systematically using a scientific (creative) problem-solving caring process; humanistic-altruistic values; promoting and accepting expressions of positive and negative feelings; instilling and enabling faith and hope; allowing for existential-phenomenological spiritual dimensions; cultivation of sensitivity to one's self and other; providing a supportive, protective, corrective mental, social and spiritual environment; and cultivating sensitivity to one's self and others (Watson, 2007). These factors move thinking from the more curative realm to one in which the caring of self and others in the moment is a treatment unto itself.

Implications for Nursing Education

Watson's theory of caring and the practices of caring have been used as a model for clinical practice and as a curriculum framework. The goal of the caring curriculum is to create an educational experience in nursing that is more in accord with true education and consistent with the professional nursing philosophy and values that are an integral part of contemporary nursing practice, research, and education. Bevis and Murray (1990) described the caring curriculum model as providing education for professional nursing that emphasizes analytical, problem-solving, and critical-thinking skills.

Content and student learning experiences must be based on the science of human caring and grounded in and derived from the actual reality of lived experience as ascertained from phenomenology rather than merely the content that nurse educators have traditionally taught or the content as they believe it should be. Although theory traditionally has been taught to inform practice, in the new models, theory and practice are viewed as informing each other. A restructured focus of learning is based in clinical practice and uses content as the substance to actively involve students in scholarly endeavors.

Caring theory is also well described in practice. Mitchell (2005) lays out the assumptions underlying caring theory as used to develop a model of clinical practice that considers patient and staff perspectives. It can also be used as a framework for nursing leadership (Britt Pipe, 2008). Incorporation of caring concepts in the curriculum can lay a solid foundation for how future practice is perceived and realized.

Faculty implementing a caring curriculum work to discover ways to eliminate adversarial relationships with students; faculty also strive to maintain open, honest, caring, and supportive relationships. It is within this context that faculty create a climate and structure that promotes the desired learning environment. Faculty develop and model the spirit of inquiry that helps students to develop maturity in their learning and cognitive abilities. Students are guided as they examine information, concepts, and principles, and as they struggle with uncertainty (Bevis, 1989). The content selected is basic to what is needed in accord with the program's philosophy and desired graduate outcomes. Faculty focus their efforts on helping students see beyond the information presented to discern the underlying assumptions.

To provide students with an in-depth educative learning experience, faculty function in different roles and become experts in learning and in the subject matter. Frequent use of instructional strategies that facilitate active learning, such as the use of questioning and dialogue, is important. Faculty-initiated dialogues with students focus on developing the attributes of intellectual curiosity, caring, caring roles, ethical ideals, and assertiveness. Dialogues occur within the context of a spirit of inquiry and should stimulate and enhance faculty and student learning as meanings of the content are explored.

Students assume responsibility for active learning and seek support and guidance from faculty. It is important that students shift their conception of faculty as authority figures to that of colleagues in the learning enterprise because students are expected to function as active participants in the decision-making structure. Changes in the faculty's relationship with students promote an energized climate in which faculty become allies with students. Students' active engagement in the teaching–learning process allows more opportunities for faculty to observe increases in students' self-esteem, self-confidence, and competence. Students experience an increase in their internal motivation and sense of responsibility.

Interpretive Pedagogies

Interpretive pedagogies focus on exploring, deconstructing, and critiquing experiences. They embrace multiple epistemologies, ways of knowing, and practices of thinking (Diekelmann, 2001). The pedagogies are methods to use when the educational emphasis is to understand or appreciate the nature of experience. The interpretive pedagogies empower the student, decenter authority, encourage social action, and construct new knowledge. Two interpretive pedagogies are discussed here: phenomenology and narrative pedagogy.

Phenomenology

Phenomenology is a philosophy and a qualitative research method nurse educators use to study the lived human experience. It is an inductive, descriptive approach used to explain the phenomenon of the human experience (Omery, 1983). Phenomenology is concerned with communicating understandings of meanings of phenomena and offers multiple approaches to examine problems at any system level. It involves reflection and discourse through a dialogue of language and experience of caring about phenomena from which meanings are transformed into themes that capture the phenomenon that one is trying to understand (Van Manen, 1990). When applied in nursing education and clinical practice, phenomenology can be used to gain understanding of the phenomena that are the focus of nursing in clinical practice. The phenomenon of concern of nursing includes nurses themselves as students and practitioners and, of course, their patients. The concerns include, but are not limited to, human experiences such as pain, suffering, loss, grief, and hope (Taylor, 1993).

Premise

Phenomenology offers a way to describe the nature of nursing practice in actual practice settings; it is a flexible and fluid pedagogy that is situated in the entire universe of professional nursing as viewed through a holistic lens. This view enables perception of the gestalt of the lived experience of nurses and patients. The physical and social environments merge into a personal, intimate, and holistic experience. A phenomenological approach establishes a view that shifts the focus from a technical, skills orientation to one that is concerned with the whole human being. Phenomenology has been used by nurse scholars such as Benner (1984), Tanner et al. (1993), Bevis (1989), and Diekelmann (2001). The goal of phenomenology is to understand human experience—the hows and whys in which events are experienced.

Implications for Nursing Education

Phenomenology can be used in the classroom; in clinical practice; and in any other situation in which patients, nurses, and nursing students are the phenomena of interest. Faculty and students have unique opportunities to gain knowledge and learn new skills from all subjects. Patients, expert clinicians, students, and faculty all have a story to unfold. Phenomenology clearly acknowledges the value of the students in making meaning out of stories while promoting trust, creativity, and inquiry. These learning experiences have the potential to promote a more in-depth understanding and enhance the caring aspects of students' clinical practice

When using a phenomenological approach to teaching, faculty select phenomena from professional literature that is relevant to the course content and explore them in the classroom. Faculty can also demonstrate ways in which aspects of a patient's or nurse's lived experience can be elicited through the use of open-ended and probing questions. Guest speakers may enhance classroom learning experience by sharing their own personal knowledge of the lived experience of patients or themselves. Faculty can use a variety of teaching–learning strategies, including clarified nursing perspectives, nursing prose, logs, case studies, anecdotal recordings, dialogue, fictional and autobiographical accounts of experience, responses to art, and artistic expression.

In clinical practice settings, expert nurse clinicians are active in the learning process. Faculty guide and show students how to learn from the expert clinician. Faculty assume responsibility for identifying, negotiating, and collaborating with the expert clinicians who guide and mentor students' learning experiences in clinical practice. In addition, faculty initiate discussion and debate, offer critiques without judgments, and guide the agenda without controlling it. Faculty become listeners and responders and enter into dialogues with students. The climate provides opportunities for students to become empowered.

The role of the student is to make meaning out of information. Students must be self-directive in seeking out what they want and need to learn from the expert clinician or faculty.

Narrative Pedagogy

Narrative pedagogy uses conventional, phenomenological, critical, and feminist pedagogies. Narrative pedagogy is a commitment to practical discourse in which knowledge is gained through the experiences of teachers, students, and clinicians. It is the collective interpretation of common experience that encourages shared learning. It is not intended to replace other types of teaching but has true application as a complementary pedagogy in nursing courses (Walsh, 2011).

A 12-year study produced nine themes from interview texts obtained from teachers, students, and clinicians (Diekelmann, 2001). The experience of learning and teaching is articulated in the common and shared experiences of what is really important in nursing education. The concernful practices of schooling, learning, teaching outlined by Diekelmann (2001, p. 57) are as follows:

- Gathering: Bringing in and calling forth
- Creating places: Keeping open a future of possibilities
- Assembling: Constructing and cultivating
- Staying: Knowing and connecting
- Caring: Engendering community
- Interpreting: Unlearning and becoming
- Presencing: Attending and being open
- Preserving: Reading, writing, thinking, and dialoguing
- Questioning: Meaning and making visible

Ironside (2003) conducted a qualitative study of nursing faculty and students to find out what teaching (or learning) in a narrative pedagogy classroom was like. Two themes were discovered. One was thinking as questioning to discover what else there is and what other ways there are to think of the topic versus finding the "best" answer. The other theme related to the capacity for preserving uncertainty and fallibility. Developing thinking like this in nursing students is beneficial, considering the massive amount of incoming information, diverging views, and chaos that defines clinical practice in the twenty-first century. In another qualitative study, Ironside (2006) found that using narrative pedagogy encourages dialogue and interpretation in a community of learning. The focus was on finding meaning to nursing practice and exploring alternate views.

Premise

Narrative pedagogy is the dialogue and debate among and between teachers, students, and clinicians that questions both what is concealed and what is revealed. We come to know one another through our narratives (Brown, Kirkpatrick, Mangum, & Avery, 2008). The nine themes listed earlier exemplify concernful practices of schooling, learning, and teaching.

Implications for Nursing Education

Faculty construct activities for content and skills acquisition through encouraging meaning making in students relative to stories about experience. This can be done through the narratives of others—for example, viewing and discussing a movie, presentation, or a book (McAllister et al., 2009). Gazarian (2010) describes how students can use digital media to tell their stories. This strategy makes use of the visual and musical aspects of computers. Through listening and responding to stories and personal perceptions, knowledge is developed in context. Sheckel and Irosnide (2006) conducted a phenomenological study on how student thinking is affected by use of narrative pedagogy. A subtheme of cultivating interpretive thinking emerged, exemplified by students' discussion of what it meant to be able to make their own clinical assignments. Questions and discussion around stories enact narrative pedagogy as a means for shifting thinking from what is known to what is important and needs to be known.

The concernful practices offer a climate of productive dialogue among and between clinicians, teachers, and students. Faculty must develop an understanding and skill in using the nine themes of concernful practices to expose the hidden understandings and provoke new possibilities in nursing education. Faculty must also understand the nature of the interpretive pedagogies in contrast to and along with conventional pedagogy. Faculty will likely engage in personal and professional introspection because the nine concernful practices will illuminate both positive and negative attributes. Students share the responsibility for discourse and deconstruction with clinicians and faculty.

Narrative pedagogy fits well with aspects of both constructivism and cognitive learning and may be viewed from a complexity science perspective regarding learning that is interactive, adaptable, creative, builds capability, less predictable and always evolving (Mitchell, Jonas-Simpson, & Cross, 2013; Fraser & Greenhalgh, 2001).

Neuroscience, Brain-Based, and Deep Learning and Multiple Intelligence

In the past, the brain was thought to develop only before birth and childhood. However, it is now known that the brain continues to develop and adapt throughout life as a result of learning. These changes can be observed by neuroscientists through various direct imaging techniques. The ability of neural circuitry to change in structure and function is called *neuroplasticity* (Kalia, 2008). Changes in the growth of neural branches and number of synapses are enhanced by learning that focuses on "the four major areas of neocortex (Sensory, back-integrative, front-integrative and motor)" (Zull, 2006, p. 5). This can be accomplished through learning that incorporates understanding and comprehension, abstract thought, and creative building and experimenting. Repetition can speed processing time through neural networks. Additionally, emotions serve to modify neuron signals and strengthen the orbitofrontal cortex (involved in executive brain function) (Cozolino & Sprokay, 2006; Zull, 2006). The direct connection between learning and brain development provides more evidence of the importance and influence of the teaching–learning process that occurs within nursing educational settings. Three theories based on concepts of neuroscience are presented here: brain-based learning, deep learning, and multiple intelligences (MI).

Neuroscience is also providing new insight into how the brains of young learners may differ from their older counterparts. Generation Z and Millennials will begin to make up larger portions of the nursing student population. Auerbach, Buerhaus, and Staiger (2011) conducted a national study and determined that the population of young people, ages 23 through 26, who are entering the registered nursing workforce has been steadily rising since 2002. Prensky (2001) has dubbed those born after 1980 as "digital natives." They have grown up in a world of 24/7 access to information, entertainment, and communication. They use technologies constantly to access up to 600 channels of TV; surf the Internet; play complex, fast-paced, highly visual video games; and engage in all types of social media. The rapid and ongoing use of such technologies affects the neuroplasticity of the brain, specifically chemical processing and development of some neural networks (Bradley Ruder, 2008; Prensky, 2001). These learners are used to multitasking and moving attention quickly from one thing to another. Young learners may also seem impatient at times and are used to immediate results. They are used to learning and sharing with others. Nurse educators can use educational theories, such as a social constructivist approach to ensure their active engagement. Their short attention span, need for immediate feedback, and diverse stimulation, as well as their proficiency in using various technologies, can be used by nurse educators who incorporate technology in their classrooms. This may include Internet videos or group exercises in which information on the Internet must be obtained and used. Revell and McCurry (2010) noted the need to adopt the use of technologies, such as personal response systems in the classroom, to promote the critical thinking, communication skills, and engagement of young learners.

Brain-Based Learning

The concept of brain-based learning arose through research in neuroscience, psychology, and biology during the last 30 years and focuses on optimal conditions for the brain to learn (Connell, 2009; Gulpinar, 2005; Jensen, 2008). The field has evolved, as evidenced by other names it has acquired, such as *nurturing the brain, neuroscience and education,* and *educational neuroscience* (Petitto & Dunbar, 2009). Early work in the area was noted with Gardner's (1993) MI and right–left hemisphere brain function. Complex and interconnected functions in the brain work to process incoming information from memory or outside senses and route for immediate action, elimination, or further processing and storage. The way the brain learns is affected by multiple factors, including time of day, nutrition, and stress (Jensen, 2008). Twelve principles of brain learning have been advanced by Caine and Caine (1991). Three of these include the idea that the learning brain continues to develop patterns and reconstruct itself, emotions are essential to pattern development, and learning can be enhanced through nonthreatening challenges.

Emotional thought is also related to cognitive function and involves multiple areas of the brain and several processes of decision making, memory, and learning. Thoughts trigger emotions and can be influenced by external information or body sensations (Immordino-Yang & Damasio, 2007). Emotions in learning have been used to further understand connections such as cognitive patterning (Craig, 2003), motivation, and actual engagement and effort (Immordino-Yang & Damasio, 2007).

Neuroscience indicates that brains learn differently at different ages. Working memory capacity may be similar for simple tasks, but younger learners maintain more working memory when tasks become more complex. Inhibitory control (blocking distracting interferences), cognitive processing speed, and long-term memory storage may be less than that of younger learner peers (Reuter-Lorenz & Park, 2010). This represents challenges for faculty working with adult learners that could, potentially, span three or four generations. Metaanalytical research conducted by Gozuyesil and Dikicl (2014) examined 31 studies and the effect of academic achievement using brain-based learning. The results indicated higher academic achievement in those who had been exposed to brain-based learning.

Premise

Learning may be maximized by enhancing the conditions under which the brain learns best:

- Relaxed alertness: a learning environment of high challenge and low threat
- Orchestrated immersion of learners in authentic, complex, multiple experiences
- Active, regular processing of experiences to develop meaning (Caine & Caine, 1991)

Brain-based learning is effective in further developing learning pathways and deeper learning. It encourages a more holistic view of how the brain, body, and environment affect learning.

Implications for Nursing Education

Brain-based learning is fostered through activities that require knowledge construction and connection to previous knowledge. Examples include authentic case studies that adapt based on new content and initial responses; simulation exercises; group projects; in-depth, multifaceted exploration of a patient; and reflection on how and why decisions are made. Any setting can foster brain-based learning that encourages interaction, authentic experiences, and learning challenges balanced in a low-threat environment. It is important for faculty to create and maintain a learning environment that engages learners and encourages expression of the "how and why" of thinking. As the "orchestrator," faculty need to design learning experiences that help learners to make connections. Faculty need to understand that each learner is unique; learners attend to and process information in different ways. It is helpful to consider learner diversity and learning style. It is up to the faculty to set the learning environment tone by demonstrating caring, valuing, and trust (Jensen, 2000). Enthusiasm and organization can be helpful in stimulating student motivation to learn. Faculty must also be cognizant of how various age differences can affect the learning brain with regard to areas such as amount and sequencing of content and repetition. Having positive feelings (emotions) and motivation to learn will increase a student's capacity to take in and process information. Coming to class or clinical prepared and well rested can positively influence both emotion and motivation.

Deep Learning

Deep learning (vs. surface learning) is learning to understand and create meaning (Smith & Colby, 2007). Learners become more persistent and able to contend with more challenging learning situations (Majeski & Stover, 2007). Whittman-Price and Godshall (2009) discussed deep, strategic, and surface learning. Surface learning is usually extrinsically motivated and involves memorizing information, often for tests. Deep learning, in contrast, is intrinsically motivated and involves a desire to learn in order to understand. Strategic learning is a combination of deep and surface learning, with students being goal oriented and doing what is necessary to achieve their goals.

Premise

Deep learning is an intentional, intrinsically motivated strategy to understand and connect knowledge to create new meaning and actions. Deep learning is related to cognitive and information processing theories in which learning from short-term memory is transferred to long-term memory with repetition and practice.

Implications for Nursing Education

Deep learning can be fostered in classroom or clinical settings that offer the time and space for interactive discourse. Faculty can create opportunities for students to learn facts and concepts for application in clinical settings. Case studies, unfolding case studies, and simulation and clinical learning experiences facilitate deep learning. Concept mapping also promotes deep learning (Hay, 2007). Students need to regularly assess their learning and be actively engaged in the learning process with peers and teachers. Students benefit through a more conceptual understanding that fosters meaning and relevance (Clare, 2007).

Multiple Intelligence

Gardner (1983) challenged the classical view of intelligence and posited that there is a plurality of intellects. The idea of MI began with a preliminary list of seven constructs: bodily-kinesthetic, visual-spatial, verbal-linguistic, logical-mathematical, musical-rhythmic, interpersonal, and intrapersonal (Gardner, 1983). Two additional intelligences have been added: naturalist and existential (Bowles, 2008; Moran, Kornhaber & Gardner, 2006). The theory suggests that individuals differ in the intelligence profiles they are born with and that profiles work in harmony, changing as influenced by experience and learning throughout life. Incorporating the MI in designing and executing instruction enhances student learning (Holland, 2007).

Premise

Every human being has a unique intelligence profile and expresses the intelligences in varying degrees. Although in any one person, one or more of the intelligences may be demonstrated at a higher operant level than the others, it is in the working together of the intelligences that a person solves problems and interacts with the environment. The goal of education is to develop all intelligences in a holistic way.

Implications for Nursing Education

Although not a prescriptive theory, MI provides a framework for understanding intelligence that can benefit both students and teachers. Faculty can empower students to recognize their own unique gifts to the nursing encounter by acknowledging profiles of problem-solving abilities that consider more than the narrow range of verbal-linguistic and logical-mathematical abilities traditionally associated with intelligence quotient testing. MI may be helpful in tapping into student creativity. Qualities identified in all of the categories can contribute to an optimal patient encounter in a practice profession such as nursing. Because most intelligence tests tap only the logical-mathematical and verbal-linguistic intelligences, students enter nursing with documentation that only partially identifies preparation for nursing. Faculty has the opportunity, using the MI theory, to focus on each student's unique profile and to use students' strengths to enhance contributions to practice and the profession.

The student can use the MI theory for self-evaluation and for the evaluation of others. Because there is no hierarchy in the MI theory, no intelligence is thought to be of higher value than any other. The student may enjoy the recognition of untested, undocumented, yet affirmed abilities that can contribute to his or her success in nursing. Students can find direction for within-nursing vocations, as well as other social choices, by giving attention to their personal profiles. A broader, more comprehensive view of the intelligences that nurses, students, faculty, and other health care professionals bring to the learning encounter can contribute to greater understanding of potential nursing interactions. The complexity of MI and individual profiles mirrors the complexity of holistic nursing. Specific and broadened attention to course and clinical learning goals relative to the constructs in the MI theory may contribute to greater student success and satisfying professional performance.

Summary

The main focus of the educational experience is the learner as active participant in transaction with the teacher, peers, and the larger environment. Students are given considerable control over the development of learning experiences, and they construct and create knowledge. Faculty assume a primary role as designers of the learning environment and learning experiences in a shared governance approach with students and others contributing to the learning climate. Faculty continue to learn as they teach, thus evolving in their educational philosophy and teaching style.

The learning theories and frameworks presented in this chapter provide a guide for faculty to use within the four steps of the teaching–learning process. Each theory or framework has varying degrees of usefulness depending on the faculty's philosophy about teaching; the philosophy that guides the curriculum; the setting and climate in which the teaching is to occur; student characteristics; and the purpose, nature, and content of the course. Within these contextual variables, faculty need to weigh the advantages and disadvantages of each theory or framework and select those that are most appropriate.

The shift to the learning paradigm ensures that learners will construct and create knowledge and faculty serve as designers, facilitators, coaches, guides, and mentors. For most learning experiences in higher education and for nursing in particular, behavioristic principles have limited relevance. Current and emerging concepts and principles in the neuroscience of learning, cognitive, humanistic, and adult learning theories and Perry's model for intellectual and cognitive development, as well as those included in the interpretive pedagogies, patterns of knowing, narrative pedagogies, and caring, are consistent with the thrust of a learning paradigm to guide nursing education. There is constant interaction as faculty create the environment and contextual learning experiences and the student assumes control over learning through active engagement.

REFLECTING ON THE EVIDENCE

1. Missildine, Fountain, Summers, and Gosselin (2013) found mixed results in a study comparing traditional lecture (n = 53), lecture and lecture capture back-up (n = 53) (audio save of lecture for student download), and the flipped classroom (n = 53) (usual class lecture as homework and real-time class for interaction and application of learning) on academic performance and student satisfaction. Students in the flipped classroom scored higher on course examination averages in the flipped classroom than in the traditional lecture or lecture and lecture capture backup groups, but were less satisfied than those in the other two approaches. What educational theories explain the results of greater academic performance? How can educational theory inform the nurse educator regarding student engagement and motivation?
2. Findings and recommendations from the national Carnegie National Nursing Education Study centered

REFLECTING ON THE EVIDENCE—CONT'D

around nursing education's failure to continually connect what is being taught to prior learning in liberal arts and science courses, and the need to develop in students integrative, multiple ways of thinking as a way to practice in today's dynamic and chaotic health care environments. What educational theories focus on previous knowledge and experience to build new knowledge? How would a typical nursing lecture be different when using this theory in action?

3. The increased complexity and diversity of patients and the health care system are driving force for nurses to be able to adapt, learn, and function effectively within health care teams. What learning theories might the nurse educator use in working with students in an interprofessional course aimed at improving the quality of health care through interdisciplinary communication, collaboration, and understanding of roles?

REFERENCES

Adams, P. (2006). Exploring social constructivism: Theories and practicalities. *Education, 34*(3), 243–257.

Anderson, J. R. (1980). *Cognitive psychology and its implications.* San Francisco: W. H. Freeman.

Anderson, J. R. (1985). *Cognitive psychology and its implications* (2nd ed.). San Francisco: W. H. Freeman.

Auerbach, D. I., Buerhaus, P. I., & Staiger, D. O. (2011). Registered nurse supply grows faster than projected amid surge in new entrants ages 23–26. *Health Affairs, 30,* 2286–2292.

Ausubel, D. P. (1960). The use of advance organizers in the learning and retention of meaningful verbal material. *Journal of Educational Psychology, 51*(5), 267–272.

Ausubel, D. P. (1978). *Educational psychology: A cognitive view* (2nd ed.). New York: Holt, Rinehart & Winston.

Bahn, D. (2001). Social learning theory: Its application in the context of nurse education. *Nurse Education Today, 21*(2), 110–117.

Bandura, A. (1977). *Social learning theory.* Englewood Cliffs, NJ: Prentice Hall.

Benner, P. (1984). *From novice to expert.* Menlo Park, CA: Addison-Wesley.

Benner, P., Sutphen, M., Leonard, V., & Day, L. (2010). *Educating nurses: A call for radical transformation*: *Vol. 15.* New York: John Wiley & Sons.

Bevis, E. O. (1989). *Toward a caring curriculum: A new pedagogy for nursing.* New York: National League for Nursing.

Bevis, E. O., & Murray, J. P. (1990). The essence of the curriculum revolution: Emancipatory teaching. *Journal of Nursing Education, 29*(7), 326–331.

Bowles, T. (2008). Self-rated estimates of multiple intelligences based on approaches to learning. *Australian Journal of Educational & Developmental Psychology, 8,* 15–26.

Bradley Ruder, D. (2008, September–October). The teen brain. *Harvard Magazine,* 8–10.

Brandon, A., & All, A. (2010). Constructivism theory analysis and application to curricula. *Nursing Education Perspectives, 31*(2), 89–92.

Britt Pipe, T. (2008). Illuminating the inner leadership journey by engaging mindfulness as guided by caring theory. *Nursing Administration Quarterly, 32*(2), 117–125.

Brown, S. T., Kirkpatrick, M. K., Mangum, D., & Avery, J. (2008). A review of narrative pedagogy strategies to transform traditional nursing education. *Journal of Nursing Education, 47*(6), 283–286.

Caffarella, R. S., & Barnett, B. G. (1994). Characteristics of adult learners and foundations of experiential learning. *New Directions for Adult and Continuing Education, 62,* 29–42.

Caine, R. N., & Caine, G. (1991). *Making connections: Teaching and the human brain.* Retrieved from, http://www.eric.ed.gov/PDFS/ED335141.pdf.

Chickering, A. W., & Gamson, Z. F. (1987). Seven principles for good practice in undergraduate education. *AAHE Bulletin, 3,* 7.

Clare, B. (2007). Promoting deep learning: A teaching learning and assessment endeavour. *Social Work Education, 26*(5), 433–446.

Connell, J. D. (2009). The global aspects of brain-based learning. *Educational Horizons, 88,* 28–39.

Cozolino, L., & Sprokay, S. (2006). Neuroscience and adult learning. *New Directions for Adult and Continuing Education, 110,* 11–19.

Craig, D. L. (2003). Brain-compatible learning: Principles and applications in athletic training. *Journal of Athletic Training, 38*(4), 342–349.

Diekelmann, N. (2001). Narrative pedagogy: Heideggerian hermeneutical analysis of lived experiences of students, teachers, and clinicians. *Advances in Nursing Science, 23*(3), 53–71.

Elsbach, K. D., Barr, P. S., & Hargadon, A. B. (2005). Identifying situated cognition in organizations. *Organization Science, 16*(4), 422–433.

Fosnot, C. T. (1996). *Constructivism: Theory, perspectives and practice.* New York: Teachers College Press.

Frank, C. (2005). Teaching and learning theory: Who needs it? *College Quarterly, 8*(2), n2. Retrieved from, http://www.collegequarterly.ca/2005-vol08-num02-spring/frank.html.

Fraser, S. W., & Greenhalgh, T. (2001). Coping with complexity: Educating for capability. *BMJ, 323*(7316), 799–803.

Frisch, N. C. (1990). An international nursing student exchange program: An educational experience that enhanced student cognitive development. *Journal of Nursing Education, 29*(1), 10–12.

Gardner, H. (1983). *Frames of mind.* New York: Basic Books.

Gardner, H. (1993). *Multiple intelligences: The theory in practice.* New York: Basic Books.

Gazarian, P. K. (2010). Digital stories: Incorporating narrative pedagogy. *Journal of Nursing Education, 49*(5), 287–290.

Goddu, K. (2012). Meeting the challenge: Teaching strategies for adult learners. *Kappa Delta Phi, 48*(4), 169–173.

Gozuyesil, E., & Dikicl, A. (2014). The effect of brain-based learning on academic achievement: A meta-analytical study. *Educational Sciences Theory & Practice, 14*(2), 642–648.

Grippin, P., & Peters, S. (1984). *Learning theory and learning outcomes.* Lanham, MD: University Press of America.

Gulpinar, M. (2005). The principles of brain-based learning and constructivist models in education. *Educational Sciences Theory & Practice, 5*(2), 299–306.

Hay, D. B. (2007). Using concept maps to measure deep, surface, and non-learning outcomes. *Studies in Higher Education, 32*(1), 39–57.

Hean, S., Craddock, D., & O'Halloran, C. (2009). Learning theories and interprofessional education: A user's guide. *Learning in Health and Social Work, 8*(4), 250–262.

Hilgard, E. R., & Bower, G. H. (1966). *Theories of learning.* New York: Appleton-Century-Crofts.

Holland, F. (2007). Bringing the body to life: Using multiple intelligence theory in the classroom. *SportEx Dynamics, 14*(Oct), 6–8.

Immordino-Yang, M. H., & Damasio, A. (2007). We feel, therefore we learn: The relevance of affective and social neuroscience to education. *Mind, Brain, and Education, 1*(1), 3–10.

Ironside, P. (2003). New pedagogies for teaching thinking: The lived experiences of students and teachers enacting narrative pedagogy. *Journal of Nursing Education, 42*(11), 509–516.

Ironside, P. M. (2006). Using narrative pedagogy: Learning and practising interpretive thinking. *Journal of Advanced Nursing, 55*(4), 478–486.

Jackson, L., & Caffarella, R. S. (1994). *Experiential learning: A new approach.* San Francisco: Jossey-Bass.

Jensen, E. (2000). *Brain-based learning: The new science of teaching and training* (rev. ed.). San Diego: The Brain Store.

Jensen, E. (2008). *Brain-based learning: The new paradigm of teaching* (2nd ed.). Thousand Oaks, CA: Corwin Press.

Kalia, M. (2008). Brain development: Anatomy, connectivity, adaptive plasticity, and toxicity. *Metabolism, 57,* S2–S5.

Knowles, M. S. (1980). *The modern practice of adult education.* Chicago: Follett.

Knowles, M. S., Holton, E. F., & Swanson, R. A. (2005). *The adult learner: The definitive classic in adult education and human resource development.* Burlington, MA: Elsevier.

Lasater, K., Mood, L., Buchwach, D., & Dieckelmann. (2015). Reducing incivility in the workplace: Results of a three-part educational intervention. *The Journal of Continuing Education in Nursing, 1*(46), 15–26.

Lewin, K. (1951). *Field theory in social science.* New York: Harper & Row.

Mager, R. F. (1962). *Preparing instructional objectives.* Palo Alto, CA: Fearon.

Majeski, R., & Stover, M. (2007). Theoretically based pedagogical strategies leading to deep learning in asynchronous online gerontology courses. *Educational Gerontology, 33*(3), 171–185.

McAllister, M., John, T., Gray, M., Williams, L., Barnes, M., Allan, J., et al. (2009). Adopting a narrative pedagogy to improve the student learning experience in a regional Australian university. *Contemporary Nurse, 32*(1–2), 156–165.

Missildine, K., Fountain, R., Summers, L., & Gosselin, K. (2013). Flipping the classroom to improve student performance and satisfaction. *Journal of Nursing Education, 52*(10), 597–599.

Mitchell, G. (2005). Advancing the practice of nursing theory: Evaluating nursing as caring. *Nursing Administration Quarterly, 18*(4), 313–319.

Mitchell, M. L., & Courtney, M. (2005). Improving transfer from the intensive care unit: The development, implementation, and evaluation of a brochure based on Knowles' adult learning theory. *International Journal of Nursing Practice, 11*(6), 257–268.

Mitchell, G., Jonas-Simpson, C., & Cross, N. (2013). Innovating nursing education: Interrelating narrative, conceptual learning, reflection, and complexity science. *Journal of Nursing Education and Practice, 3*(4), 30–39.

Moran, S., Kornhaber, M., & Gardner, H. (2006). Orchestrating multiple intelligences. *Educational Leadership, 64,* 23–27.

Omery, A. (1983). Phenomenology: A method for nursing research. *Advances in Nursing Science, 5*(2), 49–63.

Packer, M. J., & Goicechea, J. (2000). Sociocultural and constructivist theories of learning ontology, not just epistemology. *Educational Psychologist, 35*(4), 227–241.

Peer, K. S., & McClendon, R. C. (2002). Sociocultural learning theory in practice: Implications for athletic training educators. *Journal of Athletic Training, 37*(4), S136–S140.

Perry, W. G. (1970). *Forms of intellectual and ethical development in the college years: A scheme.* New York: Rinehart & Winston.

Peterson, G. (2005). Medical and nursing students' development of conceptions of science during three years of studies in higher education. *Scandinavian Journal of Educational Research, 49*(3), 281–296.

Petitto, L., & Dunbar, K. N. (2009). Educational neuroscience: New directions from bilingual brains, scientific brains, and the educated mind. *Mind Brain Education, 3*(4), 183–197.

Phillips, J. M., & Vinton, S. A. (2010). Why clinical nurse educators adopt innovative teaching strategies: A pilot study. *Nursing Education Research, 31*(4), 226–229.

Piaget, J. (1970a). Piaget's theory. In P. H. Musen (Ed.), *Carmichael's manual of psychology* (pp. 703–752). New York: Wiley.

Piaget, J. (1970b). *Structuralism.* New York: Basic Books.

Piaget, J. (1973). *To understand is to invent: The future of education.* New York: Grossman.

Powell, K. C., & Kalina, C. J. (2009). Cognitive and social constructivism: Developing tools for an effective classroom. *Education, 130*(2), 241–250.

Prensky, M. (2001). Digital natives, digital immigrants, part 1. *On the Horizon, 9*(5), 1–6.

Reuter-Lorenz, P. A., & Park, D. C. (2010). Human neuroscience and the aging mind: A new look at old problems. *The Journal of Gerontology Series B: Psychological Sciences and Social Sciences, 65B*(4), 405–415.

Revell, S. M. H., & McCurry, M. K. (2010). Effective pedagogies for teaching math to nursing students: A literature review. *Nurse Education Today, 33*(11), 1352–1356.

Rule, A. C. (2006). Editorial: The components of authentic learning. *Journal of Authentic Learning, 3*(1), 1–10.

Sanders, D., & Sugg, D. (2005). Strategies to scaffold student learning: Applying Vygotsky's zone of proximal development. *Nurse Educator, 30,* 203–207.

Sanders, D., & Welk, D. S. (2005). Strategies to scaffold student learning: Applying Vygotsky's zone of proximal development. *Nurse Educator, 30*(5), 203–207.

Sargeant, J. (2009). Theories to aid understanding and implementation of interprofessional education. *Journal of Continuing Education in the Health Professions*, *29*(3), 178–184.

Sheckel, M. M., & Irosnide, P. M. (2006). Cultivating interpretive thinking through enacting narrative pedagogy. *Nursing Outlook*, *54*(3), 159–165.

Skinner, B. F. (1953). *Science and human behavior*. New York, NY: Macmillan.

Slavin, R. E. (1988). *Educational psychology: Theory into practice* (2nd ed.). Englewood Cliffs, NJ: Prentice Hall.

Smith, T. W., & Colby, S. A. (2007). Teaching for deep learning. *The Clearing House*, *80*(5), 205–210.

Sthapornnanon, N., Sakulbumrungsil, R., Theeraroungchaisri, A., & Watcharadamrongkun, S. (2009). Social constructivist learning environment in an online professional practice course. *American Journal of Pharmaceutical Education*, *73*(1), 10.

Tanner, C., Benner, P., Chelsa, C., & Gordon, D. R. (1993). The phenomenology of knowing the patient. *Image*, *25*(4), 273–280.

Taylor, B. (1993). Phenomenology: A way to understanding nursing practice. *International Journal of Nursing Studies*, *30*(2), 171–179.

Torre, B., Daley, B., Sebastian, J., & Elnicki, M. (2006). Overview of current learning theories for medical educators. *The American Journal of Medicine*, *119*(10), 903–907.

Tulving, E. (1985). How many memory systems are there? *American Psychologist*, *40*(4), 385–398.

Valiga, T. M. (1988). Curriculum outcomes and cognitive development: New perspectives for nursing education. In E. Bevis (Ed.), *Curriculum revolution: Mandate for change* (pp. 177–200). New York: National League for Nursing.

Van Manen, M. (1990). *Researching lived experience: Human science for an action sensitive pedagogy*. Albany, NY: State University of New York Press.

Vianna, E., & Stetsenko, A. (2006). Embracing history through transforming it: Contrasting Piagetism versus Vygotskian (activity) theories of learning and development to expand constructivism within a dialectical view of history. *Theory & Psychology*, *16*, 81–108.

Vygotsky, L. (1986/1962). *Thought and language*. Cambridge, MA: MIT Press.

Walsh, M. (2011). Narrative pedagogy and simulation: Future direction for nursing education. *Nurse Education in Practice*, *11*, 216–219.

Watson, J. (1989). Transformative thinking and a caring curriculum. In E. O. Bevis & J. Watson (Eds.), *Toward a caring curriculum: A new pedagogy for nursing* (pp. 51–60). New York: National League for Nursing.

Watson, J. (2007). Watson's theory of human caring and subjective living experiences: Carative factors/caritas processes as a disciplinary guide to the professional nursing practice. *Texto & Contexto-Enfermagem*, *16*(1), 129–135.

Weinstein, C. E., & Meyer, D. K. (1991). Spring cognitive learning strategies and college teaching. In R. J. Menges & M. D. Svinicki (Eds.), *New directions for teaching and learning: College teaching: From theory to practice* (pp. 15–25). San Francisco: Jossey-Bass.

Whittman-Price, R. A., & Godshall, M. (2009). Strategies to promote deep learning in clinical nursing courses. *Nurse Educator*, *34*(5), 214–216.

Wittrock, M. C. (1977). Learning as a generative process. In M. C. Wittrock (Ed.), *Learning and instruction* (pp. 621–631). Berkeley, CA: McCrutchan.

Wittrock, M. C. (1986). Students' thought processes. In M. C. Wittrock (Ed.), *Handbook of research on teaching* (pp. 297–314). New York, NY: Macmillan.

Wittrock, M. C. (1992). Generative learning processes of the brain. *Educational Psychologist*, *27*(4), 531–541.

Zull, J. E. (2006). Key aspects of how the brain learns. *New Directions for Adult and Continuing Education*, *110*, 3–9.

14 Managing Student Incivility and Misconduct in the Learning Environment*

Susan Luparell, PhD, APRN, ACNS-BC, CNE, ANEF
Jeanne R. Conner, MN, APRN, FNP-C

On today's campuses of higher education, there appears to be increasing incidence of incivility among students (Clark & Springer, 2007; Luparell & Frisbee, 2014). When preparing a learning environment for students and faculty, how can faculty ensure that it is one that is safe and productive for all, one in which a quality teaching and learning experience can be provided? This chapter introduces developmental, legal, and risk management issues related to classroom learning environments and methods to minimize student conduct that disrupts learning. Instructional strategies are discussed to assist faculty in achieving a robust and engaging learning environment through management of the students' actions.

Management of actions includes student in-class behaviors and extends to out-of-class course-related activities, both on- and off-campus internships, clinical, and practicum, as well as online learning experiences. Specifically, this chapter explores methods to nurture and support learning and describes effective responses for situations in which student behavior could disrupt the learning environment with an emphasis on (1) a continuum of student misconduct, (2) preventative strategies, (3) proactive response strategies, and (4) effective use of campus resources.

The learning outcomes of this chapter include gaining an understanding of problem or disruptive student behavior and an understanding of specific steps faculty can take to minimize disruptions in the learning environment. The content of this chapter is based on case law, statutory law, research, and more than 20 collective years of experience working with college students and college student misconduct. As a cautionary note, it is strongly recommended that faculty consult with the administrators responsible for student conduct at their institution, their immediate supervisor, campus police, and campus legal counsel regarding issues specific to their institution.

Incivility in the Higher Education Environment

Most experienced faculty will tell you that they derive pleasure from working with students much of the time. However, on occasion, interactions between students and faculty may be somewhat uncomfortable, slightly challenging, or even distressing. Despite the "ivory tower" moniker, the academy, as a microcosm of society, is not immune to the problems of society. Incivilities of various types and among various individuals can and do occur in higher education. However, this is an aspect of the teaching role that tends to surprise novice faculty and befuddles even experienced faculty.

Both faculty and students have reported that incivility is a moderate problem in nursing education (Altmiller, 2012; Clark, 2008b; Mott, 2014). In a seminal study, Lashley and de Meneses (2001) found that all faculty who responded to a survey of student misconduct in nursing had experienced students being late, inattentive, or absent from class, and more than 90% reported student cheating as a problem. Faculty occasionally experience more serious episodes of misconduct, including verbal or physical abuse, albeit less frequently (Luparell, 2004; Williamson, 2011). Stress in both faculty and students has been identified as contributing significantly to uncivil behavior in nursing education (Clark, 2008a).

*The authors acknowledge the contributions of Karen M. Whitney, PhD, to previous editions of this chapter.

Although the majority of this chapter addresses how student misbehavior can be managed, it is important that faculty have an appreciation for the overall context in which misconduct and incivility occur. Student misconduct and incivility rarely occur in a vacuum. In both the general workplace and in nursing education, experts suggest that incivility is reciprocal in nature (Altmiller, 2012; Clark, 2008a; Porath & Pearson, 2012). If student misbehavior is viewed as a form of communication, it necessitates that we view it in a broader context that includes student interactions with faculty and the learning environment.

There is evidence to suggest that faculty play a pivotal role in establishing classroom behavioral norms and also may contribute to the problem in a variety of ways. In another landmark study, Boice (1996) concluded that faculty are the most crucial initiators of incivility in the classroom. Poor teaching skills may lead to student frustration and misbehavior. Additionally, lack of instructor willingness to address classroom incivility sends a message that such behavior is acceptable.

Furthermore, students sometimes experience incivility at the hands of faculty (Clark, 2008b; Marchiando, Marchiando, & Lasiter, 2010). Example behaviors that students may identify as uncivil on the part of faculty can be found in Box 14-1.

Although it is tempting to focus on student misconduct and incivility from a narrow perspective, it is prudent to avoid doing so. Poor student behavior and incivility, although never appropriate, may be influenced by a broad spectrum of variables, including stress levels and lack of general civility within the environment (Levine, 2010). Additionally, lack of teaching acumen by faculty may serve to increase student stress and frustration. Although this chapter provides a starting point for managing misbehavior and incivility when it occurs in the classroom, the thoughtful educator should consider multiple variables when considering how to best prevent and manage conduct problems in the classroom environment.

BOX 14-1 Uncivil Faculty Behaviors

- Unresponsive to student needs
- Targeting students, attempting to weed out
- Setting students up to fail
- Encouraging students to leave program
- Unprofessional behavior
- Defensive behavior
- Verbal abuse: berating, belittling, yelling, name-calling
- Threatening failure
- Favoritism, unfair treatment
- Rigid expectations for perfection
- Scare tactics
- Violations of due process
- Arrogance
- Making unannounced course changes

(Data from Altmiller, 2012; Del Prato, 2013; Mott, 2014)

A Continuum of Misconduct

In considering student conduct, one size does not fit all. It is important to examine each incident in terms of the behaviors observed and reported. It is also vital to use a framework from which to evaluate student behavior. With few exceptions, institutions of higher education develop policies or documents to support and inform expectations of civil behavior and conduct; these are described in many ways, such as a Student Code of Conduct, an Honor Code, Student Rights and Responsibilities, or some other variation. These policies provide the filter through which one takes a set of observed and reported behaviors and considers the extent to which a specific situation may or may not violate a code of conduct.

For purposes of analyzing student behaviors, all behaviors fall within one or more of the following three categories: (1) annoying acts, (2) administrative violations, and (3) criminal conduct (Fig. 14-1). It is possible that a single behavior, such as stealing a test, can be both an administrative violation and criminal conduct. It is also possible that a behavior repeated over time, such as interrupting a lecture repeatedly, can be considered both an annoying act and an administrative violation. Occasionally a lecture disruption might be annoying, but the behavior moves from annoying to a violation of campus

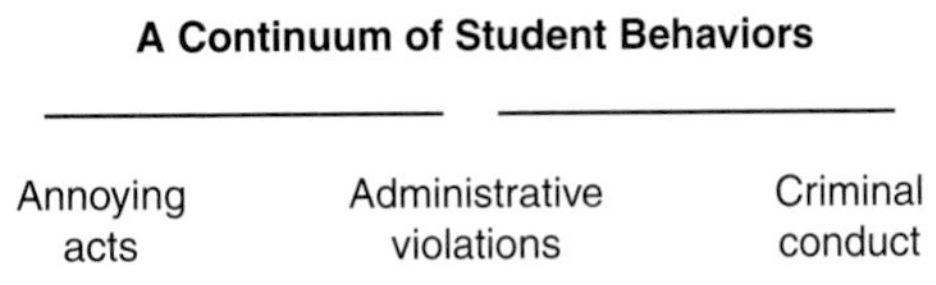

A Continuum of Student Behaviors

Annoying acts — Administrative violations — Criminal conduct

Figure 14-1 A continuum of student behaviors.

policy if the disruptions persist after the student has been counseled that the behavior exceeds reasonable limits. Regardless of where the behavior may lie on the continuum, it is critically important to create a teaching approach wherein faculty are in a position to observe student behaviors objectively. The focus should be on actions and not on emotion, rumor, or innuendo. Furthermore, it is important that faculty remain cognizant of student behaviors and their potential effect on learning in order to, at the earliest opportunity, consider the extent to which student actions fall within this framework. Awareness is the first step in managing the learning environment. Box 14-2 lists examples of student misconduct that fall within the categories of annoying acts, administrative violations, and criminal conduct.

BOX 14-2 Examples of Student Misconduct in the Classroom

ANNOYING ACTS

- Sleeping in class
- Talking in class
- Discourteous
- Uncooperative
- Late to class
- Poor hygiene
- Eating, drinking
- Pagers, cell phones
- Early exits

ADMINISTRATIVE VIOLATIONS

- Dishonesty; false accusations or information; forgery; alteration or misuse of any university document, record, or identification
- Disorderly conduct
- Actions that disrupt the academic process
- Failure to comply with directions of authorized university officials
- Cheating, plagiarism, fabrication

CRIMINAL CONDUCT—ALSO CAN BE CONSIDERED ADMINISTRATIVE VIOLATIONS

- Threats of violence against self or others
- Actions that endanger one's self or others in the university community
- Physical or verbal abuse
- Possession of firearms
- Conduct that is lewd, indecent, or obscene
- Intimidation, harassment, stalking
- Alcohol or drug possession or sale
- Theft

Annoying Acts

Annoying acts are behaviors that may not be desired but do not violate an administrative code of conduct. Annoying acts are usually included in the institution's policy informing the student of behaviors that are or are not expected of the student. Student conduct policies can address poor interpersonal communication skills, such as monopolizing class discussion, and discourteous, abrasive, aggressive, or hard-to-get-along-with behaviors. Annoying acts may also include poor time- or life-management skills, entering class late or leaving class early, or repeated excuses for poor performance. From a developmental perspective, addressing annoying behaviors in the learning environment offers a tremendous opportunity to assist the student toward professional comportment.

It is important for the educator to be mindful of the manner used to communicate with a student regarding annoying behaviors. In confronting students regarding annoying behaviors, faculty are keeping small problems small and possibly avoiding an escalation of behaviors along the continuum. The risk management level is low, but over time these types of behaviors can escalate. Although these behaviors are at the more benign end of the continuum, it is best to document any observed behaviors and interactions with students regarding their conduct.

The key in responding to annoying behaviors is to keep grounded in the learning experience, even though the behavior is annoying to you. When talking with students about annoying behaviors, focus on the importance of the learning environment and on the goal of meeting or exceeding the course learning objectives. You are not simply asking the student to be polite or thoughtful; you are exploring with the student how his or her behavior is not serving him or her, you, or the rest of the learning community. Based on these authors' experience, most likely once faculty have met with a student who displays annoying behavior, brought these behaviors to the attention of the student, and suggested new behaviors, no further misconduct will occur. In fact, coaching sessions can often lay the foundation for a productive teaching–learning–mentoring relationship.

From a professional educational standpoint, it is important to note that these annoying acts, left unchecked, may subsequently manifest themselves in the professional workplace. Clearly and consistently holding students accountable for their actions has an immediate effect on the individual as a learner and a future effect on the individual in his or her professional life.

Administrative Violations

Administrative violations are behaviors that violate an administrative code of conduct. Administrative violations include a variety of behaviors that significantly disrupt the learning process, such as acts of intimidation or harassment. These behaviors may be motivated by a desire to gain an academic advantage through scholastic misconduct, such as cheating, plagiarism, or fabricating results. Because codes or policies of student conduct are unique to each institution, it is strongly recommended that faculty acquaint themselves with their institution's code to know when a student may have violated policy. Chapter 3 further discusses the ethical issues related to academic dishonesty.

From a developmental perspective, there may be an opportunity to assist the student, but this will depend on the incident and the student's disposition and attitude for change. For instance, an incident involving an alcohol-impaired student coming to an on-campus class that has a zero tolerance for such behavior would limit faculty's ability to work with the student in a coaching capacity. If faculty have reason to believe that a student has violated the campus student code, the best approach is to document the faculty's observations, when reasonably possible talk with the student, and engage the student to fully understand the situation. If after talking with the student it continues to appear that a violation has occurred, then documentation of the student's behavior should be referred to the appropriate administrative officer as prescribed by campus policy.

It is important to communicate with the student regarding any allegations of misconduct. In confronting students regarding possible violations, the sooner you confront the student, the better. It might be advisable to contact your department chair to assist you in talking with the student. In confronting the student immediately, you avoid an escalation of behaviors along the continuum. The risk management level is moderate but over time these types of behaviors can escalate and increase the administrative severity and the possibility of the behavior violating local, state, or federal law. These behaviors should be documented, as should interactions with students regarding their conduct. Faculty should expect that the incident will be referred to the appropriate administrative office for disciplinary review.

Criminal Conduct

Criminal conduct can be characterized as behaviors that violate local, state, or federal criminal law. Criminal conduct includes a variety of behaviors that significantly disrupt the learning process, such as threats or acts of violence, stalking, intimidation, harassment, possession of firearms, drugs, alcohol, or theft. Because local and state laws can vary and the application of the law to college populations can vary as well, it is strongly recommended that faculty acquaint themselves with the practices at their institution. It is also recommended that faculty discuss these legal issues with their department chair and fellow colleagues so that they become familiar with the historical context and institutional practice.

Title IX of the Education Amendments of 1972 prohibits discrimination based on sex, including harassment and the continuum of sexual violence. Historically, Title IX has been inconsistently enforced on campuses across the nation, with the issue often clouded because of drug or alcohol use by those involved. Guidance in the application of Title IX states that sexual violence "refers to physical sexual acts perpetrated against a person's will or where a person is incapable of giving consent due to the victim's use of drugs or alcohol" (United States Department of Education, 2011). To promote a safe learning environment and comply with Title IX, faculty should act on and report all suspected incidents of sex discrimination or violence in a timely manner, regardless of whether the victim chooses to report the incident to law enforcement.

From a developmental perspective, acts that are determined to be criminal allow very little opportunity to assist the student and should be quickly relegated to campus and local law enforcement personnel for investigation and disposition. For instance, an incident involving one student threatening to injure a fellow student limits faculty's ability to work with the student in a coaching capacity. If faculty have reason to believe that a student has acted criminally, the best approach is to document their observations and immediately report the observations to the appropriate campus law enforcement personnel.

When criminal conduct is suspected, it is important for faculty to inform their immediate supervisor (e.g., department chair) of the incident and contact campus law enforcement. Each situation will dictate the faculty's role regarding any further engagement with the student regarding her or his behavior. In many cases, as the student's instructors, faculty may know the student best and could become a vital resource as to the most constructive approach to take with the student to minimize any threat of violence or disruption to the student and to the greater learning community. The risk management level is high and all exchanges with the student should be carefully coordinated with campus law enforcement and the campus office responsible for student conduct to limit an escalation of criminal conduct.

The campus administration may further hold the student accountable for an administrative violation of the student code of conduct following an investigation of the alleged behavior. It is important to understand that a university or college cannot and should not insulate the student from being held accountable for criminal actions. These behaviors should be well documented. Faculty should expect that the incident will be referred to the appropriate administrative unit for disciplinary review. Pursuing a single incident through multiple levels of the university as well as pursuing both criminal and administrative action is not considered double jeopardy; rather it is a result of multiple jurisdictions properly responding to a single behavior.

Proactive Response Strategies

With an emphasis on preventing inappropriate behavior altogether, this section describes a series of actions that faculty can implement when managing a learning environment. These strategies can be applied to learning in a conventional classroom, in off-campus settings, and in online learning environments. It is also recommended that faculty within a department discuss these strategies and adopt common practices. Students will notice common practices from class to class, which helps to reinforce these strategies (Jones & Philp, 2011, p. 22).

Forewarning in the Course Syllabus

An important first step in managing the learning environment is taking early action to prevent problematic behavior. This can be done in a variety of ways, including being attentive to creating a climate of civility from day one of class. Novice faculty tend to assume that college students intrinsically understand professional behavioral expectations of them. This may be a false assumption. It is imperative that appropriate behavior be explicitly described, both in the syllabus and on the first day of class.

In the course syllabus, faculty should express their goals and expectations for the learning environment. The program or institution may also have specific expectations or policies that faculty are required to insert into syllabi. The syllabus is a performance agreement between faculty and students. As such, it is an opportunity to express the ground rules and guidelines for engagement. This is the time that faculty should outline student behaviors that matter most to them as educators. Faculty should keep the discussion positive and indicate the behaviors they wish to see demonstrated by students. Faculty should also connect these behaviors to the achievement of the learning outcomes established for the course.

For example, if students arriving to class on time and remaining through the entire class period is an important component of the learning environment, then express this expectation in the syllabus and also indicate the rationale for this expectation. For all expectations, it is also recommended that faculty provide students with a way to manage these expectations. If a student knows that he or she will not be able to arrive at a class on time, what should the student do? Should the student not attend at all? Should the student call faculty in advance of the class and discuss the need to arrive late? Is there a place (e.g., the back row of the class) that has been designated as an area where students who arrive late or must leave early should sit so as not to disrupt the learning of others?

Clearly stating expectations in writing to students from the first day together helps students understand the behaviors faculty expect from the outset. This approach also provides faculty with a guide in case a student acts in a manner that has been previously determined unacceptable. As instructors, faculty are in a position to set standards that students must meet. These standards may be both academic and behavioral. The key is that they are clearly expressed and consistently expected of all students.

The syllabus is historically the document that articulates the basic relationship between student and instructor. Although a syllabus cannot present text for every concern, including text that expresses "the ground rules" or the rules of engagement between the instructor and students is often one way to create an environment designed to minimize conflict. Three types of suggested text are offered for your consideration in Box 14-3. The examples offered are suggestions and should be customized to support the established culture and values of your particular program and university or college.

Reviewing the Institutional Code of Conduct

With expectations clearly outlined in the syllabus, the first class meeting of the semester is a time to outline behavioral expectations for the course. In addition to sharing faculty expectations particular to the course, it is also appropriate to inform students about any policies that the institution has established to guide student conduct. It is recommended that faculty briefly address the sections of the institutional student conduct policy that have meaning for the specific learning objectives of the

BOX 14-3 Examples of Text for the Syllabus

TEACHING–LEARNING PHILOSOPHY

My expectation is that you are a self-motivated learner. By the end of the semester you will have invested your time, energy, and resources to complete this course and I want you to be successful. My responsibility as your instructor is to provide a context and environment that supports your learning through mindful, intentional curriculum that guides your investigations and learning. I expect you to be an involved, active member of this learning community who will contribute with thorough preparation, active discussion participation, and timely participation in course activities. I further expect that you will treat everyone, including the instructor, with respect and civility. Learning in this course takes place through lectures, readings, written analysis, reflective discussions, critical reflection, and written assignments.

CLASS EXPECTATIONS

This course will be most successful when all participants commit to developing a learning community in which the beliefs of all may be discussed in an open, civil, and understanding environment. Everyone will be expected to consider multiple perspectives, engage in critical reflection, and take intellectual risks built on one's confidence in the course content. Class activities will focus on critical analysis of (1) course readings, (2) case study scenarios, (3) group work, and (4) research findings. Your personal experiences are important but require critical reflection and analysis. Hence the ability to interact with the material in a personal and self-reflective manner is essential.

PROFESSIONAL EXPECTATIONS

Becoming a professional is not simply a matter of possessing a degree. Becoming a professional is agreeing to a set of standards of behavior now, as a student, that models the behavior that will be expected of you once you complete your professional program.

1. Be on time. Arrive 10 minutes prior to your expected time and be prepared to begin class or lab. Leave with plenty of time in case you encounter delays.
2. Be present every day! Your instructor has created specific lesson plans with the expectation that you will be present every class day. On what should be a rare occasion, it is imperative that if you are unable to keep your commitment, you contact your instructor as soon as possible. Ask the instructor what is the best way for you to communicate with them. Write down his or her e-mail or phone number and have it with you at all times.
3. Be professional! Maintain a professional attitude and be positive! You never get a second chance to make a first impression.
4. Know what is expected of you every day. Read your syllabus. Note all course obligations on your calendar and check your calendar daily.
5. Leave your cell phone off and out of sight. Focus on being present in the class and with your work.
6. Collegiality. Now, as a student, and in the future, as a professional, you will interact with and work extensively with your peers and colleagues. Work to be a positive influence and a productive colleague to your peers.
7. Ethics. As a student, learn and reflect on the ethical expectations of the profession and begin reflecting on your current daily decisions within an ethical context. Realize that the decisions and choices you make every day build on your ability to make decisions and actions on behalf of others you will be responsible for in the future.
8. Collaboration. As a professional you will collaborate with patients, family members, and other professional colleagues in providing care. As a student today you will be expected to collaborate in a positive, civil, and mutually beneficial way that will build your skills and understanding of working with groups of people to achieve a common goal.

course. This is the time for faculty to describe their expectations and interpretations of the code. It is also appropriate for faculty to provide positive examples of the behavior they wish to see exhibited by the students and engage the students in a discussion about these expectations. One exercise is to ask the students to describe annoying or disruptive behaviors they have seen from their fellow classmates in other classes and to talk about how important it is that each person agree to not act in a manner that disrupts learning in the classroom.

Being Transparent

Another way in which faculty can minimize problematic behavior is to be as transparent as possible with students regarding development of assignments and rationale for decision making and grading. Open communication about how the course has been developed and how decisions have been made serve to decrease student perceptions that an instructor's actions are arbitrary or even malicious. Evidence suggests that students may potentially respond disruptively when they disagree with grading decisions, when they receive an unsatisfactory clinical grade, or when they receive a failing grade for a course (Luparell, 2004). Perceptions that an instructor acts in an arbitrary manner, especially where grades are concerned, may result in a student misbehaving out of frustration.

Establishing a Trusting Environment

A trusting relationship between student and faculty is essential to creating an environment in which students can mature professionally (Shanta & Eliason, 2014). Faculty frequently need to deliver critical feedback that is constructive in nature. It is false to assume that students understand the benevolent and professional motives behind providing such feedback; they are often unprepared to receive feedback that is not wholly positive. Consequently, it is beneficial to elucidate the purpose of constructive feedback in students' professional development. A sample script for initiating this discussion can be found in Box 14-4. Once the underlying basis of trust has been established, a more conducive environment for the give and take of constructive feedback is created.

BOX 14-4 Elucidating the Role of Trust in Giving Constructive Feedback

Providing you with feedback on your performance and progress is a crucial component of this course. While often that feedback will be positive and address your strengths, at times I may need to share constructive feedback that focuses on areas that are not as well developed. I am willing to trust that you want this feedback to meet your educational goals. I ask that you trust that my sole motivation for giving you this feedback is to help you be successful in your development.

Providing Effective Behavioral Feedback

Students often are unaware of how their behaviors are perceived. In a trusting environment in which the student's professional development is a priority, faculty have a responsibility to provide concrete and specific feedback regarding behaviors that may impede a student's progress. A template for crafting such a discussion has been shared elsewhere (Luparell, 2007a) and may be found in Box 14-5. It is important to note that the script provides students with the choice to continue the behavior or not, based on whether they are concerned with the outcomes of their behavior. Students almost always choose to discontinue the annoying behavior. However, if the behavior continues you will need to address it more assertively by requesting unequivocally that it stop.

Know Who to Contact for Consultation

Sooner or later faculty will need to seek consultation regarding a student's behavior. There are important legal underpinnings that must guide faculty when addressing student misbehavior. See Chapter 3 for a more detailed discussion of the legal implications associated with disciplinary action for student misbehavior. In particular, students retain their constitutional rights of free speech and due process and these rights must be considered when addressing student misconduct. However, most novice nurse educators are not well-acquainted with the legal aspects of education. For this reason, it is important to seek assistance from knowledgeable individuals at the outset.

Every college or university has designated individuals who respond to issues regarding student behavior. There are no consistent titles or standardized credentials, and every institution, through its history, context, mission, vision, values, and goals, has constructed individualized approaches to how student behavior is managed. It is best if faculty

BOX 14-5 Sample Script for Giving Feedback Related to Problematic Behavior

Hi ______,

Thank you for coming in to see me. Remember the first day of class when we talked about the role of trust in giving feedback? I have some feedback to share with you now that may be a bit difficult to hear. Please remember that I'm sharing it with you so you can successfully meet your goal of becoming a competent nurse. When you do __________, it leaves me with the impression that ______.

If I have that impression, it's likely that others may have it as well. If you are okay with people drawing this conclusion about you, then keep on doing what you are doing. If you are not comfortable with people potentially drawing this conclusion, you may want to consider a change.

The following is an example of the script put to use with a student who does not put good effort into completing postclinical paperwork:

Hi Mary,

Thank you for coming in to see me. Remember the first day of class when we talked about the role of trust in giving feedback? I have some feedback to share with you now that may be a bit difficult to hear. Please remember that I'm sharing it with you so you can successfully meet your goal of becoming a competent nurse. When you turn in your clinical packet so insufficiently completed, it leaves me with the impression either that you really don't understand what is going on with your patient or that you are a bit of a slacker. If I have that impression, it's likely that others may have it as well. If you are okay with people drawing the conclusion that you really don't understand what you are doing or that you are a slacker, then keep on doing what you are doing. If you are not comfortable with people potentially drawing this conclusion, you may want to consider a change.

reacquaint themselves annually with the key people on campus who should be consulted regarding student behavior concerns. Consultants can include staff from such offices as the dean of students, counseling, advising, student health services, student ombudsman, student advocate, faculty professional development, student affairs, student life, human resources, or the campus police. Faculty are encouraged to inquire of their faculty colleagues and administrators as to which offices and staff have provided helpful counsel in the past, depending on the student situation. Faculty should also know who is responsible for administering the institutional student code of conduct. It is helpful to have established a working relationship with these individuals in advance of contacting them with a particular student concern. The key point is that, as instructors, faculty are supported in responding to student conduct in the classroom and have the institutional support of other professionals with specialized expertise in handling student issues.

Know When to Call for Consultation

Just as important as knowing who to call for consultation is knowing when to call for consultation and when to refer an unresolved matter to others. Quite often faculty dwell on an unresolved matter with a student much longer than necessary, which is distracting to the teaching and learning experience for the entire class. Let us assume that a faculty member has outlined during the first class the behaviors that are expected from her or his students to facilitate learning. Let us further assume that discussion of behavioral expectations also included identification of the student conduct code, with statements detailing how the code provides institutional support for the faculty's expectations. If the faculty member has outlined student behavior expectations in the syllabus, met with the student, and made the student aware that his or her behavior is not meeting the standard that has been set for the class, and the student either refuses or is unable to change the behavior to meet the expected standard, then the faculty member should immediately consult with others, such as the department chair, to identify other ways to work with the student or to request a referral to another office on campus. As mentioned earlier, the timing of a referral also depends on the unique circumstances and the continuum of behaviors observed. If at any time faculty feel their safety or the safety of others is at risk, then campus law enforcement should immediately be contacted. If, on the other hand, faculty are responding to an annoying act, then they may wish to meet with the student on repeated occasions to address a variety of issues that are adversely affecting the student's academic success.

Documentation and Communication

It is important for faculty to keep notes of student behaviors that have been observed. Faculty may observe behaviors that are not desired but that do not violate the established classroom standard or the campus student code. One reason to note these "below the radar" behaviors is that they can escalate to a level that would ultimately violate the classroom standard or the campus student code. At that point, it would be helpful when faculty meet with a student to be able to note the specific patterns of behaviors observed. Students are often surprised faculty have taken note of problematic behaviors and want to talk with them about their conduct.

Keeping personal notes may also be helpful if faculty need to refer an incident to others. The information important to document includes time, day, and place where the behavior was observed. It is also important to use descriptive and not evaluative statements. To say that the student was "rude" is not helpful; however, to document that "the student has arrived late to four of the last six classes, which disrupted the class lecture when the student attempted to locate a seat in class" is helpful, because it is specific and allows the faculty to talk with the student in a way that focuses on student behaviors and not on how the faculty may feel about those behaviors.

There is often a misunderstanding among faculty and staff throughout colleges and universities regarding documentation and communication of students' behaviors and students' privacy rights. These misunderstandings center around an interpretation of federal legislation called the Family Educational Rights and Privacy Act (FERPA). Pursuant to FERPA (United States Department of Education, 2007), faculty and staff may and, in fact, should share information about a student when a "legitimate educational interest" exists. Matters of classroom management, student conduct or misconduct, and behaviors of concern fall within a legitimate educational interest. The Department of Education acknowledges there is a balance between students' rights to privacy and the university's responsibility to ensure stability and public safety. As such,

> The University [may] disclose education[al] records without a student's prior written consent under the FERPA exception for disclosure to school officials with legitimate educational interests. A school official is a person employed by the University in an administrative, supervisory, academic or research, or support staff position (including law enforcement unit personnel and health staff); a person or company with whom the University has contracted as its agent to provide a service instead of using University employees or officials (such as an attorney, auditor, or collection agent); a person serving on the Board of Trustees; or a student serving on an official committee, such as a disciplinary or grievance committee, or assisting another school official in performing his or her tasks.

Therefore you should communicate with your department chair when you become aware of possible student behavioral concerns. It is good practice to keep the department chair updated as to any documentation, meetings, or other actions regarding student behavior issues.

Discipline as an Educational Experience

Faculty may want to simply eject a student from a class, because the faculty is offended, annoyed, or feels that the student has acted in a disrespectful manner; however, it is vitally important for faculty to frame their interactions with the student within an educational framework. Setting standards of conduct within a learning environment is part of the educational and professional preparatory experience. Students learn that there are standards of conduct as well as consequences to not meeting these standards, which contributes to their preparation for their postdegree work. Developing the discipline and focus to arrive to class on time will contribute to students' ability to effectively complete work-related duties and helps increase their understanding of the importance of collegiality, connectedness, and teamwork as a means toward achieving a quality working environment. The integrity required to ethically complete laboratory work by submitting only the results that they have personally calculated and not use the work of other students is the same integrity that will be required of graduates when they are in the workforce completing work-related reports.

Responding to Student Misconduct

When faculty have reason to believe that a student may be acting inappropriately, there are six steps to use when responding to allegations of misconduct:

1. *Gather and document information.* The information should objectively describe the student's actions and note the date, time, and others who were present.
2. *Engage and confront the student about behaviors observed.* At the earliest time possible, meet

with the student privately to discuss the behaviors that have been observed. This meeting will inform the student of faculty concerns, allow the student to express his or her perspective on the situation, and provide an opportunity for the student to understand how the behavior affects others and is disrupting the learning outcomes of the course. The script provided earlier in the chapter may be helpful here.

3. *Focus on the behavior.* Faculty should always focus on what the student did and not be swayed by ancillary aspects, such as the extent to which one knows or likes the student or the student's academic record. For instance, high-achieving students are just as likely to plagiarize as average students. It is important to be consistent in what is expected from students.
4. *Outline required new behaviors.* The purpose of meeting with the student is to first explore with the student concerns about her or his behavior. If after talking with the student the concerns remain valid, then the second goal of the meeting is to discuss with the student how the behavior should change in the future. Working with the student to change any annoying acts provides the greatest opportunity for a collaborative discussion between the student and the faculty. Any administrative violations of the code of conduct should be documented and forwarded to the appropriate administrative office and, depending on campus policy, may be followed up administratively in addition to actions the faculty has discussed with the student. All criminal conduct should be immediately forwarded to the appropriate campus office and may limit faculty's ability to outline new behaviors.
5. *Outline consequences of compliance and noncompliance.* Faculty interactions with the student should conclude with the hope that the student will choose to make different choices and will choose to comply with the standards that faculty and the campus have established. However, it is also important to be clear with the student that, should he or she fail to comply and continue to disrupt the learning environment, there will be additional follow-up that may include further sanctions.
6. *Refer unresolved or risky cases to other campus resources.* If at any time faculty are working with a student and it comes to their attention that the student's misconduct is not being resolved as planned, or if there is evidence that the incident may escalate in terms of level of disruption or safety to either the faculty or other students, the situation should automatically be referred to other campus resources.

Campus Resources

As stated previously, it is recommended that faculty become familiar with the services, programs, and personnel who staff their institution's campus support resources before they actually need their assistance. Campus resources can include counseling services, student health services, police, department chair, dean of students, and services for students with disabilities. Depending on the history and context of the institution, there may be other support services, including campus ministries and specialized centers for specific populations of students such as women, people of color, or gay, lesbian, or transgender students. Regarding behaviors of concern that rise to the level of safety for individuals or groups, universities have increasingly established formal committees that convene to conduct a broad review of a student's behavior in order to coordinate a comprehensive and organized response. Coordination of a team of professionals who can work together to assess threats and identify problems is preferred to individual faculty working alone. It is best to have multiple offices come together on a case-by-case basis and form a team to assess the situation and achieve the desired results. One easy way to develop relationships with these support services is to invite personnel from one or two of these offices to present introductory information about their offices to faculty within the nursing program and to explore how and when students should be referred as a part of the program's faculty professional development activities.

Implications for Practice

Novice faculty are frequently unprepared for the diverse challenges that arise in classroom management. It is important to recognize early that you are likely to experience some degree of student misconduct in your teaching career. *Thus it is wise to consider in advance how you might respond in specific situations.* Working with students effectively and managing the classroom learning environment in a manner that meets or exceeds the learning objectives of the course requires instructors to consider how they will approach the management of the learning environments for which they have accepted responsibility. Faculty may find it helpful to consider their emotional assets as discussed in Goleman's (2005) work on emotional intelligence. His work is a helpful guide for developing the faculty's role as a learning facilitator and developing strategies for engaging students in interventions regarding their conduct.

Additionally, because it is tempting to ignore inappropriate behavior and avoid or delay having difficult conversations with students, it may be helpful for faculty to consider various ethical imperatives that serve as a compelling rationale for action. For example, most nursing education programs have established objectives or standards related to professional behavior. Additionally, we are reminded in the Code of Ethics for Nurses (American Nurses Association, 2001) that educators are responsible for ensuring that our students demonstrate "commitment to professional practice prior to entry" (p. 13) into practice. When students consistently behave inappropriately, there is an argument to be made that they do not meet the standard of professionalism.

Unwillingness or inability to address poor behavior may have more far-reaching implications than have previously been acknowledged. Horizontal violence and disruptive behavior are unfortunate phenomena in health care and have been linked to negative patient outcomes (Institute for Safe Medication Practices, 2013; Shanta & Eliason, 2014). Faculty frequently express concern that poorly behaving students may subsequently behave poorly as practicing nurses, and evidence exists to support this concern. Physicians, for example, who have been disciplined for unprofessional behavior are more likely to have displayed problem behavior as students (Papadakis et al., 2005). More recently, Luparell and Frisbee (2014, unpublished data) conducted a large national study to explore nursing faculty knowledge of poorly behaving or uncivil students who went on to demonstrate uncivil or unprofessional behavior as practicing nurses. One third of the faculty respondents (n = 1869) reported knowing of a former badly behaving student who went on to demonstrate bad behavior in practice.

When managing the learning environment, faculty are setting both learning and behavioral expectations. In setting these expectations, faculty must also monitor and evaluate how these expectations are fulfilled. As such, faculty's own self-awareness becomes important when considering the extent to which students meet the standards that have been set. It is important that faculty observe themselves and recognize their feelings as they engage with students. As the instructor, faculty have administrative power over the student and the responsibility to act civilly, objectively, and consistently.

To effectively manage the learning environment, faculty need to appropriately and effectively manage their own emotions. Nursing faculty have reported experiencing negative emotions when subjected to student incivility, including feelings of decreased self-esteem, a loss in their confidence as teachers, resentment related to the time involved in documenting student misconduct incidents, and a loss of motivation to teach (Luparell, 2007b). It is paramount that faculty be cognizant of their own feelings about students and what is behind these personal responses to student behavior. Of course, the ultimate responsibility of faculty is to find ways to manage their emotions so that they do not interfere with the learning environment. Feelings such as fear, anxiety, anger, and sadness can cause faculty to avoid engaging students. Failing to engage or confront students limits faculty ability to manage the learning environment. These feelings can also skew faculty observations of student behavior. If a faculty member believes that a student is acting inappropriately, and remains reluctant to engage the student in a discussion about these behaviors, the faculty's feelings may be an underlying issue that needs to be addressed as well. Campus faculty teaching and professional development services can be a valuable resource in assisting faculty to develop strategies for effective student conferences.

As faculty engage with their students in learning experiences, a key to effective management is maintaining sensitivity to others' feelings and concerns and the ability to consider others' perspectives. Awareness of generational differences in understanding and response to behavioral expectations and consequences may assist faculty in engaging with students in a positive manner (Lake, 2009). Clark and Springer (2007) conducted a study of nursing faculty and students that indicated that students and faculty had different perceptions of what constituted uncivil behavior on the part of students *and* faculty. Baxter and Boblin (2007) also stated that nursing faculty and students may disagree on what constitutes dishonest behavior, especially in the classroom. When confronting a student about behavior and how it appears that the behavior is disrupting the learning environment, appreciating the differences in how people perceive and respond to situations will be helpful when communicating with students about what constitutes appropriate behavior in the learning environment. These differences in perceptions between faculty and students further illustrate the importance of faculty being explicit about the behaviors that are expected of students at the very initiation of the learning experience.

Online teaching includes a number of misconduct and incivility issues that may manifest in particular ways because of the lack of face-to-face interaction among participants. Faculty can integrate increased social presence and instructor–student interaction within completely online courses through a variety of means, including the use of short videos or podcasts prepared by the instructor so that students may see and hear the instructor actually discuss course concepts, timely discussion forum responses to student postings, and emails to students to provide individualized feedback or encouragement. Online instructors are encouraged to address incivility in the learning environment promptly and to hold offenders accountable (Clark, Ahten, & Werth, 2012).

The Faculty–Student Learning Relationship

Faculty often ask what their rights and responsibilities as instructors are and what rights and responsibilities students have as learners. Rights and responsibilities are guided by constitutional law, state law, and institutional policy. Private and public colleges and universities have been treated differently by the courts in that private institutions are seen more as private corporate entities and public institutions are considered to be agents of the government (Kaplin & Lee, 2006). Regardless of the type of institution, see Box 14-6 for an example of the rights and responsibilities that are generally held as good practice when working with students in a learning setting.

BOX 14-6 Conduct Guidelines and Grievance Procedures for Students

STUDENTS HAVE THE RIGHT TO:

- Expect confidentiality of personal information (with exception of directory information).
- Appeal any University status (i.e., scholastic suspension, financial aid suspension, conducts sanction, etc.).
- File a grievance against appropriate university employees or processes.
- Voice dissent of University decisions and processes.
- Have support to pursue changes to University policy.

FACULTY HAVE THE RESPONSIBILITY TO:

- Provide students with timely information regarding important aspects of the course, including students' obligations and responsibilities concerning both academic and personal conduct.
- Be prompt and well-prepared for class meetings and be timely and fair in grading assignments and exams.
- Refrain from considering personal information such as race, religion, age, and political beliefs in matters of academic evaluation.
- Be available to students and post liberal office hours at hours convenient to students.

STUDENTS HAVE THE RESPONSIBILITY TO:

- Be prompt, well-prepared, and regular in attending classes.
- Submit honest representations of one's own work and in a timely fashion.
- Act in a respectful manner toward other students and instructors in a way that does not detract from the learning experience.
  - Respect the personal and property rights of others.
  - Meet the course and behavior standards as defined by the instructor.
- Seek assistance from the instructor and other appropriate student resources as needed.
- Enjoy and participate in University programs.

Adapted from the *Montana State University Conduct Guidelines and Grievance Procedures for Students*. Available at www.montana.edu/policy/student_conduct/ and http://www.montana.edu/deanofstudents/studentrights.html

If an institution or program does not have clearly established expectations for the behaviors of students and faculty, these policies should be developed (Clark & Springer, 2007). In addition to faculty development activities, student development activities should also be provided by the institution to assist students in coping with the multiple stressors many are facing in their lives and to help students identify appropriate and inappropriate behaviors.

Lastly, when contemplating the consequences of student incivility directed at faculty, program leaders should contemplate the general well-being of the faculty workforce. Student incivility has been weakly correlated to decreased job satisfaction in one preliminary study (Frisbee, 2013). Additionally, new evidence suggests that more than a few nursing faculty have left teaching positions because of unpleasant interactions with students (Luparell & Frisbee, 2014, unpublished data).

Summary

Faculty have more contact time with students than anyone else in the educational setting. Faculty are the key to developing quality learning environments that allow for the civil exchange of information and ideas. Faculty and administrators must be able to recognize the early warning signs of student misconduct such as unhealthy obsessions and specific verbal clues—expressions of hopelessness, direct or indirect threats, or suicidal language—and then report them. Working with a team of campus professionals and faculty to effectively engage troubled students is a critical aspect to classroom management. When a student is struggling in a class or is affected by drugs or alcohol or by financial or relationship problems, faculty are often instrumental to successfully assisting students. When a student's behavior interferes with the educational process or campus safety, the institution can consider a range of options in response. This chapter provided some insight into those options.

This chapter provided a brief summary of developmental, legal, and risk management considerations of student misconduct and learning. Additionally, specific actions were presented that can be used to reduce in-class disruptions and maintain a well-managed learning environment, allowing both the instructor and students to meet their learning objectives in a civil manner. The goal of this chapter is to help future faculty gain an understanding of problem or disruptive student behavior, in addition to an understanding of specific steps and available professional resources one can use to minimize disruptions in a learning environment.

CASE STUDIES FOR FURTHER DISCUSSION

The following three case studies illustrate the continuum of student misconduct behaviors, the developmental opportunities, and the instructional management risks that faculty may experience when managing the learning environment.

Annoying Acts

The Situation: Alexandra

Alexandra is a first-semester student who wants to talk with you before, during, and after class, often about personal, non–course-related items. Alexandra appears emotionally needy and does not appear to have any friends in class. Lately she has started interrupting others during in-class discussion. The other students don't listen to her and have asked not to be in her lab group.

At the point that Alexandra's behavior begins to disrupt your ability to lecture in class and the students' ability to learn, you need to meet with her. At the end of one class session you ask her to come to your office. During your meeting with Alexandra, you let her know that you value her as a student and that you have enjoyed getting to know her but that recently you have noticed that she has begun interrupting students during class discussion. You ask her about her studies and how she feels the class is progressing. She mentions that she is having a tough time making friends in her program and does not know what to do, and that at times she feels very alone and isolated. You let her know that her comments are valuable, but that she also needs to allow other students to be heard. You point out that listening is a part of learning and that you would like her to wait and allow her fellow students time to make their points in class. You also let Alexandra know that making friends is important and studying in groups is helpful to learning. You suggest that Alexandra talk with a counselor at the campus counseling center to gain some ideas on how to develop these friendships on campus. As a follow-up to your meeting, you set a time to meet in 3 weeks to talk about her work in class and her overall progress in the program.

CASE STUDIES FOR FURTHER DISCUSSION— CONT'D

Administrative Violations

The Situation: Adam

It is the middle of the semester and it has become common for Adam to dominate the conversation in class. He has often become angry and visibly agitated and he uses incendiary language when interacting with other students. He is constantly challenging the material you present. When he is not present, the class is more productive and more relaxed. You realize that you have avoided talking with Adam about his behavior. You talk with him, describe his behaviors in class, and talk about how you would like him to participate in class discussion in the future and the importance of working cooperatively with his fellow students. Adam begins to argue with you and refuses to consider your request that he reflect on his own conduct. He blames other students who have "disrespected" him. During the next class, Adam's behavior escalates and is disruptive to the point that you are not able to cover the material planned for that day. You decide to forward a referral to your department chair for review and advice as to next steps.

The department chair receives your documentation and informs you that two other faculty have sent similar reports about Adam over the last year. The department chair contacts the dean of students' office and forwards all three referrals for review and action. Adam's lack of cooperation makes it difficult to approach him developmentally and his response pushes the situation to a level that violates administrative policies. The risks to manage are increasing as well, which makes it important to involve other campus offices.

The department chair, associate dean, and you meet with Adam. A behavioral contract is drawn up between the department chair and Adam. Adam agrees to adhere to the standards set in your class, and his conduct is being referred to the dean of students for administrative review as a violation of the student code of conduct.

Criminal Cases

The Situation: Cathy

Cathy is a senior in her last year of the program. You have taught Cathy before in a previous class and you are surprised that she has almost completed the program, because she has been a chronically weak student and has difficulty working with others in a clinical setting.

About three weeks into the semester a student reports to you that Cathy is very angry with a fellow student in class and has vandalized the student's car in order to "get even." You contact your department chair, who contacts the campus police and the dean of students' office.

The police investigate the allegations and criminal charges are brought against Cathy by the police. The dean of students initiates administrative disciplinary proceedings and Cathy is placed on disciplinary probation until she completes her degree. Cathy is moved to another class and is told to have no contact with the student whose car she vandalized. A condition of Cathy's probation is to attend counseling.

REFLECTING ON THE EVIDENCE

1. From a student perspective, faculty are central to the learning experience. Many of our students spend the greatest amount of time in class interacting with faculty. As such, faculty have the opportunity to cultivate relationships with students and are often in the best position to become aware of inappropriate conduct. How can faculty in a nursing program collectively cultivate an environment that positively contributes to learning and proactively responds to student misconduct?
2. As faculty, you have became aware that during the ninth week of the semester, one of your students went from performing quite well with good attendance, submitting all assignments on time and well done, and displaying a generally collegial demeanor to suddenly missing class, not turning in weekly assignments, and not returning e-mails. What is the best way to respond to this student?
3. While grading a lab assignment you notice that four students appear to have submitted identical work to the extent that you have become concerned that the students may have presented other people's work as their own. What is the best way to approach this situation? What could you have done to avoid or minimize this type of incident?
4. Under what circumstances do you ask for help in responding to possible student misconduct?

REFERENCES

Altmiller, G. (2012). Student perceptions of incivility in nursing education: Implications for educators. *Nursing Education Perspectives*, *33*(1), 15–20.

American Nurses Association. (2001). *Code of ethics for nurses with interpretive statements*. Washington, DC: American Nurses Publishing.

Baxter, P., & Boblin, S. (2007). The moral development of baccalaureate nursing students: Understanding unethical behavior in the classroom and clinical settings. *Journal of Nursing Education*, *46*(1), 20–27.

Boice, B. (1996). Classroom incivilities. *Research in Higher Education*, *37*(4), 453–486.

Clark, C. M. (2008a). The dance of incivility in nursing education as described by nursing faculty and students. *Advances in Nursing Science*, *31*(4), E37.

Clark, C. M. (2008b). Faculty and student assessment of and experience with incivility in nursing education. *Journal of Nursing Education*, *47*(10), 458.

Clark, C. M., Ahten, S., & Werth, L. (2012). Cyber-bullying and incivility in an online learning environment, part 2. *Nurse Educator*, *37*(5), 192–197.

Clark, C., & Springer, P. (2007). Incivility in nursing education: A descriptive study of definitions and prevalence. *Journal of Nursing Education*, *46*(1), 7–14.

Del Prato, D. (2013). Students' voices: The lived experience of faculty incivility as a barrier to professional formation in associate degree nursing education. *Nurse Education Today*, *33*, 286–290.

Frisbee, K. (2013). *The relationship between incivility, job satisfaction, and intent to leave among nursing faculty* (Unpublished doctoral dissertation.) Cleveland, OH: Case Western Reserve University.

Goleman, D. (2005). *Emotional intelligence*. New York: Bantam Books.

Institute for Safe Medication Practices. (2013). Unresolved disrespectful behavior in healthcare: Practitioners speak up (again), Part 1. *ISMP Safety Alert Newsletter/Nurse Advise-ERR*, *11*(10), 1–4.

Jones, G., & Philp, C. (2011). Challenging student behavior. *Perspectives: Policy and Practice in Higher Education*, *15*(1), 19–23.

Kaplin, W. A., & Lee, B. A. (2006). *The law of higher education* (4th ed.). San Francisco: Jossey-Bass.

Lake, P. (2009). Student discipline: The case against legalistic approaches. *Chronicle of Higher Education*, *55*(32), A31–A32.

Lashley, F. R., & de Meneses, M. (2001). Student civility in nursing programs: A national survey. *Journal of Professional Nursing*, *17*(2), 81–86.

Levine, P. (2010). Teaching and learning civility. *New Directions for Higher Education*, *152*, 11–17.

Luparell, S. (2004). Faculty encounters with uncivil nursing students: An overview. *Journal of Professional Nursing*, *20*(1), 59–67.

Luparell, S. (2007a). Dealing with challenging student situations: Lessons learned. In M. H. Oermann & K. T. Heinrich (Eds.), *Challenges and new directions in nursing education: 5. Annual review of nursing education* (pp. 101–110). New York: Springer.

Luparell, S. (2007b). The effects of student incivility on nursing faculty. *Journal of Nursing Education*, *46*(1), 15–19.

Luparell, S., & Frisbee, K. (2014). *Do uncivil nursing students become uncivil nurses?* In Paper presented at National League for Nursing Education Summit, Phoenix, AZ.

Marchiondo, K., Marchiondo, L. A., & Lasiter, S. (2010). Faculty incivility: Effects on program satisfaction of BSN students. *Journal of Nursing Education*, *49*(11), 608–614.

Mott, J. (2014). Undergraduate nursing student experiences with faculty bullies. *Nurse Educator*, *39*(3), 143–148.

Papadakis, M. A., Teherani, A., Banach, M. A., Knettler, T. R., Rattner, S. L., Stern, D. T., et al. (2005). Disciplinary action by medical boards and prior behavior in medical school. *New England Journal of Medicine*, *353*(25), 2673–2682.

Porath, C. L., & Pearson, C. M. (2012). Emotional and behavioral responses to workplace incivility and the impact of hierarchical status. *Journal of Applied Social Psychology*, *42*, E326–E357. http://dx.doi.org/10.1111/j.1559-1816.2012.01020.x.

Shanta, L. L., & Eliason, A. R. M. (2014). Application of an empowerment model to improve civility in nursing education. *Nurse Education in Practice*, *14*, 82–86.

United States Department of Education. (2007, October). *Balancing student privacy and school safety: A guide to the Family Educational Rights and Privacy Act for colleges and universities.* Retrieved from, http://www2.ed.gov/policy/gen/guid/fpco/brochures/postsec.html.

United States Department of Education. (2011, April). *Dear colleague letter: Sexual violence.* Retrieved from, http://www2.ed.gov/about/offices/list/ocr/letters/colleague-201104.html.

Williamson, M. M. (2011). *Nurse educators' lived experiences with student incivility* (Doctoral dissertation). Retrieved from ProQuest Dissertations & Theses Full Text, ProQuest Dissertations & Theses Global (903973569) (Order No. 3478640).

15 Strategies to Promote Student Engagement and Active Learning*

Janet M. Phillips, PhD, RN, ANEF

Adopting teaching strategies to promote student engagement and active learning is a vital component of the faculty role. An abundant amount of research shows that students who are engaged in active learning are more likely to meet learning outcomes (National Survey of Student Engagement [NSSE], 2013) and apply the concepts in the practice setting (Blau & Snell, 2013). However, a study of a subset of nursing students who participated in the NSSE study found that undergraduate nursing students do not perceive themselves as being engaged in student-centered and interactive pedagogies, compared with students in other academic disciplines (Popkess & McDaniel, 2011). This creates a challenge for nursing faculty in terms of providing learning experiences that capture students' interest and engage them in active learning. This chapter provides evidence for the benefits of student engagement and offers a description of specific teaching strategies to promote active learning that can be used across all levels of nursing education and in a number of learning environments.

Student Engagement

The theory of student engagement has its roots in Astin's theory of student involvement (1999). The words *engagement* and *involvement* have become synonymous in the educational literature over time. The main premise is that highly involved students are more likely to learn academically and develop personally. There are five basic elements of the theory. First, *involvement* and *engagement* refer to the investment of physical and psychological energy in learning. Second, involvement and engagement occur along a continuum with different degrees of involvement at varying times. Third, involvement and engagement have both quantitative (i.e., hours studying) and qualitative (i.e., measurement of comprehension) aspects. Fourth, the amount of student learning is directly influenced by the quality and quantity of student involvement and engagement. Finally, the effectiveness of education is directly related to increasing students' involvement and engagement in the learning process.

Student engagement is based on Chickering and Gamson's (1987) seven principles of good practice in undergraduate education. According to Chickering and Gamson, if educators are able to facilitate student learning through these principles, students are more likely to meet learning outcomes. These principles are: (1) encourage contact between students and faculty, (2) develop reciprocity and cooperation among students, (3) encourage active learning, (4) give prompt feedback, (5) emphasize time on task, (6) communicate high expectations, and (7) respect diverse talents and ways of learning.

Different types of student engagement activities produce a variety of learning outcomes, emphasizing active participation in the learning process. For example, students who have frequent interaction with faculty are most satisfied with their learning experience and show greater learning outcomes (Hill, 2014; Lundberg, 2014). Students are more likely to be able to cope with the stresses of academic life if they are engaged in academic support systems (Bruce, Omne-Ponten, & Gustavsson, 2010). Student engagement can easily be measured through direct observation and measurement of a variety of academic engagement activities such as the number of hours studying, meeting course competencies, and student satisfaction surveys,

*The author acknowledges the work of Connie J. Rowles, DNS, RN, in the previous editions of the chapter.

among other factors (National Survey of Student Engagement, 2013).

The student engagement theory is applicable to nursing education because it directs attention away from the subject matter and teaching technique and toward the motivation and behavior of the student, taking into account its application to nursing practice. This is in line with transformational teaching, today's view of the psychology of learning, wherein it is the responsibility of the student to be active and engaged in the learning process, and the nurse educator uses a variety of teaching and learning experiences to become a facilitator or guide in the education process (Benner, Stuphen, Leonard, & Day, 2010; Slavich & Zimbardo, 2012). Active learning, a foundational component of Astin's (1999) theory based on Chickering and Gamson's (1987) seven principles of good practice in undergraduate education, is fundamental to student learning and requires student engagement.

The Evidence for Student Engagement

Evidence for the effect of engagement in higher education on student learning has been established through the NSSE (2013). In 14 years, surveys to 1500 colleges and universities in the United States and Canada have measured "student participation in programs and activities, providing estimates of how students spend their time and what they gain from attending college" (p. 6). Student engagement behavior is associated with desired outcomes of colleges. Results of the annual NSSE report (2013) of 335,000 students' engagement were categorized into five quality indicators. First, *academic challenge* illuminated the relationship between emphasizing higher-order learning and courses that students perceive as focusing on more complex topics, challenging their thinking skills. Second, *learning with peers,* or collaborative learning, enhanced student success by facilitating incentives to learn, shared comprehension of material, and support from peers. Third, *experiences with faculty* affected students' cognitive growth, development, and retention. Effective teaching practices included courses taught with clarity and organization and student feedback that is prompt and formative. Fourth, the *campus environment* showed that student interaction with a variety of individuals on campus, such as student services, academic advisors, and administrators, have a positive influence on learning outcomes. Fifth, *high-impact practices* (learning community, service-learning, or research with a faculty member) were found to increase knowledge, skills, and personal development, and students who used these practices stated that they were more satisfied with their educational experience. Lastly, *topical modules* (additional questions on topics of interest) showed that academic advising promoted student persistence and success through guiding students to programs and events that promote engagement. *Learning with technology,* the final module, showed that use of technology was positively related to student engagement and higher-order learning.

In a large-scale study of 438,756 community college student engagement (Community College Survey of Student Engagement [CCSSE], 2014), a number of benchmarks were established showing the relationship of engagement to learning outcomes. First, *active and collaborative learning* led to students learning based on their participation in class, interacting with other students, and learning outside of the classroom. In addition, learning was correlated with the number of terms enrolled and credit hours completed. The second benchmark, *student effort,* showed that students who spent the time necessary to learn content (time on task) were able to apply themselves to the learning process. The third benchmark, *academic challenge,* in which students engaged in challenging intellectual and creative work such as evaluation and synthesis, were most consistently associated with positive academic outcomes such as persistence, grade point average, and degree completion. The fourth benchmark, *student–faculty interaction,* measured the extent to which students and faculty communicate about academic performance, career plans, course content, and assignments, revealing that students had broad effective learning and persistence toward achievement of their educational goals. Lastly, the benchmark for *support of learners* demonstrated that students performed better and were more satisfied with their learning at colleges where their success was valued, and where positive working and social relationships existed among various demographic groups.

The engagement literature reveals four research perspectives for organizing teaching strategies (Zepke & Leach, 2010): (1) engaged students are intrinsically motivated and want to achieve their learning objectives autonomously or with others; (2) students and teachers engage with each other and respond to learning when the environment is creative, active, and collaborative; (3) institutions provide support that is conducive to learning with welcoming institutional cultures providing a variety of support services; and (4) students work together with their institution to develop social and cultural learning as active citizens. These evidence-based perspectives can be helpful in designing and adopting teaching and learning strategies for student engagement and active learning.

Adopting Teaching Strategies for Student Engagement

Faculty are influenced by a number of variables when selecting teaching strategies for active learning (Phillips & Vinten, 2010). Based on Everett Rogers' (2003) diffusion of innovations model, faculty are more likely to adopt teaching strategies that are compatible with their teaching needs, values, and experiences; whether they can be "tried out" before they are adopted; and whether it is more advantageous to students' learning needs than other teaching strategies. This evidence-based study sheds light on some of the variables that influence educators in adopting teaching strategies and can be taken into consideration when faculty are adopting them for student engagement and active learning.

Teaching Strategies

Bloom's revised taxonomy (Anderson & Krathwohl, 2001) can be used to categorize teaching strategies to promote student engagement. The knowledge dimension (or the kind of knowledge to be learned) is composed of four knowledge types: (1) factual, (2) conceptual, (3) procedural, and (4) metacognitive. *Factual knowledge* refers to the basic content students must know to be familiar with a discipline or to solve problems in it. *Conceptual knowledge* refers to the relationships between the basic fundamentals within a larger configuration enabling them to function together. *Procedural knowledge* refers to skills, techniques, and methods needed for specific disciplines. *Metacognitive knowledge* is the awareness of one's own cognition in addition to cognition in general. Learning objectives and outcomes for the knowledge types can be created using the six cognitive process dimensions of Bloom's revised taxonomy: (1) remember, (2) understand, (3) apply, (4) analyze, (5) evaluate, and (6) create. (See Chapter 10.)

Examples of select teaching strategies for student engagement are listed alphabetically in the four knowledge types (Anderson & Krathwohl, 2001) in the following sections, and may be used across classroom, laboratory, clinical, and online environments. Specific teaching strategies for simulations may be found in Chapter 18, technology-supported in the connected classroom may be found in Chapter 19, teaching at a distance in Chapter 20, and teaching online in Chapter 21.

Factual Knowledge

Factual knowledge represents the basic elements students must know to be acquainted with a discipline or solve problems in it. This knowledge is acquired through a combination of lecture, peer learning, seminar and small- or large-group discussions, and team-based learning (TBL).

Lecture

A lecture is an oral presentation bridging verbal communication with writing and newer media technologies to provide flexible, adaptable, robust, and contemporary methods to deliver content. Lecture is a teaching tool used by an educator to provide learning content using overarching themes that organizes material in an interesting way.

Teaching Tips

Students learn in various ways, so add activities to the lecture that stimulate all learners. Increased student participation can be achieved if there are a variety of novel activities offered during the lecture, such as videos, case studies, audio Podcasts, or student-led mini lectures. Use of visual aids, electronic handouts, electronic feedback systems, and study guides allow students to follow the sequence of the lecture. Prelecture assignments can enhance student engagement and active learning such as group assignments, interprofessional activities, e-book readings, and online modules, as seen in the flipped classroom pedagogical model (see "Flipped Classroom" later in this chapter, and in Chapter 19.).

Advantages and Disadvantages

Lecturing is a time-efficient strategy for covering complex material, raising further student questions that lend themselves to other teaching strategies. However, maintaining student concentration during the lecture may be challenging. When presented without student engagement activities, lectures may cause a decrease in student involvement in learning. Also, it may be time consuming for faculty to develop novel activities and resources for students.

Evidence

See Cavanagh (2011); Friesen (2011); and Young, Robinson, and Alberts (2009).

Peer Learning

Peer learning is a reciprocal learning activity whereby students share mutually beneficial knowledge, ideas, and experiences, allowing learning to move from independent to interdependent methods. These strategies probably work best with small groups and can be used online or in class.

Teaching Tips

A clear connection must be made between the objectives and the strategy or students will think the activity is not a good use of their time. Create a possible list of topics or allow students to choose what they are interested in to promote active student learning. Creating relevance to the learning objectives will increase student learning. Informal meetings between faculty and students may help clarify and structure questions used to promote in-class discussion.

Advantages

Peer learning provides a point of reference from which to explore concepts from multiple points of view, including theoretical and practical; promotes reflection and critical analysis; activates truth seeking; enhances affective learning and caring; and increases contextual learning. Many strategies may be used, including student interest groups, peer review of student work, group tests, digital storytelling, and peer mentoring.

Disadvantages

Peer learning requires faculty to continually focus on the relevancy of peer assignments because students may feel as if they are not learning what they need to know from their peers. Faculty may need to assist learners to focus or refocus on concepts being discussed throughout the course. Student evaluation may be challenging if not all students are participating equally. And quiet students may need encouragement, whereas assertive students may try to monopolize the group. Guidelines are necessary for the learning activities.

Evidence

See Christiansen and Bell (2010); Cooper, Martin, Fisher, Marks, and Harrington (2013); and Priharjo and Hoy (2011).

Seminar and Small or Large Group Discussions

A seminar is a meeting for an exchange of ideas in some topical area; it may also mean a guided discussion of concepts. Interprofessional assignments can enhance student engagement and active learning, but a clear connection of the seminar discussion to the course objectives is necessary or students may perceive the seminar as an inefficient use of their time. This structure can be completed in the classroom or online, synchronously or asynchronously.

Teaching Tips

Energy, creativity, and planning by the teacher and the students are required for effective use of a discussion strategy. Clear guidelines are needed so a vocal person (student or teacher) does not dominate the discussion. Student preparation time may be reduced by having students rotate as discussion facilitators so the individual student is responsible for in-depth preparation of only a few topics. The teacher is a part of the group, sometimes acting as a participant, a consultant, or the leader.

Advantages

Discussion format allows for active student engagement with content. Collaborative, cooperative learning; peer sharing; and dialogue facilitate comprehension and practical application of concepts. It allows teachers to act as role models for concept clarification and expert problem solving. Articulation improves in discussion, as do thinking skills. Limited development time is required for teachers, but planning is still necessary to ensure effectiveness. Discussion does not typically require additional supplies such as handouts or audiovisuals, and students can learn group problem-solving techniques.

Disadvantages

The structure requires that students possess adequate knowledge for active discussion and comprehension. It may require a great amount of student preparation time or may allow a student to "slip through" without sufficient knowledge or thinking skills. Students may require instruction in how to participate in seminars.

Evidence

See Bristol and Kyarsgaard (2012); Forrester and Huston, (2014); and Henningsohn and Dolk, (2014).

Team-Based Learning

In TBL, teams of students are created to enhance student engagement and the quality of learning outcomes. Students may work in teams online or in class. Interprofessional teams enhance active learning and student engagement.

TBL groups must be properly formed and managed. Students are accountable for the quality of their individual and group work and must receive frequent and timely feedback. Team assignments must promote both learning and team development (Michaelsen, Parmelee, McMahon, & Levine, 2008).

Teaching Tips

Keep group sizes at five to seven participants. Students stay in the same team for the duration of the course. Students are expected to prepare before the start of class and join their team at the beginning of the class time. Set clear expectations for grading with a rubric for either individual or group grades.

Advantages

A TBL strategy can be used in large classes to give students the actual experience of working in a team. The group becomes accountable for learning and increases student involvement in course content.

Disadvantages

TBL requires shifts of roles of faculty and student. It requires faculty time to learn the technique and students require orientation to a different way of learning. Student scheduling issues may complicate group assignments. TBL may increase student stress if group conflict occurs.

Evidence

See Clark, Nguyen, Bray & Levine (2008); Fatmi, Hartli, Hillier, Campbell, and Oswald (2013); Michaelsen and colleagues (2008); and Ofstad and Brunner (2013).

Conceptual Knowledge

Conceptual knowledge uses interrelationships among the basic elements within a larger structure that enable them to function together. The main forms of conceptual knowledge teaching are argumentation, debate, structured controversy, and dilemmas; cooperative learning, collaborative learning, and group assignments; mind mapping and concept mapping; flipped classroom; role play; and simulation (see Chapter 18).

Argumentation, Debate, Structured Controversy, and Dilemmas

Techniques focusing on argumentation, debate, structured controversy, and dilemmas engage the process of inquiry or reasoned judgment on a proposition aimed at demonstrating the truth or falsehood of something. These techniques involve the construction of logical arguments and oral defense of a proposition, and require the recognition of assumptions and evidence and use of inductive and deductive reasoning skills. They allow identification of relationships.

Teaching Tips

Argumentation and similar strategies work best on issue- or topic-related assignments for conceptual knowledge. For the purpose of forming productive debate teams, it is helpful for students to know each other. Faculty should introduce the basic topics and structure the debate format early in the course to allow students adequate preparation time. Debate teams usually consist of five students: two students debate for the topic, two debate against the topic, and the fifth acts as the moderator. Debates follow a specified format, including opening comments, presentation of affirmative and negative viewpoints, rebuttal, and summary (Fuszard, 2004). Encouraging students to debate the opposite of their personal opinion may increase student learning. This format may be completed online or in the classroom. Interprofessional teams will enhance student engagement and active learning. These in-class strategies may be well suited for the flipped classroom (see "Flipped Classroom" later in this chapter).

Advantages

Argumentation techniques develop analytical skills and the ability to recognize complexities in many health care issues. They broaden student views of controversial topics. And these techniques develop communication skills and increase student abilities to work in groups.

Disadvantages

Argumentation techniques require a fairly high level of knowledge about the subject on the parts of both those presenting the debate and the audience. They may require teaching students the art of debate. The technique require increased student preparation time. It can create anxiety and conflict for students because of the confrontational nature of debate, and students without adequate public speaking skills may also have increased anxiety. There is a high time cost for students to work in groups.

Evidence

See Choe, Park, and Yoo (2014); Fuszard (2004); and Garity (2009).

Cooperative Learning, Collaborative Learning, and Group Assignments

Teams of learners work on assignments and assume responsibility for group learning outcomes. This can be implemented in the classroom or online.

Teaching Tips

Design meaningful assignments that can be accomplished by small groups (a group of three to five heterogeneous [in ability, gender, ethnic status, experience, etc.] students is ideal). Teach or verify groups' understanding of team roles and group process; assign or ask group to designate a "leader," "recorder," "reflector," "reporter," and other roles as necessary. Structuring the group with students who are not homogenous may increase the potential for greater student learning. Allow adequate time for reporting and processing of group work.

Advantages

Cooperative learning and similar activities promote active and reflective learning and encourage teamwork. They provide opportunity for students to become accountable for their own and others' work; group dynamics skills can be used. Large learning assignments and projects can be accomplished efficiently.

Disadvantages

Students may resist frequent use of group assignments. There is a possibility that not all students will participate equally. Student scheduling issues may complicate preparation of group assignments, and student stress may increase if group conflict occurs.

Evidence

See Forrester and Huston (2014), Suwantarathip and Wachadee (2014), and Wyatt and colleagues (2010).

Mind Mapping and Concept Mapping

Mapping strategies involve learning complex phenomenon by diagramming the concepts and subconcepts. Mind mapping puts the central concept in the center of the page with related concepts surrounding the main concept. Concept maps are visual–structural diagrams that help students organize diverse elements of a larger topic. They are good for group assignments, especially interprofessional groups with divergent conceptual knowledge.

Teaching Tips

Mapping strategies can be used to enhance conceptual knowledge and retention of learning outcomes. This teaching method is frequently used in clinical settings, but is also effective in the classroom and online. Students can organize patient data prior to entering an actual patient encounter and then add to the map correlating new and existing data to better understand the clinical presentation of the patient. Grouping specific class content can also provide students with examples of mind mapping. Concept map software may be helpful when using this technique (Martin, 2009). Concept mapping can be an effective strategy for students with many types of learning styles.

Advantages

Mapping strategies encourage better understanding and recall of complex phenomena, and are especially effective in stimulating long-term recall of like concepts. They require active involvement by the students in designing the maps to enhance conceptual thinking processes. They help students recognize similarities and differences among concepts, help clarify relationships between concepts, help link new information with information previously learned, and help students organize information and relate theories to practice. They enhance problem-solving skills. The method appeals to the visual learner. Software is available for mapping assignments.

Disadvantages

Mapping strategies may take longer initially until both faculty and students understand how to organize the concepts. They may not appeal to concrete or auditory learners. Both faculty and students may need to learn how to use mapping before this method can be used effectively.

Evidence

See Daley and Torre (2010); Harrison and Gibbons (2013); Ho, Kumar, and Velan (2014); and Martin (2009).

Flipped Classroom

The flipped classroom is a pedagogical model whereby students conduct significant preclass preparation, and traditional in-class time is reserved for discussion and problem-solving of the relevant topics. The model is used in a number of health professions education to address the gap between didactic education and clinical practice performance. It employs asynchronous learning activities such as preclass video lectures, reading assignments, practice problems, and the use of technology-based resources. In the classroom, interactive, group-based problem-solving teaching and learning strategies are used.

Teaching Tips

Structure the activities of the flipped classroom in detail ahead of time. Use a variety of asynchronous or synchronous learning activities outside of the classroom to keep students interested. Provide ways for students to be held accountable for preclass work that has been completed. Bridge the didactic content with application to practice during the in-class sessions. Provide postclass reflection activities for students to connect the asynchronous and synchronous learning for application to practice.

Advantages

The flipped classroom allows student to be prepared for in-class conceptual knowledge, and thinking and learning activities and their application to practice. Students work at their own pace in self-directed preclass assignments. A variety of teaching and learning activities address students' various learning styles. Peer interactions are improved, and there is increased student–faculty interactions.

Disadvantages

The flipped classroom may provide challenges to faculty who are accustomed to traditional lecture-style teaching. Faculty development opportunities may be needed to learn about the flipped classroom pedagogical model. It requires time to structure in-class and classroom activities, and requires ongoing assessment of teaching and learning. Students may not like the extra work required outside of the classroom.

Evidence

See Baepler, Walker, and Driessen (2014); Kim, Kim, Khera, and Getman (2014); Tune, Sturek, and Basile (2013).

Role Play

Role play is a dramatic approach in which individuals assume the roles of others. It may be scripted; unscripted, spontaneous; or semi-structured interactions that are observed by others for analysis and interpretation of learning outcomes. This strategy can be used in class or online.

Teaching Tips

Faculty need to plan thoroughly for role play, but they also need to be prepared to monitor and modify student actions and reactions if necessary. Situations that involve conflicting emotions provide good scenarios for role playing. Typical organization of the role play involves briefing, setting the stage, and explaining the objectives, which is usually the shortest stage; running, acting out the role play, which may take from 5 to 20 minutes; and debriefing, discussion, analysis, and evaluation of the role-playing experience, which may last 30 to 40 minutes or more.

The debriefing is the most important stage of the role play, so students can clarify actions and alternative decisions can be explained, observation skills can be enhanced, and other interpersonal reactions can be anticipated. Videotaping or audiotaping of the role play may aid in the debriefing stage. The technique works best with small groups of students so all those not involved in the role play can become active observers. Students should be encouraged to respond naturally to the role play and avoid insincere acting. Criticism should be directed to the behaviors exhibited in the role play and not to specific students.

Advantages

Role play increases observational skills, improves decision-making skills, and increases comprehension of complex human behaviors. It provides immediate feedback about the interpersonal and problem-solving skills used in the role play and provides a nonthreatening environment in which to try out unfamiliar communication and decision-making techniques. Role play is good for adult learners because of the connection to real-life situations and active participation. It does not generate extra costs because props, handouts, and so on are typically not used.

Disadvantages

Students may be reluctant to participate if they do not feel as if it reflects real-life situations, and is seen as simply *play-acting*. There is a high time cost for faculty to develop scenarios. Faculty who like to be in charge of the learning environment may be frustrated by this method. Stereotypical behavior can be reinforced, and role play can be a costly use of class time if it is not planned appropriately.

Evidence

See Lewis and colleagues (2013); McEwen, Stokes, Crowley, and Roberts (2014); Rao and Stupans (2012).

Procedural Knowledge

Procedural knowledge involves how to do something, methods of inquiry, and criteria for using skills, algorithms, techniques, and methods. Teaching strategies relating to procedural knowledge are algorithms, demonstration, games, imagery and mindfulness, posters, self-learning modules, simulation (see Chapter 18), and writing.

Algorithms

Algorithms are a step-by-step approach for clinical decision-making based on evidence. This refers to any course in which frequent practice is required for student mastery of content, in which rules aid in problem solving, or in which the content can be broken into concrete stages. This strategy may be completed online or in class, and is well suited for peer or interprofessional learning in pairs or groups.

Teaching Tips

Assess content for appropriate use of algorithms as a teaching strategy. Develop an algorithm and accompanying student explanations of how to use it. Allow 6 to 8 hours for the development of the first algorithms. Additional algorithms on similar content typically take less time to develop.

Advantages

An algorithm shows students how to “spot” the most relevant information for problem solving; it develops reliable, complex problem-solving abilities even in novice students and decreases the amount of one-on-one instruction often required when teaching problem-solving techniques. It is effective in teaching complex procedures that involve many steps. When used with case studies, it may enhance learning. It saves student time in trying to remember and understand complex phenomena, and is especially helpful for students with little clinical experience. It is effective in promoting learning and adherence to best practices.

Disadvantages

The teacher must clearly define the steps or students will not be able to complete the task accurately. Students may need to be taught how to use algorithms in problem solving. The development of algorithms can be time consuming for faculty. Algorithms cannot substitute for clinical reasoning in decision-making in practice.

Evidence

See Buchko and Robinson (2012); Fabrellas and colleagues (2013); Jablonski, DuPen, and Ersek (2011); and Rathbun and Ruth-Sahd (2009).

Demonstration

Students show learning outcomes through such things as projects, presentations, or learning objects, revealing to what degree they have met the learning objectives. Typically, demonstration is both a learning experience for the student and a means of evaluating academic progress by the educator. This strategy should be used for complex mental or psychomotor skill acquisition. It is suited for online and in-class assignments, and is well suited for interprofessional learning.

Teaching Tips

Have students show the steps of the process clearly, from start to finish. Ask students to go through the process a second time, showing the rationale and allowing time for questions. Provide for immediate, individual, supervised practice sessions. Video recordings may be used for student review before and after the demonstration. Demonstrations may be planned, implemented, reviewed, and revised through online videos.

Advantages

Visibly showing a process often aids in retention. Complex skills become more understandable as a result of the demonstration, and demonstration allows an expert to model the skill. Tailored performance feedback enhances retention and procedural knowledge is enhanced for future problem-solving and metacognitive knowledge.

Disadvantages

Students have differing levels of skill acquisition abilities. Students who quickly master skills may become uninterested while the others are practicing. Mastering psychomotor skills is usually very stressful for many students and requires adequate faculty supervision, space, supplies, and equipment to provide realistic practice sessions. There is a high faculty workload involved in supervision of student practice times and a high cost of supplies and equipment may limit the amount of practice time available to students.

Evidence

See Chang, Chou, Tehrerani, and Hauer (2011); Day, Iles, and Griffiths (2009); and Fakih, 2013.

Games

An educational game is a learning activity with rules involving chance showcasing the players' knowledge or skill in attempting to reach a specific learning outcome. This strategy may be completed online or in class, and is suited for interprofessional "ice breaker" assignments. Gaming software is available for online use.

Teaching Tips

Use a gaming method for reinforcement of knowledge rather than introduction of new knowledge. An open learning environment is crucial to learning with gaming. Faculty must back out; the learning is student to student in this method. Debriefing after the game is critical so students clearly connect the game with the important concepts. If faculty do not value gaming as a teaching strategy, they may unconsciously sabotage the game.

Advantages

Gaming increases student engagement and cognitive and affective learning, improves retention, is fun and exciting, increases learner involvement, motivates the learner, and can help connect practice experiences to theory. Students can learn from each other through the experience of the game; it is good for adult learners who take more responsibility for their own learning. Learners can receive immediate feedback in a learning situation and can also see the immediate application of theory to practice. Learning from gaming lasts longer when compared with learning from traditional lecture.

Disadvantages

Gaming may be threatening to some learners who may feel exposed if they are unsure of the answer. It may be time consuming and may be costly to purchase or develop. It may be difficult to evaluate the level of learning achieved through gaming if several players are involved. It may require a greater amount of space. It should have introductory and summary sessions, and faculty must set guidelines so the game remains educational.

Evidence

See Blakely, Skirton, Cooper, Allum, and Nelmes (2009); Blakely, Skirton, Cooper, Allum, and Nelmes (2010); Boctor, 2013; and Grimley, Green, Nilsen, Thompson, and Tomes (2011).

Imagery and Mindfulness

Imagery and mindfulness include mental picturing, diagramming, or rehearsal before the actual use of the information in practice. The best use is in combination with other strategies (e.g., with physical practice in psychomotor skill acquisition).

Teaching Tips

Create a scenario that mimics a real-life situation. Use the scenario to demonstrate effective use of imagery. Relaxation techniques provide a good example of how to use imagery techniques. A supportive classroom environment is needed for the effective use of this strategy. This technique may be helpful for stress reduction for students and its application to nursing practice.

Advantage

Imagery and mindfulness techniques provide superior learning of psychomotor skills when imagery is combined with physical practice. It may lead to the development of therapeutic and holistic nursing skills in practice.

Disadvantages

Individuals have varying levels of innate imagery skills, so some students may need to be taught how to conduct imagery. It does not provide a substitute for physical practice of a skill. Using imagery and physical practice of the skill will require more student study time than if only physical practice is used. Stress and performance fears may interfere with the productive use of imagery. It may require faculty development to implement imagery strategy.

Evidence

See Brady, O'Connor, Burgermeister, and Hanson (2012); Grossman, Deupi, and Leitao (2014); White, 2014.

Poster

A poster is a visual representation of learning outcomes. This project may be completed online, is well suited for peer or interprofessional learning, and provides opportunities for dissemination of knowledge.

Teaching Tips

Students may need instructions about how to design a poster. Clear guidelines of the expected poster contents, as well as evaluation techniques will need to be developed and presented to students. Poster quality may be enhanced when artistic concepts are incorporated in the poster design. Software is available for creating visually pleasing posters.

Advantages

Students can convey complex ideas through posters and making posters can facilitate student creativity. Assessment of students' knowledge can be showcased through the use of posters. Students can receive feedback from peers as well as faculty. Students get a sense of achievement from producing posters. The skills developed in the production of a poster may be valuable for students after graduation. Posters can be used to showcase student work publically in professional conferences or student poster displays. Evaluation of posters by faculty or peers can be completed quickly using guidelines or grading rubrics.

Disadvantages

Faculty time is required to develop a poster assignment and evaluation techniques. The assignment can be frustrating to students who are not visual learners.

Evidence

See Briggs (2009), Christenbery and Latham (2012), and Sterman and colleagues (2013).

Self-Learning Modules

Self-learning modules include information on one concept presented according to a few specific objectives in a format that allows skipping of a section if the student has previously mastered the content. A module typically includes self-checks (pretests, posttests) of student learning throughout the self-contained module. This format is ideal for the flipped classroom preclass assignments (see "Flipped Classroom" earlier in this chapter) before in-class meetings for foundational knowledge.

Teaching Tips

A self-learning module has many distinct sections. It can be used for a single class period, an entire course, enrichment, or remedial learning. Also, it may be created online and used in blended learning teaching modalities. Students may complete the modules in preparation for in-class learning objectives.

Advantages

A module is good for adult learners who may have limited study times; it gives students options of when and where learning will occur. Learning can occur without the presence of the teacher and is flexible according to learner needs. Modules are good for teaching psychomotor skills. They have been found to enhance learning over combined lecture and discussion methods. It is an effective method of learning for intrinsically motivated students.

Disadvantages

Students may procrastinate and not complete work in a timely manner. The module may be costly in faculty time to prepare and update.

Evidence

See Cusack and O'Donoghue (2012); Garcia, Greco, and Loescher (2011); and Hsu and Hsieh (2011).

Writing

Writing encourages learning through documentation of ideas in, for example, scholarly papers, informal journals, poems, and letters. Interprofessional scholarly writing may increase student engagement and active learning for dissemination of knowledge.

Teaching Tips

Teaching students how to write may increase the quality of student papers. Structure the writing assignment with final grading in mind. Assess the paper in its entirety rather than concentrating on grammar and style issues. Peer review of drafts may stimulate thinking and critiquing skills. Specific grading criteria decrease the amount of subjective grading. Time spent on grading can be decreased with a grading rubric. Increasing complexity in writing experiences through the curriculum increases the effect on stimulating higher-order thinking. Providing flexibility in topic selection for written assignments recognizes individual student learning needs and empowers students. Teacher review of student drafts allows early assessment of student thinking and processing of the material and allows for early intervention if problems are detected.

Many forms of writing can be used, such as journals, formal papers, creative writing assignments (e.g., poems or book reports), summaries of class content, letters to legislators and nurse administrators, and research critiques. Mentoring, reflection, and time to learn the different skills are suggested. Partnerships with students, faculty, and librarians may increase information literacy and online searching skills needed for writing academic papers. Writing manuscripts for publication involves more advanced academic writing skills; additionally, more specific instruction may be necessary.

Advantages

Writing stimulates higher-order thinking through active involvement with the literature, learning to judge the quality of the literature, organizing interpretation of the literature into logical sequences, and learning to make judgments based on what was learned. Students can discover their own beliefs and values when writing. Nurses write in many formats, and writing projects in an educational setting allows for learning different mediums and styles. Knowledge gained from the writing assignments can give confidence and helps to empower students in their own ideas. Writing improves communication skills.

Disadvantages

Grading writing assignments can be subjective. Many students may feel unprepared to complete writing assignments, which may lead to students' increased frustration and stress. Students must understand the importance of learning through writing, or writing assignments will be viewed as superfluous work. There may be a high time cost for students to complete the writing assignments depending on how the assignment is structured. There is typically a high time cost for teachers to grade. Faculty development may be needed before choosing this type of teaching strategy.

Evidence

See Beck, Blake-Campbell, and McKay (2012); Nevid, Pastva, and McClelland (2012); Troxler, Vann, and Oremann (2011).

Metacognitive Knowledge

Metacognitive knowledge is knowledge of cognition in general, as well as awareness and knowledge of one's own cognition. This strategy can be used in several formats: case study, interprofessional education (IPE), portfolio and e-portfolio, problem-based learning (PBL), questioning and Socratic questioning, reflection journal writing, and simulation (see Chapter 18).

Case Study

Case studies represent an in-depth analysis of a real-life situation as a way to illustrate class content. They apply didactic content and theory to real life, simulated life, or both. This strategy is well-suited for interprofessional or peer-group learning, may be completed online or in class, and may be used as a preclass assignment for the flipped classroom (see "Flipped Classroom" earlier in this chapter).

Teaching Tips

A well-designed case that illustrates the most important learning outcomes is critical to the success of learning with this method. Unfolding case studies are those that progress or "unfold" over time. They can offer real-life clinical situations that are progressively revealed, allowing students to build on previous knowledge, connecting theory to practice.

Before the assignment, analyze the case with the intent of determining the potential ways in which students could analyze the case, but be prepared for student questions and comments that previously have not been considered (e.g., be able to say, "I don't know" or "I haven't considered that before," if necessary). A safe, open, nonthreatening learning environment is crucial for active student participation.

At the conclusion of the assignment, provide a summary of the most important points and sources for more in-depth study. Assist in students' comprehension of critical concepts with the use of tools such as concept maps, chalkboards, flip charts, or PowerPoint slides.

Advantages

Case studies stimulate metacognitive knowledge, retention, and recall. Associating the practical with the theoretical helps many students recall important information. Problem solving can be practiced in a safe environment without the threat of endangering a patient. Case studies are especially helpful for adult learners who desire peer interaction, support for prior experience, and validation of thinking. An experienced nurse can readily devise a case study example from actual patient encounters.

Disadvantages

Case studies are more effective when used with complex situations that require problem solving; they are not appropriate when concrete facts are the only content. Developing cases is a time-consuming skill for many, and the option of published cases should be considered. Case studies require the use of good questioning skills by the faculty. Poor student preparation may result in less learning. They may frustrate students who desire content to be presented through more direct strategies such as lecture.

Evidence

See Dutra (2013); Garcia and colleagues (2011); and West, Usher, and Delaney (2012).

Interprofessional Education

In IPE "two or more professions learn with, from and about each other to improve collaboration and the quality of care" (Centre for the Advancement of Interprofessional Education, 2014). This strategy can be completed online or face-to-face.

Teaching Tips

Strong leadership is needed with the interest, knowledge, and experience to champion IPE. Detailed planning is complex and must include organizational support and equal representation of faculty from each professional program. IPE facilitation requires in-depth understanding of interactive learning methods, knowledge of group dynamics, enthusiasm for IPE teaching and learning, the ability to role-model and mirror collaborative learning, and flexibility to creatively use professional differences within groups. IPE evaluation needs to be ongoing to assess for effectiveness and revisions to improve the learning experience for all stakeholders. Students need to be oriented to IPE and its principles, value, and expected outcomes. Faculty development is needed to understand the principles of IPE and how it is embedded into the curricula across disciplines. (See also Chapter 11)

Advantages

Outcomes have shown to increase knowledge, skills, and attitudes of collaborative skills and their application to professional practice. Students will meet IPE skills in collaboration to meet workplace demands for collaborative practice teams outlined to improve health systems through calls from professional organizations (Chapter 11). IPEs may increase future teamwork and collaboration in the workplace.

Disadvantages

Planning for IPEs takes considerable time and energy. Long-term sustainability may depend on a few key enthusiasts. Organizers must arrange regular meetings to consider all perspectives of IPE; when differences arise between groups they need to be discussed and resolved. Ongoing work among groups is required to evaluate, revise, and discuss the IPE. Some students may be uncomfortable talking to those from other professions, particularly if they do not understand discipline-specific jargon. Longitudinal research studies are needed regarding the outcomes of IPE to improve systems of care.

Evidence

Hobgood and colleagues (2010); McKay, Sanko, and Shekhter (2014); and Reeves, Tassone, Parker, Wagner, and Simmons (2012).

Portfolio and E-Portfolio

A portfolio is a collection of student work showcasing learning, achievement, and personal and professional development. Documentation of student skills from prior courses or life experiences can be used for assessing learning outcomes for a course or program, or for professional development. This may be completed electronically (e-portfolio).

Teaching Tips

Students may need an orientation about how to construct a portfolio. A content outline should provide the framework for the portfolio but not limit student creativity. Assessment of portfolios can be complex and difficult. The novice may want to seek consultation from experts for assistance. Guidelines for the portfolio construction and evaluation must be clear.

Advantages

Portfolios typically provide high student motivation because they control learning. Motivated students typically learn more. Portfolios help educators understand individual student goals and aspirations. They encourage student reflection on learning. Independent, self-confident, and self-directed students will excel with this method.

Disadvantages

Portfolios must be combined with reflective strategies to encourage student ownership of learning. They require alternative ways of thinking about the learning process by both educators and students. Students with low self-confidence will need much faculty assistance. The time involvement may be high for students in development of portfolios and for faculty in evaluation of portfolios. Unless students clearly see the objective of a portfolio, the work involved may be viewed as busywork.

Evidence

See Garrett, MacPhee, and Jackson (2013); Karlowicz (2010); Ryan, 2011.

Problem-based Learning

PBL uses clinical problems and professional issues as the focus for integrating all of the content necessary for clinical practice. It is a highly structured and learner-centered method of teaching and learning. Real-life problems are the basis of the initial learning content. Learning is student-initiated, usually in groups. Faculty members are facilitators of student learning. The five steps in the PBL process include analysis of problems, establishment of learning outcomes, collection of information, summarizing, and reflection. PBL is usually used as an approach to the entire curriculum, rather than focusing on separate disciplines or nursing specialties. This strategy can be completed online or in the classroom, and it can be used for interprofessional or peer learning.

Teaching Tips

Develop realistic, comprehensive clinical problems that will prompt and advance intended learning outcomes. The case problem presented is typically accomplished through several scenes containing complex but realistic information that requires the students to process the available information into categories. Faculty workload can increase significantly, particularly during the development stages. PBL requires close collaboration between various disciplines if the case or curriculum is interdisciplinary. Orient students to the PBL approach and allow sufficient time for students to research the problem and discuss answers. Groups of six to nine students are most effective for PBL.

Advantages

PBL fosters active and cooperative learning. Students use skills of inquiry and metacognitive thinking, as well as peer teaching and peer evaluation. The problem can be developed in paper-and-pencil or electronic formats. Students often work in teams or groups. PBL can be used in interdisciplinary learning environments to develop roles and competencies of each discipline. Contextual learning motivates students and increases the ability to apply knowledge in clinical situations. It increases student responsibility for self-directed and peer learning and develops flexible knowledge that can be applied to different contexts. This learning method develops lifelong learning skills.

Disadvantages

PBL involves faculty time in developing the problem situation. Extensive time is needed for faculty to learn to use PBL. Students require orientation to the role of the learner in a PBL setting, and must work through potential discrepancies in expectations and goals for learning. Student learning seems to be connected to the effectiveness of the case as well as the functioning of the group. It is difficult to use as a teaching technique when the class size is large.

Evidence

See Choi, Lindquist, and Song (2014); Lin Lu, Chung, and Yang (2010); Martyn, Terwijn, Kek, and Huijser (2014).

Questioning and Socratic Questioning

Questioning is an expression of inquiry—an interrogative sentence, phrase, or gesture—that invites or calls for a reply. Socratic questioning involves probing questioning to analyze an individual's thinking. This strategy can be completed online or in the classroom. When using IPE methods, be sure that all students know the "language" of the profession and refrain from using profession-specific jargon or slang.

Teaching Tips

Allow sufficient time to construct thought-provoking questions. Faculty need to be prepared to facilitate the discussion that should follow a good questioning period. Student learning is enhanced if a preclass assignment that will lead to adequate student preparation is designed. Questioning can be used spontaneously, as an exploratory strategy, or with issue-specific content. An open, trusting classroom environment is needed. Design questions to assess the various domains of learning. Appropriate phrasing of questions is required so that students do not feel demeaned by the questioning experience. Peer learning can take place with guided peer questioning.

Advantages

Questioning promotes metacognition about conclusions to be drawn, increases interaction between students and faculty, and promotes discussion from multiple points of view. It allows students to discuss concepts from their own experiences and discloses underlying assumptions. Questioning increases the articulation of evidence, stimulates students to ask higher-order thinking questions, and promotes a higher level of problem-solving skills. Learning is transferred from the classroom to the clinical environment and promotes thinking skills to enhance test-taking abilities.

Disadvantages

Questioning presumes a comprehensive knowledge of content. Preclass preparation by student and faculty must be thorough. Students cannot rely on a simple recitation of facts.

Evidence

See Lakdizaji, Abdollahzadeh, Hassankhanih, and Kalantrai (2013); and Carvalho-Grevious (2013).

Reflection and Journal Writing

Through this strategy students detail personal experiences and connect them to learning outcomes. The most frequent use of journaling is connecting classroom theories and curriculum objectives to actual practice situations. Oral and written reflections are equally as effective. This strategy may be completed online, and is suited for group, peer, or interprofessional learning assignments.

Teaching Tips

Set clear expectations for journal writing so that students know what is expected. Using different approaches to journal writing (e.g., writing learning objectives, summary of the experience, a diary, and focused argument) may increase student interest in the assignment. Thoughtful feedback (not necessarily lengthy feedback) from the teacher is important to student learning. Group discussions about the journals and what students are saying may increase learning for all students. Using specific thought-provoking questions in the journal enhances metacognitive thinking. Students may need to be taught how to conduct reflective exercises. Reflective journals are most often not graded with a letter grade. If so, grading rubrics will set clear expectations and provide guidelines for grading uniformly.

Advantages

Reflection promotes learning from experiences and helps students learn how to transfer facts from one context to another. It encourages students to think about clinical experiences in relation to didactic course content. Student-centered learning is especially valuable to adult learners. Reflection is helpful in demonstrating how to become a lifelong learner. It stimulates metacognitive thinking and provides a feedback loop between teacher and student so teaching emphasis can be modified to enhance student learning. It can be used for all levels of nursing education.

Disadvantages

Educators may want to revert to the expert role rather than concentrating on the students' experiences; student-directed learning may frustrate some teachers and may stimulate unresolved conflict within some students. Faculty need to direct student learning through questioning and discussion that may cover topics in which they are not prepared. Students may see it as only a required exercise and not take the time to make appropriate use of the learning opportunity. There is a high time cost for faculty to construct reflection guidelines, read student reflections, and help individual students process their reflections; there is a high time cost for students to complete reflections.

Evidence

See Garrity (2013); Kuo, Turton, Su-Fen, and Lee-Hsieh (2011); McMillan-Coddington, (2013); Muncy (2014); and Sherwood & Horton-Deutsch (2012).

Summary

Student engagement is founded on Astin's (1999) theory of student involvement and on the principles of Chickering and Gamson's (1987) seven principles of good practice in education, which include: (1) encourage contact between students and faculty, (2) develop reciprocity and cooperation among students, (3) encourage active learning, (4) give prompt feedback, (5) emphasize time on task, (6) communicate high expectations, and (7) respect diverse talents and ways of learning. Evidence of the learning outcomes of student engagement over the years can be seen in research conducted by NSSE (2013) and CCSSE (2014). Student engagement can be seen in a number of quality indicators leading to improved learning, which include (1) academic challenge, (2) learning with peers, (3) experiences with faculty, (4) the campus environment, (5) high-impact learning experiences, (6) academic advising, and (7) learning with technology.

Bloom's knowledge dimensions consists of four major types of knowledge: (1) factual, (2) conceptual, (3) procedural, and (4) metacognitive. When selecting teaching strategies, nurse educators may use this framework as a guideline in choosing the appropriate strategy for the knowledge dimensions. A number of select strategies are listed in this chapter, with the advantages and disadvantages of each, in relation to the knowledge types. The evidence is growing to explicate the use of student engagement and active learning strategies, and nurse educators will want to be discerning about the nature of the evidence in choosing the best fit for the learning environment to prepare graduates at all levels for the complexities of today's health care system.

REFLECTING ON THE EVIDENCE

1. As the evidence for student engagement and active learning continues to grow, how will nurse educators discern which evidence is best?
2. As learner-centered curricula continue to become adopted by nurse educators, what further research is needed to enhance student engagement and active learning?
3. Using Bloom's revised taxonomy of educational objectives (Anderson & Krathwohl, 2001), how can nurse educators use the knowledge dimensions as a framework for student engagement and active learning?

REFERENCES

Anderson, L. W. & Krathwohl, D. R. (Eds.), (2001). *A taxonomy for learning, teaching, and assessing: A revision of Bloom's taxonomy of educational objectives.* New York: Longman.

Astin, A. W. (1999). Student involvement: A developmental theory for higher education. *Journal of College Student Development, 40*(5), 518–529.

Baepler, P., Walker, J. D., & Driessen, M. (2014). It's not about seat time: Blending, flipping, and efficiency in active learning classrooms. *Computers and Education, 78*, 227–236.

Beck, S., Blake-Campbell, B., & McKay, D. (2012). Partnership for the advancement of information literacy in a nursing program. *Community and Junior College Libraries, 18*(1), 3–11. http://dx.doi.org/10.1080/02763915.2012.651957.

Benner, P., Sutphen, M., Leonard, V., & Day, L. (2010). *Educating nurses: A call for radical transformation.* Stanford, CA: Carnegie Foundation for the Advancement of Teaching.

Blakely, G., Skirton, H., Cooper, S., Allum, P., & Nelmes, P. (2009). Educational gaming in the health sciences: Systematic review. *Journal of Advanced Nursing, 65*(2), 259–269. http://dx.doi.org/10.1111/j.1365-2648.2008.04843.x.

Blakely, G., Skirton, H., Cooper, S., Allum, P., & Nelmes, P. (2010). Use of educational games in the health professions: A mixed-methods study of educators' perspectives in the UK. *Nursing and Health Sciences, 12*, 27–32. http://dx.doi.org/10.1111/j.1442-2018.2009.00479.x.

Blau, G., & Snell, C. (2013). Understanding undergraduate professional development engagement and its impact. *College Student Journal, 47*, 689–702.

Brady, S., O'Connor, N., Burgermeister, D., & Hanson, P. (2012). The impact of mindfulness meditation in promoting a culture of safety on an acute psychiatric unit. *Perspectives in Psychiatric Care, 48*(3), 129–137. http://dx.doi.org/10.1111/j.1744-6163.2011.00315.x.

Bristol, T. J., & Kyarsgaard, V. (2012). Asynchronous discussion: A comparison of larger and smaller discussion group size. *Nursing Education Perspectives, 33*(6), 386–390.

Boctor, L. (2013). Active-learning strategies: The use of a game to reinforce learning in nursing education. A case study. *Nurse Education in Practice, 13*, 96–100.

Briggs, D. J. (2009). A practical guide to designing a poster for presentation. *Nursing Standard, 23*(34), 35–39.

Bruce, M., Omne-Pontén, M. (2010). Active and emotional student engagement: A nationwide, prospective, longitudinal study of Swedish nursing students. *International Journal of Nursing Education Scholarship, 7*(1), 1–18.

Buchko, B., & Robinson, L. E. (2012). An evidence-based approach to decrease early post-operative urinary retention following urogynecologic surgery. *Urololgic Nursing, 32*(5), 260–273.

Carvalho-Grevious, M. (2013). Breaking the cycle of shame: Socratic teaching methods to enhance critical thinking. *Journal of Baccalaureate Social Work, 18*(1), 77–94.

Cavanagh, M. (2011). Students' experiences of active engagement through cooperative learning activities in lectures. *Active Learning in Higher Education, 12*(23), 23–33. http://dx.doi.org/10.1177/1469.

Centre for the Advancement of Interprofessional Education. (2014). *Definition of interprofessional education*. Retrieved from, http://caipe.org.uk/about-us/the-definition-and-principles-of-interprofessional-education/.

Chang, A., Chou, C. L., Teherani, A., & Hauer, K. E. (2011). Clinical skills-related learning goals of senior medical students after performance feedback. *Medical Education, 45*, 878–885. http://dx.doi.org/10.1111/j1365-2923.2011.04015.x.

Christenbery, T. L., & Latham, T. G. (2012). Creating effective scholarly posters: A guide for DNP students. *Journal of the American Association of Nurse Practitioners, 25*(1), 16–23.

Christiansen, A., & Bell, A. (2010). Peer learning partnerships: Exploring the experience of pre-registration nursing students. *Journal of Clinical Nursing, 19*, 803–810. http://dx.doi.org/10.1111/j.13652702.2009.02981.x.

Chickering, A. W., & Gamson, Z. F. (1987, March). Seven principles for good practice in undergraduate education. *AAHE Bulletin, 39*(7), 3–7.

Choe, K., Park, S., & Yoo, S. Y. (2014). Effects of constructivist teaching methods on bioethics for nursing students: A quasi-experimental study. *Nurse Education Today, 34*(5), 848–885. http://dx.doi.org/10.1016/j.nedt.2013.09.012.

Choi, E., Lindquist, R., & Song, Y. (2014). Effects of problem-based learning vs. traditional lecture on Korean nursing students' critical thinking, problem-solving, and self-directed learning. *Nurse Education Today, 34*(1), 52–56. http://dx.doi.org/10.1016/jmedt.2013.02.012.

Clark, M. C., Nguyen, H. T., Bray, C., & Levine, R. E. (2008). Team-based learning in an undergraduate nursing course. *Journal of Nursing Education, 47*(3), 111–117. Community College Survey of Student Engagement (CCSSE). (2014). 2014 cohort key findings. Retrieved from, http://www.ccsse.org/survey/survey.cfm.

Cooper, J. R., Martin, T., Fisher, W., Marks, J., & Harrington, M. (2013). Peer-to-peer teaching: Improving communication techniques for students in an accelerated nursing program. *Nursing Education Perspectives, 34*(5), 349–350.

Cusack, T., & O'Donoghue, G. (2012). The introduction of an interprofessional education module: Students' perceptions. *Quality in Primary Care, 2*(20), 231–238.

Daley, B. J., & Torre, D. M. (2010). Concept maps in medical education: An analytical literature review. *Medical Education, 44*, 440–448. http://dx.doi.org/10.1111/j.1365-2923.2010.03628.x.

Day, T., Iles, N., & Griffiths, P. (2009). Effect of performance feedback on tracheal suctioning knowledge and skills: Randomized controlled trial. *Journal of Advanced Nursing, 65*(7), 1423–1431.

Dutra, D. K. (2013). Implementation of case studies in undergraduate didactic nursing courses: A qualitative study. *Biomedical Central Nursing, 12*(1), 15–23. http://dx.doi.org/10.1186/1472-6955-12-15.

Fabrellas, N., Sanchez, C., Juve, E., Aurin, E., Monserrat, D., Casanovas, E., et al. (2013). A program of nurse algorithm-guided care for adult patients with acute minor illnesses in primary car. *Biomedical Central Family Practice, 14*(61), 1–7.

Fakih, M. G. (2013). Peripheral venous catheter care in the emergency department: Education and feedback led to marked improvements. *American Journal of Infection Control, 41*(6), 531–536.

Fatmi, M., Hartli, L., Hillier, T., Campbell, S., & Oswald, A. E. (2013). The effectiveness of team-based learning on learning outcomes in health professions education. *Medical Teacher, 35*(12), 1608–1624. http://dx.doi.org/10.3109/0142159X.201384980.

Friesen, N. (2011). The lecture as a transmedia pedagogical form: A historical analysis. *Educational Researcher, 40*(95), 95–102. http://dx.doi.org/10.3102/0013189X11404603.

Forrester, R., & Hutson, K. (2014). Balancing faculty and student preferences in the assignment of students to groups. *Journal of Innovative Education, 12*(2), 131–147. http://dx.doi.org/10.1111/dsji.12029.

Fuszard, B. (2004). *Innovative teaching strategies in nursing education* (3rd ed.). Gaithersburg, MD: Aspen.

Garcia, S. P., Greco, K. E., & Loescher, L. J. (2011). Teaching strategies to incorporate genomics education into academic nursing curricula. *Journal of Nursing Education, 50*(11), 612–618.

Garity, J. (2009). Fostering nursing students' use of ethical theory and decision-making models: Teaching strategies. *Learning in Health and Social Care, 8*(2), 114–122. http://dx.doi.org/10.1111/j.1473-6861.2009.00223x.

Garrett, B. M., MacPhee, M., & Jackson, C. (2013). Evaluation of an e-portfolio for the assessment of clinical competence in a baccalaureate nursing program. *Nurse Education Today, 33*(10), 1207–1213. http://dx.doi.org/10.1016/jnedt.2012.06.015.

Garrity, M. K. (2013). Developing nursing leadership skills through reflective journaling: A nursing professor's personal reflection. *Reflective Practice, 14*(1), 118–130. http://dx.doi.org/10.1080/14623943.2012.732940.

Grimley, M., Green, R., Nilsen, T., Thompson, D., & Tomes, R. (2011). Using computer games for instruction: The student experience. *Active Learning in Higher Education, 12*(45), 45–56. http://dx.doi.org/10.1177/1469787410387733.

Grossman, S., Deupi, J., & Leitao, K. (2014). Seeing the forest for the trees: Increasing nurse practitioner students' observational and mindfulness skills. *Creative Nursing, 20*(1), http://dx.doi.org/10.1891/1078-4535.20.1.67.

Harrison, S., & Gibbons, C. (2013). Nursing student perceptions of concept maps: From theory to practice. *Nursing Education Perspectives, 34*(6), 395–399. http://dx.doi.org/10.5480/10-465.

Henningsohn, L., & Dolk, A. (2014). The medical exhibition seminar. *The Clinical Teacher, 11*(3), 219–224. http://dx.doi.org/10.1111/tct.12095.

Hill, L. H. (2014). Graduate students' perspectives of effective teaching. *Adult Learning, 25*(2), 57–65.

Ho, V., Kumar, R. K., & Velan, G. (2014). Online testable concept maps: Benefits for learning about pathogenesis of disease. *Medical Education, 48*(7), 687–697. http://dx.doi.org/10.1111/medu.12422.

Hobgood, C., Sherwood, G., Frush, K., Hollar, D., Maynard, L., Foster, B., et al. (2010). Teamwork training with nursing and medical students: Does the method matter? Results of an interinstitutional, interdisciplinary collaboration. *Quality and Safety in Health Care, 19*(6), e25. http://dx.doi.org/10.1136/qshc.2008.031732.

Hsu, L., & Hsieh, S. (2011). Effects of a blended learning module on self-reported learning performances in baccalaureate nursing students. *Journal of Advanced Nursing, 67*(11), 2435–2444. http://dx.doi.org/10.1111/j.1365-2648.2011.05684.x.

Jablonski, A. M., DuPen, A. R., & Ersek, M. (2011). The use of algorithms in assessing and managing persistent pain in older adults. *American Journal of Nursing, 111*(3), 34–43.

Karlowicz, K. A. (2010). Development and testing of a portfolio evaluation scoring tool. *Journal of Nursing Education, 49*(2), 78–86. http://dx.doi.org/10.3928/01484834-20090918-07.

Kim, M. K., Kim, S. M., Khera, O., & Getman, J. (2014). The experience of three flipped classrooms in an urban university: An exploration of design principles. *Internet and Higher Education, 22*, 37–50.

Kuo, C., Turton, M., Su-Fen, C., & Lee-Hsieh, J. (2011). Using clinical caring journaling: Nursing student and instructor experiences. *Journal of Nursing Research, 19*(2), 141–149. http://dx.doi.org/10.1097/JNR.0b013e31821aala7.

Lakdizaji, S., Abdollahzadeh, F., Hassankhanih, H., & Kalantrai, M. (2013). Impact of guided reciprocal peer questioning on nursing students' self-esteem and learning. *Iranian Journal of Nursing and Midwifery Research, 18*(4), 285–289.

Lewis, D., O'Boyle-Duggan, M., Chapman, J., Dee, P., Sellner, K., & Gorman, S. (2013). Putting words into action: Using role play in skills training. *British Journal of Nursing, 22*(11), 638–644.

Lin, C., Lu, M., Chung, C., & Yang, C. (2010). A comparison of problem-based learning and conventional teaching in nursing ethics education. *Nursing Ethics, 17*(3), 373–382. http://dx.doi.org/10.1177/096973309355380.

Lundberg, C. A. (2014). Peers and faculty as predictors of learning for community college students. *Community College Review, 42*(4), 79–98. http://dx.doi.org/10.1177/0091552113517931.

Martin, K. (2009). Computer-generated concept maps: An innovative group didactic activity. *Nurse Educator, 34*(6), 238–240.

Martyn, J., Terwijn, R., Kek, M., & Huijser, H. (2014). Exploring the relationships between teaching, approaches to learning and critical thinking in a problem-based learning foundation nursing course. *Nurse Education Today, 34*(5), 829–835. http://dx.doi.org/10.1016/j.nedt2013.04.023.

McEwen, L., Stokes, A., Crowley, K., & Roberts, C. (2014). Using role play for expert science communication with professional stakeholders in flood risk management. *Journal of Geography in Higher Education, 38*(2), 277–300. http://dx.doi.org/10.1080/03098265.2014.911827.

McKay, J., Sanko, J., Shekhter, I., & Birnback, D. (2014, April). Twitter as a tool to enhance student engagement during an interprofessional patient safety course. *Journal of Interprofessional Care*, http://dx.doi.org/10.3109/13561820.2014.912618 online.

McMillin-Coddington, D. (2013). Reflection through journal writing to educate registered nursing students on patient care. *Teaching and Learning in Nursing, 8*(2), 63–67. http://dx.doi.org/10.1016/jteln.2012.09.004.

Michaelsen, L. K., Parmelee, D. X., McMahon, K. K., & Levine, R. E. (2008). *Team-based learning for health professions education*. Sterling, VA: Stylus.

Muncy, J. (2014). Blogging for reflection: The use of online journals to engage students in reflective learning. *Marketing Education Review, 24*(2), 101–114. http://dx.doi.org/10.2753/MER1052-8008240202.

National Survey of Student Engagement (NSSE). (2013). *NSSE annual results 2013: A fresh look at student engagement*. Retrieved from, http://nsse.iub.edu/html/annual_results.cfm.

Nevid, J. S., Pastva, A., & McClelland, N. (2012). Writing-to-learn assignments in introductory psychology: Is there a learning benefit? *Teaching of Psychology, 39*, 272–275. http://dx.doi.org/10.1177/0098628312456622.

Ofstad, W., & Brunner, L. (2013). Team-based learning in pharmacy education. *American Journal of Pharmaceutical Education, 77*(4), 1–11.

Phillips, J. M., & Vinten, S. A. (2010). Why clinical nurse educators adopt innovating teaching strategies: A pilot study. *Nursing Education Perspectives, 31*(4), 226–229.

Popkess, A. M., & McDaniel, A. (2011). Are nursing students engaged in learning? A secondary analysis of data. *Nursing Education Perspectives, 32*(2), 89–94.

Priharjo, R., & Hoy, G. (2011). Use of peer teaching to enhance student and patient education. *Nursing Standard, 25*(20), 40–43.

Rathbun, M. C., & Ruth-Sahd, L. A. (2009). Educational innovations: Algorithmic tools for interpreting vital signs. *Journal of Nursing Education, 48*(7), 395–400.

Rao, D., & Stupans, L. (2012). Exploring the potential of role play in higher education: Development of a typology and teacher guidelines. *Innovations in Education and Teaching International, 49*(4), 427–436.

Reeves, S., Tassone, M., Parker, K., Wagner, S., & Simmons, B. (2012). Interprofessional education: An overview of the key developments in the past three decades. *Work, 41*(3), 233–245. http://dx.doi.org/10.3233/WOR-201201298.

Rogers, E. M. (2003). *Diffusion of innovations* (5th ed.). New York: Free Press.

Ryan, M. (2011). Evaluating portfolio use as a tool for assessment and professional development in graduate nursing education. *Journal of Professional Nursing, 27*(2), 84–91. http://dx.doi.org/10.1016/jprofnurs.2010.09.008.

Sherwood, G., & Horton-Deutsch, S. (2012). *Reflective practice: Transforming of nursing and improving outcomes.* Indianapolis: Honor Society of Nursing, Sigma Theta Tau International.

Slavich, G. M., & Zimbardo, P. G. (2012). Transformational teaching: Theoretical underpinnings, basic principles, and core methods. *Educational Psychology Review, 24*(4), 560–608. http://dx.doi.org/10.1007/s10648-012-9199-6.

Sterman, E., Ross, B., Russell, S. L., Aizley, C., Viellette, E. L., Suplicki, L., et al. (2013). Impact of different educational methods on nursing knowledge and satisfaction. *Journal for Nurses in Professional Development, 29*(1), 2–7.

Suwantarathip, O., & Wichadee, S. (2014). The effects of collaborative writing activity using Googledocs on student writing abilities. *Turkish Journal of Educational Technology, 13*(2), 148–156.

Troxler, H., Vann, J. C., & Oremann, M. H. (2011). How baccalaureate nursing programs teach writing. *Nursing Forum, 46*(4), 280–288.

Tune, J. D., Sturek, M., & Basile, D. P. (2013). Flipped classroom model improves graduate student performance in cardiovascular, respirator, and renal physiology. *Advances in Physiology Education, 37,* 316–320. http://dx.doi.org/10.1152/advan.00091.2013.

West, C., Usher, K., & Delaney, L. (2012). Unfolding case studies in pre-registration nursing education: Lessons learned. *Nurse Education Today, 32,* 575–580.

White, L. (2014). Mindfulness in nursing: An evolutionary concept analysis. *Journal of Advanced Nursing, 70*(2), 282–294. http://dx.doi.org/10.1111/jan.12182.

Wyatt, T. H., Krauskopf, P. B., Gaylord, N. M., Ward, A., Huffstutler-Hawkins, S., & Goodwin, L. (2010). Cooperative m-learning with nurse practitioner students. *Nursing Education Perspectives, 31*(2), 109–113.

Young, M. S., Robinson, S., & Alberts, P. (2009). Students pay attention: Combating the vigilance decrement to improve learning during lectures. *Active Learning in Higher Education, 10*(41), 41–55. http://dx.doi.org/10.1177/14697874081000194.

Zepke, N., & Leach, L. (2010). Improving student engagement: Ten proposals for action. *Active Learning in Higher Education, 11*(3), 167–177. http://dx.doi.org/10.1177/1469787410379680.

16 Multicultural Education in Nursing*

G. Rumay Alexander, EdD, MSN, BSN, FAAN

More than classrooms are flipping these days. The profound changes in the nation's demographics are creating new realities for nursing faculty. With a projection of 50% of the population being composed of minorities by 2050, academic institutions will increasingly be made up of groups of people who are disproportionately represented among the educationally underserved, and are currently underrepresented among academic high achievers throughout the educational pipeline (Pederson-Clayton & Pederson-Clayton, 2008).

Furthermore, a large body of social science research indicates that higher education is not immune from the inequities that occur in American society. Most of this research focuses on the experiences and outcomes of college and university students and indicates that Latino/a, African American, and Native American students have lower rates of college enrollment and retention than white students (Status and Trends in the Education of Racial and Ethnic Minorities (2008); Steele, 2010). These attrition rates require faculty to design curricula and courses to meet the needs of all students and initiate support systems to ensure student success.

After growing by 3.2 million between 2006 and 2011, college enrollment in the United States has declined for the past 2 years (Bauman, 2014). Specific minority groups, including Hispanics, African Americans, and Asians, also experienced an increase in enrollment between 2007 and 2012, but minority enrollment did not increase in the 2012–2013 school year. Two-year institutions have been most affected by this decline, but 4-year colleges and graduate schools also have been affected (Bauman, 2014). These changes are reflected in nursing schools as they attempt to recruit, enroll, and retain a student body reflective of the community in which the graduates will practice.

Although the nation's student population is becoming more diverse, the majority of full-time faculty positions continue to be filled by white men and women. From 1997 through 2007, for example, the percentage of students of color enrolled in U.S. colleges and universities climbed from 25% to 30%, but the percentage of full-time faculty positions held by people of color increased only slightly—from 13% in 1997 to 17% in 2007 (Ryu, 2010). Women of color, in particular, continue to be underrepresented. In 2007, women of color held only 7.5% of full-time faculty positions. Moreover, the percentage of women of color declined steadily with rising academic rank. Women of color composed 10% of instructors and lecturers, 10% of assistant professors, 7% of associate professors, and only 3% of full professors (Ryu, 2010).

Narratives collected by Muhs, Niemann, Gonzalez, and Harris (2012) reveal that not only the demographics but the culture of academia is distinctly white, heterosexual, and middle and upper-middle class. These increases in the diversity of the population and of nursing, even while faculty remain primarily white, female Baby Boomers, have implications for creating an inclusive learning environment given that biases in academia still exist despite noble efforts for their elimination.

Both the Sullivan Commission (2004) report on *Diversity in the Healthcare Workforce* and the landmark nursing report of the Institute of Medicine (Institute of Medicine [IOM], 2010), *The Future of Nursing: Leading Change, Advancing Health* clearly point out the need

*The author acknowledges the work of Lillian Gatlin Stokes and Natasha Flowers in previous editions of the chapter.

for increasing diversity in the health care workforce. The IOM recommends that the country double the number of nurses with doctorates; doing so will support more nurse leaders, promote nurse-led science and discovery, and contribute to better care for patients by having more educators in place to prepare the next generation of nurses. Increasing the diversity in academic programs will increase diversity in the workforce as well as prepare students for civic engagement and global understanding.

Demographic data for students enrolled in nursing programs tend to mirror that of the society at large. However, with the publication of position papers and policy statements calling attention to the need to increase the diversity of nursing students (American Association of Colleges of Nursing [AACN], 1997, 2013; National League for Nursing, 2009), recent enrollment data (AACN, 2015) indicate that in 2014, approximately 30% of the students at each level of BSN, MSN, and doctoral (PhD/DNP) programs represent minorities, a steady increase since 2004. There has also been an increase in male students to 11% from 9% in 2004. Nursing organizations have also provided an impetus for creating inclusive academic programs and have curriculum and policy guidelines with statements about developing cultural competency (http://www.nln.org/about/position-statements/nln-reflections-dialogue/read/dialogue-reflection/2009/01/02/reflection-dialogue-3---a-commitment-to-diversity-in-nursing-and-nursing-education-january-2009 http://www.aacn.nche.edu/publications/position/diversity-and-equality) and implementing culturally competent care.

The purpose of this chapter is to provide guidance about creating a learning environment for nursing faculty, staff, and students that embraces inclusivity. The chapter begins with a definition of *multicultural* and *inclusive education,* and then describes how faculty can create an inclusive environment for teaching and learning. The chapter also offers strategies for creating culturally responsive academic programs, curricula, and courses, with examples of instructional strategies and approaches essential to addressing diversity in the classroom and across the curriculum.

Multicultural Education

Multicultural education refers to teaching practices that incorporate values, beliefs, and perspectives of students from different cultural backgrounds. Multicultural education shares the same premise of addressing student learning outcomes and success as cultural competence does in addressing health disparities. Table 16-1 describes the differences between these two concepts.

Multicultural education has challenged educators and educational administrators to consider equality and inclusion for the benefit of all students. Banks (2007) outlined what he called the five dimensions of multicultural education. These dimensions include (1) content integration, (2) knowledge construction, (3) equity pedagogy, (4) prejudice reduction, and (5) empowering school culture and social structure. Although not developmental, these five critical components of multicultural education emphasize planning and action steps in empowering cultural groups in the classroom setting. Opening the classroom to dialogue, providing opportunities for students to learn diverse perspectives (e.g., non-Western perspectives), and supplying opportunities for reflection can greatly enhance students' learning, which ultimately can support the provision of quality care.

Faculty must first develop cultural knowledge, cultural sensitivity, and skills, and become culturally competent themselves. Yoder (1996) suggests that when responding to student diversity, faculty move on a continuum from not having an appreciation of cultural diversity and denying that diversity influences the teaching–learning process to "mainstreaming" in which faculty are culturally aware, but attribute problems to the student's lack of awareness of the dominant culture and expect the students to conform to that culture. In the next phase, "nontolerant," educators create barriers for students, but as they move to "struggling," educators find ways to adapt to individual student needs. In the final stage, faculty have a greater cultural awareness and value diversity. Here, faculty encourage students to maintain their cultural identity while functioning biculturally.

Cultural Knowledge

Cultural knowledge is the attainment of factual information about different cultural groups. Having cultural knowledge is important for faculty and students in the classroom and in clinical areas. Faculty can plan assignments for students to assess their own cultural knowledge. There are a variety of conceptual models and frameworks that faculty can use

TABLE 16-1 Multicultural Teaching and Teaching for Cultural Competence

	Multicultural Teaching	Teaching for Cultural Competence
Focus	Creating curriculum and using instructional strategies and material to support diverse students (e.g., equity)	Assisting students to learn about their own values, beliefs, and attitudes and those of individuals from other cultural backgrounds
Process	Developmental, a continuum	Developmental, a continuum
Knowledge Assessment	Takes cultural background and attitudes, learning styles, biases, prejudices, and needs into account in planning for teaching and learning	Takes cultural background, attitudes, values, and beliefs into account to promote cultural understanding
Learning Environment	Focuses on learning for diverse students, equity pedagogy Promotes respect for and among all students Ensures instructional materials are free of bias; facilitates use of extracurricular activities to assist student learning	Focus on varied aspects of culture in relation to patient care Promotes understanding and respect for all human variations Ensures inclusion of content about various cultures
Instruction	Allows student more responsibility and choices for learning Uses multiple ways of conveying information to facilitate student understanding	Promotes understanding Uses multiple strategies and approaches to facilitate knowledge acquisition
Teaching Strategies	Groups, instructional media, games, journals, ethnographies, guest speakers, panels, role play, textbooks, simulations, articles, discussion, reflection	Role play, games, vignettes, case studies and groups, media, popular books, visits to museums and other community settings, panels, interviews, storytelling, experiential immersion, exchange experiences, service learning, ethnographies, workshops, educational programming, engagement
Assessing Progress	Observe student engagement Curriculum and program review Course evaluation	Measurement of knowledge of cultural concepts (e.g., cultural awareness and cultural sensitivity, cultural competence), course evaluation, student evaluation of extent of perceived cultural competence
Evaluation	Student evaluation of course and instruction Faculty and student self-evaluation Peer evaluation of faculty; evidence of inclusive teaching External review of curriculum for multicultural education Student and alumni review of curriculum and instruction	Testing (multiple choice), writing, role playing discussions, simulation, abilities to provide appropriate cultural care

to assist students in acquiring cultural knowledge. For example, Giger and Davidhizar (2008) developed a transcultural assessment model that includes five components: communication, time, space, health beliefs and practices, and environment. Such a model can help students learn about themselves and other individuals by using these components as a framework for assessment, as well as for special assignments and points of reference in less formal conversations. Additional models designed for nursing are Leininger's (1993) Cultural Care Theory; Purnell and Paulanka's (2008) model for cultural competence; and Campinha-Bacote's (1999) model, The Process for Cultural Competence and Delivery of Healthcare Services, which incorporates cultural knowledge, awareness, skill, desire, and encounters.

As knowledge is shared, and as students seek to learn new knowledge about specific cultural groups, faculty can ensure that students have knowledge of the concept of heterogeneity (e.g., variety, diversity, and differences in subgroups) as contrasted with the concept of homogeneity (sameness). Although there is a tendency to classify individuals within an ethnic group as one group, the truth is that there are "multiple culturally similar" but not culturally homogeneous ethnic subgroups" (Aponte, 2009). An understanding of the differences must be manifested through the manner in which questions are phrased. The underlying point is to not make assumptions; in making cultural assessments faculty should ask open-ended questions rather than direct questions.

Cultural Understanding, Cultural Sensitivity, and Cultural Skills

Cultural understanding is the recognition that there are multiple perspectives, multiple truths, multiple solutions, and multiple ways of knowing. In other words, students develop insights and learn that "one culture does not fit all." To assess students' cultural understanding, faculty should plan activities that have the potential for students to demonstrate an understanding of different cultures. In addition to clinical practice, students can actively engage in discussion groups, for example, through case studies, vignettes, role playing, essay writing, responses to questions, panel discussions, and games. A student who has an appropriate cultural understanding will recognize when values, beliefs, and practices of individuals are not compromised. As with other attributes of cultural competence, measurement for understanding can be sought through self-assessment, tests, feedback from essays and other written assignments, role playing, and engagement in games.

Cultural sensitivity develops as faculty and students come to appreciate, respect, and value cultural differences. Because cultural sensitivity is not easily developed through classroom learning activities, using clinical exchange experiences in a different part of the city or in different areas within the United States is an effective strategy. Here, students have an opportunity to establish personal relationships with people who are from socioeconomic classes or cultural groups that are not the same as theirs. As a follow up to these experiences, faculty can provide leading questions or points that will help students feel comfortable engaging in conversations.

Cultural skill relates to effective performance, for example, in communicating with others. Skill development in the area of communication can be enhanced through the use of interviews and visual media, the latter of which can be shown in segments and as time permits for discussion and evaluation of the effectiveness and ineffectiveness of the communication or interview techniques. Faculty can provide feedback following role plays, small-group exercises, discussions of case presentation, as well as permit students to self-assess. Evidence of skill development will be exhibited when beliefs, values, and practices are integrated into plans, when communication is effective, and when appropriate assessments and interventions are made. Cultural competence is by nature a skill evidenced through skill sets.

Cultural Competence

Because faculty are role models and cultural agents, they must possess necessary knowledge, skills, and attitudes to facilitate inclusive teaching and guide students to provide culturally competent care. It is equally important for faculty and students to have an awareness and understanding of their personal beliefs and how these may affect teaching and learning and patient care. See Table 16-2 for a tool to assess personal cultural competence.

Nunez (2000) describes cultural competence as the capacity to function effectively as an individual and an organization within the context of the cultural beliefs, behaviors, and needs presented by consumers in their communities. Purnell and Paulanka (2008) defined cultural competence as developing an awareness of one's own existence, thoughts, and environments without letting it influence others from different backgrounds; demonstrating awareness and understanding of the patient's cultural background; respecting and accepting cultural differences and similarities; and providing congruent care by adapting it to the patient's cultural health care beliefs, values, and norms. Campinha-Bacote, Yahie, and Langenkamp (1996) defined cultural competence as "a process, not an end point, in which the nurse continuously strives to achieve the ability to effectively work within the cultural context of an individual, family, or community from a diverse cultural and ethnic background" (pp. 1–2). This implies that one continuously strives to achieve. Therefore it can be considered to be developmental as well as a journey.

In addition to these definitions, cultural competence has been described as existing on a continuum. Each provides a beginning point for faculty as they direct efforts to facilitate cultural competence understanding among students. Burchum (2002) identified eight attributes of cultural competence: cultural awareness, cultural knowledge, cultural understanding, cultural sensitivity, cultural interaction, cultural skill, cultural competence, and cultural proficiency. Likewise, Lister (1999) identified seven terms classified as a taxonomy: (1) *cultural awareness,* (2) *cultural knowledge,* (3) *cultural understanding,* (4) *cultural sensitivity,* (5) *cultural interaction,* (6) *cultural skill,* (7) *cultural competence.*

Wells (2000) proposed a model of cultural competence that incorporates two phases: cognitive and affective. The cognitive phase involves acquiring knowledge

TABLE 16-2 Assessing Personal Cultural Competence

Ask specific questions relating to each of the attributes.	
Awareness	Am I aware of my personal biases, stereotypes, and prejudices toward cultures that are different than my own? To what extent am I aware?
Knowledge	Do I have factual information of the similarities and differences between and among varying cultural groups, specifically regarding their health care practices, beliefs, and traditions?
Understanding	Do I understand that there are a variety of cultural factors that may contribute to why my students, peers, classmates or patients may react the way they do? To what extent do I understand?
Sensitivity	Am I sensitive enough to convey to others that I appreciate, respect, and value their cultural differences? To what extent do I demonstrate sensitivity?
Cultural Interaction	Do I make deliberate efforts to make personal contact with individuals who are from a cultural group different than my own? Do I read books, articles, or watch movies, etc., and intellectually reflect on what I saw, read, or heard? To what extent? Do I take advantage of exchange programs in my school such as study-abroad programs or mission trips that would take me to environments of people within my community that have a culture different from my own? Do I frequent cultural establishments in my community?
Cultural Skill	Do I possess the skill sets to effectively communicate with my patients when I conduct a cultural assessment and a physical assessment that will provide evidence that I am appropriate, efficient, and safe? To what extent?
Cultural Competence	Do I demonstrate competence to the extent that I could in my teaching about or giving patient care? Identify the following outcomes that provide evidence of: • Facilitating or providing care that respects the values, beliefs, and health practices of the patient as well as being safe and satisfying care. • Integrating cultural beliefs, values, languages, and health practices of others in assessment plans and actual care. • Examining the influence of culturally tied beliefs and practices on individual health care needs. • Meeting cultural needs of individuals and their families. • Incorporating cultural aspects of health and illness during assessments and communication and in actual care. • Applying national standards to facilitate the provision of appropriate care to individuals and families.

whereas the affective phase relates to changes in attitudes and behaviors. Both of these are considered to be developmental. In viewing the concept on a continuum, there is progression from lack of or limited knowledge to cultural knowledge and then awareness. Characteristics of the affective phase are the development of cultural sensitivity, cultural competence, and cultural proficiency. The components of cultural competence are similar in each of these models.

Preparing a culturally competent graduate is a goal of all nursing programs. To achieve this goal, instruction and activities should be directed toward the meanings, development of cultural confidence, attributes, assessment, instructional strategies, resources, and evaluation.

The Inclusive Learning Environment

Learning environments can be unequal power spaces, but when faculty adopt an "inclusive excellence" framework, they view everyone in the academic program or course as a resource on the topic at hand while at the same time recognizing that students' perspectives will vary based on their personal experience with the topic (Bleich, MacWilliams, & Schmidt, 2014; Pederson-Clayton & Pederson-Clayton, 2008). Inclusive learning environments are places in which thoughtfulness, mutual respect, multiple perspectives, varied experiences, and academic excellence are valued and promoted. This is largely due to the fact that the faculty and students work together to create and sustain an environment in which everyone feels safe, supported, and encouraged to express her or his views and concerns. In the classroom, content is presented in a manner that reduces all students' experiences of marginalization and, wherever possible, helps students understand that individual experiences, values, and perspectives influence how they construct knowledge in any field or discipline.

To create an inclusive learning environment, everyone in the school is responsible for making students feel welcome and comfortable. Managing dynamics that go beyond fitting in if one is different from the majority to messages of belonging and safety are crucial. The admission to schools of nursing of diverse populations of students directly affects factors such as the learning environment of the educational unit (campus-wide and the school of nursing), the social environment, and recruitment (and retention). Therefore concerted efforts must be made to direct interventions that will have positive effects for all students.

Because most of the interaction among students and faculty occur in the classroom and clinical agencies, faculty must be prepared to create a learning environment there that is sensitive to the dynamics of student interaction, recognize and manage microaggressions and gender and linguistic biases, and understand racial and ethnic differences in students' learning style. Refer to Box 16-1 for strategies to create a welcoming and inclusive classroom.

BOX 16-1 Strategies to Create a Culturally Inclusive Teaching and Learning Environment

- Introduce each other in a way that all students can get to know something about the faculty, their class colleagues, and the diversity of experience in the class.
- Inform students of the faculty's approach to teaching and learning. Include some information about your own cultural origin and any cross-cultural teaching and learning experiences you may have had over time.
- Ask students what form of address they prefer. Use inclusive language that doesn't assume Western name forms—*family* name, not *last* name; *given* name, not *Christian* name. Students from more formal educational cultures, where status differences related to age or educational qualifications are important, might be uncomfortable addressing teaching staff by their given names. A compromise can be for students to use your title and given name (e.g., Professor Marie, Dr. Ivan).
- Include discussions of privilege because it broadens the discussion of race and issues of power, both explicit and implicit.
- During silences, ask students to write down anonymously what they are feeling at the moment and why. Point to the similarities and differences between the responses to elicit discussion.

Classroom Dynamics

One of the major barriers to learning for minority students is fear of participating in class and experiencing rejection from their classmates. In the classroom, faculty must be aware of students' backgrounds and response patterns and how classroom norms and rules are forms of power. Payne's classic book *A Framework for Understanding Poverty* (2005) is an excellent resource summarizing the major hidden rules—the unspoken cues and habits that differ among the classes of poverty, middle class, and wealth. Students who have experienced poverty have at least two sets of behaviors from which to choose—one for the street and one for the school or work settings. Students from the middle class value work and achievement while students from wealth emphasize financial, social, and political connections. When faculty understand these behaviors and the hidden rules and power differentials, they can structure the classroom to overcome these differences.

Capitalizing on the opportunity from the beginning to create a welcoming environment will neutralize to a great degree the stress that comes with the feeling of not belonging. A caring pedagogy makes allowances for behaviors that are exhibited by students in the classroom even during moments of silence. It is especially important to stay learner-driven and therefore student-centered. This calls for an astute awareness of the adaptations that may be needed while simultaneously complementing participatory learning.

Microaggressions

Microaggressions, which are reported to be common, are defined by Sue and colleagues (2007) as "brief and commonplace verbal, behavioral, or environmental indignities, whether intentional or unintentional, that communicate hostile, derogatory, or negative racial slights or insults toward people of color" (p. 271). In addition to race, they are reported to be perpetuated on the basis of gender, sexual orientation, religious beliefs, and ability status. Refer to Table 16-3. The effect of continuing microaggressions to exclude the person of difference is real. Individuals experiencing these microaggressions have expressed feelings of lessened self-confidence and productivity (Mays, 2009). The implication is for educators to think about any method of verbal exchange so as to eliminate statements that might be perceived as microaggressions.

TABLE 16-3 Examples of Microaggressions

Culture and Learning	Statement or Behavior	Perceived Meaning of Statement
Ethnicity and Race	When I look at you, I don't see color. There is only one race: the human race Being ignored in the classroom.	Denial of individual's racial and ethnic experiences. Denial of individual's ethnic and cultural being. Students from certain cultural groups are not valued.
Gender	Anyone can succeed, man or woman, if he or she works hard.	No acknowledgement of unfair benefits because of gender.
Ability	You are so articulate. You are a credit to your race and community.	People of color may perceive this statement as negative and demeaning rather than positive and uplifting.

When microaggressions occur, faculty or anyone present has the responsibility to manage the incident. The goal is to preserve the dignity of those involved:

- Be open to discussing, exploring, and clarifying what is felt and seen. In other words, "pay attention to the tension."
- Do a check-in. Watch body language and indications that students have checked out. This will do much to engender trust and to positively seal a caring relationship.
- Offer a simple "I'm sorry," which is all that may be called for in many instances.
- Reduce ambiguity and uncertainty, and make the invisible visible.
- Use the opportunity to educate all members of the community. Education holds one of the primary keys to combating and overcoming the harm that microaggressions deliver.
- Indicate at the outset that anyone present could unintentionally or intentionally commit these acts, especially through the language we use.

Managing the situation when one is involved as either the target or perpetrator requires particular acumen. Faculty and students can be open to exploring the possibility that one has acted in a biased fashion and controlling defensiveness. This involves suspending interpretation of behavior for those who challenge views, and becoming aware of values, biases, and assumptions about human behavior.

When faculty or students are working in a team when microaggressions occur, they should manage the process, not the content. This occurs by acknowledging the accuracy of statements when appropriate, helping individuals see the difference between intention and effect, and encouraging individuals to explore how their feelings may be saying something about them and enlisting the aid of others on the team by asking them what they see happening. When courage shows up, it is important for faculty to recognize, validate, and express appreciation for the individual's willingness to take a risk and to hold a courageous dialogue. By doing so, faculty model healthy relationship behaviors.

Gender and Linguistic Bias

Everyone is capable of bias and therefore is not and cannot be all-knowing and completely objective; this is true also for members of the scientific community as well as faculty and staff in nursing programs. Thus for faculty, understanding their own biases as well as their students' beliefs and biases is a component of cultural due diligence and a prerequisite to establishing an inclusive learning environment.

In a class with diverse students, it is prudent as well as necessary for faculty to be attentive to responses by anyone in the class that may be perceived as dismissive or minimizing. Unconscious bias plays a part in the way faculty and students are perceived by others. Faculty and students can determine their biases by taking assessment tools, which can be a springboard for getting in touch with personal subconscious biases in a safe manner. The results can be transformative in terms of self-awareness. These online tests are easily accessible at https://implicit.harvard.edu/implicit/takeatest.html.

Promoting equity in teaching also means that teachers are aware of subconscious biases and differential treatment. As psychologist Claude Steele's (2010) research indicates, even the fear that one will be judged according to extant stereotypes can depress academic performance. Examples of bias include gender bias and reactions to students who are culturally and linguistically diverse (CALD).

Research on gender bias in classrooms has supported tendencies for teachers to interact with one gender more than another (Salter, 2004). Specifically in classrooms with predominantly majority students, there is a tendency for teachers to interact with white male students more than they interact with women and men of color. With this awareness, teachers should make concerted efforts to provide equal treatment by engaging all students. This includes the quiet student who speaks up infrequently. Deliberate actions can be taken to accomplish this by devising a system for engaging students regardless of gender or ethnicity. One frequently used technique is placing index cards in an accessible manner where individuals can write their comments or questions anonymously. This provides insights on where students are struggling with concepts or have concerns that must be addressed.

With increasing numbers of male students in nursing programs, gender dynamics become important, and it is essential to deploy gender-neutral language unless specificity of gender affects the lesson being taught or the point being made.

Faculty may also have a bias for students who are culturally and linguistically diverse (CALD). In fact, language differences is a key source of discrimination on the part of faculty, students, and patients, causing students for whom English is not their first or only language to feel devaluated (Smith & Smyer, 2015). English language learner (ELL) students, also known as CALD students (Fuller, 2013), must be able to learn, write, take tests, and communicate with classmates and patients in two languages, first translating the concepts or communication into their own language and then back into English. If a student has an accent, challenges in communications may arise between the ELL student and other students or between the ELL student and faculty; class participation that requires verbal responses may be a challenge. In such situations, faculty may refer students to accent reduction or modification programs. Carr and Dekemel-Ichikawa (2012) reported favorable results for international students who participated in an accent-modification course.

Assumptions and beliefs undergird all interactions with others. For example, non-verbal behaviors such as frowns, furrowed brows, and intense concentration may not be deliberate behaviors; rather, their use may be related to efforts to try to capture what is being voiced by the student, and faculty and students should seek to understand the meaning of the behavior rather than make assumptions about it. Unless clarified, these non-verbal behaviors may have an effect on students' future participation in discussions and classroom interactions. They may refrain from participation or not respond to or ask questions because of the panicky feelings they may experience at having to speak in class.

Efforts can be made to address some of these differences by incorporating strategies to improve linguistic competence such as the use of assignments for reading with a study guide, for writing (including brief written assignments, accepting paper drafts, and ongoing writing), and for speaking and listening (Guttman, 2004).

Faculty can pay attention to techniques that are used for questioning, for example, asking "why" and "how" questions and encouraging and requesting students to "take risks" at no cost and to explore "possibilities." Questions framed in an open manner tend to be less intimidating than those that give the impression that only one answer is possible. Waiting up to 10 to 12 seconds for a reply provides an opportunity for students to formulate and translate their thoughts from their native language to English.

An additional way to engage students in language use is to use a learning activity that requires them to write a question related to the assignment each week and ask them to read the question in class or small peer group. This activity has a high potential for opening dialogue, decreasing shyness, and enhancing community building with the class.

Furthermore, faculty must be willing to address students' affective issues that influence their feelings about English. According to Halic, Greenburg, and Paulus (2009), graduate students from various countries outside the United States who participated in a phenomenological study about their language identity expressed major concerns about how faculty and peers perceived them as they developed a stronger grasp of the English language. Also, these students shared their own notions of English as a barrier and a "channel of access" given their interactions in classroom settings (Halic et al., 2009, p. 82).

It is not uncommon in informal settings for students to share personal feelings of exclusion or isolation. Opportunities should be provided for informal conversations outside of the classroom.

The use of "gatherings" as a support strategy has been reported to be beneficial for CALD students, as well as for other underrepresented students (Stokes, 2003). This support initiative provides a forum for students to openly discuss issues and concerns in a supportive nonacademic environment. As a result, students have increased confidence in their abilities and may make more frequent participation in informal and more formal classroom activities, including discussions.

Faculty must also be aware of students' use of voice registers. According to Payne (2005), every language in the world has five registers. Joos (1967) found that it is socially acceptable to go down one register in the same conversation. However, to drop two registers or more in the same conversation is to be socially offensive. Faculty must be sensitive to the subtleties in student vocalizations and the voice registers they use; for example, in some cultures, it may be appropriate to be what might be considered by the dominant culture as "soft spoken" or "loud."

Learning Styles

Recent evidence indicates that students' learning styles may also differ by race and ethnicity (see Chapter 2). For example, using the Kolb Learning Style Inventory, Fogg, Carlson-Sabelli, Carlson, and Giddens (2013) reported that there were distinct differences in learning style based on self-identified racial ethnic group: there was a good likelihood that African American students were assimilators, whites were convergers, Hispanics and Latinos were accommodators, and Asian Americans were divergers. These findings are significant in light of the underrepresentation of minority students in nursing education. Using multimodal methods of learning may help students regardless of learning style. Because learning styles are not static and can change over time, faculty can assist students with the identification of their learning style and conduct sessions for students to optimize their learning style throughout the nursing curriculum (Kyprianidou, Demetriadis, Tsiatsos, & Pombortsis 2012).

Another area in which there are reported cultural differences is the need for context, or the amount of background information students need to facilitate their learning (Giddens, 2008). American Indian students and students from Asia, Japan, Saudi Arabia, and Spain tend to require more context. For students from these high-context cultures, meaning comes from the environment, is more human oriented, and is sought in relationships between the ideas expressed in the communication process. These students benefit from learning activities such as story telling and description. On the other hand, students from Anglo or European cultures tend to require little context to support their learning, These low-context students place meaning in exact verbal descriptions or direct forms of communication, and benefit from having limited amount of detail and enrichment for learning.

Students from different cultures also vary in their preferences for having faculty present and for studying alone versus studying in groups. Some students have the implicit expectation that faculty will transmit all the knowledge; they may be reluctant to raise questions, but instead will memorize information as presented (Amaro, Abriam-Yago, & Yoder, 2006). This hierarchical perspective can affect the manner in which students respond to classroom activities.

In classrooms in the United States, students are expected to be active learners, to participate in group activities, to ask questions, and to openly express thoughts. On the other hand, the responses of Asian students to classroom activities such as group exercises may not be highly regarded because the "authoritative figure" is not primary and center. Group and team work also may not be an effective approach for all students. Self-organizing groups work well, but can leave those who are perceived or seen as different left out, with a sense of not being wanted or welcome. Faculty must ensure that cliques do not form when they or students make group or team assignments.

Developing Inclusive Excellence in Academic Institutions, Programs, Curricula and Courses

To meet the needs for diversity in nursing education and to prepare a workforce that is representative of the diversity of patients to be served, administrators, staff, and faculty must build a culture of inclusivity at the institutional level as well as within the school of nursing, and develop academic programs that embrace the strengths of all members of the academic community. Additionally, the school must be able to recruit, retain and graduate a diverse student body and support a culture of inclusivity in its programs, curricula, and courses.

Institutional Values

Developing a culture of inclusivity begins at the institutional level and is made visible through explicit values for diversity and inclusivity; practices and procedures that support recruitment and retention of faculty, staff, and students from underrepresented populations; and policies that hold no tolerance for acts of discrimination. Whereas a diverse culture is open to a variety of perspectives, beliefs, cultures, religions, and sexual orientations, an inclusive culture brings this variety into the decision-making structures, academic programs, and classrooms; embraces it; and removes barriers to full engagement in the mission of the institution (Bleich et al., 2014).

Bleich and colleagues (2014) have identified six strategies that accelerate the development of an inclusive organization: (1) improve admission process; (2) reduce invisibility of underrepresented faculty, staff, and students; (3) create communities of support and ensure that promotion and tenure structures are balanced; (5) eliminate exclusion; and (6) stand against tokenism. Additionally, colleges and universities and their schools of nursing must have statements about their commitment to diversity and inclusivity as well as specific campus conduct policies and procedures for discrimination related to age, gender, race, color, national origin, disability, and veteran status, among other factors. (See also Chapter 3).

Academic Programs

To establish inclusive learning environments at the school level, administrators and faculty can first assess their current environmental support for inclusion (Table 16-4). Inclusive academic programs also have programs to support recruitment, retention, and graduation of underrepresented students. These programs also have a dedicated office of diversity and a dean or director of diversity.

Recruitment

To obtain a diverse student population, the school of nursing must be involved in active recruitment efforts. Recruitment of underrepresented minority students or a "diversity pipeline" program can begin as early as grade school at a time when students are making career choices. These programs involve sharing information about nursing as a career such as "shadow a nurse" activities or clubs that focus on nursing careers. Another strategy is to prepare high school students for certified nursing assistant positions with the intent of transitioning these graduates to nursing programs (Colville, Cotton, Robinette, Wald, & Waters, 2015). Other programs include establishing partnerships or academic transition programs between high schools, BSN, and graduate programs that streamline the curricula to facilitate admission and progression in the next level of academic preparation. Financial support and scholarships dedicated to underrepresented

TABLE 16-4 Services to Support an Inclusive Academic Program

Advertising Materials	Should be recruitment and diversity friendly; brochures, leaflets, pamphlets, bulletins, and websites should reflect diversity. Advertisement materials are frequently examined as students and their family and faculty are searching for a school or seeking employment
Campus and Nursing Programs	Should promote services that are needed by diverse populations. Academic and student services should be welcoming and reflect the potential population for the campus or school. Provide a variety of services, including mentors and peer tutors, writing centers, inviting study areas, libraries, and equipment with representative population holdings. Enact gender-neutral and culturally appropriate language in policies. For recruitment and retention, provide faculty role models, diverse staff and student populations (including men). Provide academic services inclusive of mentors and peer tutors.
Classroom	Should be designed for multipurpose use and diverse ways of learning; movable tables, chairs, and desks are useful for peer-to-peer interaction and small-group work.
Social Environment	Plan events to bring students of diverse populations together for socialization and learning. Bring prominent and renowned speakers from a variety of ethnic groups and special program offerings.

minority students also aid in recruitment. In a study of the success of diversity pipeline programs, Brooks-Carthon, Nguyen, Chittams, Park, and Guevara (2014) found that mentorship and academic and psychosocial support were associated with increased enrollment and graduation for students participating in these programs. They also noted that only 20% of nursing programs in their study reported having diversity pipeline programs.

Program admission criteria can also affect recruitment efforts. Admission requirements that depend solely on achievement test scores and grade point averages may restrict minority student application and acceptance rates, and limit the school's opportunities for experiencing the benefits of having a more diverse student body. Some schools are taking a more holistic view of admission criteria and have added interviews, essays, academic readiness, and potential for success as a student and professional as other admission criteria to a holistic admission process (Urban Universities for Health, 2014).

Retention

Once underrepresented minorities are admitted, nursing schools must also have programs in place to ensure student success. Barriers to success include lack of financial support, decreased family support, lack of cultural competence, poor preparation for college, insufficient basic technology skills, and lack of role models. Success programs seek to help students overcome these barriers. Success programs can include early identification of students at high risk for failure, mentoring, advising, study skills and test-taking skills programs, peer tutoring, use of social workers, writing centers, and empowerment sessions. Persistence and perseverance has been noted as one powerful aspect of students' completion of a nursing program (Nadeau, 2014).

Preparation for Graduation and Transition to Practice

As students approach graduation, other strategies can be employed to prepare students for transition to practice. Here licensing exam or certification exam preparation courses are helpful in preparing students to pass these exams. Capstone courses, internships, and elective courses can prepare students for the realities of employment. Residency programs have proved successful in facilitating transition to practice and retention to the employment setting. Other courses within the curriculum focus on leadership, career, and professional development, and prepare students to be lifelong learners and active members of professional nursing organizations.

The Curriculum

Diverse cultural content should be integrated throughout the curriculum. The multicultural model designed by Banks and Banks (2004, 2006) can be adapted to all levels of the curriculum. Bagnardi, Bryant, and Colin (2009) describe the experience of integrating Banks and Banks' model throughout an undergraduate curriculum. Students should learn to apply various nondominant perspectives (Morey & Kitano, 1997). As Banks and Banks suggest, instructors must move beyond the initial level of integrating cultural artifacts such as names and holidays to an integrative level where students obtain more substantive information about cultural groups (Banks & Banks, 1993, 2004). Educators should make concerted efforts to exhibit attitudes of positive portrayal of diversity and indicate that diversity is valued. Exposing students to various cultural norms, health beliefs, practices, and a balanced assignment of reviewing articles and research written or conducted by faculty of color and members of the lesbian, gay, bisexual, transgender (LGBT) community, or covering topics of concern to the marginalized is a feasible first step in diversifying the curriculum. Underwood (2006) used an inquiry approach to facilitate enhanced knowledge and sensitivity related to culture and health. A student assignment was to write three questions about an ethnic group of the student's choice. The themes that emerged from these questions were used to structure the course.

The expected curricular outcomes should be clearly identified and should guide didactic content, student assignments, and evaluation. In this way, students' progress toward cultural competence can be monitored and assessed as students move through the curriculum. The curriculum provides a framework for mapping and a set of criteria for evaluation. The results of the evaluation should exemplify the attainment of specific knowledge, skills, and attitudes.

Course Design

A thorough course analysis is a significant component of multicultural course transformation. The modification itself can present in various ways. A first step is to identify the expected outcomes. For example, after articulating that one goal for a course is to increase knowledge of bias and ethnocentrism as it relates to the study of various cultural groups, a faculty member may determine that the course's content includes various examples of cultural groups. However, the course may not facilitate opportunities for open and equitable exchanges of ideas and values. Therefore the transformative work may begin in the area of instruction for classroom as well as clinical practice.

Syllabus

The syllabus should be welcoming and convey inclusiveness. Because the syllabus is a contract with accompanying legal ramifications, faculty should ensure that the language used shows respect for differences and equity of opportunity (Chapter 10). Most syllabi have references to disability services and sexual harassment and bullying policies, but often religious observance policies are missing. Having a religious observance policy in place and including it prominently in the syllabus sends a tangible cue of respect for all religious holidays given that most college campuses follow the Christian calendar. The policy should indicate that it is the student's responsibility to inform the faculty member of religious holidays that conflict with any exams, project due dates, or assignments so that other reasonable arrangements can be negotiated. By doing so, students get practice for the work world where such responsibilities will be theirs as well (see Box 16-2).

> **BOX 16-2 Example of a Religious Observances Policy From University of North Carolina School of Nursing**
>
> The School of Nursing recognizes and respects that many religions have days of the year and celebrations they honor. By University policy, students are authorized up to two excused absences each academic year for religious observances required by their faith. To assure reasonable accommodations and appropriate alternative assignments, when a student needs to miss classes, exams, clinical experiences, and/or written assignments due to a religious observance, he/she must notify the course coordinator in writing about the conflict two weeks in advance of the date requested or as soon as possible if the date occurs within the first two weeks of the semester.
>
> Reprinted with permission from University of North Carolina Chapel School of Nursing.

Course Materials and Instructional Resources

As educators choose instructional resources to support teaching and learning, they should pay careful, close attention to implicit and explicit cues, wording, stereotypes, or generalizations. This also may mean that a variety of materials, articles, and media should be used to make up for deficits of limited information and examples in textbooks. Faculty should also examine teacher-made course materials for inclusion, exclusion, and bias. For example, course syllabi, handouts, worksheets, and evaluation instruments may inadvertently be written with culture or gender bias.

Additionally, special documentation such as books and web resources that include photos or illustrations may not include adequate racial, ethnic, or gender representation. To facilitate the availability of more unbiased instructional materials, evaluation and feedback should be provided to authors, with suggestions to include content that supports a transformed curriculum. The use of a guide similar to the one developed by Byrne, Weddle, Davis, and McGinnis (2003) can be useful in the assessment of instructional materials as well as in helping faculty evaluate and create new products.

Learning Activities

When students and faculty engage, four cultural encounters are involved: being a student, being a faculty member, learning in the academic institution or clinical practice setting, and being in a given country or region. If alliances are formed in a mutually respectful way, learning takes place in a bidirectional manner. Systems then can be developed to ensure that students have opportunities to engage in learning activities with peers from different racial and ethnic groups, peers with age variations, and peers who are both male and female. In addition to student interaction, a diverse mix of experts from the community can be used for classroom activities as appropriate. These individuals, experts in their own right, are often willing to be involved in the education of students. Faculty should take advantage of the willingness of these individuals and use them to enhance inclusivity.

In the classroom, learning activities should be planned to facilitate knowledge acquisition and interaction and collaboration of diverse groups of students. Because all encounters are cultural encounters, each of these variations brings different experiences and perspectives. In other words, in the classroom faculty must move from lectures to activity and variety that promote an opportunity to interact with each other; seek understanding; and establish respect for diverse ways of learning, opinions, beliefs, and attitudes.

As cultural agents and role models, faculty can take actions that bridge gaps between students' cultures of origin and the campus culture. Culture, like genetics, has a group definition but individual expression. The implication here is to provide a variety of learning activities that appeal to varying styles of learning, and for students to understand how their own learning style preferences affect their learning. There is evidence that cognitive and psychological traits affect learning styles, academic performance, and the engagement of students.

Using a variety of strategies and learning opportunities is particularly helpful to promote cultural understanding and competence (see also Chapter 15). Faculty can assign students to write short papers describing themselves and then reflect on the descriptions. Encouraging students to accept invitations from individuals from a different ethnic or cultural group to special events such as weddings, graduations, parties, and rite of passage ceremonies can broaden perspectives.

Students and faculty should take advantage of programs both on campus and in the community. When faculty accompany students, they can encourage a shared, common experience whereby faculty can talk individually with students and explain what the student is seeing, learning, and possibly experiencing. Faculty can make a list of cultural events and establishments such as ethnic restaurants and special museums to share with students.

Promoting reflection among students increases self-awareness. Faculty can engage students by designing written assignments, such as journaling logs or learning diaries. Personal letters written by and for the student have a dual purpose of addressing personal fears, feelings, assumptions, and expectations about a planned experience or about different racial and ethnic or age groups, and later reflecting on the identified written content in preparation for writing a major paper. The connecting link between the initial letter and the reflection could be a service learning experience. Students can read the letters after the experience and reflect on the initial letter in terms of similarities to and differences from their previous thoughts, feelings, and assumptions, thus providing an avenue for deeper reflection, meanings, and considerable learning. The letter strategy, used for 5 years in a course for beginning students, resulted in noted improvement in the quality and specificity of papers and enhanced learning as identified by students (Stokes, Linde, & Zimmerman, 2008).

Clinical Practice Courses

Emphasis should be placed on inclusive teaching and learning not only in classroom settings but in clinical practice settings as well. As attention is given to making curricular and content changes, opportunities must also be provided for clinical practice so that knowledge is reinforced, skills are developed, and changes in attitudes occur. (See also Chapter 17.) The clinical setting is a place where cultures collide and research confirms that the experiences can be challenging. One study by Welch, Harvey, and Robinson (2010) identified that there is a mismatch of perceptions and expectation of knowledge, clinical skills, and level of performance between those of the majority, be they academia or stakeholders, and those of the minority. Other studies concur that students participating in clinical experiences in a different cultural context required higher levels of support to enable them to perform at the expected levels (Boughton, Halliday, & Brown, 2010; Gerrish & Griffith, 2004; Jeong et al., 2010; Walker, 2009).

Communication is an important skill in clinical practice. To address the diversity of communication approaches, faculty can encourage students to actively observe different ways of communicating by summarizing news articles, watching television programs, and listening to the local news. When doing so, faculty should direct students to observe eye contact and mention that faculty and students with a Eurocentric background prefer eye-to-eye contact and often view others who do not look them in the eye as dishonest. Faculty can also use video clips, with examples of communication interactions between health care team members, and develop opportunities to practice different communications styles through the use of simulations and interprofessional simulations with the health care team members.

Helping students develop culturally appropriate therapeutic communication skills is equally important. Harvey, Robinson, and Frohman (2013) emphasize the importance of communication skills and highlight that the development of conversational strategies and patterns can aid all students to perform at the expected level. The authors note, however, that it can be difficult for students to change lifelong cultural ways of communication to meet the expectations of other cultures.

When selecting clinical placement sites, faculty should plan to use both in-patient and community-based facilities. Faculty should make concerted efforts to ensure that one in every five patients selected for student clinical learning experiences is from a different cultural group. Checklists or databases can be established for students and faculty to monitor and track the gender, age, racial and ethnic makeup, and socioeconomic status of patients assigned for care. When using these tracking systems, faculty should take the time to explain the systems being used and the rationale for their use with students.

By visiting urban areas or specific cultural districts, faculty can provide opportunities for students to view areas of the community that are different from their own, and conduct an organizational climate audit as part of their assignment. For example, grocery stores, storefronts, houses of worship, health clinics, and businesses could be among the destinations. Often manufacturing plants and waste sites may be close to housing communities of the underserved. Students can be directed to books, movies, and stage plays that depict an image of life as experienced by varied cultures. To make these worthwhile experiences, faculty can assist students in developing focus points that can direct their observations, conversations, and discussions before and following the experience.

Immersion Experiences

Immersion experiences are another beneficial approach to integrate content, engage students, and afford opportunities for reflection and the development of cultural competence. Faculty can use immersion experiences in several ways. One experience can be service learning with agencies that serve culturally diverse patients or those that have a specific patient population. The benefits of such experiences are multifaceted (Hunt, 2007). Caffrey, Neander, Markle, and Stewart (2005) conducted a study to evaluate the effect of integrating cultural content in an undergraduate curriculum on students' self-perceived cultural competence and to determine whether a 5-week clinical immersion in international nursing had additional effects on students' self-perceived cultural competence. The results of the study revealed a larger gain of self-perceived cultural competence for students who engaged in the immersion experience.

Another form of immersion is through the use of ethnographies. *Ethnography* refers to a written presentation of qualitative descriptions of human social information based on fieldwork. Brennan and Schulze (2004) engaged students in reading ethnographies. The activity was followed by a written assignment of an analysis of the reading. Presentations and discussions of the analysis were made in groups. Results of the ethnographic analyses indicated that students were immersed in the culture. Group discussion of the analyses was beneficial in providing a multicultural experience for all participants. Experiences can also occur through spending time and engaging with specific cultural groups within the United States (e.g., special populations) and abroad.

Online Courses

The use of the online courses and programs has increased the array of educational offerings available to students. Online courses can offer quality instruction to remote students, reach underserved populations, respond to the diverse learning styles of and paces at which students learn, break down barriers of time and space, and give access to students with different languages and cultures.

Yet despite all these advantages, there are cultural issues at play that can affect teaching and learning. Recognizing that instructional design cannot be culturally neutral is a first step in the process of becoming more culturally competent. Joos (1967) identified a number of potential issues: content, multimedia, writing style, writing structure, and web design. Hanna and De Nooy (2004) studied the validity of four assumptions some people may have about how culture is present in cyberspace: (1) the Internet removes cultural differences, (2) the Internet is a direct access to cultural differences, (3) communication over the Internet is similar to communication in other forms, and (4) computer-mediated communication influences cultural and genre-related communication. Overall, the authors found that the first three assumptions were difficult to validate as culture is discernible in online content and communication. The same applies in website and e-mail communications. Clear norms and netiquette (network etiquette) must be established at the outset of the course to indicate key principles, such as respect for diversity. An initial challenge is that in online courses visual cues as to gender and race of both students and faculty are absent. Faculty can seek to overcome this by requesting that students post their photos (and that faculty do likewise) or by using voice thread technology for students to post introductions and short comments. If instructors are able to recognize the capability of students to construct their own knowledge and apply prior experience and their own culturally preferred ways of knowing to the task, then it is likely that a more culturally sensitive online classroom will be created.

In addition, the roles of the student and the instructor in an online course may raise cultural issues. For instance, in some cultures it is considered inappropriate for students to question the instructor or the knowledge being conveyed in the course. The co-creation of knowledge and meaning in an online course, coupled with the instructor's role as an equal player in the process, may be uncomfortable for a student from this type of culture. Conversely, a student whose culture is more communal, and where group process is valued, may feel uncomfortable in a course where independent learning is the primary mode of instruction.

Faculty can devise strategies to facilitate cultural engagement in online classrooms. For example faculty can employ approaches to help students understand cultural differences such as discussing the cultural differences in online classroom dynamics in the United States in comparison with other cultures prior to the first days of class. To enhance open communication in the online classroom using developmental approaches such as structured group exercises, permitting students to present written assignments verbally in small groups and progressing to the point at which the fear of participating in discussions is overcome have been reported as highly successful in achieving this aim. Games are another widely used medium for engaging students and encouraging participation.

Online courses and experiences have the additional potential for linking classrooms for the purpose of establishing cultural exchanges through the use of virtual experiences. Additionally, faculty teaching online courses can facilitate students' awareness of their own beliefs and those of others by posing questions that require students to reflect on their values, beliefs, or culture and contrast them with those of other members in the class (Flowers, 2002). Online surveys and journals are two strategies for prompting these discussions. (See also Chapter 21.)

Evaluation of Learning Outcomes

Evaluation of all students must be fair and equitable. When evaluating underrepresented minority students, faculty must follow best practices in evaluation such as having clear learning outcomes, providing opportunity for learning and practice, and providing clear guidelines for evaluation. Tests, written work, and clinical performance as evaluation strategies must be developed with the diversity and language abilities of the students in mind. (See also Chapters 22, 23 and 24.)

Teacher-made tests are often a source of unintentional multicultural bias. Faculty should review these tests to eliminate references to the nurse as *she,* to remove any cultural stereotyping, to avoid the use of American slang, and to use language that would be understood by all students to test fairly (Ukoha, 2004). If tests are biased because of poorly written questions, faculty evaluation of student competency will be distorted (Hicks, 2011).

One way to avoid these test errors is to have colleagues take the teacher-made test; often colleagues can provide new insights because they have a fresh set of eyes and are more likely to find test construction errors. Experts also recommend writing test questions to reduce linguistic bias that can occur with multiple-choice questions (Bosher & Bowles, 2008; Lujan, 2008), unnecessary language complexity, and construct-irrelevant variance. Linguistic modification is a process by which the language load of test items is reduced semantically and syntactically while the content and integrity of the items are maintained. For highly vulnerable students, every test becomes a test of language proficiency. To a greater degree than their native English–speaking peers, nonnative English speakers must process the language of tests and negotiate the cultural expectations embedded in them.

When faculty write tests, they must consider word frequency; word length; sentence length; and linguistic structures such as passive voice constructions, long noun phrases, long question phrases, prepositional phrases, conditional clauses, and constructions that are negative, abstract, or impersonal. (See also Chapter 24.) Sentence completion, items asking for priority actions without bolding or highlighting, or using clauses and unclear wording are frequently cited as issues for many students (Bosher, 2009). Lampe and Tsaouse (2010) reviewed questions in a selected textbook publisher's test bank and found significant linguistic bias. All of the questions were in sentence completion format, priority questions did not use bolding or highlighting to emphasize important words, and 20% of the questions had embedded clauses. All of these occurrences can have an adverse effect on a student's test scores, their self-worth, and ultimately their successful matriculation in a program. See Box 16-3 for the identification and revision of culturally biased multiple-choice examination items.

When evaluating written work, faculty must consider the needs of students for whom English is not the first language and provide opportunity for students to receive feedback and review of their work prior to grading. Grading rubrics should be used to clarify the elements of the written work that will be evaluated.

Clinical performance evaluation also depends on having clearly stated learning outcomes and opportunity to practice. When evaluating students from diverse cultures, faculty must take into consideration the challenges involved when any student is giving care to a patient that is from a different culture than theirs.

Summary: I Hope You Dance

The increasing enrollments of diverse student populations in nursing programs provide opportunities for educators to be engaged in changes and to use current knowledge of multicultural education, equity pedagogy, and life experiences of diverse students to create a rich learning environment so that all students have an equal chance to achieve academically and professionally. Faculty must develop curriculum and course requirements that explicitly state goals for cultural competency. Given that all encounters are cultural encounters and therefore teaching opportunities, faculty must develop inclusive learning environments in which all students are welcome, learn from each other, become empowered, manage differences, avoid bias, and learn to provide competent cultural care to their patients.

The use of teaching–learning strategies that incorporate concepts of equity, inclusiveness, and active engagement can also affect positive learning. Cultural competence may be used as an exemplar for applying some of the principles of multicultural education while at the same time facilitating an understanding of its value in quality care. By exemplifying cultural

BOX 16-3 Guidelines for Linguistic Modification of Classroom Tests

LINGUISTIC

Each multiple-choice question (MCQ) should have a clear and focused question that can be understood and answered without looking at the responses. Use the question format (rather than completion).

Avoid unnecessary information that is not required to answer the question.

Use the active rather than the passive verb voice; use direct verbs to avoid confusion.

Avoid the use of negatives (e.g., *not, except, incorrect*) in the question.

Avoid using imprecise terms (e.g., *frequently, appropriate, few, many, some*).

Do not use trick questions in which students are asked to identify the incorrect response rather than the correct answer.

When using the best answer format, words such as *most, first,* and *best* should be bold-faced, underlined, and capitalized (e.g., ***MOST***).

Ensure that test items are independent of one another.

Avoid complex MCQs that have a range of correct responses and ask students to select from a number of combinations of these responses, known as *multiple-multiples* or *K-type MCQs*.

STRUCTURAL

Questions, options, and directions should be written in clear, unambiguous language. Test items should be easily understood on the first reading.

Use adequate spacing and consistent formatting throughout the test.

All items should be grammatically correct and free from typographical and spelling errors. All options should be grammatically consistent with the stem and parallel in style and form.

CULTURAL

Nursing items should use the same terminology used in coursework and textbooks, as well as common words for everyday items (e.g., use *toilet* instead of *commode*).[19]

Avoid items that test knowledge of nonessential dominant culture (examples are presented in Table 16-2).

Eliminate names, stereotypes, and unnecessary gender distinctions in test items.

Avoid using humor in the question or options.

BOX 16-4 Dance Professor Dance

Professor you don't know me but I am sure that you have seen me around.
Who am I? What do I look like? Well that's not important right now.
I am truly amazed by all of your certifications and nursing degrees.
I see you each day as I sit and listen attentively to you speak.
Boldly I begin to think, that may be me someday.
A prolific nurse educator with diverse knowledge, flare, and no-nonsense ways.
Professor you don't know me but I am sure that you have seen me around.
Who am I? What do I look like? Well that's not important right now.
At first it seems that you wanted me here but as time passed it became crystal clear.
Today when I approach you I feel instantly rejected.
I start to think no, this cannot be true of all of you.
Professor you don't know me but I am sure that you have seen me around.
Who am I? What do I look like? Well that's not important right now.
I sit in your class day to day and we have even stood side-by-side.
I make no excuse for my silky caramel complexion,
long black wavy hair or even my urban style.
The grades I earn speak for themselves
and my nursing skills are always above the rest.
It's true I know what you see in me
is not your vision of the trailblazing nurse of the 21st century.
Professor you don't know me but I am sure that you have seen me around.
Who am I? What do I look like? Well that's not important right now.
Please remember that I not only see you as a disseminator of nursing knowledge.
Unfortunately what you cannot see is that you truly are the mentor and I the mentee.
Together we dance invisibly.
Professor you don't know me but I am sure that you have seen me around.
Who am I? What do I look like? Well that's not important right now.
I too represent the future and plan to become
the new Nightingale, Peplau, Roy, or the prolific Wykle.
Now please do not be ashamed that you overlooked my talent, worth, and skill.
Do not look back at the past.
Look ahead to change your perspective this academic year.
Once again there I will sit in your class listening to you teach.
Professor let's not again begin our mentor-mentee dance invisibly.

Courtesy of Lorrie R. Davis-Dick, EdDc, MSN, RN-BC.

competence as a process or a journey, both academic leaders and students will realize that lifelong learning is inherent and a requirement for teaching, learning, and preparing graduates to work in a society that includes multiple diverse groups.

Principles of inclusive excellence suggest faculty give consideration to the four major course components: managing the environment, content, instructional strategies, assessment of student knowledge, and classroom dynamics. This is particularly important as long as there are power inequities as in the workplace, the world place, and academia.

Lorrie Davis Dick, who is African American, in her insightful poem "Dance Professor Dance" (see Box 16-4) sums up the request and desires of all students, which is to remember that success and achievement are either race-, ethnicity-, generational-, or sexual identity–specific goals.

REFLECTING ON THE EVIDENCE

1. How can faculty assess their own readiness to develop and implement a multicultural and inclusive curriculum?
2. What is the state of the science for multicultural education in nursing?
3. Are instructional materials appropriate for a multicultural curriculum? To what extent do textbooks support inclusiveness? Are course materials reflective of diversity? Are tests free of gender, culture, religious, and ethnic bias? Can course policies be implemented fairly for all students?
4. To what extent are the instructional strategies used in an inclusive classroom evidence-based?
5. To what extent do I:
   a. support diverse learning styles in my classroom?
   b. seek to incorporate evidence-based teaching strategies?
   c. encourage discussions from various perspectives?
   d. embrace inclusivity in my pursuit of pedagogy?

REFERENCES

Amaro, D., Abriam-Yago, K., & Yoder, M. (2006). Perceived barriers for ethnically diverse students in nursing programs. *Journal of Nursing Education, 45*(7), 247–254.

American Association of Colleges of Nursing (AACN). (1997). *Diversity and equality of opportunity.* Retrieved from, http://www.aacn.nche.edu/publications/position/diversity-and-equality.

American Association of Colleges of Nursing (AACN). (2013). *Policy Brief, 2013: The changing landscape: Nursing student diversity on the rise.* Retrieved from, http://www.aacn.nche.edu/government-affairs/Student-Diversity-FS.pdf.

American Association of Colleges of Nursing (AACN). (2015). *New AACN Data Confirm Enrollment Surge in Schools of Nursing.* Retrieved from, http://www.aacn.nche.edu/news/articles/2015/enrollment.

Aponte, J. (2009). Addressing cultural heterogeneity among Hispanic subgroups by using Campinha-Bacote's Model of Cultural Competency. *Holistic Nursing Practice, 23*(1), 3–12.

Bagnardi, M., Bryant, L., & Colin, J. (2009). Banks multicultural model: A framework for integrating multiculturalism into nursing curriculum. *Journal of Professional Nursing, 25*(4), 234–239.

Banks, J. A. (2006). *Multicultural education: Goals and dimensions.* Center for Multicultural Education: University of Washington, College of Education. Retrieved from, http://education.washington.edu/.

Banks, J. (2007). *Educating citizens in a multicultural society* (2nd ed.). New York: Teachers College.

Banks, J., & Banks, C. (1993). *Multicultural education: Issues and perspectives.* Boston: Allyn & Bacon.

Banks, J. A., & Banks, C. A. M. (2004). *Handbook of research on multicultural education.* San Francisco: Jossey-Bass.

Bauman, K. (2014, October 6). Q&A with census analyst. *The daily tarheel.* p. 9.

Bleich, M., MacWilliams, B., & Schmidt, B. (2014, September 10). Advancing diversity through inclusive excellence in nursing education. *Journal of Professional Nursing.* published online. Retrieved from, http://dx.doi.org/10.1016/j.profnurs.2014.09.003.

Bosher, S. D. (2009). Removing language as a barrier to success on multiple-choice nursing exams. In S. D. Bosher & M. D. Pharris (Eds.), *Transforming nursing education: The culturally inclusive environment* (pp. 264–266). New York: Springer.

Bosher, S., & Bowles, M. (2008). The effects of linguistic modification on ESL students' comprehension of nursing course test items. *Nursing Education Perspectives, 29*(3), 165–172.

Boughton, M., Halliday, L., & Brown, L. (2010). A tailored program of support for culturally and linguistically diverse (CALD) nursing students in a graduate entry masters of nursing course: A qualitative evaluation of outcomes. *Nurse Education in Practice, 10,* 355–360. http://dx.doi.org/10.1016/j. nepr.2010.05.003.

Brennan, S., & Schulze, M. (2004). Cultural immersion through ethnography: The lived experience and group process. *Journal of Nursing Education, 43*(6), 285–288.

Brooks-Carthon, J., Nguyen, T., Chittams, J., Park, E., & Guevara, J. (2014). Measuring success: Results from a national survey of recruitment and retention initiatives in the nursing workforce. *Nursing Outlook, 62*(4), 259–267.

Burchum, R. (2002). Cultural competence: An evolutionary perspective. *Nursing Forum, 37*(2), 5–15.

Byrne, M., Weddle, C., Davis, E., & McGinnis, P. (2003). The Byrne guide for inclusionary cultural content. *Journal of Nursing Education, 42*(6), 277–281.

Caffrey, R., Neander, W., Markle, D., & Stewart, B. (2005). Improving the cultural competence of nursing students: Results of integrating cultural content in the curriculum and an international immersion experience. *Journal of Nursing Education, 44*(5), 234–240.

Campinha-Bacote, J. (1999). A model and instrument to address cultural competence in health care. *Journal of Nursing Education, 38*(5), 203–207.

Campinha-Bacote, J., Yahie, T., & Langenkamp, M. (1996). The challenge of cultural diversity for nurse educators. *Journal of Continuing Education in Nursing, 27*(2), 59–64.

Carr, S. M., & Dekemel-Ichikawa, K. (2012). Improving communication through accent modification: Growing the nursing workforce. *Journal of Cultural Diversity, 19*(3), 79–84.

Colville, J., Cotton, S., Robinette, T., Wald, H., & Waters, T. (2015). A community college model to support nursing workforce diversity. *Journal of Nursing Education, 54*(2), 65–71.

Flowers, N. (2002). Inclusive teaching online. In D. Billings (Ed.), *Conversations in e-learning* (pp. 197–201). Boston: Jones & Bartlett.

Fogg, L., Carlson-Sabelli, L., Carlson, K., & Giddens, J. (2013). The perceived benefits of a virtual community: Effects of learning style, race, ethnicity, and frequency of use on nursing students. *Nursing Education Perspectives, 34*(6), 390–394.

Fuller, B. (2013). Evidence-based instructional strategies: Facilitating linguistically diverse nursing student learning. *Nurse Educator, 38*(3), 118–121.

Gerrish, K., & Griffith, V. (2004). Integration of overseas registered nurses: Evaluation of an adaptation programme. *Journal of Advanced Nursing, 45,* 579–587. http://dx.doi.org/10.1046/j.1365-2648.200302949.x.

Giddens, J. (2008). Achieving diversity in nursing through multicontextual learning environments. *Nursing Outlook, 56*(2), 78–83.

Giger, J., & Davidhizar, R. (2008). *Transcultural nursing: Assessment and intervention* (5th ed.). St. Louis: Mosby.

Guttman, M. (2004). Increasing the linguistic competence of the nurse with limited English proficiency. *Journal of Continuing Education in Nursing, 35*(6), 264–269.

Halic, O., Greenburg, K., & Paulus, T. (2009). Language and academic identity: A study of the experiences of non-native English speaking international students. *International Education, 38*(2), 73.

Hanna, B., & De Nooy, J. (2004). Negotiating cross-cultural difference in electronic discussion. *Multilingua: Journal of Cross-Cultural and Interlanguage Communication, 23*(3), 257–281.

Harvey, T., Robinson, C., & Frohman, R. (2013). Preparing culturally and linguistically diverse nursing students for clinical practice. *Journal of Nursing Education, 52*(7), 365–370.

Hicks, N. A. (2011). Guidelines for identifying and revising culturally biased multiple-choice nursing examination items. *Nurse Educator, 36*(6), 266–270.

Hunt, R. (2007). Service-learning: An eye-opening experience that provokes emotion and challenges stereotypes. *Journal of Nursing Education, 46*(6), 277–281.

Institute of Medicine (IOM). (2010). *The future of nursing: Leading change, advancing health.* Washington, DC: National Academies Press.

Jeong, S. Y., Hickey, N., Lvett-Jones, T., Pitt, V., Hoffman, K., Norton, C. A., et al. (2010). Understanding and enhancing the learning experiences of culturally and linguistically diverse nursing students in an Australian bachelor of nursing program. *Nursing Education Today, 31*, 238–244. http://dx.doi.org/10.1016/j.nedt. 2010.10.016.

Joos, M. (1967). The styles of the five clocks. In R. D. Abrahams & R. C. Troike (Eds.), *Language and culture diversity in American education.* Englewood Cliffs, NJ: Prentice-Hall.

Kypriandou, M., Demetriadis, S., Tsiatsos, T., & Pombortsis, A. (2012). Group formation based on learning styles: Can it improve students' teamwork? *Educational Technology Research & Development, 60*(1), 83–110. http://dx.doi.org/10.1007/s11423-011-9215-4.

Lampe, S., & Tsaouse, B. (2010). Linguistic bias in multiple-choice test questions. *Creative Nursing, 16*(2), 63–67. Retrieved from, http://dx.doi.org/10.1891/1078-4535.16.2.63.

Leininger, M. (1993). Culture care theory: The relevant theory to guide nurses functioning in a multi-cultural world. In M. Parkes (Ed.), *Patterns of nursing theories in practice* (pp. 105–121). New York: NLN Press.

Lister, P. (1999). A taxonomy for developing cultural competence. *Nurse Education Today, 19*(4), 313–318.

Lujan, J. (2008). Linguistic and cultural adaptation needs of Mexican American nursing students related to multiple-choice tests. *Journal of Nursing Education, 47*(7), 327–330.

Mays, R. (Presenter). (2009, December 4). Multicultural education in nursing a [Web seminar presented at the New Jersey Nursing Initiative, Faculty Preparation Program, Princeton, New Jersey: Robert Wood Johnson Foundation].

Morey, A. I., & Kitano, M. K. (1997). *Multicultural course transformation in higher education: A broader truth.* Boston, MA: Allyn & Bacon.

Muhs, G. Y., Niemann, Y. F., Gonzalez, C. G., & Harris, A. P. (2012). *Presumed incompetent: The intersections of race and class for women in academia.* Boulder: University Press of Colorado.

Nadeau, J. (2014). Listening and responding to the voices of Latina prenursing students. *Nursing Education Perspectives, 35*(1), 8–13.

National League for Nursing. (2009). *A commitment to diversity in nursing and nursing education.* Retrieved from, http://www.nln.org/aboutnln/reflection_dialogue/refl_dial_3.htm.

Nunez, A. (2000). Transforming cultural competence into cross-cultural efficacy in women's health education. *Academic Medicine, 75*(11), 1071–1075.

Payne, R. K. (2005). *A framework for understanding poverty* (4th rev ed). Highland, TX: Aha! Process, Inc.

Pederson-Clayton, A., & Pederson-Clayton, S. (2008). Making excellence inclusive in education and beyond. *Pepperdine Law Review, 35*(3), 611–648.

Purnell, L., & Paulanka, B. (2008). *Transcultural health care: A culturally competent approach* (3rd ed.). Philadelphia: FA Davis Company.

Ryu, M. (2010). *Minorities in higher education: Twenty-fourth status report.* Washington, DC: American Council on Education.

Salter, D. (2004). *Gender bias in college classrooms: A study of the interactions between psychological and environmental types.* Retrieved from, http://www.ed.psu.edu/seta/NAWE.htm.

Smith, A., & Smyer, T. (2015). Black African nurses educated in the United States. *Journal of Nursing Education, 54*(2), 72–78.

Status and Trends in the Education of Racial and Ethnic Minorities. (2008). *National center for education statistics.* Retrieved from, https://nces.ed.gov/pubs2010/2010015/index.asp.

Steele, C. M. (2010). *Whistling Vivaldi and other clues to how stereotypes affect us.* New York: W.W. Norton and Company.

Stokes, L. (2003, July/August). Gatherings as a retention strategy. *Association of Black Nursing Faculty (ABNF) Journal, 14*(4), 80–82.

Stokes, L., Linde, B., & Zimmerman, M. (2005, 2008). *Instructional strategy for learning communities.* (Unpublished documentations.).

Sue, D. W., Capodilupo, C. M., Torino, G. C., Bucceri, J. M., Holder, A. M. B., Nadal, K. L., et al. (2007). Racial microaggressions in everyday life. *American Psychologist, 62*(4), 271–284.

The Sullivan Commission. (2004). *Missing persons: Minorities in the health profession (Report of the Sullivan Commission on Diversity in the Healthcare Workforce).* Washington, DC: Author.

Ukoha, R. (2004). Evidence-based multicultural teaching methods. *Nursing Educator, 29*(1), 10–12.

Underwood, S. M. (2006). Culture, diversity and health: Responding to the queries of inquisitive minds. *Journal of Nursing Education, 45*(7), 281–286.

Urban Universities for Health. (2014, September). *Holistic admission: Findings from a National survey.* Retrieved from: http://urbanuniversitiesforhealth.org/media/documents/Holistic_Admissions_in_the_Health_Professions.pdf.

Walker, L. (2009). The complex ethics of nurse migration. *Kai Tiaki Nursing New Zealand, 15*(7), 2.

Welch, A., Harvey, T., & Robinson, C. (2010). Effective transition for international nursing students undertaking the one-year program leading to nursing registration in Australia. In: *Paper presented at the 16th Qualitative health Research conference. Vancouver, British Columbia.*

Wells, M. (2000). Beyond cultural competence: A model for individual and institutional cultural development. *Journal of Community Health Nursing, 17*(4), 189–199.

Yoder, M. (1996). Instructional Responses to ethnically diverse nursing students. *Journal of Nursing Education, 35*, 315–321.

17 Teaching in the Clinical Setting*

Paula Gubrud, EdD, RN, FAAN

The health care system is ever changing and the Patient Protection and Affordable Care Act (PPACA) (Patient Protection and Affordable Care Act, 2014) challenges faculty to prepare students for future roles and to practice in a health care system that is patient-centered, wellness-oriented, community- and population-based, and technologically advanced. Clinical settings within a variety of health care systems have also become highly complex. Clinical learning occurs in actual health care environments and laboratory settings where students apply their acquired knowledge and skills as they think critically, make clinical decisions, and acquire professional values necessary to work in the practice environment. The purpose of this chapter is to describe the environments for clinical teaching and learning, how the curriculum relates to clinical teaching, roles and responsibilities of clinical teachers, and teaching methods and models that facilitate learning in clinical environments.

Practice Learning Environments

The environment for practicum experiences may be any place where students interact with patients and families for purposes such as acquiring needed cognitive skills that facilitate clinical reasoning and decision-making as well as psychomotor and affective skills. The practicum environment, also referred to as the *clinical learning environment* (CLE), is an interactive network of forces within the clinical setting that influence students' clinical learning outcomes. The environment also provides opportunities for students to integrate theoretical nursing knowledge into nursing care, cultivate clinical reasoning and judgment skills, and develop a professional identity (O'Mara, McDonald, Gillespie, Brown, & Miles, 2014). The CLE introduces students to the expectations of the practice environment, as well as the roles and responsibilities of health care professionals. To accomplish these outcomes, a variety of experiences are required in multiple settings. These settings may be special venues within schools of nursing or within acute care settings or communities. It is essential that practice environments be supportive and conducive to learning so that students will develop the qualities and skill abilities needed to become competent professionals (O'Mara et al., 2014). The following section describes these settings. Included among these are practice learning centers such as learning labs, acute and transitional care, and community-based environments.

Clinical Learning Resource Centers

To foster a nonthreatening and safe learning environment, the practice learning center is used at several stages of students' learning. These centers encourage guided experiences that allow students to practice and perfect a variety of psychomotor, affective, and cognitive skills such as critical thinking and clinical reasoning before moving into complex patient environments. Simulation is one example of a teaching method used in the practice learning center. This method is increasingly used to evaluate knowledge acquisition as well as skill sets (Jeffries, 2014).

Simulation

According to the National Council of State Boards of Nursing (NCSBN, 2005), "simulation is a teaching strategy used to validate the complex and comprehensive skill required of health care professionals."

*The author acknowledges the work of Lillian Gatlin Stokes and Gail Kost in the previous editions of this chapter.

Simulation-based learning is designed to replicate the reality of the clinical environment to provide participants with opportunities to practice and refine clinical reasoning, skilled procedures, and interprofessional collaboration. Schiavenato (2009) also states, "The human patient simulator (HPS) or high-fidelity mannequin has become synonymous with the word *simulation* in nursing education" (p. 388). The explosion of simulation as a standard clinical learning activity is evident in the literature and a recent multisite study validates the use of this modality in clinical education (Hayden, Smiley, Alexander, Kardong-Edgren, & Jeffries, 2014). This study included 10 prelicensure sites and used a three-group quasiexperimental research design. The control group had traditional clinical experiences with no more than 10% of their time spent in simulation. One experimental group had 25% of their clinical time in simulation, and the other experimental group spent 50% of their clinical time in simulation. The study began with the first clinical courses and used multiple measures to assess participants' nursing knowledge and clinical competency throughout the entire program of study. Study participants also rated how their learning needs were met in both simulation and in the clinical environment. Study results found no significant differences between all groups among assessment measures. The study validates simulation as high-quality clinical learning experience that can be used to replace a significant number of traditional clinical hours.

Virtual Clinical Practica

Given the challenges of finding sufficient clinical experiences for students, faculty are exploring the use of virtual clinical experiences made possible by online technologies that can create virtual clinical environments (Knapfel, Moore, & Skiba, 2014) and use existing technologies such as electronic intensive care units and telehealth capabilities to create opportunities for clinical experiences focused on providing opportunities to practice critical thinking, clinical reasoning, communication, and teamwork as a member of the interprofessional team (Sepples, Goran, & Zimmer-Rankin, 2013). The virtual clinical practicum (VCP) is designed to provide a live clinical experience to nursing students from a distance. Students gain clinical experience and practice skills and clinical judgment using telehealth technologies in which students observe a nurse taking care of a patient in a clinical setting without going to the actual clinical site, or as a registered nurse in masters doctoral programs who are learning to provide the care. The students can interact with the nurse, other members of the interprofessional team, and the patient using telehealth technology. The VCP process is developing as a potential solution in response to limited clinical practice sites as well as limited clinical experts, and for specific populations such as acute care pediatric patients. VCP provides needed clinical learning opportunity, especially in rural areas. (See Chapter 21 for further discussion of virtual environments.)

Acute and Transitional Care Environments

Acute and transitional care environments provide clinical experiences for undergraduate and graduate students preparing for advanced practice roles. Experiences in these environments enable undergraduate students, in particular, to exemplify caring abilities and practice the use of cognitive, psychomotor, and communication skills as they interact with patients and their families. These environments have become increasingly complex. A recent multisite study found that the complexity relates to factors such as extensive use of technology (e.g., electronic health records), rapid patient and staff turnover, high patient acuity, and complex patient needs (McNelis et al., 2014). These sites are suitable for learning experiences that focus on providing care in complex clinical settings, but faculty must consider the level of the student, the focus of the experience and the increased risk to patient safety when students have clinical assignments in these units.

Clinical Cases, Unfolding Case Studies, Scenarios, and Simulations

Simulated experiences that provide opportunities for students to integrate psychomotor, critical thinking, and clinical reasoning decision-making skills are equally valuable in assisting students to critically evaluate their own actions and reflect on their own abilities to apply theory to practice. The use of the high-fidelity HPS is one example of using realistic scenarios to prepare students for clinical experiences, substitute for unavailable or unpredictable clinical experiences, or enhance clinical experiences in a safe environment. The use of HPS helps transition the student from the classroom to the practicum environment. Students' learning with the HPS method can be enhanced, patient care can be optimized, and patient safety can be improved. Additional benefits may include enhanced learning in a risk-free environment, promotion of interactive learning, repeated practice of skills, and immediate faculty or tutor feedback. (See Chapter 18 for additional discussion.) Cases, unfolding case studies, and scenarios are lower fidelity strategies but are equally helpful in preparing students for clinical experiences and bridging the gap between classroom and practice (Benner, Sutphen, Leonard, & Day, 2010; McNelis et al., 2014).

Community-Based Environments

The health care delivery system and implementation of the PPACA is continuing to shift nursing practice from acute care hospital environments to the outpatient and community settings. These changes have resulted in care provided through the medical home model (Henderson, Princell, & Martin, 2012) and an increased use of community agencies such as ambulatory, long-term, home health, and nurse-managed clinics; hospice; homeless shelters; social agencies (e.g., homes for battered women); physicians' offices; health maintenance organizations; and worksite venues and summer camps.

The use of technology such as video conferencing, wireless remote communication, information systems, and online courses has made it possible for clinical experiences in a community-based environment to occur at a distance. The transition to community-based teaching requires the faculty to ensure that learning opportunities available in the clinical placement allow the student to achieve the learning objectives. Faculty must adapt clinical learning experiences and incorporate skills used to develop competency with new technology and modify teaching methods (Bisholt, Ohlsson, Kullén Engström, Sundler Johansson, & Gustafsson, 2014). Additionally faculty must adapt to methods of clinical supervision such as being accessible by mobile phone and texting.

Establishing appropriate and sufficient learning experiences in the community may be difficult and challenging. These challenges often relate to economic constraints and the changes in nurse staffing patterns, with a resultant lack of time for professionals to facilitate skill development and serve as role models. These challenges may require faculty to be creative in their use and selection of resources within these environments and to consider establishing partnerships with the service agencies. Using community-based settings creates opportunity for critical thinking, understanding the health care system, and development of communication skills. Faculty can provide other experiences using simulation or the clinical learning laboratory to assist students to develop proficiency in skills traditionally performed in the acute care setting.

Learner-Centered Clinical Education Environment

Every health care environment and specific unit within these environments has a culture. The culture of the immediate environment affects teaching and learning (O'Mara et al., 2014). For example, the culture or patterns of actions and behaviors of the health care professionals can be observed in their attitudes, interactions, teamwork, and commitment to quality and safe patient care. Staffing levels, acuity of patients, anxiety of staff, and workload can influence these actions and behaviors. These aspects of the culture of the environment can in turn influence the time staff has to devote to students. The culture of the environment may also result in behaviors related to lateral violence. Lateral violence is often observed, witnessed, and verbalized by students. These verbalizations provide an opportunity for faculty to implement strategies and assist students with processing what they may be seeing, hearing, and feeling, and thus lessen the effects of these behaviors on students' learning. For example, faculty can hold debriefing sessions, listen to students' perceptions, and make concerted efforts to balance students' feelings and thoughts by using appropriate strategies to soften, yet not deny, the reality of the culture.

Selecting Health Care Environments

Regardless of the practice environment, faculty are responsible for selecting appropriate CLEs within health care agencies and other organizations such as schools and social service agencies. Faculty must be aware of what particular systems are in place within the program to negotiate contracts that are congruent with the philosophies of the school of nursing and the agency, as well as those that specify the rights and responsibilities of both. Determinations must be made about regulation and accreditation status, adequacy of staff, the patient population for needed experiences, expected course outcomes, and whether or not the practice model is compatible for intended uses and curriculum needs. In addition, the adequacy and availability of physical resources (e.g., conference space) for students and faculty should be determined. Finding a practice environment that meets all specified needs is becoming a challenge because of factors associated with the delivery of health care. For example, rapid patient turnover often means faculty have to select available patients rather than those that best meet students' learning needs. This limitation in patient availability can create opportunities for faculty to be creative in the manner in which learning experiences are selected and teaching strategies used. Regardless of the limitation, the role of the faculty is to assist students in making learning connections focused on application of content presented in the classroom to clinical practice. Dual clinical and classroom assignments for faculty may assist in making those necessary connections between clinical and classroom. "The very strength of pedagogical approaches in the clinical setting is itself a persuasive argument for intentional integration of knowledge, clinical reasoning, and skilled know-how and ethical comportment across the nursing curriculum" (Benner et al., 2010, p. 159). Thus faculty have a significant role in helping students to make the necessary connections between clinical and classroom experiences as they learn to think and act like a nurse (Tanner, 2002), in spite of limitations for clinical learning in the health care environment.

Building Relationships with Personnel within Health Care Agency Environments

The ability of the clinical faculty to facilitate students' learning can be enhanced when an effective working relationship is established within the clinical agency. Effective relationships begin with effective communication, which must be practiced in an ongoing manner to maintain relationships and facilitate learning (Dahlke, Baumbusch, Affleck, & Kwon, 2012). This requires having an understanding of the environment and the roles of the individuals within the environment, adapting teaching approaches to the situation, and establishing relationships aimed toward enhancing the educational experience. These elements do not exist in isolation but are patterned to dovetail with or complement other roles. Information should be shared continually, clearly, and consistently about goals, competencies, and expected outcomes; the level of students; practice expectations; the clinical schedule; and related information. Such information enables staff to assist with identification of appropriate experiences for students.

Inasmuch as clinical faculty have the primary responsibility for teaching and guiding students in the clinical environment, others often assist in the process. Therefore the sharing of expectations with the staff is critical. Ensuring an orientation to the practicum environment and having students engage with staff early in the clinical experience promote positive student–staff interaction and provide opportunities for role clarification and the development of collegial relationships. A consistent demonstration of awareness of the mission and values of the agency through actions that are inherently respectful is crucial. Follow-up communication provides an avenue for those within the practice environment to keep abreast of changes.

Clinical Practicum Experiences across the Curriculum

Understanding the Curriculum

The curriculum, composed of a series of well-organized and logical entities, guides the selection of learning experiences and clinical assignments, organizes teaching–learning activities, and informs the measurement of student performance. The manner in which the curriculum is organized guides the planning of learning experiences in a logical, rational sequence. The curriculum is designed to build on prior knowledge and to reinforce the application of learning. While this description of curriculum relates to process, this does not preclude faculty's use of creative and innovative methods in clinical environments. Creative methods have a high potential to motivate students and facilitate construction of knowledge to be applied in practice. Studies focused on perceptions of both clinical instructors and students indicate understanding the whole curriculum is a critical aspect of clinical instruction (Bisholt et al., 2014; Dahlke et al., 2012; Wyte-Lake, Tran, Bowman, Needlemann, & Dobablian, 2013). As students progress and engage in varied practicum experiences, it is faculty's responsibility to interpret the curriculum and to describe the relationships between course competencies and practicum experiences.

Understanding the Student

Clinical experiences provide opportunities for students to practice the art and science of nursing, which enhances their ability to learn. To maximize these experiences, faculty must have full knowledge and understanding of each student (see also Chapter 2). The nursing student population is culturally diverse and includes members of varied age groups, many ethnic and racial groups, and an increasing number of men. This population is also likely to include persons with (or without) prior degrees from a variety of disciplines, as well as those who possess many different health care experiences and technological skill levels. In addition, students differ in their learning styles, levels of knowledge, and preferences for learning experiences; therefore faculty must make concerted efforts to balance the students' learning needs, interests, and abilities when selecting clinical experiences without losing sight of the curriculum and expected competencies and outcomes. Such action can be facilitated by making an assessment of the knowledge, culture, and skills of the learner. Such an assessment helps the faculty determine whether students possess the cognitive, critical thinking, clinical reasoning, decision-making, psychomotor, and affective skills needed for the experiences.

Understanding the Clinical Environment

The clinical environment has been described as a place where students synthesize the knowledge gained in the classroom and make applications to practical situations. Chan (2002) describes the CLE as "the interaction network of forces within the clinical setting that influences student learning outcomes" (p. 70). A number of forces affect expected learning outcomes, including the availability of staff for supervision and coaching, and the degree of student-centeredness exhibited by the clinical teachers (Chan, 2002; Newton, Jolly, Ockerby, & Cross, 2012). Additionally, opportunities available for students to pursue individual learning outcomes define the effectiveness of the clinical environment (Newton et al., 2012). The extent to which the clinical environment values nurses' work and provides an adaptive culture that embraces innovation, creativity, and flexible work practices also are important aspects that set the stage of effective learning (Newton et al., 2012). These forces, coupled with the need to adjust to an environment that requires an integration of thinking skills and performance skills, often result in increased anxiety among students. Creating a supportive clinical environment involves comprehensive orientation of students to the environment, ensuring they are prepared to perform necessary skills and encouraging creative and critical thinking (Ganley & Linnard-Palmer, 2010). Creating an environment where students are expected to succeed also reduces student anxiety (Ganley & Linnard-Palmer, 2010).

Traditionally, clinical rotations have consisted of short blocks of time spent on a unit caring for a patient or two, mostly performing nursing skills with little or no time dedicated to focus on integration of theory, application of critical thinking, and clinical reasoning. Often there is minimal focus on providing feedback or effective evaluation of the interventions performed. Additionally, the focus of the CLE is often focused on the operational aspects of the unit. Nursing staff are expected to meet productivity goals and are caring for patients that are extremely ill with multiple health care needs in complex and dynamic organizations. Nurses intuitively want to be good role models and nurture students but often do not have the time to do so. Faculty must balance the operational needs of the unit with the importance of ensuring that students receive feedback and have the opportunity to focus on daily learning goals related to clinical course outcomes.

Regardless of location of the practice setting, faculty and staff should provide an environment in which caring relationships are evident. The clinical practice environment should be a place where students feel that they are accepted and their contributions are appreciated by individuals with whom they interact (Chan, 2002). Attributes of staff such as warmth, support in obtaining access to learning experiences, and willingness to engage in a teaching relationship are considered helpful.

Selecting Clinical Practicum Experiences

Practicum experiences refer to all activities in which students engage in the practice of nursing. Such experiences are essential for knowledge application, skill development, and professional socialization. Practicum experiences are selected and planned to provide students with opportunities to work across settings and manage care for varied populations with emphasis on applying theory content from the classroom to the clinical experiences. Clinical experiences should include an emphasis on the nursing roles related to health promotion and disease prevention. Selection of practicum learning experiences requires all faculty to be knowledgeable about clinical education and have a sound understanding of the curriculum, the learners, and the learning environment.

The practicum experiences should also help students prepare for outcomes in a progressive, developmental manner. Experiences with patients from diverse populations and with different levels of wellness should be provided. Faculty should take advantage of opportunities to use their creative talents, clinical skills, and expertise to ensure that all students have opportunities to interface virtually or directly with a variety of patient populations.

As faculty begin to plan the clinical experience, it is essential to determine the goal of the particular clinical experience for that day. For the beginning student, focused clinical experiences in which the student is to focus on specific objectives and to achieve specific competencies incorporating individual learning needs requires faculty to create focused, goal-oriented learning activities (Gubrud-Howe & Schoessler, 2009). In a focused clinical learning activity, instead of providing all required care for one or two patients, students can focus on becoming proficient at a particular skill by practicing that skill for several patients. For example, students may interview several patients to work on communication skills, perform vital sign assessments on multiple patients to develop this particular skill set, or focus on learning standards of care in a specialty area. Organizing learning experiences allowing students to assign and delegate care or give and receive reports are other examples of focused clinical learning activities. The purpose of focused clinical learning is to design clinical learning experiences focusing on repetitive practice related to a particular skill set. Focused experienced should integrate students' individual learning needs and focus on course outcomes.

Other learning goals may emphasize facilitating students' ability to synthesize information, integrate didactic and clinical knowledge, develop clinical reasoning and judgment skills, and plan care for groups of patients (Benner et al., 2010; Tanner, 2010). Here, assignments that involve planning care for patients with complex needs and for multiple patients are appropriate. These *integrative* clinical experiences prepare students for transition to practice and typically occur toward the end of the program.

The selection of experiences should be consistent with the desired course and curriculum outcomes, which may be multiple and specific to the nursing program. For example, the expected outcomes for students in an undergraduate degree nursing program are different than those for students in a graduate degree program. Therefore the learning experiences and clinical environment that are selected and the practice opportunities that are offered to students should be congruent with the program outcomes.

Interprofessional Clinical Education

Learning to collaborate with the many health care groups involved in patient care can be a daunting task. Through these experiences, nursing students can learn to work collaboratively with a variety of health disciplines. Therefore students should be provided with opportunities to work as members of interprofessional teams and in practice environments where practice models are used for joint planning, implementation, and evaluation of outcomes of care. The goal of interprofessional education is to foster development of teamwork competencies while enhancing contribution to each profession.

Interprofessional simulations may assist students in health care disciplines such as nursing, medicine, pharmacy, and respiratory therapy to learn about the clinical management of a variety of patients. Several recent studies demonstrate interprofessional simulations may improve patient care through shared learning, development of collaborative team functioning, and shared knowledge creation leading to trust and thoughtful decision making (Bandali, Craig, & Ziv, 2012; Reese, Jeffries, & Engum, 2010; Smithburger, Kane-Gill, Kloet, Lohr, & Seybert, 2013; Strouse, 2010).

Nursing faculty are increasingly participating in teams and designing interprofessional clinical courses and learning experiences. Successful course development and implementation depend on faculty's commitment to the goal of interprofessional practice and a wide range of additional factors. For example, educators must demonstrate professional respect and role clarity. Educators must also have the ability to secure clinical facilities and develop schedules for clinical experiences that are compatible with the concurrent coursework and curriculum progression in each discipline. Other factors include identification of content and experiences with similarities, differences, and overlaps, as well as clarification of autonomy and role interdependency. Success depends on the ability to identify philosophical similarities and differences in clinical practice and to establish clear communication through avenues such as frequent interdisciplinary clinical conferences.

An expected outcome of interprofessional education is increased future collaboration among professionals (Interprofessional Education Collaborative Expert Panel, 2011). The assumption is that students who are taught together will learn to collaborate more effectively when they later assume professional roles in an integrated health care system. Rewards and benefits of interprofessional practice and education include clearer understanding of roles and better employment opportunities for graduates. The long-term outcome is improved access to care, quality care, and increased patient satisfaction and safety. (See also Chapter 11.)

Evaluating Experiences

Students are required to demonstrate multiple behaviors in cognitive, psychomotor, and affective domains. Consequently, clinical faculty must evaluate students in each of these areas. The evaluation must be both ongoing (formative evaluation) to assist students in learning and terminal (summative evaluation) to determine learning outcomes. Constructive and timely feedback, which promotes achievement and growth, is an essential element of evaluation. For a discussion of clinical performance evaluation, refer to Chapter 25.

Scheduling Clinical Practicum Assignments

Although faculty schedule clinical practicum experiences to promote learning, there is ongoing dialogue about the best way to schedule experiences, with emphasis placed on the length of the experiences (hours per day, number of days per week, number of weeks per semester), the timing of the experiences in relation to didactic course assignments, and student needs. Faculty should consider course goals related to both theory and clinical courses and integration of theory content with clinical experiences when making scheduling decisions.

When the learning goal is to integrate students into a clinical setting or when the students are working with a preceptor, students may work the same shift as the nurse with whom they are paired. Many acute care hospitals have a 8-hour shift option, whereas others have only 12-hour shifts. Giving students the opportunity to work the 12-hour shift affords the full scope of practice in any given nurse's day. Students are able to quickly see and experience the role of the nurse. In one small study of senior nursing students in a second degree program working a 12-hour shift, Rossen and Fegan (2009) found that benefits included that students felt accepted by staff, had better socialization, and experienced a realistic work environment; disadvantages included decreased teaching time from the faculty. Although a shorter clinical day allows for skill acquisition, there is little time for the development of extensive critical thinking, clinical reasoning, and evaluation of care. It is equally important that students be exposed to the unit's structure, operations, and culture.

Although results of research about outcomes and student satisfaction with timing and scheduling of clinical experiences offer some guidance, faculty also must consider additional variables such as availability of patients, clinical facilities, course schedules, and student needs. Scheduling is frequently influenced by the desire to have concurrent classroom and clinical experiences so that knowledge can be transferred and applied immediately. Clinical scheduling can be further complicated by the need to coordinate schedules of students from more than one school of nursing. Thus, ideal scheduling may not be a reality.

Effective Clinical Teaching

Clinical teaching must use multiple instructional techniques and teaching tactics to develop and adapt to the environment in which students have opportunities. The clinical instructor should implement activities aimed to foster mutual respect and support for students with each other while they are achieving identified learning outcomes. Faculty who teach in practicum environments are the crucial links to successful experiences for students.

Research about clinical teaching over time consistently indicates that effective clinical teachers are clinically competent, communicate clear expectations, are approachable, and can coach students through difficult patient situations (Dahlke et al., 2012). Additionally, students indicate effective clinical teachers have knowledge of the clinical environment and curriculum, make clinical learning enjoyable through supportive actions, express empathy, and communicate passion for the profession). Making clinical learning enjoyable involves helping students connect theory to practice and applying clinical reasoning while using a patient-centered approach to addressing problems (Dahlke et al., 2012).

Being knowledgeable and being able to share practice wisdom with students in clinical settings is essential. Such knowledge includes an understanding of the theories and concepts related to the practice of nursing. Equally important is an ability to convey the knowledge in an understandable manner. Karuhije (1997) directs attention to three discrete teaching domains that will facilitate acquisition of the teaching skills needed to foster success in clinical settings: instructional, interpersonal, and evaluative. *Instructional* refers to approaches or strategies used to facilitate a transfer of knowledge from didactic to practicum. Strategies may include questioning and peer or patient teaching. Faculty should be cognizant that the type of questions can cover a range during exchanges with students. Faculty should also be mindful of the manner in which questions are constructed to facilitate positive effects on learning. Questions that ask students to analyze and synthesize information, to make clinical judgments, to evaluate outcomes of care, or to propose alternative courses of action result in more learning than simple recall. In clinical practice, factors such as the nature of the situation and available time are likely to influence the types of questions raised.

Effective clinical teaching requires educators to coach students as they learn clinical reasoning and judgment. Clinical reasoning is a "complex process that uses cognition, metacognition, and discipline-specific knowledge to gather and analyze patient information, evaluate its significance, and weigh alternative actions" (Simmons, 2010, p. 1151). Clinical judgment is the outcome of the clinical reasoning process and is defined as "an interpretation or conclusion about a patient's needs, concerns or health problems and/or the decision to take action (or not), and to use or modify standard approaches, or to improvise new ones as deemed appropriate by the patient's response" (Tanner, 2006, p. 204). Clinical reasoning occurs when an individual has the ability to reason about the details of a particular clinical situation and identify what is salient (Benner et al., 2010; Tanner, 2006). Effective and efficient clinical reasoning is derived from knowing the patient, grasping baseline data, and understanding the case (Gillespie & Patterson, 2009). Clinical reasoning requires knowledge, skills, and abilities grounded in reflection. Clinical reasoning is supported by an individual's capacity for self-regulation and leads to the development of expertise (Kuiper, Pesut, & Kautz, 2009).

Beginning students struggle with the ability to engage in clinical reasoning required to make sound judgments. The novice student does not have the ability to identify the subtle or relevant cues seen in a patient whose health condition is changing and for whom complications are beginning to occur. Faculty can assist students in identifying these subtle and relevant cues and start to collaborate with other health care professionals to provide the interventions needed to anticipate potential problems and consider the options aimed toward eliminating or treating complications (Cappelletti, Engel, & Prentice, 2014). (See Box 17-1).

Coaching and Giving Feedback

Coaching students to help them develop clinical competency requires giving students feedback. *Feedback*, an essential element in teaching and learning, is described as information communicated to students as a result of an assessment of an action by students (Wells & McLaughlin, 2014). Feedback, when properly delivered, has a high potential for learning and achievement. In clinical practice where assessments need to be made about the extent to which clinical competencies are met, clinical faculty have a variety of opportunities to offer feedback in response to performance behaviors relating to psychomotor as well as cognitive and affective actions. Regardless of the action, key considerations should be practiced. These considerations are *specificity, timing, consistency, continuity*, and *approach*. Approach is important because of its capacity to alleviate anxiety and enhance engagement.

Because of the variations in needs of students, each clinical experience provides opportunities for feedback. It is imperative that feedback not be given only at documented, scheduled times for formative and summative evaluations. Faculty should be cognizant of those actions that require immediate interaction and those for which feedback can be delayed until a short time later, but not too much later. Methods must be identified to maintain data for timely sharing both strengths and challenges with students, for example. Faculty should create an efficient system for making brief written or electronic anecdotal or mental notes. The delivery of feedback can take multiple forms and depends on the situation. Face-to-face, time-sensitive, brief conferences (e.g., a few minutes) or electronic conversations or dialogue are examples.

BOX 17-1 Clinical Reasoning

Subtle Changes and Complications	Relevant "Cues"	Anticipated Collaborative Interventions	Anticipated Outcomes
Pulmonary edema	• Breath sounds (crackles, wheezing)	• Semi- or high Fowler's position	• Decreased shortness of breath
	• Coughing	• Implement call orders related to low O_2	• Increase FiO_2 and PaO_2
	• FiO_2 % decreased • PaO_2 decreased	• Using SBAR, contact physician to obtain orders	• Normotensive • Increased U/O
	• Shortness of breath	• Anticipate the following:	• No accessory muscle use
	• Cyanosis	• Diuretic: (e.g., Lasix)	• Clear breath sounds
	• Tachypnea • Orthopnea	• Chest X-ray • Decrease IV fluids	• No arrhythmias associated with low K+
	• Anxiety	• Give K+ if low	
	• Accessory muscle use		
	• Blood-tinged sputum		
	• Hypertension or hypotension		

Regardless of the method of delivery, guiding principles must be applied and the learning intent of feedback should be provided. Knowing how to give feedback regarding clinical performance and written clinical assignments is an important element of teaching. One method is to point out positive aspects of performance as well as areas that require improvement. Some situations may provide an opportune time to role-model. For example, if a student fails to integrate communication while performing a procedure, faculty can fill in the missing words. Such action may (or may not) alert the student to an "aha" learning moment: "I failed to communicate. . . ." The faculty interjecting could have a lasting outcome. See Chapter 25 for information about assessing clinical learning and the delivery of feedback.

Debriefing and guided reflections are forms of feedback often used immediately following a clinical experience, nursing rounds, simulation, or presentation to determine the extent to which expectations were met and identify any areas of concern (Overstreet, 2010). In the process of making determinations, the discussion often evolves into identifying areas needing improvement. Although debriefing sessions generally take place in group settings (e.g., in clinical conferences), it is not uncommon for sessions to occur on a one-on-one basis. Faculty may take the lead by posing specific questions and listening to responses to guide further discussion. Students assume an active role in debriefing sessions and can take the lead in initiating the process (Dreifuerst, 2012).

Effective clinical teachers are expected to have expertise in the "art" of teaching. Equally important are teacher behaviors that facilitate learning and support students in their acquisition of nursing skills. Empirical evidence correlates specific teaching methods with enhanced student learning. A recent study suggests effective clinical teaching involves the ability to optimize the environment to provide meaningful learning experiences focused on predetermined objectives (Gubrud-Howe & Schoessler, 2009). Facilitation of cooperative learning, active engagement, and the use of a variety of methods for learning has been reported to be highly effective (Dahlke et al., 2012). Common examples of cooperative strategies are peer teaching and pairing students for student-to-student instructions. Other effective behaviors include sharing anecdotal notes, using objective language when giving feedback, probing to help students self-correct misunderstandings, and communicating expectations clearly.

Effective Clinical Teaching Behaviors and Attitudes

Teaching behaviors that facilitate students' development in higher-order thinking skills include prompts to help students recognize the salient cues in a situation, prioritization, retrieval, and application of theoretical and factual knowledge from coursework. Most importantly, effective clinical instruction focuses on helping students to think contextually with intent to understand the unique characteristics of the patient's situation at hand (Benner et al., 2010). Included among motivational strategies are discussing course goals and relating them to the practicum arena, exhibiting enthusiasm about the profession, discerning student expectations, establishing reward systems, and trying new and different teaching strategies. Strategies that facilitate thinking modalities also include logic models (Ellerman, Kataoka-Yahiro, & Wong, 2006), case studies, and concept mapping. These strategies can be used in the classroom as a way to prepare students for clinical practice and to bridge the gap between didactic courses and clinical learning experiences.

Teacher behaviors relating to interpersonal skills are reported to affect student outcomes. Behaviors such as showing respect for students and treating students with respect (Dahlke et al., 2012), correcting mistakes without belittling), and being supportive and understanding are helpful.

Nursing students experience stress and anxiety in clinical learning situations (Elliott, 2002; Lo, 2002; Timmins & Kaliszer, 2002). Negative relationships with faculty can contribute to anxiety (O'Mara et al., 2014). The effective clinical teacher recognizes students' need for supportive and collegial relationships and develops an interpersonal style that promotes a collegial learning environment; O'Mara et al., 2014). Positive relationships are nurturing and can enhance learning. Caring behaviors and a caring environment are also essential (O'Mara et al., 2014).

The literature points to the importance of building relationships between students and teachers. It is believed that the quality of their interaction affects learning outcomes (Tanner, 2005). Concepts that facilitate the building of relationships may include the following: connections, caring, compassion, mutual knowing, trusting and respecting, availability, knowledge, confidence, and communicating (Gillespie, 2002). By knowing the students' strengths, challenges and individual goals, faculty are prevented from making assumptions and reacting to students' misunderstandings or poor performance. Making assumptions regarding student intent or motivation may be perceived by students as being disrespectful. Making connections to identity early in the relationship assists faculty in determining the elements needed to meet students' learning needs (Dahlke et al., 2012; O'Mara et al., 2014).

Teacher confidence is another factor that enhances learning; teachers who lack confidence actually create distance between themselves and the students they teach). This hinders the sense of knowing and the possible connections that may have formed. A part of teacher confidence is a foundation of knowledge. When clinical teachers use their expertise to support learning, the teacher–student relationship is strengthened.

Cook (2005) engaged in a study to explore perceptions of teacher behaviors that invite trust and create student anxiety. The findings indicate that teachers need to be aware of how their behaviors can be negatively perceived by students, thus influencing the anxiety that occurs during the clinical experience and ultimately affecting learning. Senior clinical faculty should serve as role models and mentor junior clinical faculty to create a legacy of effective clinical teaching. Additional characteristics of effective teachers are listed in Box 17-2.

Preparing Faculty for Clinical Teaching

The preparation and development of faculty for clinical teaching are not as widely discussed and documented as the preparation of students for clinical learning. Studies indicate that the exposure of faculty to evidence-based teaching strategies and learning theory is minimal (Dahlke et al., 2012; McNelis et al., 2014). Krautscheid, Kaakinen, and Warner (2008) directed efforts to facilitate a reversal in this trend. A clinical faculty development

BOX 17-2 Characteristics of Effective Clinical Teachers

1. Create an environment that is conducive to learning that requires:
    - Knowledge of the practice area
    - Clinical competence
    - Knowledge of how to teach
    - A desire to teach
2. Be supportive of learners. Such support requires:
    - Knowledge of the learners
    - Knowledge of the practice area
    - Mutual respect
3. Possess teaching skills that maximize student learning. This requires an ability to:
    - Diagnose student needs
    - Learn about students as individuals, including their needs, personalities, and capabilities
4. Foster independence and accountability so that students learn how to learn.
5. Encourage exploration and questions without penalty.
6. Accept differences among students.
7. Relate how clinical experiences facilitate the development of clinical competence.
8. Possess effective communication and question skills.
9. Serve as a role model.
10. Enjoy nursing and teaching.
11. Be friendly, approachable, understanding, enthusiastic about teaching, and confident with teaching.
12. Be knowledgeable about the subject matter and be able to convey that knowledge to students in their practice areas.
13. Exhibit fairness in evaluation.
14. Provide frequent feedback.

program, developed to help faculty practice teaching by analogy and reflect on clinical teaching, was implemented. With this program, clinical teaching simulations were used to allow faculty to practice, teach, and receive immediate feedback. Scenarios were used to facilitate the process. As a result of the clinical teaching simulations, faculty reported being more reflective as teachers and practitioners and identified the importance of facilitating a safe learning environment in the clinical practice setting.

Expert clinicians often have a desire to teach in the practicum area. Providing the faculty development needs of expert clinicians can be challenging. It can be very difficult to equip clinicians with teaching skills required to be an effective clinical teacher for those faculty who also maintain full-time clinical practices. Some have been preceptors and to fully attain the skills needed to make the transition to a new role as clinical teachers, further instruction, coaching, and guidance is required. These individuals should be encouraged and provided with information about where and how they can engage in activities that will facilitate their acquisition of the knowledge and skills required for the clinical teaching role. Some schools have developed modules for that purpose.

One method for meeting the challenge of educating clinical teachers is to use an online course to orient clinicians who are making the transition from the role of expert clinician to that of clinical teacher (Reid, Hinderer, Jarosinski, Mister, & Seldomridge, 2013). Essential topics include teaching–learning theory, critical thinking, how to deal with challenging students, and making patient assignments. Because being an excellent clinical nurse does not mean that the nurse will be an excellent teacher, Cangelosi, Crocker, and Sorrell (2009) developed a Clinical Nurse Educator Academy to prepare clinicians for clinical teaching. After analyzing reflective papers at the end of the academy, the authors found that the nurses were enthusiastic about the educator role, but that the frustration from lack of mentoring indicates a need for ongoing development of the educator role.

In summary, effective clinical teachers are knowledgeable and know how to convey concepts to students in effective ways, are clinically competent, coach students to develop clinical reasoning and judgment, exhibit interpersonal skills that positively influence students' learning, and establish collegial relationships that often last well beyond a specific course or program. Clinical faculty also need to be oriented to and developed for the role. Research is likely to continue in this area.

Preparing Students for Patient Care

Teaching for patient care should involve orderly and logical actions taken to accomplish particular educational goals. The actual selection and use of a particular strategy should be based on expected outcomes, principles of learning, and learner needs. This section focuses on several strategies commonly used in clinical teaching: patient care assignments, clinical conferences, nursing rounds, and written assignments.

Students come to the health care environment not really understanding the culture of confidentiality. It is imperative that students know and understand the Health Insurance Portability and Accountability Act of 1996 (HIPAA) privacy and security regulations. It is the role of faculty to instruct students on the need to implement the HIPAA rules and regulations in all patient encounters. They are designed to protect the patient's right to privacy. Students should be informed of what they can and cannot do in relation to confidentiality, and these instructions must be enforced.

Patient Care Assignments

Patient care provides students with opportunities to integrate, synthesize, and use previously learned knowledge and skills. Some nursing courses require students to prepare in advance for their clinical experience. Advance preparation commences with making clinical assignments, which may be the responsibility of the clinical teacher, the teacher and student together (especially useful for beginning students), the student alone, the student with guidance from the teacher, or the nursing and health care staff or preceptors. Allowing students some input into selecting clinical assignments encourages them to be self-directed as well as to choose experience on the basis of their personal learning needs. Refer to Box 17-3 for other suggestions for making assignments.

The selection of clinical assignments by students in collaboration with others has several benefits. It provides opportunities for students to select experiences that are based on personal learning needs, to experience a degree of control over their education, and to interact with practicing professionals during the process of selecting experiences. The extent to which students are permitted to self-select experiences depends on the goals or expected outcomes of the program, the philosophy of the specific clinical teacher, and the availability of resources in the clinical environment to assist students (i.e., to answer questions and provide guidance in patient selection).

Involvement of the clinical faculty is important when students select their experiences. For example, faculty serve as resource advisers and sources of emotional support, communicate goals and intended outcomes, assist students in assessing the congruency between personal learning needs and course objectives, facilitate planning the experiences, collaborate with students as they strive to meet goals, and evaluate accomplishments. Making clinical assignments can be a challenge for clinical faculty. Novice faculty are often at a loss in terms of knowing where to begin. This is where mentoring by senior-level or expert faculty is helpful.

BOX 17-3 Tips for Making Assignments

New faculty often are at a loss in knowing where to begin. The following tips should assist new faculty to enhance their comfort level in implementing this task.

- Come to the unit with knowledge of specific student needs.
- Have an assignment sheet with a list of the students for the given day.
- Get input from those in charge and from the staff nurses.
- Talk to the nurse in charge and ask for brief suggestions about the patients on the unit. This simple act of communication is one way to build a trusting, supportive relationship with the staff on the unit, as they can be very helpful in guiding what patients will make for a good assignment.
- Make rounds and talk to all of the patients and family you plan to care for on the following day. Just a few minutes chatting can assist you in deciding whether a patient will be appropriate for a student nurse.
- Obtain patient and family permission, as this may prevent early morning assignment changes because a patient refuses to have a student.
- Consider the specialty on your particular unit. Knowing the patient population will help determine when to make assignments. For example, if it is a surgical unit, you may want to make assignments later in the afternoon because patients may be admitted late to the unit following surgery. If you make an assignment too early, you may risk the problem of a patient being reassigned to a different unit or discharged.
- Be sure that students know who the charge nurse is in case the assignments need revision when faculty are not available. Establishing a protocol for this will lessen frustration among the staff.
- Always have a backup plan. Add a couple of extra patients to the assignment sheet in case something changes when faculty are not available.

Strategies for Implementing Clinical Assignments

Clinical assignments are an integral part of nursing practicum experiences. Several strategies for making clinical assignments have been adopted for clinical teaching. The strategy used in clinical instruction is often determined by factors such as the skill level of the student, the patient acuity level, the number of assigned students, and the availability of patients and resources, including the availability of technology. Traditional and alternative strategies, such as dual assignments, multiple assignments, and clinical conferencing, are discussed.

The traditional strategy is one in which nursing students are taught in a clinical setting with a varying faculty-to-student ratio. Ratios should be determined with an aim for facilitating optimum learning, knowledge of regulatory and agency requirements, and consideration of the workflow of the unit or agency. Most importantly, consideration of patient safety and quality care is essential (Ironside & McNelis, 2010; McNelis et al., 2014). The rationale for these ratios relates to the effect of increased numbers of students on patient safety (Ironside & McNelis, 2010). From a student's perspective, this strategy involves the assignment of one student to one or two patients. The students assume responsibility for the nursing interventions needed in the care of the patient and may work alone in planning, implementing, and evaluating nursing activities.

Alternatives to the traditional method of clinical assignment are dual and multiple assignments. The dual assignment strategy (Fugate & Rebeschi, 1991) involves assigning two students to one patient. This alternative is useful when the level or complexity of care is beyond the capabilities of one student. Because students must work closely to implement care, collaboration and communication between the students are requisites for effective use of this strategy. Benefits of this strategy include improved time management, opportunities for collaboration and peer support, and fewer numbers of patients for which the faculty is responsible. When dual assignments are made, faculty have the responsibility of ensuring that each student understands his or her specific responsibility. For 2-day clinical rotations, roles may be reversed on the second day of care). Such reversal makes it possible for both students to direct care to the patient.

The strategy of multiple assignments is useful for beginning students and in situations where a limited number of patients are available. This strategy involves the assignment of three students per patient. Three roles are assumed: the doer who provides the care; the information gatherer or researcher who is responsible for obtaining information needed for the safe care of the patient; and the observer who observes the student, the researcher, the student–patient interactions, the responses of the patient to his or her care, and the family members. The observer also makes suggestions for improving care. As with dual assignments, the roles for each student must be clearly defined. Adequate time must be made available for collaboration and discussion among students and faculty.

The multiple assignment approach must meet learning objectives. Glanville (1971) conducted a study to determine the effectiveness of this method as an approach to clinical teaching. Results revealed similarity in the extent to which objectives were met and in the levels of achievement for students assigned to the multiple assignment approach and those assigned to the traditional method. VanDenBerg (1976) randomly assigned 22 first-year associate degree students to two groups, one of which used traditional assignments and one of which used multiple assignments. Results showed that students assigned to the multiple assignment group demonstrated a significant increase in nursing knowledge compared with those assigned to the traditional group.

In light of the increasing complexity of learning environments and the instability of the patient census, consistent clinical assignments and multiple placement assignments were compared to determine learning outcomes (Adams, 2002). Here, *consistent* means that students were assigned to a unit for a specific time frame or used more than one unit during the period. Quantitative measures revealed no difference in the two methods of clinical rotation. However, the perceptions of the benefit of consistent clinical assignments were positive.

In summary, faculty, staff, and students play a significant role in determining assignments. Assignments are made according to a number of factors, including course objectives, learner needs, skill level, complexity of the clinical environment, and patients' acuity. The assignments may be implemented as solo or multistudent experiences. Each has been considered beneficial in enhancing learning.

Clinical Conferences

Clinical conferences are group learning experiences that are an integral part of the clinical experience. The use of clinical conferences in nursing is common. Conferences can provide meaningful learning experiences and excellent opportunities for students to bridge the gap between theory and practice. Through conferences students can develop critical thinking and clinical decision-making skills (Wink, 1995) and acquire confidence in their ability to express themselves with clarity and logic.

Successful clinical conferences are planned. Plans for conferences should take into consideration the curriculum and the learner. An identification of the purpose, topic, process, strategies, and methods of evaluation are essential if the teacher is to be instrumental in bridging the gap between theory and clinical practice.

Types of Conferences

The conferences can include traditional preclinical, midclinical, and postclinical conferencing. As a result of advancing technology, conferences may take place through electronic media and online. As such, the rules and regulations related to HIPAA and the Health Information Technology for Economic and Clinical Health Act apply to clinical groups that use clinical conferencing by electronic media. Student groups must be aware of maintaining patient confidentiality as the group presents patient data by electronic means. Using this form of conferencing is a means of using technology while supporting the needs of students. Some may be doing clinical assignments at different sites and electronic conferencing brings students together where debriefing can occur without having to travel to a central location.

Traditional Conferences

Preclinical, midclinical, and *postclinical conferences* by nature are small-group discussion periods that immediately precede, occur during, or follow a clinical experience. Each provides opportunities for discussion. In preclinical conferences, students share information about upcoming experiences, ask questions, express concerns, and seek clarification about plans for care. Preclinical conferences also provide opportunities for faculty to correct student misconceptions, identify problem areas, assess student thinking, and identify student readiness to implement care.

Midclinical conferencing, in contrast to preclinical and postclinical conferencing, is another form of gathering students together to provide some form of midclinical debriefing. It has been found that, while doing a 12-hour clinical day, this gives students an opportunity to gather to share pertinent patient information and plan for further interventions, which may include patient teaching and discharge planning. This midclinical conference time also may help students collectively evaluate the efficacy of prior patient interventions. This exchange of data, in the form of a midconference, is a method of imparting knowledge and sharing common data with the intent of positively affecting patient care.

Postclinical conferences provide a forum in which students and faculty can discuss the clinical experiences, share information, analyze clinical situations, clarify relationships, identify problems, ventilate feelings, and develop support systems. In postclinical conferences there is interaction between the teacher and the students, which offers both a medium for learning and an exchange resulting in meaningful experiences.

Online Conferences

Online conferencing, occurring before or after clinical experiences, can assist students to come together in a virtual environment to exchange ideas, solve problems, discuss alternatives, and acquire information about issues of clinical care that occurred before or during the clinical experience (Gaberson, Oermann, & Shellenberger, 2015). See Chapter 21 for further discussion of teaching in online learning communities.

Student and Faculty Roles during Conferences

Both students and faculty have specific roles in conferences. Student should be made aware of their role as active participants. As such, they should defend choices of care, clarify points of view, explore alternatives, and practice decision making. A student may also assume the role of group leader. Faculty serve as conference facilitators by supporting, encouraging, and sharing information; posing questions and asking for alternative hypotheses; giving feedback; helping students identify patterns; and guiding the debriefing process. As conferences are facilitated, efforts should be made to ask higher-level questions that assist students in applying knowledge to clinical situations (Gaberson et al., 2015). Conferences also provide opportunities for students to apply group processes and develop team-building skills.

Evaluating the Conferences

Conferences should be evaluated in light of their effectiveness and goal accomplishment. The teacher should obtain and provide feedback regarding the extent to which goals were accomplished, the effectiveness of the teaching methods or strategies, and the degree of learning achieved. The data from the evaluation can be used for planning future conferences.

In summary, traditional and electronic conferences play a significant role in facilitating students' learning. Conferences afford opportunities for enhancing critical thinking, clinical reasoning, and decision-making skills; for creating new meaning for care issues; and for enhancing group process and team-building skills. Successful conferences are planned. Inherent in planning are identifying the purpose, selecting topics, selecting teaching methods, and conducting and evaluating these methods.

Complementary Clinical Experiences

Nursing Grand Rounds

The practice of nursing grand rounds is a teaching strategy that uses the patients' bedside for direct, purposeful experiences. These experiences may involve demonstration, interview, or discussion of patient problems and nursing care. Rounds also afford an excellent opportunity for the exchange of ideas about patient care situations, which may involve clinical faculty, students, and staff.

The use of rounds as a teaching strategy requires planning. Planning includes obtaining permission from the patient and providing information about the nature of the rounds and the role the patient will play. After the session, patient participation should be acknowledged and some form of debriefing should occur, including planning for subsequent rounds.

Concept-Based Learning Activities

Concept-based learning activities are a type of experience used recently in clinical education (Gubrud-Howe & Schoessler, 2009; Nielsen, 2009; Nielsen, Noone, Voss, & Matthews, 2013). This learning activity is designed to develop deep learning and pattern recognition of a particular health problem or medical diagnosis. Concepts are identified for students to study in the context of the patient care environment. Fluid and electrolytes is an example of a concept students may explore. Each student completes an in-depth assessment of a patient with a fluid and electrolyte problem. The pathophysiology, treatment, pharmacology, and patient response to care is explored. The faculty facilitates comprehensive discussion of each case and directs discussion so students begin to see the similarities and differences between each patient in an effort to begin to identify salient findings related to each case. The faculty help students identify unexpected findings in the patients' situation related to the concept being studied and help students recognize current or potential complications that need to be addressed. Students are not responsible for care but need to address any safety issues that emerge as they are assessing their assigned patient. This activity allows the student to focus on critical thinking about the concept being studied without the distraction of attending to tasks associated with general patient care (Nielsen et al., 2013). Communicating the focus of this assignment and learning activity with staff is essential to avoid misunderstanding of the student's role on the unit (Gubrud-Howe & Schoessler, 2009).

Written Assignments

Written assignments generally complement clinical experiences and are considered to be useful in that they facilitate development of critical thinking and clinical reasoning and they promote an understanding of content. Such assignments may include short papers, clinical reasoning papers, nursing care plans, clinical logs, journals, and concept maps. Findings from research on the use of clinical logs indicate that their use provides opportunities for students to reflect on clinical experiences, communicate with the teacher, identify mistakes and negative experiences, and learn from these experiences. See Box 17-4 for possible journaling questions.

BOX 17-4 Sample of Journaling Questions

- How did you feel about your clinical day?
- What was the best part of your clinical day?
- What did you feel most confident about?
- If you could do your clinical day over, what would you do differently?
- What were you most concerned about as related to your patient's care?
- What did you learn today that can apply to future patients with similar problems?
- What do you need to learn more about?
- Describe interactions with other professions. What went well? Describe how the interaction was or was not patient centered.
- Describe any patient quality or safety issues you had to address or manage. What goals do you have for your next clinical day?

Point-of-Care Technology and Mobile Health

Nurses are increasingly using handheld devices, electronic health records, and other point-of-care technologies in the clinical setting, and faculty must provide opportunities for students to become familiar with their use. Simulated electronic health records can be embedded in clinical simulations as preparation for their use in the clinical agency or as a substitute for learning when agency policy precludes students' use of them in the agency. Smart phones equipped with reference software enable access to clinical information; care plans; and nursing, procedure, and evidence-based practice guidelines; and can provide access to skills videos and patient teaching materials (Zurmehly, 2010). Increasingly, nurses are using software applications ("apps") on a smartphone to diagnose, monitor, and teach patients in community-based settings; students must have experience using these point-of-care and mobile health technologies as well. See Chapter 19 for information about policies for using technology in clinical settings.

Models for Clinical Education

Several models for clinical education are used to educate nursing students. These models, alternatives to the traditional model, include preceptorship, associate model, paired model, academia–service partnerships, and adjunct faculty joint appointments. These models have evolved to increase capacity for clinical placements, facilitate development of competency for today's practice, manage faculty shortages, prepare graduates to be competent for practice, and foster closer ties with clinical agencies (Delunas & Rooda, 2009; Murray, Crain, Meyer, McDonough, & Schweiss, 2010; Neiderhauser, Macintyre, Garner, Teel, & Murray, 2010; Niederhauser, Schoessler, Gubrud-Howe, Magnussen, & Codier, 2012; Nielsen et al., 2013). Given the diversity of health care settings, faculty shortage, and the need for reduced faculty-to-student ratios, new models serve to enhance effective student learning, facilitate development of clinical skills, and promote role development.

Preceptorship

Preceptorship is a teaching model in which the student is assigned to a nurse who serves as a preceptor. Preceptors are experienced nurses who facilitate and evaluate student learning in the clinical area during a specified time. Their role is intentionally implemented in conjunction with other responsibilities related to patient care in the clinical environment. The preceptor model is based on the assumption that a consistent one-on-one relationship provides opportunities for socialization into practice and bridges the gap between theory and practice. The preceptor model may be used at several levels. However, it is considered to be particularly useful for senior-level students and graduate students in advanced practice roles. Use at these levels provides opportunities for students to synthesize theoretical knowledge and apply information, including evidence-based research, in the practice environment. This method is also an excellent way for students to practice collaboration.

Theoretically, the preceptor provides one-on-one teaching, guidance, and support, and serves as a role model. In one model (Billings, Jeffries, Rowles, Stone, & Urden, 2002), the preceptor, faculty, and student form a triad to facilitate the student's acquisition of clinical competencies. The preceptor may be assigned to a student on the basis of shared learning needs. The preceptor and student meet before the first clinical experience to discuss learning styles and goals for competency attainment and the desired outcome of the clinical experience. Although faculty have ultimate responsibility for the course and students' learning outcomes, the student and preceptor are empowered to conduct formative and summative evaluations of the student's clinical performance and learning outcomes. In the Integrative Clinical Preceptor Model (Mallette, Laury, Engleke, & Andrews, 2005; Mamhidir, Kristofferzon, Hellström-Hyson, Persson, & Mårtensson, 2014), the student assumes a proactive role, not only as a student, but also as a member of the health care team. In this model, the preceptor assumes responsibilities as a clinical teacher, mentor, and role model, and faculty serve as a role model and facilitator for the preceptor and the student as well as a consultant.

Preceptors are expected to be clinical experts, to be willing to teach, and to be able to teach effectively (McClure & Black, 2013). Benefits that have been derived from preceptorships include enhanced ability to apply theory to practice, improvement in psychomotor skills, increased self-confidence, and improved socialization. Attributes of an effective preceptor are listed in Box 17-5.

BOX 17-5 Attributes of an Effective Preceptor

1. Knowledge of the patient care area
2. Effective communication skills (verbal and nonverbal)
3. Experience in a particular clinical area
4. Ability to relate to health care personnel and client
5. Honesty
6. Effective decision-making skills
7. Genuine caring behaviors
8. Leadership skills
9. Interest in professional development

Used with permission from Lewis, K. E. (1986). What it takes to be a preceptor. *The Canadian Nurse/L'infirmière Canadienne, 82*(11), 18–19.

In a preceptorship, the role of the nursing faculty transitions from direct instruction to an emphasis on facilitation and evaluation. Preceptors and faculty must work in a close relationship). Faculty provide the link between practice and education. In providing this link, faculty monitor how well the students complete assignments and accomplish outcomes. Evaluation is a collaborative responsibility of faculty, students, and preceptors but most nurse practice acts require the faculty to assume accountability for evaluating the student's attainment of learning outcomes.

The use of preceptors requires that planning be done to ensure an understanding of their role. Ideally this is facilitated through strategically planned orientation and follow-up sessions; some schools of nursing offer workshops or courses to orient preceptors to their role (McClure & Black, 2013; Smedley & Penney, 2009). These sessions provide a forum for sharing information related to the philosophical perspectives of preceptorship, expected outcomes, teaching strategies, and methods of evaluation. Because roles change for faculty, students, and preceptors, all require orientation to new roles (McClure & Black, 2013; Mallette et al., 2005).

The value of the preceptor model is generally related to providing students a sense of independence for patient care and the ability to develop a professional identity. Preceptors and clinical agencies also value the preceptor model because preceptors develop additional skill sets related to teaching and the clinical agency that stands to benefit from hiring a well-prepared graduate.

Clinical Teaching Associate

The clinical teaching associate (CTA) model involves a staff nurse who collaborates with a designated faculty member and instructs a specified number of students in the clinical area (Baird, Bopp, Schofer, Langenberg, & Matheis-Kraft, 1994; DeVoogd & Saldbenblatt, 1989). Teaching responsibilities are assumed by the CTA, who also serves as a resource person and role model. A faculty member serves as lead teacher and is responsible for supervision and evaluation of clinical learning experiences, including assignment of grades and collaboration with the CTA about assignments and experiences.

Results from a survey of nurse managers, CTAs, faculty, and students conducted to determine the effectiveness of this model were positive (Baird et al., 1994). Positive comments were presented in terms of student learning. Patient satisfaction with care was reported to be greater than with the traditional model. Nurses in the CTA role reported an increase in student confidence. Faculty reported that students were more relaxed and more self-confident. The effectiveness of the model was reported by students as allowing them to assume increased responsibility in comparison with the traditional model.

Paired Model

The paired model is designed to pair a student and a staff nurse for a practicum experience. It is an alternative to the one-patient, one-student model and is a variation of the preceptor model. This model is often used in combination with the Dedicated Education Model and in community-based setting such as an ambulatory care center or clinic. During the course, each student has a specified number of days in a paired relationship. The remaining time is spent acquiring experiences by using the traditional model. The staff nurse plans the learning experience; the faculty member oversees the experiences while creating a learning environment for students. However, most of the faculty member's time is spent in the traditional role with other students who have not been paired. To enhance the effectiveness of the paired model, it is essential that the staffing pattern be evaluated before making assignments.

Academia–Service Partnerships

The clinical teaching partnership is a collaborative model shared by service and academia settings to enhance mutual goals of developing nurses competent for practice and creating safe practice environments. Partnerships are also formed to create new models of clinical instruction and increase student and faculty capacity in nursing programs (Delunas & Rooda, 2009; Nielsen et al., 2013). Although these partnerships take different forms, they are established collaboratively and result in redesigned clinical education experiences for students and faculty as well as for the nurses at the clinical agency. Academic and service partnerships are a promising framework to address the nursing faculty shortage.

In one early partnership model, the service institution shared the resources of nurses, a clinical nurse specialist (CNS), and an academic faculty member (Shah & Pennypacker, 1992). The CNS serves as an adjunct faculty member who provides patient assignments. The academic faculty member schedules the experiences. Jointly they collaborate in evaluating assignments facilitating learning experiences and assessing students' performance. Communication is reciprocal and essential to the success of this model. The faculty member shares information about problems that may influence students' performance. The CNS keeps the faculty member abreast of current student performance. Both schedule conferences to discuss anecdotal records of students. Murray et al. (2010) report that students in their partnership model were better integrated into the clinical setting and increased levels of critical thinking and clinical decision making.

Adjunct Faculty

Adjunct faculty are health care professionals who are employed in the service setting and have a part-time academic appointment. Adjunct faculty may assume various roles, including those of preceptor, CTA, mentor, guest lecturer, and supervisor. These individuals may also collaborate on research projects. Faculty who are appointed in an adjunct capacity are registered professional nurses or professionals who are experts in areas such as clinical practice, research, leadership, management, legislation, and law.

Dedicated Education Units

Over the past decade, the dedicated education unit (DEU) model has been implemented at various universities across the country. Moscato, Miller, Logsdon, Weinberg, and Chorpenning (2007) indicate that the "DEU offers a concrete strategy to more closely connect nursing units and education programs" (p. 32). DEUs involve new partnerships among nurse executives, staff nurses, and faculty for transforming patient care units into environments designed to support learning experiences for students and staff nurses while continuing the critical work of providing quality care to acutely ill patients. Mulready-Shick, Flannagan, Banister, Mylott, and Curtin (2013) found that the DEU model facilitates stronger relationship building between nurses in academia and practice, and students report significantly more positive learning experience when compared with traditional clinical placement experiences. Universities are implementing this strategy in a variety of ways. One Midwest university uses the term *practice education partnership (PEP) units*. The PEP unit is a hospital-based unit designed to provide the student with a strong partnership between the practice and education settings. The PEP model differs from the Australian DEU model in that it works to incorporate the culture of the unit and its clinical specialty into the availability of preceptors, level of patient acuity, and other influences on the education of the student. One of the unique aspects of the PEP model is that there is continuity and consistency among preceptors, faculty, and students as they partner to learn and grow together. Preceptors are coached on preceptor competencies by attending a full-day workshop. It is at this time that the partnership between the nurse and the faculty begins. This partnership is developed over time and ultimately the student learns the role of the nurse and together the student and preceptor provide exceptional patient care.

The use of DEUs has increased significantly in the last decade (Moscato, Nishioka, & Coe, 2013). Research indicates the educational quality and competency development are significant for students receiving clinical instruction in DEUs (Dapremont & Lee, 2013; Mulready-Shick et al., 2013).

Residency Models

Recognizing that prelicensure programs may not be sufficient for preparing nurses for practice in complex health care settings, several studies and commissions (Benner et al., 2010; Institute of Medicine, 2010; Tanner, 2010) report on the need for postgraduate residencies and call for their increased use to improve transition to practice and development of leadership and population management skills. Accreditation and regulatory standards have been developed for this approach to residency. The American Association of Colleges of Nursing (AACN) developed a 12-month program designed to facilitate further development of competency and ease the transition into practice. The AACN piloted six programs in 2004 and there are now residency programs in more than 30 states (Barnett, Minnick, & Norman, 2014). The NCSBN developed a model that provides a framework for standardized transition to practice and regulatory guidelines are under consideration (Goode, Lynn, McElroy, Bednash, & Murray, 2013).

Several studies have been conducted to examine the outcomes of nurse residency programs (Goode et al., 2013). The findings suggest nurse residency programs increase overall confidence and competence particularly in the ability to organize, prioritize, communicate effectively, and provide leadership (Goode et al., 2013). Residency programs have a statistically positive influence on nurse retention rates (Goode et al., 2013). Further research is needed to determine the influence of postgraduate nurse residency programs on patient outcomes (Barnett et al., 2014).

Summary

In summary, several models for clinical education of student nurses exist. Alternative models, collaborative in nature, have evolved because of the increasing complexity of the health care environment. Among these models are preceptorships, the teaching associate model, the paired model, clinical teaching partnerships, and adjunct faculty. The nature of each model dictates the level of student that would benefit most. The paired and clinical associate models have been used for beginning students, whereas the preceptorship model is widely used for students in the upper level of their program and for graduate students. Empirical research on the effectiveness of these models has been sparse; there is a need for further evaluation of and research on these models in terms of their effectiveness on student learning and preparation for the workforce.

Clinical teaching involves student–teacher interaction in experiential clinical situations that take place in diverse and often interprofessional practice environments. These environments may include laboratory, acute care, transitional, and community sites, including homeless shelters, clinics, schools, camps, and social service agencies. Faculty must have in-depth knowledge of teaching behaviors that facilitate students' learning and development, and have complete knowledge of the culture of the practice area as well as the health care provider. Effective clinical teachers are able to plan, facilitate, and evaluate experiences using instructive, interpersonal, and evaluative strategies. These strategies facilitate faculty's acquisition of the knowledge and skills required to become nurses.

A variety of teaching methods can be used to enable students to achieve desired outcomes. Patient assignments, clinical conferences, nursing grand rounds, concept-based clinical activities, and written assignments are among these. The skill level of students, patient's acuity level, number of students, and patient care resource availability will affect the method used. Among the models suggested for educating nursing students are the traditional approach and alternatives to this model, including preceptorships, CTAs, teaching partnerships, and adjunct faculty. Practicum experiences prepare students for working in a health care system that is evidence based and patient centered. Teaching in the practicum setting blends faculty's clinical expertise with teaching skills to prepare nurses for current and future roles in an ever-changing health care system.

REFLECTING ON THE EVIDENCE

1. Choose a set of clinical teaching strategies for a group of students. What do you need to consider about the student, the setting, and the patients in order to make this decision? What evidence for practice will you draw on to make your decision?
2. What is the role of Internet-based teaching and learning in clinical teaching? Can clinical practice be learned in a fully online course?
3. What is the state of science about clinical teaching? What research questions are being asked? What methods are being used? What variables are included in the studies?
4. What are the best practices that are evidenced-based?

REFERENCES

Adams, V. (2002). Consistent clinical assignment for nursing students compared to multiple placements. *Journal of Nursing Education, 41*(2), 80–85.

American Association of Colleges of Nursing. (2010). *UHC/AACN Nurse Residency Programs.* Retrieved from, http://www.aacn.nche.edu/education/nurseresidency.htm.

Ard, N., & Valiga, T. M. (2009). Transforming clinical education in nursing. In N. Ard & T. M. Valiga (Eds.), *Clinical nursing education: Current Reflections* (pp. 227–236). New York: National League for Nursing.

Baird, S., Bopp, A., Schofer, K., Langenberg, A., & Matheis-Kraft, C. (1994). An innovative model for clinical teaching. *Nursing Educator, 19*(3), 23–25.

Bandali, K. S., Craig, R., & Ziv, A. (2012). Innovations in applied health: Evaluating a simulation-enhanced, interprofessional curriculum. *Medical Teacher, 34*, e176–e184. Retrieved from, http://dx.doi.org/10.1111/j.2365-2648.2008.04798x.

Barnett, J. S., Minnick, A. F., & Norman, L. (2014). A description of U.S. post-graduation nurse residency programs. *Nursing Outlook, 62*, 174–184.

Benner, P., Sutphen, M., Leonard, V., & Day, L. (2010). *Educating nurses: A call for radical transformation.* San Francisco: Jossey-Bass.

Billings, D. M., Jeffries, P., Rowles, C. J., Stone, C., & Urden, L. (2002). A partnership model of nursing education to prepare critical care nurses. *Excellence in Clinical Practice, 3*(4), 3.

Bisholt, B., Ohlsson, U., Kullén Engström, A., Sundler Johansson, A., & Gustafsson, M. (2014). Nursing students' assessment of the learning environment in different clinical settings. *Nurse Education in Practice, 14*, 304–310.

Bradbury-Jones, C., Irvine, F., & Sambrook, S. (2010). Empowerment of nursing students in clinical practice: Spheres of influence. *Journal of Advanced Nursing, 66*, 2061–2070.

Cangelosi, P. R., Crocker, S., & Sorrell, J. M. (2009). Expert to novice: Clinicians learning new roles as clinical nurse educators. *Nursing Education Perspectives, 30*(6), 367–371.

Cappelletti, A., Engel, J. K., & Prentice, D. (2014). Systematic review of clinical judgment and reasoning in nursing. *Journal of Nursing Education, 53*(8), 453–458.

Chan, D. (2002). Development of the clinical learning environment inventory: Using theoretical framework of learning environment studies to access nursing students' perceptions for the hospital as a learning environment. *Journal of Nursing Education, 41*(2), 69–75.

Cook, L. (2005). Inviting teacher behaviors of clinical faculty and nursing students' anxiety. *Journal of Nursing Education, 44*(4), 156–161.

Dahlke, S., Baumbusch, J., Affleck, F., & Kwon, J. (2012). The clinical instructor role in nursing education: A structured literature review. *Journal of Nursing Education, 51*(12), 692–696.

Dapremont, J., & Lee, S. (2013). Partnering to educate: Dedicated education units. *Nurse Education in Practice, 14*, 335–337.

Delunas, L. R., & Rooda, L. (2009). A new model for the clinical instruction of undergraduate nursing students. *Nursing Education Perspectives, 30*(6), 377–380.

DeVoogd, R., & Saldbenblatt, C. (1989). The clinical teaching associate model: Advantages and disadvantages in practice. *Journal of Nursing Education, 28*(6), 276–277.

Diefenbeck, C. A., Plowfield, L. A., & Herrman, J. W. (2006). Clinical immersion: A residency model for nursing education. *Nursing Education Perspectives, 27*(2), 72–79.

Dreifuerst, K. T. (2012). Using debriefing for meaningful learning to foster development of clinical reasoning in simulation. *Journal of Nursing Education, 51*(6), 326–333.

Ellerman, C. R., Kataoka-Yahiro, M. R., & Wong, L. C. (2006). Logic models used to enhance critical thinking. *Journal of Nursing Education, 45*(6), 220–227.

Elliott, M. (2002). The clinical environment: A source of stress for undergraduate nurses. *Australian Journal of Advanced Nursing, 20*(1), 34–38.

Faller, H. S., McDowell, M. A., & Jackson, M. A. (1995). Bridge to the future: Nontraditional settings and concepts. *Journal of Nursing Education, 34*(8), 344–349.

Fugate, T., & Rebeschi, L. (1991). Dual assignment: An alternative clinical teaching strategy. *Nurse Educator, 15*(6), 14–16.

Gaberson, K. B., Oermann, M. H., & Shellenberger, T. (2015). *Clinical teaching strategies in nursing* (4th ed.). New York: Springer.

Ganley, B. J., & Linnard-Palmer, L. (2010). Academic safety during nursing simulation: Perceptions of nursing students and faculty. *Clinical Simulation in Nursing, 8*(2), e49–e57. http://dx.doi.org/10.1016/j.ecns.2010.06.004.

Gillespie, M. (2002). Student–teacher connection in clinical nursing education. *Journal of Advanced Nursing, 37*(6), 566–576.

Gillespie, M., & Patterson, B. (2009). Helping novice nurses make effective clinical decisions: The situated clinical decision-making framework. *Nursing Education Perspectives, 30*(3), 164–170.

Glanville, C. (1971). Mutliple student assignment as an approach to clinical teaching in pediatric nursing. *Nursing Research, 20*(3), 237–244.

Goode, C. J., Lynn, M. R., McElroy, D., Bednash, G. D., & Murray, B. (2013). Lessons learned from 10 years of research on post-baccalaureate nurse residency program. *Journal of Nursing Administration, 43*(2), 73–79.

Gubrud-Howe, P., & Schoessler, M. (2008). From random access opportunity to a clinical education curriculum. *Journal of Nursing Education, 47*(1), 3.

Gubrud-Howe, P. M., & Schoessler, M. (2009). OCNE Clinical Education Model. In N. Ard & T. M. Valliga (Eds.), *Clinical nursing education: Current reflections* (pp. 39–58). New York: National League for Nursing.

Hall-Lord, M. L., Theander, K., & Athlin, E. (2013). A clinical supervision model in bachelor nursing education—Purpose, content and evaluation. *Nurse Education in Practice, 13*, 506–511.

Hayden, J., Smiley, R. A., Alexander, M., Kardong-Edgren, S., & Jeffries, P. (2014). The NCSBN National Simulation Study: A longitudinal, randomized, controlled study replacing clinical hours with simulation and prelicensure nursing education. *Journal of Nursing Regulation, 5*(2 Suppl.), S4S64.

Henderson, S., Princell, C., & Martin, S. D. (2012). The patient-centered medical home. *American Journal of Nursing, 122*(12), 54–59.

Institute of Medicine. (2010). *Future of nursing: Leading change, advancing health.* Retrieved from, http://www.iom.edu/About-IOM.aspx.

Interprofessional Education Collaborative Expert Panel. (2011). *Core competencies for interprofessional collaborative practice: Report of an Expert panel.* Washington. D.C: Interprofessional Education Collaborative.

Ironside, P. M., & McNelis, A. M. (2010). *Clinical education in prelicensure nursing programs.* New York: National League for Nursing.

Jeffries, P. (2014). *Clinical simulations in nursing education: Advanced concepts, trends and opportunities.* Philadelphia: Wolters Kluwer Health.

Karuhije, H. F. (1997). Classroom and clinical teaching in nursing: Delineating differences. *Nursing Forum, 32*(2), 5–12.

Knapfel, S., Moore, G., & Skiba, D. J. (2014). Second Life and other virtual emerging simulations. In P. Jeffries (Ed.), *Clinical simulations in nursing education: Advanced concepts, trends, and opportunities.* Philadelphia: Wolters Kluwer Health.

Krautscheid, L., Kaakinen, J., & Warner, J. (2008). Clinical faculty development: Using simulation to demonstrate and practice clinical teaching. *Journal of Nursing Education, 47*(9), 431–434.

Kuiper, R., Pesut, D., & Kautz, D. (2009). Promoting the self-regulation of clinical reasoning skills in nursing students. *The Open Nursing Journal, 3,* 70–76.

Lo, R. (2002). A longitudinal study of perceived level of stress, coping and self-esteem of undergraduate nursing students: An Australian case study. *Journal of Advanced Nursing, 39*(2), 119–126.

Mallette, S., Laury, S., Engleke, M. K., & Andrews, A. (2005). The integrative clinical preceptor model: A new method for teaching undergraduate community health nursing. *Nurse Educator, 30*(1), 21–26.

Mamhidir, A. G., Kristofferzon, M. L., Hellström-Hyson, E., Persson, E., & Mårtensson, G. (2014). Nursing preceptors experiences of two clinical education models. *Nurse Education in Practice, 14,* 427–433.

Massarweh, L. (1999). Promoting a positive clinical experience. *Nursing Educator, 24*(3), 44–47.

McClure, E., & Black, L. (2013). The role of the clinical preceptor: An integrative literature review. *Journal of Nursing Education, 52*(6), 335–341.

McNelis, A. M., Ironside, P. M., Ebright, P. R., Dreifuerst, K. T., Zvonar, S. E., & Conner, S. (2014). Learning in practice: A multisite, multimethod investigation of clinical education. *Journal of Nursing Regulation, 4*(4), 30–35.

Moscato, S. R., Miller, J., Logsdon, K., Weinberg, S., & Chorpenning, L. (2007). Dedicated education unit: An innovative clinical partner education model. *Nursing Outlook, 55*(1), 31–37.

Moscato, S. R., Nishioka, V. M., & Coe, M. (2013). Dedicated education unit: Implementing an innovation in replication sites. *Journal of Nursing Education, 52*(5), 259–267.

Mulready-Shick, J., Flannagan, K. M., Banister, G. E., Mylott, L., & Curtin, L. (2013). Evaluating dedication units for clinical education quality. *Journal of Nursing Education, 52*(11), 606–614.

Murray, T. A., Crain, C., Meyer, G. A., McDonough, M. E., & Schweiss, D. M. (2010). Building bridges: An innovative academic-service partnership. *Nursing Outlook, 58*(5), 252–260.

National Council of State Boards of Nursing. (2005). *Clinical instruction in pre-licensure nursing programs.* Retrieved from, http//www.ncsbn.org/Final_Clinical_Instr_Pre_Nsg_programs.pdf.

Neiderhauser, V., Macintyre, R. D., Garner, C., Teel, C., & Murray, T. (2010). Transformational partnerships in nursing education. *Nursing Education Perspectives, 31*(6), 353–355.

Newton, J. M., Jolly, B. C., Ockerby, C. M., & Cross, W. (2012). Student centredness in clinical learning: The influence of the clinical teacher. *Journal of Advanced Nursing, 68*(10), 2331–2340.

Niederhauser, V., Schoessler, M., Gubrud-Howe, P., Magnussen, L., & Codier, E. (2012). Creating innovative model of clinical nursing education. *Journal of Nursing Education, 51*(11), 603–608.

Nielsen, A. (2009). Concept-based learning activities using the clinical judgment model as a foundation for clinical learning. *Journal of Nursing Education, 48*(8), 350–354.

Nielsen, A. E., Noone, J., Voss, H., & Matthews, L. (2013). Preparing nursing students for the future: An innovative approach to clinical education. *Nurse Education in Practice, 13,* 301–309.

O'Mara, L., McDonald, J., Gillespie, M., Brown, H., & Miles, L. (2014). Challenging clinical learning environments: Experiences of undergraduate nursing students. *Nurse Education in Practice, 14,* 208–213.

Overstreet, M. (2010). E-chats: The seven components of nursing debriefing. *The Journal of Continuing Education in Nursing, 41*(12), 538–539.

Patient Protection and Affordable Care Act (PPACA). (2014). *U.S. Department of Health & Human Services, 2014.* Retrieved from http://www.hhs.gov/healthcare/rights/.

Reese, C. E., Jeffries, P. R., & Engum, S. A. (2010). Learning together: Using simulations to develop nursing and medical student collaboration. *Nursing Education Perspectives, 31*(1), 33–37. Retrieved from, http://dx.doi.org/10.1043/1536-5026-31.1.33.

Reid, T. P., Hinderer, K. A., Jarosinski, J. M., Mister, B. J., & Seldomridge, L. (2013). Expert clinician to teacher: Developing a faculty academy and mentoring initiative. *Nurse Education in Practice, 13,* 288–293.

Rossen, B. E., & Fegan, M. A. (2009). Eight- or twelve-hour shifts: What nursing students prefer. *Nursing Education Perspectives, 30*(1), 40–43.

Schiavenato, M. (2009). Reevaluating simulation in nursing education: Beyond the human patient simulator. *Journal of Nursing Education, 48*(7), 388–393.

Sepples, S. B., Goran, S. F., & Zimmer-Rankin, M. (2013). Thinking inside the box: The tele-intensive care unit as a new clinical site. *Journal of Nursing Education, 52*(7), 401–404.

Shah, H., & Pennypacker, D. (1992). The clinical teaching partnership. *Nurse Educator, 17*(2), 10–12.

Simmons, B. (2010). Clinical reasoning: Concept analysis. *Journal of Advanced Nursing, 66*(5), 1151–1157.

Smedley, A., & Penney, D. (2009). A partnership approach to the preparation of preceptors. *Nursing Education Perspectives, 30*(1), 31–36.

Smithburger, P. L., Kane-Gill, S. L., Kloet, M. A., Lohr, B., & Seybert, A. L. (2013). Advancing interprofessional education through the use of high fidelity human patient simulators. *Pharmacy Practice, 11*(2), 61–65.

Strouse, A. C. (2010). Multidisciplinary simulation centers: Promoting safe practice. *Clinical Simulation in Nursing, 6,* e139–e142. Retrieved from, http://dx.doe.org/10.1016/j.ecns.2009.08.007.

Tanner, C. (2002). Clinical education, circa 2010. *Journal of Nursing Education, 41*(2), 51–52.

Tanner, C. (2005). The art and science of clinical teaching. *Journal of Nursing Education, 44*(4), 151–152.

Tanner, C. A. (2006). Thinking like a nurse: A research-based model of clinical judgment in nursing. *Journal of Nursing Education, 45*(6), 204–211.

Tanner, C. (2010). Transforming prelicensure nursing education. *Nursing Education Perspectives, 31*(6), 347–351.

Timmins, F., & Kaliszer, M. (2002). Aspects of education programmes that frequently cause stress to nursing students—Fact-finding sample survey. *Nursing Education Today, 22*(3), 203–211.

VanDenBerg, E. (1976). The multiple assignment: An effective alternative for laboratory experiences. *Journal of Nursing Education, 15*(3), 3–12.

Wells, L., & McLaughlin, M. (2014). Fitness to practice and feedback to students: A literature review. *Nurse Education in Practice, 14*, 137–141.

Wink, D. (1993). Using questioning as a teaching strategy. *Nurse Educator, 18*(5), 11–15.

Wink, D. (1995). The effective clinical conference. *Nursing Outlook, 43*(1), 29–32.

Wyte-Lake, T., Tran, K., Bowman, C. C., Needlemann, J., & Dobablian, A. (2013). A systematic review of strategies to address the clinical nursing faculty shortage. *Journal of Nursing Education, 52*(5), 245–252.

Zurmehly, J. (2010). Personal digital assistants (PDAs): Review and evaluation. *Nursing Education Perspectives, 31*(3), 179–182.

18 Teaching and Learning Using Simulations*

Pamela R. Jeffries, PhD, MSN, RN, FAAN, ANEF
Sandra M. Swoboda, RN, MS, FCCM
Bimbola Akintade, PhD, MBA, MHA, ACNP-BC, CCRN

The complexities of the health care system coupled with a changing patient population have created a need for nursing students to be prepared to care for all types of patients in a variety of care settings. Additionally, as health care shifts to community settings, nurse educators have been challenged to find appropriate clinical sites and clinical experiences for nursing students to meet curricula competencies and required clinical experiences. Because of these challenges, nurse educators are exploring alternative strategies for clinical preparation for nursing students. Simulation offers nurses, students, and health professionals the opportunity to learn in situations that are comparable to actual patient encounters within a controlled learning environment (Alden & Durham, 2012; Katz, Peifer, & Armstrong, 2010) that supports the learners' transfer of classroom and skills laboratory knowledge to realistic patient interactions (Anderson & Warren, 2011; Halstead, 2006; Meyer, Connors, Hou, & Gajewski, 2011). Clinical simulation technology is becoming increasingly more realistic, and nursing programs are making substantial investments in equipment and learning space. As simulations and related teaching and learning strategies move into nursing programs, and evidence supports clinical simulations as an alternative to actual clinical experiences (Hayden, Smiley, Alexander, Kardong-Edgren, & Jeffries, 2014), nurse educators must be prepared to teach using this methodology.

This chapter discusses simulations as an experiential, student-centered pedagogical approach. The chapter begins with an overview of types of simulation—the purposes, challenges, and benefits of clinical simulations—and concludes with information about planning, implementing, and evaluating simulations as they are integrated into courses and curricula. The chapter emphasizes (1) the types of clinical simulations being developed and implemented in nursing programs; (2) challenges and benefits to student learning, thinking, and practice; (3) a framework and steps to consider when developing and using clinical simulations; and (4) the evaluation component to consider when implementing simulations in the teaching–learning environment.

Simulations

Simulations are activities or events, such as performing basic life support on a patient simulator to manage a cardiac arrest, that mimic real-world practice. Simulations are used when real-world training is too expensive, occurs rarely, or puts participants (or patients) at unnecessary risk. Simulations provide the opportunity for students to practice within their scope of practice, think critically, problem solve, use clinical reasoning, and care for diverse patients in a nonthreatening, safe environment. Incorporating simulations into a nursing curriculum as a teaching and learning strategy offers nurse educators the opportunity to support learners' educational needs by providing them with an interactive, practice-based instructional strategy.

Simulation Nomenclature

There are various types of simulations. The terms used to describe various aspects of the simulation experience are described here. The simulation nomenclature matrix includes *learning domains* and *tool and environmental realism.* Tool and environmental realism are further categorized into types of

*The authors acknowledge the work of Marcella Hovancsek, MSN, RN, and John Clochesy, PhD, RN, FAAN, in the previous editions of the chapter.

fidelity—low, medium, and high—and the context of the fidelity as partial or full.

Fidelity

Fidelity, or the realism of simulations, is described along a continuum—from low fidelity to high fidelity—relative to the degree to which they approach reality.

- *Low fidelity:* This type of simulation experience includes case studies to educate students about patient situations, role playing, the use of a partial task trainer or static manikin (e.g., plastic model arm to learn how to perform a venipuncture, wound care trainer for wound management) to allow students to perform a task or skill. Low-level realism is present; however, principles and concepts can still be learned using this type of simulation (International Nursing Association for Clinical Simulation and Learning [INACSL] Board of Directors, 2011).
- *Medium fidelity:* This type of simulation is technologically sophisticated in that the participants can rely on a two-dimensional, focused experience to solve problems, perform skills, and make decisions during the clinical scenario. These manikins have the ability to auscultate heart sounds and breath sounds but the chest does not rise. Some examples include VitalSim Anne and VitalSim Kelly.
- *High fidelity:* This type of simulation involves full-scale, high-fidelity human patient simulators, virtual reality or standardized patients (actress or actors portraying simulated patients that have certain health disruptions) that are extremely realistic and provide a high level of interactivity and realism for the learner (International Nursing Association for Clinical Simulation and Learning [INACSL] Board of Directors, 2011). Examples include SimMan 3G, SimNewbie, iStan, and METI HPS, as well as a birthing simulator called Victoria and her newborn infant, all of which permit the student to listen to various body sounds and can be programmed to talk and to respond to interventions performed by the students.

Partial or Full-Context Simulations

The context of simulations can be partial or full.

- *Partial task trainers:* Partial task trainers are those simulations in which a body part, plastic model, or partial manikin is used to depict a certain function and on which a student can practice a particular psychomotor skill. Examples of partial task trainers include intravenous (IV) cannulation arms and low-technology manikins that are used to help students practice specific psychomotor skills integral to patient care such as inserting urinary catheters or nasogastric tubes.
- *Full-context simulations:* These simulations include the full context of a scenario, an event, or an activity that replicates reality. For example, a static manikin with limited functions such as VitalSim Kelly is full context but medium fidelity. The full context of an event can be represented using this type of simulation in a low-fidelity manner. High fidelity, full context is a simulated learning experience using a high-fidelity simulator and immersing the participants in a realistic mock code situation or a simulated live birth.

Full-scale patient simulations using sophisticated, high-fidelity patient simulators provide a high level of interactivity and realism for the learner. Less sophisticated, but still educationally useful, are computer-based simulations in which the participant relies on a two-dimensional, focused experience to solve problems, perform skills, and make decisions during the clinical scenario. Studies have shown that the two-dimensional experience has merit in terms of positive learning outcomes and skill acquisition (Jeffries, Woolf, & Linde, 2003). Partial task training devices such as IV arms and haptic (force feedback) IV trainers are used in simulations for psychomotor skills. The learner is able to practice a skill repeatedly before performing it on a real patient. The partial task trainers typically ensure a satisfactory rate of achievement of objectives and benefit to the participant. Studies have shown that after having used these task trainers, participants demonstrate a psychomotor skill and use that skill set in the real patient environment (Engum & Jeffries, 2003). Programs or courses in which the task trainers are used include clinical laboratory courses and modules during which specific skill sets and goals need to be obtained. Another approach to learning is the use of two-dimensional CD-ROMs to provide interactive practice with skills.

Types of Simulation

Simulations variously involve role playing, standardized patients (actors), interactive videos built on gaming platforms, and manikins to teach procedures, decision making, and critical thinking in realistic environments (Ryan et al., 2010). There are a variety of technology-based simulations to support student and novice nurses. They include computer-based interactive simulations, haptic partial task trainers, and digitally enhanced manikins. Haptic trainers use force feedback to provide opportunities to develop psychomotor skills. In addition to types of simulations categorized by the equipment or manikin used, there are simulations categorized by the type of pedagogy used when implementing the simulations. These types of simulations are described in the following sections.

Hybrid Simulations

A hybrid simulation is the combination of a standardized patient and the use of a patient simulator in one scenario to depict a clinical event for the learner. For example, the simulation scenario may begin with the student performing a health history on a standardized patient who has just arrived in the emergency department after having been involved in a motor vehicle accident. As the case evolves, the activity shifts to a patient simulator because of the clinical symptoms that need to be demonstrated by the manikin to reflect reality. This is a hybrid simulation because the history is being performed on a standardized patient and then the scenario shifts to a patient simulator, where the patient is now experiencing "hypovolemic shock" that is being reflected in the vital signs and other clinical findings of the manikin. A common hybrid simulation in obstetrics involves a low-fidelity task trainer with a standardized patient for simulations of normal birth or complications such as shoulder dystocia. This can be done with a standard actor and the pelvis of a birthing simulator or with the use of the Mama Natalie, which is a low-cost, wearable device that can manually deliver a baby and placenta and simulate postpartum complications.

Unfolding Case Simulations

Another type of simulation is the unfolding case. Unfolding cases evolve over time in an unpredictable manner. An unfolding case may include three to four events that build on each other, providing students an opportunity to plan care across a clinical event, a hospitalization, a care transition or across the life span (Page, Kowlowitz, & Alden, 2010). Unfolding cases can be used to meet a variety of learning goals:

1. To demonstrate hierarchal order so the learner can follow the progression of a health problem and the related nursing care. For example, the first scenario demonstrates the patient being admitted with a head injury caused by a fall; the learner must conduct a focused neurologic assessment. The unfolding case leads to a second scenario, in which the patient experiences specific neurologic signs (e.g., severe headache, widening pulse pressure); the learner must use additional assessment skills. The third case occurs postcraniotomy and involves care of the patient after the subdural hematoma is removed.
2. To visualize and prioritize hospital trajectory and care of a patient that progresses. For example, the patient is admitted through the emergency department, with the learner performing an assessment. The second scenario depicts the patient being admitted to the progressive care unit and the third scenario is designed for the learner to prepare the patient with discharge instructions.
3. To provide the learner with a view of care transitions, showing the effect of the health disruption or disease process and nursing interventions required for a particular patient. For example, the first scenario depicts a hospitalized patient newly diagnosed with chronic obstructive pulmonary disease (COPD). The second scenario progresses to the patient having compromised gas exchange related to COPD and being managed at an ambulatory care center. The third scenario depicts end-stage disease with a focus on end-of-life care with hospice care.
4. To serve as a mechanism to include a variety of important assessments and findings where one event leads to another. For example, the first scenario focuses on hypotension and subtle findings of sepsis and the second scenario centers on the critically ill patient with sepsis and hypotension.

Several organizations have developed unfolding case studies related to particular topics that are available at no cost to faculty. Four unfolding cases that focus on older adults and address the complexity of decision making about their care can be found at http://www.nln.org/facultyprograms/facultyresources/aces/unfolding_cases.htm; unfolding cases related to patient safety can be found at the Quality and Safety Education for Nurses (QSEN) site at http://www.qsen.org.

Standardized Patients

Standardized patients are live actors trained to portray the role of a patient according to a script or clinical scenarios written by the faculty. The actors become the patients, demonstrating clinical symptoms and responses of real patients. A variation of the standardized patient instructional strategy is the use of these types of simulations to evaluate physical assessment skills, history taking, communication techniques, patient teaching, and types of psychomotor skills or objective structured clinical examination (OSCE).

In Situ Simulations

In situ simulation is a type of simulation that involves training performed in a real-life setting where patient care is commonly provided (Dismukes, Gaba, & Howard, 2006). The aim of this type of simulation is to achieve high fidelity (realism) by performing the simulations in actual clinical settings, blending and providing both a clinical and learning environment. Typically, the simulation-based experiential learning focuses on interdisciplinary professional teams. Practicing professionals are well versed in their particular field, possess a fair amount of experience, and prefer their learning to be problem-centered and meaningful to their professional lives. Adults learn best when they can immediately apply what they have learned. Traditional teaching methods (e.g., a teacher imparts facts to the student in a unidirectional model) are not particularly effective in adult learning because it is important for adults to make sense of what they experience or observe.

Virtual Simulations and Digital Platforms

Simulations can also take place in virtual environments. Increasing development in virtual patient simulation is evolving and allows the learner to interact with the patient and the virtual environment where the patient is responsive to interventions through a digital media platform. An example of this platform is Second Life, a virtual world accessible by the Internet that enables its users to interact with each other through avatars. In this simulated world, users can explore, meet other users, socialize, participate in individual or group activities, and create services for one another or travel throughout the world. The software is a three-dimensional modeling tool that attempts to depict reality for the users. Second Life is used as a platform for education by many institutions, such as colleges, universities, libraries, and government entities. For the top 10 health care–related virtual reality applications, go to http://scienceroll.com/2007/06/17/top-10-virtualmedical-sites-in-second-life/.

There are other platforms whereby software programs replicate clinical practice and respond to learner interactions; some provide written feedback to the learner with suggestions and evidence as feedback. Simulation through game-based learning can be independently performed or moderated and this type of simulation helps prepare students for the clinical setting and allows the learner to make decisions and interact with a patient with real-time response in a safe learning environment.

Cook (2012) designed and evaluated a virtual world simulation for family nurse practitioner students and also created a primary care pediatric simulation for use by family nurse practitioner students in Second Life. Seefeldt et al. (2012) used Second Life to allow pharmacy, nursing, physical therapy, occupational therapy, and physician assistant students to interact around a mock patient case. The pilot study examined the feasibility of using Second Life as a means to foster interprofessional education (IPE). Students overall found the platform useful; however, there were technical difficulties in using the platform and students lacked the necessary knowledge and skills to use the platform. Farra, Miller, Timm, and Schafer (2013) found out that virtual environments can be used as a learning strategy for nursing students to practice and hone their disaster response and management skills. The study found that students were able to retain the knowledge after the simulation and there was an overall positive response to the use of the virtual platform.

Purpose of Simulations

Clinical simulations in nursing education can be used for many purposes, for example, as a teaching strategy or for assessment and evaluation, or as an avenue to encourage IPE. However, one of the most important reasons that educators use simulations is to provide experiential learning for the student. Students can be immersed in a simulation where they can actually portray the primary nurse, a newly employed nurse in orientation, or whatever role within the scope of nursing practice the learner is assigned.

Simulations as Experiential Learning

The use of simulation corresponds with a shift from an emphasis on teaching to an emphasis on learning (Dunn, 2004; Jeffries, 2005) in which the faculty facilitate learning by encouraging students to discover, or construct, knowledge and meaning. Kolb (1984) and others (Sewchuck, 2005; Svinicki & Dixon, 1987) suggest that the experiential learning cycle is a continuous process in which knowledge is created by transforming experience. Individuals have a concrete experience, they reflect on that experience (reflective observation), they derive meaning (abstract conceptualization) from the experience, and they try out or apply (active experimentation) the meaning they've created, thus continuing the cycle with another concrete experience.

When making a shift in approach from a focus on teaching to a focus on learning, goals of the educational programs serve as the framework for the development of specific learning activities. For example, both nursing students and novice nurses entering professional practice find it difficult to transfer theoretical knowledge into clinical practice. The use of simulation allows students to experience the application of theory in a safe environment where mistakes can be made without risk to patients.

The use of highly realistic and complex simulation may not always be an appropriate educational approach. In some situations, beginning students can use low-fidelity simulation to work on attainment of foundational skills, including effective communication with patients, psychomotor skill performance, and basic assessment techniques. With task trainers or standard manikins, students can practice procedural skills and caregiving in a safe environment that allows them to make mistakes, learn from those mistakes, and develop confidence in their ability to approach and communicate with patients in the clinical setting. In addition, students benefit from the opportunity to work with technologically sophisticated equipment such as clinical information systems and hemodynamic monitoring systems in the educational setting before encountering such equipment in the clinical setting.

Advanced practice nursing students benefit from high-fidelity simulations that are complex, realistic, and interactively challenging experiences that support them in developing and practicing leadership abilities, teamwork, and decision-making skills. With patient simulators, for example, students can practice complex assessment skills in their area of clinical practice. Faculty can create scenarios and program equipment to simulate serious clinical situations such as respiratory arrest or aberrant cardiac rhythms that may require an emergent response. Simulations are also appropriate to prepare psychiatric nurse practitioners. As students respond to these more complex situations, they demonstrate their abilities to establish priorities, make decisions, take appropriate action, and work successfully as part of a team (Reese, Jeffries, & Engum, 2010). Within the simulated environment, advanced students also can demonstrate application of learning because they are no longer merely acquiring knowledge and skills. Students learn from the simulated practice without the need for faculty stepping in to correct and control the situation. High-fidelity simulation affords all students the opportunity to experience a baseline set of clinical scenarios, including those that are uncommon or rare, and to practice skill sets repeatedly until they develop a routine and process for safe patient care (Reising & Hensel, 2014).

Simulations as a Teaching–Learning Strategy

Nurse educators have used low-fidelity simulation such as manikins, role play, and case studies as a teaching–learning strategy for decades. The introduction of high-fidelity simulation (in the form of affordable, portable, and versatile human patient simulators) in the late 1990s transformed health care education and is now one of the foundational strategies in the preparation of health care professionals not only for teaching, but also for assessment and evaluation, developing interprofessional team skills, and for clinical substitution and make up for missed experiences.

Simulations Used for Assessment and Evaluation of Learning

Given the widespread use of simulations, there is also the potential for using simulations for assessment and evaluation of student learning. Using simulation for assessment and evaluation of learning should be integrated into the larger process of planning, implementing, assessing, and evaluating learning. Faculty should identify the purpose of the assessment or evaluation early in the process to ensure the evaluation is relevant and evaluates the learning outcomes for which it is intended (Adamson, 2014). Although more traditional forms of assessment continue to be employed—for example, pretesting and posttesting using multiple-choice tests—simulation-based assessments are increasingly being used in the evaluation process, both in a formative manner, as part of an educational activity or training, or in a summative manner, as part of a graduation or certification process.

When simulations are being used for assessment or evaluation, the activities fall into two broad categories—"low-stakes" and "high-stakes" situations—depending on the significance of the evaluation (Boulet & Swanson, 2004). Low-stakes assessments are situations in which the simulation is used by the learner and faculty to mark progress toward personal, course, or program learning goals. High-stakes assessments include licensing and certification examinations, credentialing processes, and employment decisions (Jeffries, Hovancsek, & Clochesy, 2005). Simulation technologies used for assessment range from case studies and standardized patients (e.g., OSCEs) to haptic task trainers and high-fidelity human simulators.

As with any type of assessment, faculty must consider the issues of validity and reliability. For assessments in low-stakes or learning situations, construct and concurrent validity should be addressed. Construct validity is the degree to which an assessment instrument measures the dimensions of knowledge or skill development intended. Concurrent validity is determined by evaluating the relationship between how individuals perform on the new assessment (in this case a simulation) and the traditional (standard) assessment instrument. An assessment with high concurrent validity, for example, is one in which the learner's simulator assessment score is comparable to his or her score when performing the same examination on a standardized patient scored by using a checklist.

Predictive validity is required for simulations used in assessments in which licensure, certification, or employment are at stake. Determining predictive validity in high-stakes assessment is a complex process. Predictive validity is the extent to which performance on a particular simulation predicts future performance, such as clinical decision making or psychomotor skills. Evaluating predictive validity requires that, in addition to current performance, the clinical skill or decision making of specific individuals be tracked over time. There has been little research and evidence-based information specifically focused on quantifying the effect of simulation-based assessment activities on student or practitioner learning.

Simulations also are being used to assess and evaluate students' clinical skill competencies and clinical decision-making capabilities. Using standardized patients to assess the clinical skills of medical students and residents has become widespread (Chambers, Boulet, & Gary, 2000). OSCEs are clinical examinations that vary in format but mostly include a set period for the student to assess and interact with a standardized patient, an actor or actress hired to portray a certain type of patient with a specific diagnosis and clinical symptoms. Wilson, Shepherd, and Pitzner (2005) used the low-fidelity human patient simulator to acquire and then assess nurses' health assessment knowledge and skills. The use of the low-fidelity manikins proved to be an effective tool to assess for health assessment skills. Miller, Leadingham, and Vance (2010) used the human patient simulator to meet learning objectives across core nursing courses.

When using simulations as an assessment mechanism, the nurse educator should also consider the improvement in the use of standardized patients, the sophistication of computer-based evaluation techniques, the use of newer physiologic electromechanical manikins, and the fidelity of immersive haptic devices. Because of these advances, nurse educators are now better able to assess learning, promote a better educational effort, improve academic courses and programs, and ultimately prepare students to provide quality, competent and safe patient care.

Simulations Used in Interprofessional Education

Conventionally, nursing and other health care education as a whole is delivered on a uniprofessional basis, eliminating the reality of everyday interprofessional collaborative clinical practice. IPE is bridging that gap (Alinier, Harwood, & Harwood, 2014). *IPE* can be defined as two or more professions that work together and learn from and about one another in an effort to improve collaborative practices and the overall quality of patient care (Newton, Bainbridge, & Ball, 2014). (See also Chapter 11.) In Canada, IPE to improve interprofessional collaborative practice has been documented for more than 50 years, but in terms of research, it has gained popularity in the last 15 years. Currently, most health education programs are beginning to embed IPE into their curricula, thus increasing attention to continuing professional development. There are many advantages of IPE, including breaking down both real and perceived barriers between different clinical aspects, enhancing interprofessional cohesiveness and awareness, and providing an opportunity to develop mutual respect among members of an interdisciplinary team. Within an interprofessional team, an important element of providing safe and effective patient care is knowledge and understanding of other professionals' roles and skills (MacDonald et al., 2010). A study by Alinier et al. (2014) investigated the knowledge and perceptions of immersive clinical simulation in undergraduate health care IPE. The study showed that students acquired knowledge, became familiar with other professions, and developed a better appreciation of interprofessional learning even with limited interprofessional simulation experiences. During the debriefings, discussions highlighted the importance and value of interprofessional training by students, especially when well contextualized and facilitated through exposure to realistic scenarios. Even though it is widely agreed that collaborative practice among health care professionals improves quality of care and patient outcomes, evidence-based and innovative suggestions as to how this should be accomplished are lacking. Current literature is limited in providing strategies that foster interprofessional collaborative learning in an easily adoptable and implementable way. Additional research is needed in IPE to quantify its effects on theoretical and clinical practice applications and the ability for nursing students and the integration of novice nurses into clinical practice.

Simulations Used for Clinical Substitution and Clinical Make-up

Simulations are currently being used in clinical settings to substitute for real clinical time for various reasons. For some schools of nursing, the issue of finding quality, appropriate clinical sites is a challenge for faculty, particularly in specialty areas such as pediatrics or maternal health (Hayden, Kegan, Kardong-Edgren, & Smiley, 2014; Meyer et al., 2011). Nurse educators have substituted clinical time in many cases for time in the simulation area to provide nursing students appropriate clinical experiences that are developed and implemented through clinical simulations. In some instances, schools of nursing are labeling clinical times as "off-campus" clinical for actual experiences in health care institutions and "on-campus clinical" when the clinical experience is obtained in the simulation laboratory. At New York University, adult health courses are being delivered with 50% off-campus clinical (real clinical time) and 50% on-campus clinical to help with their clinical faculty shortage and competition for clinical sites (Richardson, Goldsant, Simmons, Gilmartin, & Jeffries, 2014).

In some schools of nursing, clinical simulations are being used for "clinical make-up" days for those students missing clinical because of illness, weather, or other unforeseen causes. There can be an entire "clinical day" set up in the simulation lab for clinical hours. Some nurse educators use virtual simulations (computer-based learning) that has a debriefing component and scoring to meet clinical make-up hours when needed and when the content fits with the curriculum needs.

A landmark multisite study done by the National Council of State Boards of Nursing (NCSBN) explored the clinical competency of new graduates on their transition to practice based on their participation in either a control group, a group that substituted 25% of real clinical hours for simulations, or a group that substituted 50% of their clinical hours for simulation (https://www.ncsbn.org/index.htm). The study report stated,

> substantial evidence [demonstrates] that up to 50% simulation can be effectively substituted for traditional clinical experience in all prelicensure core nursing courses under conditions that are comparable to those described in the study. These conditions include faculty members who are formally trained in simulation pedagogy, an adequate number of faculty members to support the student learners, subject matter experts who conduct theory-based debriefing, [and] equipment and supplies to create a realistic environment. (Hayden, Smiley, Alexander, Kardong, & Jeffries, 2014, p. S38)

The NCSBN also stated that the State Boards of Nursing should feel assured about the validity of simulation programs if nursing schools have enough dedicated staff members and resources to maintain the program in an ongoing basis. These findings are significant for the nurse educator community because too often quality clinical sites are difficult to find; health care agencies are limiting the amount of practice and procedures students can actually perform in the clinical setting; and, the client census is diminishing in the acute care settings such that clinical experiences are limited and focus only on the acute care population.

Challenges and Benefits of Using Simulations

Simulations can offer nurse educators and health care providers a significant educational method that meets the needs of today's learners by providing them with interactive, practice-based instructional strategies. Implementing and testing the use of simulations in educational practice has both challenges and benefits.

Most of the challenges of using clinical simulations center on educators' preparation for using simulations and interprofessional simulations. Before using simulations as a learning strategy, the faculty must have:

1. A firm foundation in experiential learning
2. Clear learning objectives for the simulation experience
3. A detailed design taking into account that an educator facilitates learning (versus tells the learner)
4. Sufficient time for learners to experience the simulation, to reflect on the experience, and to make meaning of the experience
5. Faculty development in the area of simulation pedagogy; the teaching strategy is student-centered, which for many is a paradigm shift in teaching
6. Strategic ways to quantify and document clinical simulation hours towards licensure or certification
7. When using IPE simulation, there must be alignment of student clinical placements across the professions; preparation of all faculty and preceptors involved; commitment from all professions to making IPE experiences a priority; and adequate financial, human, and space resources. (See also chapter 11)

The benefits of using simulations include:

1. *Active involvement of students in their learning process.* By interacting with the simulation, examples, and exercises, the learner is required to use a higher order of learning rather than simply mimicking the teacher role model. Decision-making and critical thinking skills are reinforced through this teaching modality.
2. *More effective use of faculty in the teaching of clinical skills and interventions.* In a simulated experience, faculty members have an opportunity to observe students more closely and to allow students to demonstrate their potential more fully. The feedback or debriefing by faculty is a powerful learning tool.
3. *Increased student flexibility to practice based on their schedules.* The learner can access the simulation at his or her convenience and is not required to practice the skills in front of an instructor, although that option remains available for those who need extra instruction or reinforcement. The learner can revisit a skill several times in an environment that is safe, nonthreatening, and conducive to learning.
4. *Improved student instruction.* Student instruction is improved through better consistency of teaching; increased learner satisfaction in both the classroom and the clinical setting; the opportunity for safer, nonthreatening practice of skills and decision making; and a state-of-the-art learning environment.
5. *Effective competency check for undergraduates, new graduates, or new nurses going through orientation.* The simulation experience provides a competency check of the participants' knowledge, skills, and problem-solving abilities in a nonthreatening, safe environment.
6. *Correction of errors discussed immediately.* Students can learn by being immersed in their learning experience and then being debriefed after the encounter on what was right and what needed to be done differently.
7. *Standardized, consistent, and comparable experiences for all students.* Educators can create consistent, standardized teaching activities so that all students in a clinical

course can experience an important clinical event, assessment activity, or other essential clinical learning encounter.

8. *Opportunities for collaboration and IPE.* This provides an avenue for safe and effective patient care through knowledge and understanding of other professionals' roles and skills that all students in a clinical course can experience.

As educators are incorporating simulations into their courses and into the nursing curriculum, major challenges and benefits have been noted. Faculty must consider both challenges and benefits as the simulation pedagogy is adopted into courses and the nursing curriculum.

Planning to Use Simulations

Using simulations as a teaching–learning strategy requires advance planning. Planning should consider the need for resources, the overall curriculum, preparation of the student, and faculty development.

Resources

Operationalizing simulation requires physical space and equipment, the use of different types of simulation equipment and technology (manikins, virtual reality, Skype, electronic health records), faculty, and support staff. The physical space must be large enough to accommodate teaching and learning space, office space for faculty and staff, storage space, debriefing space, and, if used, space for video recording. Well-resourced spaces may mimic an acute care setting or operating room suite. Resources also include support staff who assist faculty in managing the equipment, and supporting the audiovisual technology.

Curriculum Considerations

A needs assessment and analysis should be performed to understand the intricacies of the curriculum in general and how the specific courses intersect with each other. Examining specific course content and the clinical site placements gives a broad overview of the types of experiences students are exposed to and how objectives are met. Further examination of QSEN competencies, national patient safety goals, the NCSBN Licensure Examination blueprint, the Institute of Medicine Initiatives, and standardized testing results can help design and pattern content for simulation. In thinking *who* the learners are, *why* they learn, *what* they learn, and *how* they learn, a schematic design for each course can be developed to determine how the goals of theory, simulation, and clinical are interconnected and where simulation would be appropriate.

Preparing the Student

Simulation is likely a learning strategy that is a new experience for the student. Faculty must orient the student to the use of the equipment and to his or her role as an active and engaged learner. Students must understand the learning goals, what assignments they should complete or information to have at hand during the simulation, how the simulation relates to the reality of clinical practice, and the significance of the debriefing session. If the simulation is being used for assessment or evaluation, faculty must provide an opportunity for students to become familiar with the equipment, and make clear the rubrics that will be used to judge performance.

Simulation supports students' learning needs in a variety of ways. For example, simulations may offer a flexible, accessible opportunity to practice skills and interventions when student schedules permit. The learner can access the simulation at his or her convenience and not be required to practice the skills in front of an instructor, although that option can remain available for those who need extra instruction or reinforcement. Simulations also offer an opportunity to practice a selected skill set a number of times in an environment that is safe, nonthreatening, and conducive to learning. Simulations also provide exposure to real-life clinical experiences for students before caring for a specific type of patient in a specific type of clinical setting, thus giving them confidence when in the actual clinical setting.

Faculty Development

Educators prepared in the use of simulations are essential to the success of integrating simulations across the curriculum. However, unlike the traditional classroom setting, the faculty role when using simulations is no longer teacher-centered but rather is student-centered, with the educator assuming the role of a facilitator in the student's learning process. The educator's role during the simulation process varies, depending on whether the simulation is being conducted for learning or evaluation purposes. Educators must provide learner support as needed throughout the simulation and facilitate or guide the debriefing at the conclusion of the experience. If the simulation is being conducted for evaluation purposes, the teacher's role changes to that of an observer and rater/grader.

When using simulations for the first time, faculty must feel comfortable with the simulations they are using. Pretraining on simulation pedagogy and debriefing is essential (National League for Nursing, 2015). Faculty may require assistance with simulation design, use of the technology, and setting up equipment for the activity. Whei Ming and Juestel (2010) found that novice faculty members needed assistance to operationalize the critical thinking learning objectives in a clinical simulation. To assist faculty, the educators developed a series of questions that provide direction about the specific thought processes involved in the application of the nursing process through the use of clinical simulations (Table 18-1).

Schools of nursing have found it helpful to send faculty to an orientation course or develop their own orientation to develop faculty for using simulations in their teaching. These courses include information about designing and using scenarios, the role of the faculty, and how to conduct the debriefing. Faculty experience a simulation first-hand as they participate in these courses.

Designing Simulations

Simulations should be carefully planned. The process of designing, implementing, and evaluating a simulation to support learning in nursing education is best done using a systematic, organized approach. To help nursing educators and researchers in this

TABLE 18-1 Critical Thinking Learning Objectives and Core Questions to Ask in Clinical Simulations

Critical Thinking Learning Objectives	Core Questions
Assess client to collect relevant data. • Identify cues and make inferences. • Validate data.	• What are the possible problems in this situation that need to be solved? On what evidence have you based your inferences?
	• Is your evidence valid? What factors may alter the accuracy of the data? How would you validate each item of evidence?
	• Why are these items relevant? How are they related?
Diagnose actual and potential client health needs.	• Are the clustered data sufficient to support each diagnosis? What additional data do you need?
• Cluster data. • Draw diagnostic conclusions.	• Are there different possibilities for clustering these data? Are there other alternative diagnoses that may fit different ways of clustering?
	• What other data are needed to rule these possibilities in or out?
Plan care based on identified client health needs. • Set priorities.	• What are the most important problems that need to be solved? On what criteria did you base your decision?
• Predict outcome criteria. • Generate solutions (interventions).	• What are the expected outcomes of the problem?
	• What are the possible interventions for the problem described?
	• What are the possible risks and benefits involved in each intervention?
Implement plan of care. • Test solutions.	• When do you assess the client's response to each intervention? What are the desired responses to the intervention?
Evaluate progress toward attainment of outcomes. • Perform a criterion-based evaluation.	• If an adverse reaction happened, what would you do next? Why?
Self-critique thinking strategies used to reach decisions.	• What were the factors influencing your thinking?
• Self-regulate thinking.	• What would you do differently in a different situation?

From Whei Ming, S., & Juestel, M. (2010). Direct teaching of thinking skills using clinical simulation. *Nurse Educator, 35*(5), 197–204.

developmental process, a simulation framework (Jeffries, 2005) has been developed to identify the components of the process and their relationship to guide the design, implementation, and evaluation of these activities.

The Simulation Model

A framework (Fig. 18-1) has been designed by a national group organized by the National League for Nursing to assist educators in outlining the first steps of simulation development to provide a consistent and empirically supported model to guide the design and implementation of simulations as well as the assessment of learning outcomes when using simulations (Jeffries, 2005, 2012). Within the framework, five design features for developing a clinical simulation scenario are described. A simulation template used as a guide to develop the clinical simulations can be found at the Simulation Innovation Resource Center (SIRC) website at http://sirc.nln.org/.

When developing the scenario, the design features are considered within the development process. For example, problem-solving components are considered in the scenario progression writing. Faculty can consider one or two problem-solving components designed in the scenario to be implemented by the novice students and three or four decision-making components for the more advanced student, perhaps to facilitate and emphasize prioritization at this level. After the simulation template is completed, it is advised that the scenarios be peer reviewed by content experts to ensure that evidence-based practices are being incorporated into the scenario and to confirm accuracy and that the content is up to date for today's health care world. Finally, the scenario must be pilot-tested with targeted end users so that educators can ensure that the scenario is at the correct level for the learner and can review the scenario for sufficient decision-making points and cues to engage the students in the simulation. A variety of resources exist

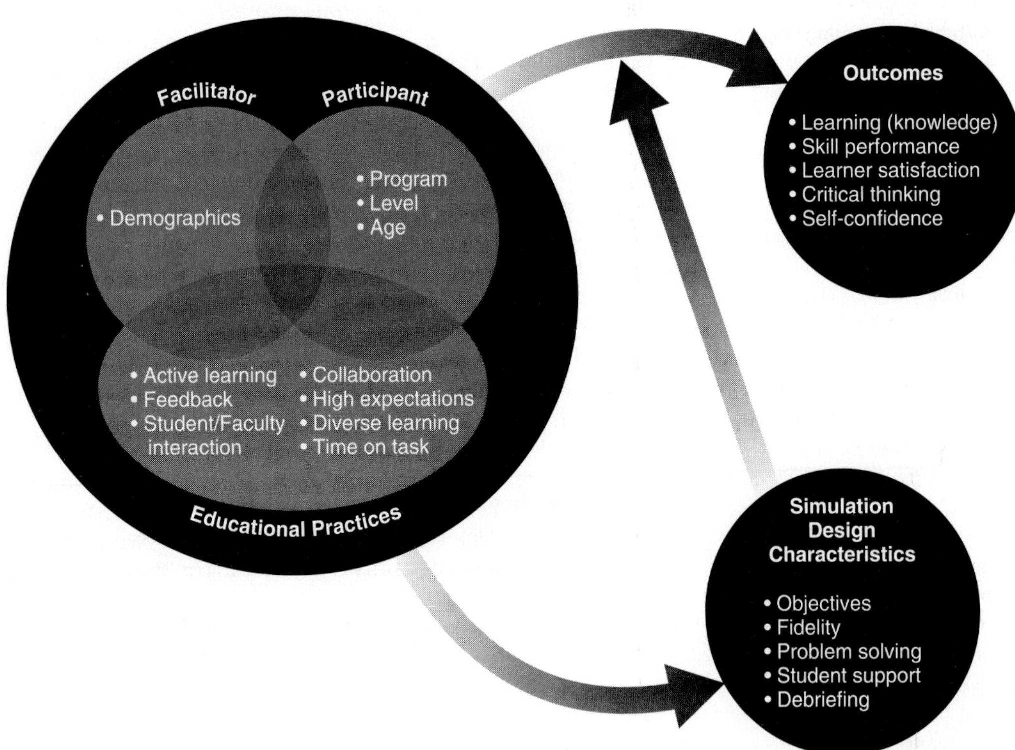

Figure 18-1 Simulation model. Jeffries, P. R. (2012). *Simulations in nursing education: From conceptualization to evaluation* (2nd ed.). Philadelphia: Lippincott, Williams and Wilkins. (Used with permission.)

to provide educators with knowledge and skills on developing simulation scenarios, including regional and national workshops, conferences, instructor courses, and several publications (Campbell & Daley, 2008; Guhde, 2011; Jeffries, 2007; Simulation Innovation Resource Center [SIRC], n.d.).

Evidence-based Debriefing and Reflection

Debriefing is one of the key design features to consider when developing a simulation (see Fig. 18-1). Debriefing is a process by which educators facilitate learners' reflection or reexamination of clinical encounters (Dreifuerst, 2009, 2012). Ideally, debriefing should be twice as long as the scenario and involves active participation from all learners (caregivers to observers), where the learners do most of the talking. The debriefing environment should be a safe environment where learners can engage in meaningful discussion. Debriefing in the context of simulation involves reflective observation and abstract conceptualization. Reflective observation has its roots in Gestalt psychology and in the works of Lewin (1951); Schön (1987); Diefenbeck, Plowfield, and Herrman (2006); and Kolb (1984). Kolb (1984) and others (Sewchuck, 2005; Svinicki & Dixon, 1987) suggest that the experiential learning cycle is a continuous process in which knowledge is created by transforming experience. Individuals have a concrete experience, they reflect on that experience (reflective observation), they derive meaning (abstract conceptualization) from the experience, and they try out or apply (active experimentation) the meaning they have created, thus continuing the cycle with another concrete experience. Debriefing encompasses the cognitive domain assessing knowledge; the kinetic domain assessing skill and action; and the affective domain, or how the learner felt or interacted with the patient or other staff.

The role of faculty in facilitating simulation exercises is to support participants in the reflection and debriefing process. Objectives of debriefing include the opportunity for the learners to describe what the experience was like for them; this includes a release of emotional tension about the experience, a guided review of the patient and objectives, the identification and sorting of thinking, and reinforcement of teaching and correction of misconceptions. Debriefing is an opportunity to reference real-life experiences, normalize behaviors, and acknowledge emotions.

Debriefing strategies are varied and several models are used in the simulation setting (Cheng et al., 2014; Simon, Rudolph, & Raemer, 2009; Waznonis, 2014). The National League for Nursing in its Vision Statement, Debriefing Across the Curriculum, recommends that faculty use evidence-based resources to develop their skills in debriefing (National League for Nursing, 2015). The Debriefing Assessment for Simulation in Healthcare (DASH) tool is designed to evaluate and develop the debriefing skills of the facilitator. This tool evaluates the facilitators' ability to conduct debriefings following specific behaviors. It is an evidence-based tool designed according to how people learn and change in experiential learning and was vetted by an expert panel at Harvard (http://www.harvardmedsim.org/_media/DASH_Bibliography_2011.pdf). Table 18-2 depicts one debriefing model (Overstreet, 2010).

Facilitators face challenges in debriefing, including blame-setting for performance, statements such as "this wouldn't happen in real clinical," learners who are open with dislike about the learning environment, learners who are hostile and defensive or who are self-critical and defeated based on performance. Facilitators provide a safe, nonjudgmental environment and coach students to reflect on what they saw, heard, and experienced. All debriefings should be well planned and structured. The key for faculty during debriefing is not to provide more information or to lecture on the "correct" way or answer, but to guide students along the path of reflection. Open-ended questions, silence, and pauses help elicit feedback from learners and encourage active participation. Identification of a "take-away" message or transfer of learning to other situations should be included (Lusk & Fater, 2013).

Implementing Simulations

Once the simulation is designed, faculty members are ready to implement it into the nursing course. The following guidelines may be useful to educators implementing simulations into their nursing courses:

1. Make sure specific objectives match the implementation phase of the simulation. When faculty design a simulation, the objectives and nature of the simulation should be clearly defined for the students and facilitator. Furthermore, if the simulation is designed, for example, around the care of an

TABLE 18-2 Components for Debriefing Nursing Students Using the Ee-Chats

Debriefing Component	Educator Action/Activity/Strategy
E—Emotion	Faculty need to address learners' emotions that have been stimulated during the simulation encounter; encourage the students to translate emotions into words.
e—Experience	Faculty can briefly share their experiences or stories; inform the students how the expert would have handled the situation—but be brief, this is only one small part of debriefing.
C—Communication	Educators should talk less and students more; students also can observe your verbal and nonverbal messages; the debriefing should be a positive experience.
H—Higher Order of Thinking	Students should be encouraged to reflect in, on, and beyond the simulation encounter they have experienced; how will this experience translate into the clinical one?
A—Accentuate the Positive	Educators need to be positive when conducting a debriefing—reframe and rephrase your questions into inquiry-time ones, not blaming. Focus on behaviors that are professional and essential.
T—Time	Allow students time to formulate their responses and reflections. Embrace silence.
S—Structure	Debriefing time should focus on the encounter, the events, actions, and behaviors demonstrated in the simulation.

From Overstreet, M. (2010). Ee-chats: The seven components of nursing debriefing. *The Journal of Continuing Education in Nursing, 41*(12), 538–539.

insulin-dependent patient, then the scenario should be created using problems typically encountered and the problem-solving skills needed for that patient's care. The simulation should focus on the objectives and not on potential co-morbidities or extraneous issues.

2. Set a time limit for the simulation and the debriefing encounter and then adhere to it. Too often instructors observe that in simulations students are immersed for a specific time limit but are not able to accomplish all of the assessments and interventions the instructor had desired. At times instructors may let the scenario proceed beyond the specific time frame; however, if the simulation is scheduled for 20 minutes, the encounter needs to be 20 minutes. If students do not achieve the objectives desired, the reflective observation time can be spent on their experiences and the meaning they make of them.
3. Implement an appropriate orientation of students to the simulation labs where they will be interacting with the simulators. This is an important step to help eliminate the anxiety and fear of the unknown associated with initial exposure to simulation as a whole. It is also important to engage in a confidentiality agreement with the students that makes debriefing a safe environment for students and faculty, and lastly, implement a fiction contract where students are expected to treat the simulation environment as they would a true clinical encounter.
4. In undergraduate nursing programs, it is advisable to make assignments so students know their specific roles during the simulation. Unless developing or testing team leadership skills, students need roles (e.g., nurse, observer, family member) assigned before encountering the simulation to bring organization to the experience. If roles are not assigned, students waste time trying to decide what role to play. In advanced practice nursing programs, role delineation may be handled by the students. It is conceivable that advanced practice nurses can come together to determine specific roles and responsibilities. This may also be a good topic to investigate during postsimulation debriefing.
5. Avoid interrupting the simulated encounter when students are trying to problem-solve on their own. In simulation, the learners function as professionals, not as students, so they are asked to step beyond their comfort zone and interact in the scenario without someone directing them how to act. Facilitators should observe a simulation remotely, either behind a one-way mirror

or via closed-circuit television, so students cannot see facial expressions, hear comments, or see nonverbal gestures. It is best for faculty to discuss the points of concern, prioritization, and problem-solving issues during the debriefing immediately after the simulation event. If this is not done in the immediacy of the simulation, the behaviors can be forgotten or confused with other scenarios.

6. Involve a limited number of learners in the simulation experience in addition to one or two observers or recorders of the encounter. Typically, two to six students are each assigned a role in the simulation experience. The roles within the simulation need to be identified before and recognized during the simulation. For example, students can wear name tags or labels and appropriate clothing for particular roles or have certain props available to help delineate the roles. When an educator has more students than are needed to participate in the simulation, these students can be assigned an observer role.
7. Ensure that the simulation is appropriate for the learners' skill levels and cognitive ability. Although a prominent design feature when developing simulations is fidelity, simulations need to be realistic to the degree that matches the learning level of the student group. Early on in exposure to the simulation environment, students benefit from scenarios that are comparable to their didactic learning. Low- or medium-fidelity manikin and standardized patients with basic care needs offer opportunities to focus on basic skill and knowledge acquisition. Failure and anxiety in the simulation scenario can occur when the simulation objectives include skills or competencies students have not learned (e.g., IV management prior to IV curriculum or altered cardiac or lung sounds prior to cardiac or lung modules). As exposure to the simulated environment increases, learners benefit from a higher level of complexity and a mix of fidelity, including challenges found in a complex environment such as simulated emergent events that involve critical thinking, active interaction, teamwork, and collaboration with the health care team to achieve a common goal. Simulations assist students at the application level of learning to practice their decision-making, problem-solving, and team member skills in a nonthreatening environment. The environment needs to be sufficiently realistic to allow for suspension of disbelief, so that the transition of knowledge from theory to practice can be stimulated. In simulation there is no "pretend." All necessary equipment should be available and standards and protocols should be followed to mimic the clinical setting. If a patient is to take a medication, the proper steps for administration should be used.
8. When planning to incorporate simulations into the course or curriculum, ensure that faculty development is included in the planning. Faculty need to know how to conduct a simulation and a debriefing session to achieve the desired outcomes with the teaching–learning strategy. Faculty need to be prepared to design and conduct simulations in the educational setting before they are actually placed in the learning laboratory or clinical practicum with students in a simulation situation. All faculty members using this type of strategy in their classroom or clinical instruction need to be aware of and clear about the purpose of the simulation activity. At the end of the simulation, a clear summary and highlights need to be included by all instructors, particularly if there are several educators using the same simulation in a course. Discussion about simulations and how to implement them and clarity on learning outcomes for the simulation are needed and must be agreed on by faculty before implementation of the simulation. Clear delineation of the objectives of the scenario and the debriefing model should be followed by all facilitators. A predesigned concept map for each scenario can help guide facilitators for consistent debriefing.

Integrating Simulations into Courses and Curricula

Simulations can be integrated into nursing courses, laboratory experiences, and clinical courses to promote more active and experiential learning at most schools of nursing (Katz et al., 2010). As more schools adopt clinical simulations in their courses and curricula and as actual clinical experiences are becoming more difficult to obtain, some faculty and their state boards of nursing are supplementing or substituting clinical time with simulations.

More recently, following the trend in electronic communications for teaching and students' strong acceptance of online learning, more sophisticated technologies have enabled simulation approaches to transition from the classroom to a virtual platform.

Virtual simulation in online nursing education combines the pedagogy of face-to-face simulation with electronic multimedia options to produce activities that are both interactive and mediated by the learner. Virtual simulation programs can be hosted online and accessed using a choice of navigable software using learning objectives that vary from highly focused technical skills training to broader, case-based patient scenarios that require critical thinking and clinical decision making (Cant & Cooper, 2014). Some popular virtual simulation software products available for online nursing education include ArchieMD, CliniSpace, Second Life, TINA, Virtual Heroes, and vSim.

Faculty have integrated simulations in a variety of courses. Thomas, Hodson-Carlton, and Ryan (2010) used clinical simulations in a senior leadership course to better prepare and facilitate new graduates to clinical practice. Clinical scenarios were developed that incorporated students, faculty, staff, and community volunteers who role-played situations that students may encounter after graduation. Some of the issues embedded in the scenarios include staffing problems, physician interactions, patient and family communications, and crisis interventions.

Hamilton (2010) used clinical simulations during academic and clinical experiences to equip students with the skills necessary to productively cope with the stressors faced in difficult end-of-life situations. Using the End-of-Life Nursing Education Consortium materials, the educator found simulations to be an effective teaching strategy to identify anxiety levels prior to clinical experience and as a venue for exploring learning and coping styles.

Maternity simulators have been used to teach students about maternal and child health. Undergraduate faculty from a large Midwest nursing program implemented a 6-hour laboratory and virtual clinical experience for students in the maternal–newborn health rotation that incorporated various simulations (Bantz, Dancer, Hodson-Carlton, & Van Hove, 2007). This experience consisted of eight stations, including assessment of the postpartum fundus, newborn assessment and care (with a SimBaby), newborn nutrition, labor, and birth (with the Noelle birthing simulation manikin), fetal heart rate assessment and interpretation, Leopold's maneuvers, and computerized charting. According to Bantz et al. (2007), the majority of students who participated in this clinical laboratory experience indicated that they felt better prepared to provide nursing care to newborns and their mothers in the clinical site.

DeBourgh and Prion (2010) used a quasiexperimental pretest and posttest study of 285 prelicensure students to teach students fall prevention and patient safety using clinical simulations with standardized patients. The results of the teaching and research conducted concluded that the simulation learning experience provided students with knowledge and skill gains they could apply to clinical practice.

Thompson and Bonnel (2008) integrated the use of high-fidelity simulation in an undergraduate pharmacology course to provide an applied learning experience where students could make connections between learned content and clinical application. An experience of safe medication administration has been added to both pharmacology course simulations and any simulation in which the "patient" is to receive medications.

Rosenzweig, Hravnak, and Magdic (2008) developed a patient communication simulation experience for the acute care nurse practitioner students at a major university to evaluate students' perceived confidence and communication effectiveness before, immediately after completion, and 4 months after completion. Results showed that the content and methods used for the simulation experience improved students' confidence and perceived skill in communication in difficult acute care situations.

As distance education course formats proliferate in nursing curricula, simulation has been recognized as a potentially rich learning strategy. Nelson and Blenkin (2007) used online role-play simulation to provide students with the opportunity to learn professional and personal relationships in an online environment. The online learning platform provided students with a learning opportunity to deal with difficult behavior and to manage violence, abuse, and patients with dementia. To initiate the learning activity, the authors built what was called a "kickstart" episode, in which students would have to react to a significant event, for example, a patient dying. Participating students logged in and played their assigned roles, which ranged from long-term care residents to facility staff members. During the computer-based event, students role-playing as health care professionals could enter into an "interaction space (ispace)" where a threaded discussion could occur about the patient's problem. Several resources were available to students within the online simulation environment, including instruction sheets and video clips to assist the students with the care of these selected patients. Students immersed themselves in the online simulations and believed that the level of realism paralleled clinical nursing practice and offered a relevant student learning experience.

Unfolding case simulations are gaining more attention in nursing programs. Durham and Sherwood (2008) used unfolding simulated cases to teach quality and safety concepts and how these concepts are integrated into nursing practice. In addition, Batscha and Moloney (2005) used online unfolding case studies to facilitate nursing students to analyze, organize, and prioritize in novel situations. Finally, Azzarello and Wood (2006) suggest that unfolding cases can be used to evaluate students' changing mental models because they offer a practical strategy for revealing flaws in students' problem solving that would otherwise not be obvious. Unfolding cases are not limited to the traditional simulation laboratory. Innovative use of unfolding cases has the potential to transform traditional teacher-centered classrooms into interactive, engaging learning environments that support the flipped classroom (Educause Learning Initiative, 2012). The notion of the unfolding cases fit very well when teaching in the connected and "flipped" classroom (see Chapter 19).

Evaluation Considerations when Using Simulations

Evaluation of the Design and Development Phase of Simulation

To evaluate the design and development of simulations created by nurse educators, Jeffries (2005) developed the Simulation Design Scale (SDS). The purpose of this tool is to provide the educator with information and feedback that can be used to improve the simulation design and implementation. The SDS is a 20-item tool that the learner completes after participating in a simulation to provide feedback on whether the intended simulation design features were present. These features include the objectives and information, support, problem solving, feedback and debriefing, and fidelity. These are referred to as *simulation design features* because they define what a quality simulation requires if it will have a positive effect on learning outcomes. Content validity of this instrument was determined by a panel of nine nurse experts. Cronbach's alpha was computed to assess internal consistency reliability for each scale. The coefficient alpha for the overall scale was 0.94. Table 18-3 briefly describes the SDS's five components.

TABLE 18-3 Simulation Design Scale Components

Concept and Design Features	Description of Concept
Information/objectives	Clear objectives and timeframe for the simulation is information needed by the student before the simulation begins.
Problem solving/complexity	The simulation needs to be designed with problem-solving components embedded in the written scenario or case. The level of problem solving needs to be considered; for example, use simple tasks and decisions if students are in a fundamentals course versus more complex tasks if students are in an upper-level course and are 6 months away from graduating.
Student support/cues	Student support in a simulation is offered before, during, and after. Support includes providing information and direction to the student before the simulation.
Fidelity	A simulation should be as close an approximation as possible to the real event or activity that is being modeled to promote better learning outcomes.
Guided reflection/debriefing	Guided reflection reinforces the positive aspects of the experience and encourages reflective learning, which allows the participant to link theory to practice and research, think critically, and discuss how to intervene professionally in very complex situations.

From Jeffries, P. R. (2007). *Simulations in nursing education: From conceptualization to evaluation.* New York: The National League for Nursing. (Used with permission.)

Evaluation of the Implementation Phase

When simulations are implemented, particular components need to be included to ensure good learning experience, student satisfaction, and good learner performance. According to Chickering and Gamson (1987, 1991), incorporating the Principles of Best Practice in Education assists educators to implement quality teaching activities and improve student learning. As a component of the simulation model (Jeffries, 2005), those educational practices are considered very important in the implementation of simulations in the students' learning environment. To measure this component, the Educational Practices in Simulation Scale (EPSS) was developed. The EPSS is a 16-item tool that the learner completes after a simulation. This tool measures whether the best practices in education, according to Chickering and Gamson (1987), are being used in the simulation. All seven educational practices in simulation are being evaluated; however, after conducting a factor analysis on the scale, four factors were identified and several of the factors were collapsed into these four components of the scale. Therefore the elements being evaluated in the EPSS are active learning, diverse ways of learning, high expectations, and collaboration, as shown in Table 18-4. The questionnaire was tested for validity and reliability. Content validity was established through a review by nine nursing experts. The coefficient alpha was 0.92.

Evaluation of Learning Outcomes

As discussed previously, learning outcomes can be measured through low-stakes and high-stakes simulations. Outcomes are defined for the learning activity and can be measured by a well-designed clinical simulation. Research in this area is growing as educators measure the outcomes of the simulation activity desiring to close the knowledge and skills gap within academe and practice. Some instruments available for evaluation include the Laseter Clinical Judgment Rubric (Laseter, 2007) and the Seattle University Evaluation Tool, and the Creighton Evaluation Instrument (Hayden, Keegan, Kardong-Edgren, & Smiley, 2014). Limited valid and reliable grading checklists for the evaluation of high-stakes simulation exist. Scoring checklists are an emerging area of research in simulation

TABLE 18-4 Educational Practices in Simulation Scale

Components of the EPSS	Description of Components within the Scale	Examples
Active learning	Through simulation, learners are directly engaged in the activity and obtain immediate feedback and reinforcement of learning. Learning activities can range from simple to complex.	A case scenario in which an intubated patient is restless, agitated, and coughing, affecting his oxygenation status. Students can be asked to select the most appropriate intervention and describe the rationale for the intervention.
Diverse styles of learning	Simulations should be designed to accommodate diverse learning styles and teaching methods and allow students and groups with varying cultural backgrounds to benefit from the experience.	Design a scenario that has visual, auditory, and kinesthetic components.
High expectations	High teacher expectations are important for the student during a learning experience because expecting the student to do well becomes a self-fulfilling prophecy.	Set up a scenario with multiple patient problems to challenge the learner and to advance learning and skill application to the next level.
Collaboration	Collaboration is pairing students in a simulation to work together. Roles are assigned so that students jointly work on the problem-solving and decision-making skills within the simulation together.	Assign a student the role of a primary nurse and a third-year medical student the role of a physician. Place the two students in a setting where they will be confronted with a patient having postoperative complications that requires quick assessments and efficient decision-making skills to intervene appropriately with the patient.

From Jeffries, P. R. (2007). *Simulations in nursing education: From conceptualization to evaluation.* New York: The National League for Nursing. (Used with permission.)

pedagogy that have been developed and tested for validity and reliability; an example is a checklist for use during perioperative emergency simulation training (McEvoy et al., 2014). Evaluation tools for clinical simulation training are evolving.

Summary

Educators use simulations to enhance learning outcomes and promote safe patient care environments. Nursing organizations, commissions of higher education, accrediting bodies, academic institutions, and schools of nursing are seeking answers to questions about simulation design and development, teaching and learning practices, implementation processes, and associated learning outcomes. Educators and researchers must join forces to develop more rigorous research studies testing simulation outcomes. National, multisite simulation studies by nurse educators are currently being conducted to enhance understanding of the educational usefulness of nursing simulations. For example, when simulations are used as a teaching–learning intervention, are learning outcomes improved? When developing a simulation, what are the important design features of a well-executed simulation in nursing education? How can simulations be used to prepare for or replace clinical experience? How does the use of simulations contribute to advancing nursing into the next generation? Educators need to make certain they are informed about the possibilities of simulations, their usefulness in enhancing student education, and the progress of educational research efforts conducted to develop and test new models of using simulation in nursing education.

REFLECTING ON THE EVIDENCE

1. What evidence is available on the effectiveness of using simulation in support of learning?
2. When using a simulation framework, how would you construct a research project to test the framework?
3. Identify three research questions that might be addressed when studying reflective observation.
4. What is the optimal balance of simulated versus actual clinical practice in nursing education?

REFERENCES

Adamson, K. A. (2014). Evaluation tools and metrics for simulations. In P. R. Jeffries (Ed.), *Clinical simulations in nursing education: Advanced concepts, trends, and opportunities* (pp. 145–164). Philadelphia: Wolters Kluwer. chapter 12.

Alden, K. R., & Durham, C. F. (2012). Integrating reflection in simulation: Structure, content, and processes. In G. Sherwood & S. Horton-Deutesch (Eds.), *Reflective practice: Transforming education and improving outcomes* (pp. 149–168). Indianapolis: Sigma Theta Tau International.

Alinier, G., Harwood, C., Harwood, P., et al. (2014). Immersive clinical simulation in undergraduate health care interprofessional education: Knowledge and perceptions. *Clinical Simulation in Nursing, 10*, e205–e216.

Anderson, J. M., & Warren, J. B. (2011). Using simulations to enhance the acquisition and retention of clinical skills in neonatology. *Seminars in Perinatology, 35*, 59–67. http://dx.doi.org/10.1053/j.semperi.2011.01.004.

Azzarello, J., & Wood, D. E. (2006). Assessing dynamic mental models: Unfolding case studies. *Nurse Educator, 31*(1), 10–14.

Bantz, D., Dancer, M., Hodson-Carlton, K., & Van Hove, S. (2007). A daylong clinical laboratories: From gaming to high fidelity. *Nurse Educator, 32*(6), 274–277.

Batscha, C., & Moloney, B. (2005). Using PowerPoint to enhance unfolding case studies. *Journal of Nursing Education, 44*(8), 387.

Boulet, J. R., & Swanson, D. B. (2004). Psychometric challenges of using simulations in high-stakes assessment. In W. F. Dunn (Ed.), *Simulation in critical care and beyond* (pp. 119–130). Des Plains, IL: Society of Critical Care Medicine.

Campbell, S., & Daley, K. (2008). *Simulation scenarios for nursing educators: Making it real.* New York: Springer.

Cant, R., & Cooper, S. (2014). Simulation in the Internet age: The place of web-based simulation in nursing education. An integrative review. *Nurse Education Today, 34*, 1435–1442.

Chambers, K., Boulet, J., & Gary, N. (2000). The management of patient encounter time in a high-stakes assessment using standardized patients. *Medical Education, 34*, 813–817.

Cheng, A., Eppich, W., Grant, V., Sherbino, J., Zendejas, B., & Cook, D. A. (2014). Debriefing for technology-enhanced simulation: A systematic review and meta analysis. *Medical Education, 48*(7), 657–666.

Chickering, A. W., & Gamson, Z. F. (1987). Seven principles for good practice in undergraduate education. *AAHE Bulletin, 39*(7), 3–7.

Chickering, A. W., & Gamson, Z. F. (1991). Applying the seven principles for good practice in undergraduate education. *New Directions for Teaching and Learning, 47.*

Cook, M. J. (2012). Design and initial evaluation of a virtual pediatric primary care clinical in Second Life. *Journal of the American Academy of Nurse Practitioner, 24*(9), 521–527.

DeBourgh, G. A., & Prion, S. (2010). Using simulation to teach prelicensure nursing students to minimize patient risk and harm. *Clinical Simulation in Nursing, 6*(1), e1–e210.

Diefenbeck, C. A., Plowfield, L. A., & Herrman, J. W. (2006). Clinical immersion: A residency model for nursing education. *Nursing Education Perspectives, 27*(2), 72–79.

Dismukes, R. K., Gaba, D. M., & Howard, S. K. (2006). So many roads: Facilitated debriefing in healthcare. *Simulation in Healthcare, 1*(1), 23–25.

Dreifuerst, K. (2009). The essential of debriefing in simulation learning: A concept analysis. *Nursing Education Perspectives, 30*(2), 109–114.

Dreifuerst, K. T. (2012). Using debriefing for meaningful learning to foster development of clinical reasoning in simulation. *Journal of Nursing Education, 51*(6), 321–333.

Dunn, W. F. (2004). *Simulators in critical care and beyond.* Des Plaines, IL: Society of Critical Care Medicine.

Durham, C., & Sherwood, G. (2008). Education to bridge the quality gap: A case study approach. *Urological Nursing, 28*(6), 431–438.

Educause Learning Initiative. (2012). *Seven things you should know about flipped classrooms.* Retrieved from, http://net.educause.Edu/ir/library/pdf/eli7081.pdf.

Engum, S., & Jeffries, P. R. (2003). Intravenous catheter training system: Computer-based education versus traditional learning methods. *The American Journal of Surgery, 186*(1), 67–74.

Farra, S., Miller, E., Timm, N., & Schafer, J. (2013). Improved training for disasters: Using 3-D virtual reality simulation. *Western Journal of Nursing Research, 35*(5), 655–671.

Guhde, J. (2011). Nursing students' perceptions of the effect on critical thinking, assessment, and learner satisfaction in simple versus complex high-fidelity simulation scenarios. *Journal of Nursing Education, 50*(2), 73–78.

Halstead, J. (2006). Evidence-based teaching and clinical simulation. *Journal of International Nursing Association of Clinical Simulation, 2*(1), 1–6.

Hamilton, C. A. (2010). The simulation imperative of end-of-life education. *Clinical Simulation in Nursing, 6*(4), e131–e138.

Hayden, J., Keegan, M., Kardong-Edgren, S., & Smiley, R. A. (2014, July–August). Reliability and validity testing of the Creighton Competency Evaluation Instrument for use in the NCSBN National Simulation Study. *Nursing Education Perspectives, 35*(4), 244–252.

Hayden, J., Smiley, R., Alexander, M. A., Kardong-Edgren, S., & Jeffries, P. (2014a). The NCSBN National Simulation Study: A longitudinal, randomized, controlled study replacing clinical hours with simulation in prelicensure nursing education. *Journal of Nursing Regulation, 5*(2), S3–S40.

International Nursing Association for Clinical Simulation and Learning (INACSL) Board of Directors. (2011). Standards of best practice: Simulation: Standard 1: Terminology. *Clinical Simulation in Nursing, 7*(Suppl), S3–S7. http://dx.doi.org/10.1016/j.ecns.2011.05.005.

Jeffries, P. R. (2005). A framework for designing, implementing, and evaluating simulations used as teaching strategies in nursing. *Nursing Education Perspectives, 26*(2), 96–103.

Jeffries, P. R. (2007). *Simulations in nursing education: From conceptualization to evaluation.* New York: The National League for Nursing.

Jeffries, P. (2012). *Simulation in nursing education: From conceptualization to evaluation* (2nd ed.). Philadelphia: Lippincott Williams and Wilkins.

Jeffries, P. R., Hovancsek, M. T., & Clochesy, J. M. (2005). Using clinical simulations in distance education. In J. M. Novotny & R. J. Davis (Eds.), *Distance education in nursing* (2nd ed.), (pp. 83–99). New York: Springer.

Jeffries, P. R., Woolf, S., & Linde, B. (2003). Technology-based vs. traditional: A comparison of two instructional methods to teach the skill of performing a 12-lead ECG. *Nursing Education Perspectives, 24*(2), 70–74.

Katz, G. B., Peifer, K. L., & Armstrong, G. (2010). Assessment of patient simulation use in selected baccalaureate nursing programs in the United States. *Simulation in Healthcare, 5*(1), 46–51.

Kolb, D. A. (1984). *Experiential learning.* Upper Saddle River, NJ: Prentice-Hall.

Laseter, K. (2007). Clinical judgment using simulations to create an assessment rubric. *Journal of Nursing Education, 46*(11), 496–503.

Lewin, K. (1951). *Field theory in social science.* New York: Harper & Row.

Lusk, J. M., & Fater, K. (2013). Postsimulation debriefing to maximize clinical judgment development. *Nurse Educator, 38,* 16–19. http://dx.doi.org/10.1097/NNE.ObO13e318276df8b.

MacDonald, M. B., Bally, J. M., Ferguson, L. M., Murray, B. L., Fowler-Kerry, S. E., & Anonson, J. M. S. (2010). Knowledge of the professional role of others: A key interprofessional competency. *Nurse Education in Practice, 10,* 238–242.

McEvoy, M. D., Hand, W. R., Furse, C. M., Field, L. C., Clark, C. A., Moitra, V. K., et al. (2014). Validity and reliability assessment of detailed scoring checklists for use during perioperative emergency simulation training. *Simulation in Healthcare, 5,* 295–303. http://dx.doi.org/10.1097/SIH.0000000000000048.

Meyer, M. N., Connors, H., Hou, Q., & Gajewski, B. (2011). The effect of simulation on clinical performance. *Simulation in Healthcare, 6*(5), 269–277. http://dx.doi.org/10.1097/SIH.Ob013e318223a048.

Miller, C. L., Leadingham, C., & Vance, R. (2010). Utilizing human patient simulators (HPS) to meet learning objectives across concurrent core nursing courses: A pilot study. *Journal of College Teaching & Learning, 7*(1), 37–43.

National League for Nursing. (2015). *Debriefing across the curriculum.* Retrieved from, http://www.nln.org/docs/default-source/about/nln-vision-series-%28position-statements%29/nln-vision-debriefing-across-the-curriculum.pdf?sfvrsn=0.

Nelson, D. L., & Blenkin, C. (2007). The power of online role-play simulations: Technology in nursing education. *International Journal of Nursing Education Scholarship, 4*(1), 1–12.

Newton, C., Bainbridge, L., Ball, V., et al. (2014). The Health Care Team Challenge™: Developing an international interprofessional education research collaboration. *Nurse Education Today, 1,* 1–5.

Overstreet, M. (2010). Ee-chats: The seven components of nursing debriefing. *The Journal of Continuing Education in Nursing, 41*(12), 538–539.

Page, J. B., Kowlowitz, V., & Alden, K. R. (2010). Development of a scripted unfolding case study focusing on delirium in older adults. *Journal of Continuing Education in Nursing, 41*(5), 225–230.

Reese, C., Jeffries, P. R., & Engum, S. (2010). Learning together: Using simulations to develop nursing and medical student collaboration. *Nursing Education Perspectives, 31*(1), 33–37.

Reising, D., & Hensel, D. (2014). Clinical simulations focused on patient safety. In P. Jeffries (Ed.), *Clinical simulations in nursing education: Advanced concepts, trends, and opportunities.* Philadelphia: Wolters Kluwer.

Richardson, H., Goldsant, L., Simmons, J., Gilmartin, M., & Jeffries, P. (2014). Increasing faculty capacity: Findings from an evaluation simulation clinical teaching. *Nursing Education Perspectives.* Retrieved from, http://dx.doi.org/10.5480/14-1384.

Rosenzweig, M., Hravnak, M., & Magdic, K. (2008). Patient communication simulation laboratory for students in an acute care nurse practitioner program. *American Journal of Critical Care, 17*, 364–372.

Ryan, C. A., Walshe, N., Gaffney, R., Shanks, A., Burgoyne, L., & Wiskin, C. M. (2010). Using standardized patients to assess communication skills in medical and nursing students. *BMC Medical Education, 10*(24), 1–8.

Schön, D. A. (1987). *Educating the reflective practitioner.* San Francisco: Jossey-Bass.

Seefeldt, T., Mort, J., Brockevelt, B., Giger, J., Jorde, B., Lawler, M., et al. (2012). A pilot study of interprofesssional case discussions for health professions students using the virtual world Second Life. *Currents in Pharmacy Teaching and Learning, 4*(4), 224–231.

Sewchuck, D. H. (2005). Experiential learning—A theoretical framework for perioperative education. *AORN Journal, 81*(6), 1311–1318.

Simon, R., Rudolph, J. W., & Raemer, D. B. (2009). *Debriefing assessment for simulation in healthcare—Rater version.* Cambridge, MA: Center for Medical Simulation.

Simulation Innovation Resource Center (SIRC). (n.d.) *Homepage.* Retrieved from sirc.nln.org.

Svinicki, M. D., & Dixon, N. M. (1987). The Kolb model modified for classroom activities. *College Teaching, 35*(4), 141–146.

Thomas, C., Hodson-Carlton, K., & Ryan, M. (2010). Preparing nursing students in a leadership/management course for the workplace through simulations. *Clinical Simulation in Nursing, 6*(1), e1–e6.

Thompson, T. L., & Bonnel, W. (2008). Integration of high-fidelity simulation in an undergraduate pharmacology course. *Journal of Nursing Education, 47*(11), 518–521.

Waznonis, A. (2014). Methods and evaluations for simulation debriefing in nursing education. *Journal of Nursing Education, 53*(8), 459–465.

Whei Ming, S., & Juestel, M. (2010). Direct teaching of thinking skills using clinical simulation. *Nurse Educator, 35*(5), 197–204.

Wilson, M., Shepherd, C., & Pitzner, K. J. (2005). Assessment of a low-fidelity human patient simulator for the acquisition of nursing skills. *Nurse Education Today, 25*(1), 56–67.

19 The Connected Classroom: Using Digital Technology to Promote Learning

Brent W. Thompson, PhD, RN

Nursing faculty continuously face the arrival of new technologies that affect their clinical practice and teaching. There are new tools for assessing and monitoring patients, delivering medication or fluids, charting medications, and documenting patient care. In addition, new health care practices, medications, treatments, and wearable technologies are announced in the press almost daily. Nursing organizations such as the National League for Nursing (NLN) and the American Association of Colleges of Nursing (AACN) have recognized these changes and have called for curricular reforms that will embrace the use of these technologies (Morris & Faulk, 2012; National League for Nursing [NLN], 2015).

Fortunately, faculty now have new digital learning technologies to help prepare students for these changes. When they are used as part of a "connected classroom," students engage with the faculty and each other, as well as with resources and clinical practice sites beyond the classroom. The connected classroom is both a physical and virtual space in which students and faculty use digital learning technologies to prepare for the current realities of a complex and increasingly global health care system. The connected classroom assumes more importance as health care services move from acute care settings to the community. Whereas nursing students have always learned in in-patient clinical agencies, they are now also likely to have clinical experiences in home care settings, assisted living facilities, K–12 schools, senior centers, and other community practice settings, maintaining connections becomes even more important as faculty and students access the resources they need to practice away from the traditional support systems available in hospitals. Thus it is in the connected classroom that faculty can orchestrate the use of digital learning technologies to provide meaningful learning experiences for their students.

For much of the history of higher education it was the role of the teacher to bring students into a classroom, shut the door, and deliver information. No phones, computers, or even talking in class were permitted. The role of each student was to pay attention to the instructor and receive wisdom. This approach has become inadequate as the amount and availability of knowledge increases, and one person is no longer the sole source of information. To practice nursing in constantly changing environments nurses must learn how to make connections to needed resources such as experts, patients, or documents. It is now the role of nursing faculty to facilitate these connections (National League for Nursing, 2015).

This chapter discusses the forces that have led to the emergence of the connected classroom, and then describes the digital technologies that are used to facilitate teaching and learning in this environment. The chapter offers specific suggestions for effective ways to use the technologies to engage students in interactive learning. The chapter concludes by encouraging faculty to embrace the use of technology as they prepare students for practice in a complex, patient-centered, consumer-oriented, and technology-rich health care environment.

Evolution of the Connected Classroom

The need for a connected classroom has been driven by social changes that are being enabled by digital technology. These include, among many, changes in health care information technology and consumer health, the increasing use of new pedagogies and evidence-based teaching practices, and changes in nursing education driven by technology savvy students and faculty (Abel, Brown, & Suess, 2013).

Changes in Health Care Information Technology

New technologies have spawned shifts in the delivery of health care. The way the health care teams communicate, retrieve information, and make clinical decisions has been radically changed in this century. Communication, once limited to a wired phone on a desk, now takes place with providers and patients using mobile devices via voice calls, text messaging, and e-mail. Finding the latest literature once required a trip to the library, and if the needed books or articles were not available, faculty waited for them to be mailed from another library. Today, nurses retrieve evidence-based literature delivered to a mobile device. Clinical decisions that previously relied on having personal experience or experts at hand now can be made by access to decision-making algorithms and direct contact with experts in remote locations.

Electronic health records (EHRs) have become ubiquitous as health care providers shift from paper documentation. EHRs provide more than readable and easily transmitted documentation. EHRs also give nurses tools to improve assessment by reminding nurses to obtain needed data. They can also be integrated with decision-making tools to prompt for nursing interventions. Additionally, some EHRs have integrated resources such as the hospital formulary and procedure manuals.

Patients have become much more engaged in their health care, and health care is becoming more personalized, in large part because of the availability of health care technology and consumer applications. Nurses will become increasingly involved in using mobile technology for assessing patients and helping them manage their own health.

These shifts create three issues for nursing faculty. First, traditional ways of teaching are not sufficient for students to learn how to establish nurse–patient, nurse–primary provider, and nurse–nurse relationships using the newest health care technology. Second, nursing faculty must learn how to teach the use of these tools. Third, students must learn how to practice nursing with the new tools in both classroom and clinical experiences.

Pedagogical Shifts

How faculty teach has been influenced by changes in higher education, emerging evidence from nursing education research, and the increasing availability of learning technology. Two shifts have significance for nurse educators: the shift from teaching to learning and the use of the flipped classroom.

From Teaching to Learning

One of the most prevalent shifts in higher education is the move from the lecturer at the front of the room while students listen, known as "the sage on the stage," to the instructor who interacts with students to facilitate learning, or "the guide on the side." In recent years technological advancements have provided faculty new tools to engage in interactive pedagogy such as electronic case histories and concept maps (Shellenbarger & Robb, 2014), and have enabled faculty to shift their role to a guide, coach, and facilitator of learning. (See Chapter 15 for other strategies to promote engaged learning.)

The Flipped Classroom

Recent interest in the use of the "flipped classroom" is another example of a pedagogical shift. The flipped classroom is based on the idea that active learning is superior to passive learning. It is called *flipped* because the traditional method of a lecture presented to a passive group followed with homework to practice and apply learning is reversed (Hawks, 2014). In the flipped classroom the preparatory information for the class such as a lecture, reading materials, case studies, and quizzes are made available ahead of class time. Students are to come to class prepared to engage in learning through activities that practice application of the course material and to receive feedback about their progress in attaining learning outcomes set for the particular class (Hamdan, N., McKnight, P., McKnight, K., & Arfstrom, K. M. 2013).

For a flipped classroom to work, students must prepare diligently for class, and faculty must have support to learn to use technologic tools for recording lectures and implementing classroom activities (Schlairet, Green, & Benton, 2014; Silverthorn, 2006). Prior to attending class in the flipped classroom, students must understand and comprehend basic course materials and be prepared to clarify concepts and connect them to clinical practice during the class. Faculty use a variety of digital learning activities such as online case studies, virtual excursions, wikis, and blogs to engage students and ensure that students are able to reach higher levels of learning domains such as application, synthesization, and creation.

An effective flipped classroom requires a change in the culture of learning to a more student-centered approach, and that content must be intentionally chosen for what needs to be presented by the teacher (Hamdan, McKnight, McKnight, & Arfstrom, 2013). The role of the faculty is to develop the learning activities, pose clinical challenges, and guide and facilitate learning. During each class session faculty also must assess learning to be certain students have attained higher order learning outcomes. The role of the student is to assume responsibility for completing preclass preparatory assignments and assessments, and be an active participant in the class.

Access to digital technology and expertise in its use is essential in the flipped classroom. Students use digital devices to access information, use online learning activities, collaborate, work in teams, contact experts, and assess their learning and monitor their progress throughout the course. Prior to the class, faculty use digital technology to develop videocasts, podcasts, and narrated presentation slides to present course concepts (Bull, 2013). During class faculty and students use wikis, blogs, presentation software, and video clips to activate learning. Learning "analytics" such as testing software, audience response systems (ARSs) that record individual students' responses to questions, and learning management systems (LMS), as well as newer (and more expensive) software that can track student learning are integral to the flipped classroom because this software can make it possible for faculty to identify which students need assistance, track student progress, and modify learning activities during class. Students, too, can use these tools to track their progress and grades as the course unfolds.

Research on the flipped classroom indicates that it takes a great deal of preparation and technology support to create a flipped classroom (Schlairet et al., 2014; Schwartz, 2014). In one small study of nurse practitioner students in a flipped classroom, the faculty found that most students found readings and answering questions prior to class was worthwhile, and 50% of the students found listening to the prerecorded lectures were worthwhile, but not all students were totally satisfied with every aspect of flipping the classroom (Critz & Knight, 2013). In another study, Missildine, Fountain, Summers, and Gosselin (2013) compared three approaches to learning: lecture only, lecture capture with back up, and the flipped classroom with innovative learning activities during class. Results indicated that exam results were higher for students in the flipped classroom, but that students in the flipped classroom were less satisfied with this method when compared to the other approaches. A flipped classroom also can be an efficient way to provide instruction in professional development settings as students can learn at their own pace (McDonald & Smith, 2013).

Changes in Nursing Education: Students and Faculty

One of the biggest changes in nursing education is the student's experience with digital learning. Most nursing students have grown up in a digital world and are accustomed to instantaneous access to entertainment and information. They also expect immediate feedback. The new generation of students has been called *digital natives* because of their familiarity with technology (Watson & Pecchioni, 2011). Students may be more comfortable than faculty with technology. In the United States the average faculty member is older than 51 (American Association of Colleges of Nursing, 2014). Despite these generational differences, it is important for nursing faculty not to confuse technological familiarity with expertise or wisdom about how to use technology.

Another change is that students are coming to class with their own technology. The 2013 Educause survey of more than 113,000 undergraduates found that nearly every student owned a laptop, smartphone, tablet, or e-book device (Dahlstrom, Walker, & Dziuban, 2013). Most owned more than one device capable of accessing the Internet, with more than one-third owning four or more devices. Yet, although most students own these devices, fewer than 25% were required to use them in the classroom, and in many cases were banned from using the devices during class. Students are coming to class with the newest tools, but too often they have faculty who are not helping them learn to use those tools (Wilkinson, Roberts, & While, 2013).

Many curricula are adding requirements for computer literacy, information literacy, and nursing informatics. The literature shows that while faculty recognize the importance of these topics, integration into the curriculum has been slow (Button, Harrington, & Belan, 2013). Additionally, students often feel inadequately prepared for the use of technology.

Changes in nursing education require a change in the role of the faculty (National Council of State Boards of Nursing, 2011). To create a connected classroom, faculty must learn to use familiar tools in new ways, as well as to learn to integrate new tools. This can be a daunting task for faculty unfamiliar or uncomfortable with technology. It is important not to use technology for technology's sake but to achieve objectives that would be difficult to achieve without technology.

To gain experience with technology, faculty can use multiple sources. Faculty can find colleagues that have expertise with the proposed use of technology, read technology columns in nursing education journals, or attend technology conferences. Many faculty have access to technology support at their school of nursing and can access libraries that have developed extensive search tools for finding evidence-based literature.

The Connected Classroom

The connected classroom uses digital technology to connect students, faculty, experts, patients, and virtual clinical experiences to facilitate learning. The key to the connected classroom is interactivity. The connected classroom improves student engagement, increases the amount of feedback for learning, provides opportunities for application of course concepts to clinical experiences, and gives both students and faculty immediate access to information resources. If students are to learn to connect with others, they have to practice those connections. Skiba (2014a; Skiba 2014b) notes that connections are now possible via technology, among people, resources, data, and ideas. Students with mobile technology know how to connect with the world via the Internet, but at the same time, the 2013 Educause Center for Analysis and Research (ECAR) study of undergraduate use of technology (Dahlstrom et al., 2013) found that students like technology but want guidance in its use.

Establishing the Connected Classroom

Establishing the connected classroom involves not only the technological aspects of the physical setting of the classroom and connecting the classroom to the Internet, but also requires faculty and students to learn how to use interactive methods in productive ways that will enhance learning. Teaching in a connected classroom also must respect privacy of students, patients, and health care information; computer use policies must be in place to communicate these guidelines.

Creating the Learning Space for a Connected Classroom

The first consideration for creating a connected classroom is to create a learning space that encourages connections among students and the teacher. Unlike traditional classrooms with a podium for the teacher at the front of the classroom, and chairs set in rows for the students, the connected classroom is designed with movable chairs and tables for students to work in teams or alone as needed, and for the faculty to move among the students to guide learning. Although there may be wall-mounted screens, smartboards, and writing surfaces, visual displays also must be distributed around the room and be accessible by students as well as the faculty. At the same time, the classroom must be arranged to facilitate use for teleconferences, telehealth, and point-to-point conferences.

Connecting to the Internet

A key technology of the connected classroom is the availability of Wi-Fi for wireless connections to the Internet. Students and faculty need Internet access to locate literature, news, and resources. The Internet is also needed for software downloads and updates. When teaching in any classroom, faculty should first determine what access to the Internet is available and how to make the connection to the Internet using either a wired or wireless network. A wired classroom has an Ethernet connection to the local network. A 10-foot Ethernet cable can often connect a laptop to the Internet when the wireless network will not connect. If the Internet connection is wireless, faculty also need to know the name of the wireless network and the password for entry. Because students will be using the wireless network, faculty must also determine the availability of simultaneous wireless connections and how many connections are permitted. If the number is less than the number of students who will be connecting, it will be necessary to change assignments or have students work in groups.

Ensuring Technology Support

Technology support is needed for both faculty and students when technology is used in the classroom and by students when studying elsewhere on campus or at a distance (Gonen, Sharon, Offir, & Lev-Ari, 2014). Support is also needed when faculty choose software and hardware that will be used by students in or out of the classroom. Most faculty would rather concentrate on teaching than on providing technical support; planning to obtain this support is essential.

When selecting or recommending hardware, faculty should determine what user support is needed and what support the manufacturer can offer. Apple, for example, has its Genius Bars in their stores and has support available for a fee after the initial warranty period. When selecting software, particularly the reference text managers, faculty will likely need support as they assist students to install the software on their devices. Faculty should ask the vendor about their hours, length of the support term, frequency and cost of updates, and fees for support. Some software vendors provide in-class training for students and faculty.

Faculty should also check with their institution for the availability of mobile computing support. Now that most students are arriving on campus with these devices, it may be easier to find support from the school's information technology services. Some institutions require devices to be registered before being permitted wireless access, while others only require knowledge of the name of the wireless network and a user-created password. It is also advisable for faculty to know how to access support for classroom technologies before using the hardware and software in the classroom. Prior to use, faculty should practice connecting projectors, using sound amplification of computer presentations or videos, using a microphone, raising or lowering a screen, controlling the room lights, and any other technologies such as smartboards or ARSs.

Developing and Using Electronic Device Use Policies

It is important for nursing programs to have clear policies on the use of electronic devices in classroom and clinical experiences. Smartphones and tablets are useful tools but they can violate patient's and classmate's rights if used inappropriately.

In clinical settings, the cameras, microphones, and telephones in digital devices could easily violate patients' rights to privacy. Health Insurance Portability and Accountability Act rules require that no user-identifiable data leave a facility or be seen by unauthorized personnel (Thompson, 2005). The American Nurses Association (ANA) (2015) has developed guidelines for using social media that indicate that nurses must not transmit identifiable patient information, should maintain ethical nurse–patient boundaries, should keep personal and professional communication separate, and be aware that postings on social media may be viewed by employers (American Association of Colleges of Nursing, 2014).

Cleanliness of the mobile device is another concern that should be considered in policy decisions. Studies have shown that mobile devices can carry pathogens and that many health care workers are not aware that their devices are potential vectors for cross-contamination (Ustan & Cihangiroglu, 2012). Possible policy requirements include not permitting devices in isolation rooms and specifying how and when to clean a device.

Similar guidelines should be in place in the classroom. An electronic usage policy should be clearly documented and discussed before students enter areas where violations could occur. These policies should be broad enough to cover present and future technologies, have clear statements of expectation, and outline violation consequences. In the classroom there may be times faculty do not want students to have access to resource materials such as during an exam, and policies should include aspects of academic honesty.

Faculty must establish an electronic device use policy if students will be using devices in clinical or classroom settings (Box 19-1). For the clinical setting, the policy should indicate that photographs of patients or patient-identifiable information may not be stored or transmitted beyond the clinical setting. Students should be aware that clinical agency policy may override school policy. Voice calls, texts, and use of social media also should be restricted while in the clinical setting in accordance with clinical agency policies. Usage policies should also outline the judicial process for violations. Classroom electronic device policies are generally tailored to prevent disruptions and academic integrity violations.

BOX 19-1 Sample Electronic Device Policy on Use of Electronic Devices

Students are not permitted to make phone calls, send text messages or e-mails, or engage in nonclass-related Internet activity while in the clinical or classroom setting without the permission of the instructor. Taking photographs of patients is not permitted at any time. No patient-identifiable information is to be stored on the device or removed from the clinical agency. Clinical agencies or instructors may apply additional restrictions or rules. Violations of this policy will be considered a violation of Standards of Safe Clinical Practice.

From West Chester University of Pennsylvania, Department of Nursing BSN Handbook 2014–2015.

Digital Technology to Promote Learning in the Connected Classroom

There are a variety of digital learning technologies available for use in the connected classroom. These include mobile devices such as computers, smartphones, and tablets as well as presentation software, ARSs, e-books, podcasts, and wikis. When considering the use of any of these technologies, faculty must consider the intention for its use. Technologies work best when they are used with purpose and not just for novelty.

Mobile Devices

Mobile devices include laptop computers, smartphones, and tablets. The common feature of these devices is they can connect to the Internet and offer the ability to add third-party software applications. The advent of computers that are easily portable gives students direct connections to resources, the faculty, and their classmates, and also provide students an opportunity to learn to use these tools as they will use them in nursing practice.

A smartphone is a mobile computer with telephone capability. Key features are a 4- to 5-inch diagonal touch screen and connection to the Internet. Some phones now have screens larger than 5 inches that approach the size of tablets. These large phones have been given the nickname "phablets" as a portmanteau of the words *phone* and *tablet.* Most smartphones also include a web browser, a camera, and GPS capability. Another key difference from desktop or laptop computers is the dependence on wireless communication. Smartphones use Wi-Fi or cellular phone data services to connect to the Internet. They also have Bluetooth capability to communicate with nearby devices such as printers, keyboards, or even health assessment tools such as a Bluetooth-enabled blood pressure cuff. The reason smartphones are considered computers is that individual programs called applications ("apps") can be loaded and run by the user. In the same way as using a desktop computer, users can add and subtract applications ("apps"). Management of these functions requires an operating system. The operating system for nearly all smartphones is either Apple's iOS or Google's Android, with a small percentage using Windows Phone OS. Most commercial health care and nursing education software is sold with iOS and Android versions but not Windows Phone OS.

Tablet computers became more popular with the advent of Apple's iPad. Tablets share the portability of a smartphone but with a larger screen. They have computing power closer to a laptop but without the physical keyboard. All tablets come with Wi-Fi receivers for Internet connections. Some tablets are available with cellular data receivers that allow access to the Internet wherever there is cellular phone service, but these services require a monthly fee. Most tablets use either the Apple iOS or a variant of the Google Android operating system. Applications are often rewritten from smartphone apps to make best use of the larger screen. The larger screen means the display of electronic books and documents are easier to read than on a smartphone, and more closely resemble the experience of reading a paper book.

Requiring Student Use of Mobile Devices

Some nursing programs require students to own a smartphone or tablet computer. The process for deciding to require the use of a mobile device is not unlike choosing a required or optional textbook. Faculty will need to evaluate what is available, the cost for hardware and software, how the device will be used in the connected classroom and clinical experience, and how support issues will be handled (Doyle, Garrett, & Currie, 2014). Because many students have already purchased a mobile computing device, choosing one particular brand could be a problem for students who have already invested in a competing brand. Fortunately, most reference titles are available in both Apple iOS and Google Android formats.

There are several issues to consider when instituting a mobile device requirement for students. These can include cost, faculty and student lack of familiarity with the technology and its capabilities, or an unwillingness to change teaching and learning methods. These issues need to be addressed before adopting a requirement for use of mobile devices. Cost for students has become less of an issue as nearly all students now own a mobile device of some type. However, cost can be an issue if faculty are expected to use these devices themselves, and it will be necessary to plan how faculty will obtain and use these devices; a consultant or campus technology expert may be helpful during the planning process. When deciding to require the use of digital devices, faculty must consider how to provide training for faculty and students when they are first used (George, Davidson, Serapiglia, Barla, & Thotakura, (2010); Swan et al., 2013). Swan and colleagues (2013) found that students particularly liked using tablets for note taking and managing course calendars, but found that reading textbooks on the device was fatiguing. Overall, students were satisfied with tablets as a supplemental tool for their learning.

Nursing Software for Mobile Devices

There is increasing availability of software for nurses and nursing students. When considering purchase of software, faculty should be aware that smartphones and tablets have no optical disk drives; therefore all software must be installed wirelessly. Applications for the Apple iOS family of devices can be managed through iTunes on the device or on a desktop computer. Android software can be purchased through the Google Play store and other online stores such as Amazon. Many applications are free or very low cost. Some apps are free but require in-app purchase of features. Most of the reference titles are purchased via a free "bookshelf" app that manages the purchase and installation of textbooks. Apps such as the Skyscape Reader or Unbound Medicine's Nursing Central may provide free references and tools, and are available for the Apple iOS and Android operating systems. The electronic versions of the reference books are then purchased separately. Some companies, such as Pepid, also sell bundled or integrated apps that include multiple titles that are purchased through subscription.

Reference Software

Reference textbooks have always been available in print form, but electronic versions are not only more portable but can also change the way nursing care is practiced. Electronic references include drug information, laboratory test norms, medical terminology dictionaries, and guides to nursing diagnoses. Students with mobile versions of these references can put in their pocket material that previously filled a bookshelf. The cost of these references is equivalent to the print version in most cases. One important difference is that, unlike paper textbooks, electronic versions of references cannot be sold or transferred to another user. Most of these titles are sold on a subscription basis. Students buy access to updates for a period of time ranging from months to years. Faculty should check with the software provider if the application is still usable after the subscription period ends. For some titles such as drug guides, it is important that students have current subscriptions so they are up-to-date with the latest drug information. Additionally, most of these subscriptions include web-based access to the data for use on laptops or tablets via a web browser.

Mobile computers can easily hold a wide variety of other reference texts. Medical dictionaries, diagnostic and laboratory test guides, and nursing practice guides are all available for mobile digital devices. Nursing practice guides include references on nursing diagnoses, care planning, and physical assessment. These texts, like the drug guides, can be updated by the publisher. Updates require a subscription of a length that can vary from months to years. Most titles can still be used on a mobile device after the subscription ends but they will no longer be updated. Some titles will be appropriate for use after graduation and the student may wish to continue the subscription.

Drug Guides

Publishers of the major print drug guides now produce electronic versions for mobile computers that have identical information as the print guide, but offer several advantages. Finding drug information is far faster because the guide can be searched by trade or generic name by just typing a few letters in the search box. Paper guides are usually organized by generic name or by type of drug; this requires the user to search through an index just to find the drug information. Electronic versions are also updated frequently. Instead of waiting for a new addition or a printed supplement, the electronic guides can be updated daily via the Internet. Information on new drugs, black box warnings, or banned drugs is then immediately available. Some guides come with additional features such as a pill finder that displays the image of actual pills. "Pill finder guides" help students learn what the pill should look like before administering it, and can be used with patients in home care settings who may be unsure of the identity of their pills. Additional features such as drug dosage calculators and drug interaction checkers are also included in some guides.

Several free drug guides are available for nurses. These guides are regularly updated and have many useful tools built in, but they usually do not contain the drug administration information and nursing considerations contained in the subscriptions. Faculty should select an electronic health guide using the same criteria for content in the same manner as evaluating a paper guide, but also should assess the intuitiveness of the interface by practicing with familiar drug names and then evaluate how easy it is find the needed information.

Health-related Applications

Many applications are specifically designed for health care professionals. These include clinical calculators, assessment tools, specialized reference tools, and health care education apps. Other applications such as electrocardiographic monitoring, blood testing, glaucoma screening, and health assessment tools are now available or in development (Doswell et al., 2013). Clinical calculators are used for determining a child's growth percentile, the insulin needs for a patient with diabetes, or converting units of measurement. Assessment tools can speed assessment of patients using validated tools such as a pain scale, neurologic assessment, or behavior assessment. By asking the user a series of questions about the patient the tool can quickly calculate a score.

Health care applications can be obtained through the Apple iTunes app on iOS devices or with the Google Play app for Android devices and their cost is nominal. Faculty can direct students to specific applications with a link that can be used like a URL link to a web page. Students may also find applications that are useful for the needs of their particular patients.

Selection of an app for student use requires several steps. First, faculty (and students) should download and try several similar apps and evaluate their quality, ease of use, and applicability to the classroom or clinical experience (Skiba, 2014c). Faculty then must verify that the data used in the application is referenced to recent research or peer-reviewed content. The decision for purchase must be based on cost, including licensing or subscription fees, and the benefit that students will derive from its use.

Using Mobile Devices in the Connected Classroom

Having mobile devices in the classroom changes the teaching and learning environment. The devices require an investment in learning their use by faculty and students. If faculty make this investment, then mobile devices need to be used with intention to teach in a way that shifts from presenting content, to using it. Using mobile computers in the classroom provides an opportunity for students to apply the course content as they would in a real-world setting. Using learning experiences that require students to use mobile devices in class assists students learn how to find information they need, how to interpret that information, and how to apply that information to nursing practice. As the use of wearable computers approaches, it may be even more important to move to connected classroom experiences that provide practice in using these tools.

The classroom is the best place for students to learn how to use mobile resources for their own learning as well as for providing patient care. Faculty can create situations for students either individually or in small groups that require the use of their resources to plan care for a hypothetical patient. See Box 19-2 for suggestions for incorporating mobile devices into classroom instruction.

Presentation Software

Presentation software such as Microsoft PowerPoint or Apple Keynote has become commonplace in nursing classrooms. Although often considered to be a low-impact teaching strategy, when used appropriately presentation software can in fact facilitate higher order learning. Before using presentation software it is important to consider the learning outcome and the best use of the software. Will the "slides" be used to provide a script for the faculty? Will they be used to assist student learning of new concepts? Will they be used to facilitate or

BOX 19-2 Using Mobile Devices in the Connected Classroom

1. When learning pharmacology, have students use a drug guide to explain why a particular drug would be prescribed. Have students explain the benefits, risks, and administration considerations.
2. Create a vocabulary quiz in which students find the meaning of a word using their mobile dictionary.
3. Present a short case study and have students use their resources to develop the needed assessments, nursing diagnoses, and interventions.
4. Present laboratory findings for a case study. Have students use their mobile laboratory value guide to evaluate the meaning of the values and develop needed nursing care.
5. When discussing a nursing procedure, have students search the literature for evidence-based practice research on that procedure. Ask students to compare the literature with what is seen at their clinical agencies.
6. Give students real-life imperial to metric conversions. For example, present a patient case with their weight in pounds, then have students convert the weight to kilograms. Students can then apply the weight to a mg/kg drug-dosing calculation.
7. Present case assessments that are aided by the use of clinical calculators for findings such as body mass index, Glasgow coma scale, pregnancy due dates, and so on.

organize note taking? Will they be shared with students before class to aid their preparation? Are they being used to facilitate learning for students who have learning style preferences for visual learning? Will they be used to guide student interaction?

Developing and using effective presentations requires careful planning. Common errors include too much text per slide, too many slides for the length of the presentation, and color or font choices that decrease legibility.

Think visually and include images that will help students who are visual learners by keeping them focused on key concepts. Develop a "story" that has a beginning, middle, and end; builds on previous learning; and leaves students with a lasting memory of the information presented in the experience.

Not all slides need a header title followed by bullet points. If the intention of the slides is to organize the presentation, try creating slides that only have one word or an image on them; less is more. A single word or image shows students the focus of the current point of the class and prevents faculty from just reading the slides like a script. Material that requires more text than can be properly shown on a slide should be given to the student in printed form as a supplemental guide. Avoid slide "bloat," which occurs when faculty have too many slides and then must race through text-dense slides in an effort to "cover the material."

Keep in mind the learning objectives for the class. Consider what can realistically be learned in the given time. Generally, only a few objectives can be truly learned in a 1-hour class. Presentation slides need to be carefully designed to help students learn those concepts.

Rehearse presentations to be certain they can be completed within the allotted time. It is best to finish under the allotted time to leave time for questions and clarifications during the actual class. Ideally, the rehearsal should be in the room where the presentation will be done, with the same lighting and projection. Faculty can then determine the clarity of slides, the color contrasts, text clarity, and look for words that could be removed or reduced to short phrases.

Avoid using premade templates. Choose contrasting background and text colors that are legible in the lighting conditions where the class is to be held. Use contrasts such as a dark blue background with yellow text. This combination may not be ideal in a brightly lit classroom. A white background with dark black or primary color text is often more legible in a room where the lights are on for students to take notes and interact. Slides with a dark background should have text colors of a good contrast such as white or yellow.

Presentation slides can include images, videos, graphs, and interactive responses. Faculty can find images and video clips using filters on search engines. YouTube also has many videos that are of direct interest to nursing (May, Wedgeworth, & Bigham, 2013). Videos demonstrating assessment techniques, equipment operation, and therapeutic communication, for example, can be embedded into a presentation slide. Fair use rules of U.S. copyright law allow images and short videos to be used in face-to-face instruction, or online if through a course management system that emulates a face-to-face classroom.

Interactive responses can be combined with presentation software to engage the learners. Some ARSs offer software that can embed questions into a presentation or display questions as a separate application. Interactive questioning of material can help students test their knowledge. Additionally, periodic interactive questioning keeps students engaged because they have to think about the concepts and answer the teacher's questions. Embedded questions similar to those that will be used for classroom tests or licensing or certification exams can be used to prepare students to develop critical thinking and clinical decision-making skills and generate discussion. Embedded questioning moves the class from a show to be watched by a passive audience to a participatory discussion.

Hyperlinks, or URLs, to a web page or video can also be embedded into a slide. If students are also expected to connect to the hyperlink, then be sure to provide the URL as a link in the LMS or embed it into a document that can be clicked to connect.

Additional information about developing presentations and using presentation software is presented in Box 19-3.

Audience Response Systems

ARSs, often called *student response systems,* or *classroom response systems,* or *clickers* in reference to the old nickname for remote controls, have a radio-frequency receiver connected to the presenter's computer USB port. Each member of the audience has a radio transmitter that has an individual identifier. When faculty ask a question, each audience member can press his or her answer on the remote system. The receiver gathers the responses, passes them on to the preinstalled software on the presenter's computer, and the results are then displayed.

ARSs can be used to poll for opinions, pose multiple-choice questions, administer a graded quiz, or take attendance. ARSs have been shown to increase student engagement (Klein & Kientz, 2013; Revell & McCurry, 2010). Other studies have shown high student satisfaction (Berry, 2009; Lee & Dapremont, 2012; Russell, McWilliams, Chasen, & Farley, 2011). Additionally, not linking answers to individual students may reduce anxiety about selecting a "wrong" answer to an instructor's question. An anonymous ARS eliminates the need for students to raise their hand and possibly give a wrong answer. Once students respond, the ARS software can show the class how other students answered without embarrassing any student. On the other hand, linking the ARS response to a grade increases the stakes for a student, which also increases engagement.

BOX 19-3 Developing and Using Presentation Software

DEVELOPING THE PRESENTATION

- Avoid using commercial templates. Simple is better; a plain background is best.
- Use large fonts (24 point or larger) of a sans-serif font such as Arial, Helvetica, or Calibri.
- Label each screen to keep students prompted about the current topic.
- Limit punctuation (e.g., periods at end of lines).
- Avoid use of all capital letters; they are difficult to read.
- Use dark text on a light background; it is easier to see in a classroom with lights on.
- Use pictures to illustrate concepts rather than words wherever possible.
- Avoid using "clip art": it has become cliché and is rarely helpful.
- Video and audio clips are helpful. Avoid unnecessary sound effects.
- Avoid unnecessary animations or transitions unless needed.
- Fewer words and larger text will have an effect on learning. Slides are prompts and organizers, not scripts.
- Use charts to present data but keep them simple and illustrative of a major point or concept.
- Distribute the slides ahead of time by creating a handout of three to six slides per page and saving in PDF format. Students will be able to take notes and not need presentation software to view.

REHEARSING THE PRESENTATION BEFORE CLASS

- Position the screen in the middle of the classroom and the podium to the right of the screen. Arrange seats so all students can view the screen. Test readability by standing in the back of the room with the lights on as they would be in the class.
- Obtain and test the needed passcodes for Wi-Fi access.
- Test Internet links to web pages.
- If using linked video or audio clips, test the sound system and set at an appropriate volume.
- Check spelling and grammar. Use the built-in checkers.
- Time the presentation, but realize that the actual class can take more time if there are questions.

Another method of collecting anonymous responses is available through text messaging. Messaging services software is available for free or low cost that provides a number for students to text their responses. The group's answers are then displayed in a web page that can be projected for the class. A big advantage of this method is that most students have a messaging phone, and thus do not need to buy a separate transmitter. Another advantage of this method is that students can respond by typing their response as words. Their responses can then create a "word cloud" graphic of responses showing the frequency of submitted words with relative sizes. A disadvantage of this method is that it can be more cumbersome to enter long numeric strings required for responses with this method.

Obtaining student responses can also be accomplished without electronic technology. A low-cost method to gather audience responses is to create paper responses with colors or numbers that students hold up with their answers to a teacher's question. The teacher then counts the number of each response and reports the results to the class. This method only works for simple multiple choice or true–false questions, but has the advantage of having students respond before seeing how others answered. It also quickly lets the instructor see who has or has not responded and where additional teaching might be needed. This low-tech method can be effective and requires no electricity, transmitters, or Internet connection. See Box 19-4 for suggestions on using ARSs.

BOX 19-4 Using Audience Response Systems

- Be sure all faculty know how to incorporate audience response systems (ARS) questions into lectures. Encourage faculty to practice before using in a live classroom.
- If students must purchase an ARS transmitter, they expect it to be used regularly. Make it part of most classes.
- If ARS transmitters are required, establish consequences for failure to bring it to class.
- Show questions at regular intervals to keep students engaged.
- Improve student reasoning skills by asking students to explain their answer before revealing the classroom tally.
- Vary the timing of asking questions. Questions do not have to be done at the end of every lesson concept. Showing questions later in the class or even another day helps students test their retention of knowledge.
- Provide sample exam questions. These help students learn how to approach questions and learn how to reason when taking the actual exam.

e-books

Applications such as Amazon's Kindle app, Apple's iBooks, and Barnes & Noble's Nook bring electronic books to tablets (and to smartphones, although they are harder to read on the smaller screen). Several publishers of nursing textbooks have begun to offer their printed textbooks in electronic form. When requiring the purchase of electronic books, faculty should be aware that reading books on a tablet requires more battery power than dedicated e-book readers such as the Kindle or Nook.

Books can be purchased directly on the tablet and immediately downloaded. Documents in the .pdf or .doc format can also be displayed without additional software. Faculty can create documents and distribute them to students via an LMS or sent by e-mail to each student.

E-books offer many advantages and disadvantages over traditional paper textbooks (Abell & Garrett-Wright, 2014). Electronic books can be read on a dedicated device that is similar to a tablet computer but has limited functions beyond displaying text. Dedicated devices are called *e-book readers.* Examples include the Amazon Kindle, Barnes & Noble Nook, or Sony Reader. The biggest advantages of an e-book reader over a multifunction tablet computer are low power consumption, highly legible screens, lighter weight, and lower cost.

A fully charged e-book reader can be used for weeks between charges compared with hours for a tablet computer. This is because e-books use an e-ink display that is a black and white, non-glare, paperlike display. It can be more pleasant reading from an e-ink display because there is no glare from a shiny screen or white light used to light up a tablet computer. This also means that photos are rendered in pixelated shades of gray. The reduced power consumption is also a function of much slower computer processors. An e-book reader does not need the graphics capabilities and processing power of a tablet, which saves battery life. This simpler technology means that e-book readers sell for anywhere from \$50 to \$600 less than a tablet computer. For the highly cost-sensitive instructor or student, this low cost makes e-books attractive, but there are tradeoffs over using a tablet computer.

The benefits of e-books can also be a hindrance to use in education (Glackin, Rodenhiser, & Herzog, 2014). The limited screen display and slow processor severely limits graphics capability. E-books with an e-ink display cannot display a color photograph or diagram, nor display any kind of video. Most e-book devices have a small screen that can make navigating a large textbook cumbersome, particularly when combined with the slower processor and limited navigation features of e-book devices.

The limitations of e-book devices make them less desirable for nursing education. There may be settings in the community where the light weight and long battery life may be beneficial, but generally nursing educators will find more versatility with mobile computers such as smartphones and tablets. Faculty should continue to monitor the e-book device market for improvements in the technology. Larger screens, color, and faster processors may create a viable alternative to the paper version of a textbook.

Podcasts

Podcasts are compressed audio files distributed via the Internet. The term is a portmanteau of "Pod" from *iPod* and "cast" from *broadcast.* Podcasting makes it easy to distribute audio files such as lectures or panel discussions to students. As a compressed file (usually in the mp3 format), an audio file can be quickly transmitted and takes up little space even for recordings several hours in length. In contrast, music files on a CD would use hundreds of times more drive space to store on a computer or smartphone. Students can listen to podcasts on their computers, smartphones, or tablets.

Faculty can use podcasts to either prepare students in advance of class or to replace classroom lectures or discussion, which is part of the flipped classroom strategy discussed earlier (Greenfield, 2011; Johnston, Massa, & Burne, 2013; Kidd, 2014). Podcasts can also help keep students up to date when circumstances such as illness or weather interfere with class attendance. Many students use podcast recordings of lectures they attended to review the content and their notes, which has been shown to improve learning (Abate, 2013; Beard & Morote, 2010). Faculty can also use podcasts to create special presentations such as a case study of a patient, a "walk-through" of a complex task such as a physical examination, an interview with client or clinician, or discussion of an exemplar paper (Marrocco, Kazer, & Neal-Boylan, 2014).

There are several ways to make a podcast recording. To create a manageable file size for distribution, the audio file needs to be recorded in the mp3 format, which can be used by every portable audio device, smartphone, and desktop computer using either built-in software or freely distributed software. Most laptops have a microphone and recording capability. Although the laptop method requires no extra equipment, the sound quality can be low because of ambient noise. An alternative recording method is to use a dedicated mp3 recorder. These devices are the size of a deck of cards and record audio onto a removable memory card. Regardless of the method used to record, it is best to use a good-quality microphone held near the mouth while speaking. This reduces ambient noise and creates a clearer recording.

Distribution of podcasts can be public or private. Podcasts for public use require proper formatting and publicly accessible server space. Complex formatting is not required if the files are being distributed only for local use. The simplest distribution method is to use the document-posting feature of an LMS. See Box 19-5 for suggestions for making and using podcasts.

BOX 19-5 Making and Using Podcasts

- Use a laptop or dedicated mp3 recorder.
- Use a good quality microphone.
- Save files as mp3 format, mono, and 64 to 128 kilobytes per second (kbs) to save space without hurting audio quality. Lower kbs will save space but can reduce listenability of the recording.
- Give the file a meaningful name when saving to help identify the recording (e.g., Class 5-Postop-Feb28-15.mp3).
- State learning outcomes and expectations as the beginning of the podcast.
- Keep podcast segments short; listener attention span is approximately 10 minutes
- Create interactivity by posing questions or asking the student to perform a task or write an answer to a question.

Wikis

A wiki is an online space where users can enter, edit, or review a document (Honey & Doherty, 2014). It is designed to facilitate collaboration and reach a group consensus; sometimes the process is called "crowd sourcing," referring to the wisdom of the crowd rather than relying on an individual contributor. Wikipedia, the most well-known wiki, is a vast encyclopedia that is continuously updated by its users; new information is added as it arises and incorrect or outdated information is deleted. Wikipedia may be the best known wiki, but its use in nursing education may be limited. Wikipedia entries may be edited by almost anyone so there is a risk that entries may include incorrect information (Kardon-Edgren et al., 2009).

An intriguing way to use wikis in class is to use an online wiki service to create a private wiki; many LMSs (see Chapter 21) have wiki software embedded in their system. Students can be given topics to post to the wiki. For example, in a section on nursing history small groups of students each could be assigned to write about a nursing historical figure. Each member of the group would then contribute and edit the wiki. Students could evaluate the quality of information, sources used, and future needs. The wiki can be an ongoing project that is periodically updated and refined.

Another use is to have students develop a wiki for other students in their nursing program. Wikis on studying for a nursing exam, buying books, selecting mobile hardware, succeeding at a particular clinical agency, or buying uniforms are possible topics. The process of creating and editing a wiki helps both the student who edits the wiki as well as the student who reads it. Creating a wiki entry requires critical thinking, organization of ideas, and application of the principles of good writing.

Wikis can also be used to "crowd-source" a care plan. Have the class all contribute to a plan of care or a case study. Assign small groups of students with different areas of expertise to contribute to the care plan. Students then critique and edit the areas they did not work on. Faculty can then require students to identify resources they used to support their postings.

There are myriad other possible uses for wikis in nursing, such as community assessments, literature reviews, debates on ethical issues, FAQs for a clinical agency, or study guides for exams. Wiki projects can help students connect with each other, learn to critique the work of others, and learn how to justify an opinion or clinical decision. See Box 19-6 for suggestions for using wikis in the connected classroom.

BOX 19-6 Using Wikis

- Free wiki sites are available for educational use. Search for "education wikis." Sites such as Wikispaces.com allow teachers to set up their own wiki "classroom."
- Verify that all edits are recorded and can identify the student who is editing.
- Evaluate the academic quality of student-created entries for use of peer-reviewed sources.
- Consider wikis as a tool to achieve group work objectives in an online course during which students are not physically together.

Streaming Videos

Showing movies and videos has long been part of nursing education but the introduction of streaming videos simplifies their use. Videos can convey psychomotor skills, emotional situations, and patient care situations better than any other media (Edmonds, 2013). Streaming videos help engage students and encourage critical thinking (June, Yaacob, & Kheng, 2014). Videos are particularly useful for addressing learning objectives in the affective domain (May et al., 2013). A video of a patient relating an experience with a disease can help students learn empathy for others. In the psychomotor domain, watching the steps of a procedure enhances learning of those steps. In the cognitive domain, unique presentations of concepts such as those presented by the Khan Academy designed specifically for nursing students can also aid learning (http://www.khanacademy.org/test-prep/NCLEX-RN).

Steaming videos can be embedded within a presentation. Embedding videos eliminates disruption of a presentation that can occur by switching to a video player. Videos can be embedded either as a link or played as a file stored on the local computer. Playing from a link is easier and requires no storage space, but it does require an active link to the Internet. A stored video has to be downloaded and saved in a format usable by the local computer, which may cause playback problems if the presentation is done on a computer different from the computer that produced the presentation.

Streaming videos can be found on common video sites such as YouTube and Vimeo, but are also available commercially from nursing care video providers. Hard media such as DVD or Blu-Ray disks require production costs, shipping, and storage; streaming videos avoid these problems. A potential difficulty with streaming videos is that the loss of Internet access prevents the video from playing. Some streaming videos can be downloaded and saved to a USB memory stick for situations where the Internet is not available or is not of high enough speed for streaming.

Social Media

Social media are forms of electronic communication used to create online communities and share information. Social networking and media are incredibly popular; millions visit sites such as Facebook, Twitter, Instagram, LinkedIn, Pinterest, and YouTube every day. Searching social media for health-related postings as an assignment allows students to explore the concerns and knowledge of the lay population. This can be a springboard for discussions on health care issues, health policy, patient teaching, and alternative treatments. Social networks can also be used as a method for finding participants for nursing research studies (Amerson, 2011).

Social media sites are also useful for communication among students and faculty, as well as for with the general public about nursing, school, or health care issues. Facebook provides the ability to create closed groups. A closed group can be used among students as a support group. Twitter accounts can be created to generate tweets, or short news items, about events on campus or health-related topics. Instagram can be used for posts of photographs of campus events or student activities. Faculty can use blogs by using LMS discussion tools or free blogging software (Chapter 21). Social media such as Ning have also been used to promote discussion in a community health course (Drake & Leander, 2013).

Social media sites have great potential risk for privacy violations if used improperly, and there are increasing reports of violations (National Council of State Boards of Nursing, 2011). Schmitt, Sims-Giddens, and Booth (2014) suggests that social media tools can be part of the new pedagogy if used with precautions against invasions of privacy. The risks of social media can be incorporated into discussions of privacy and professionalism (Peck, 2014).

Learning Management Systems

Many institutions offer an LMS to integrate technology into a class, provide supplemental materials, manage grades, communicate with students, give quizzes, and submit assignments (Watson, 2007). The LMS can be configured to assist faculty who teach in a hybrid online/classroom course or an all-online course. An LMS can also track students' progress toward mastery of established learning objectives. Online collaboration helps students connect with each other and the teacher through LMS chat rooms. An important aspect of the LMS is that the teacher controls access and the information on the course site is restricted to authorized users. This protects the integrity of the course materials and the privacy of the students, and avoids copyright limitations for materials that could not be put on the general Internet. For example, videos or documents can be posted with access limited to enrolled students (see Chapter 21).

The Connected Clinical Experience

The connected classroom assumes greater importance as faculty design curricula that better link classroom experiences for application in clinical practice. One of the greatest advantages of using mobile devices in the clinical setting is the ability for students to bring their reference texts in a highly portable form. During the course of a clinical experience students may encounter drugs, terminology, diseases, or laboratory values they have yet to learn. Looking up information as needed is learning by doing and in a context that aids retention. Before planning to use mobile devices in clinical settings, faculty must be sure to have policies concerning their proper use.

Using Mobile Devices during Clinical Experiences

The use of mobile devices during clinical experiences can aid learning and help students apply what they are learning in the classroom (Farrell & Rose 2008; Gregory & Lowder, 2013; Secco, Amirault, Doiron-Maillet, & Furlong, 2013; Wittman-Price, Kennedy & Godwin, 2012). Students should be

BOX 19-7 Using Mobile Devices in the Clinical Setting

1. Have students use a medical dictionary when reading patient histories for any word students do not recognize. Seeing the definitions in context with a real patient situation aids learning of medical vocabulary.
2. Use an acronym guide when reading patient charts. Students can be overwhelmed by the use of acronyms in patient records. An acronym guide is one way students can become familiar with the dozens of acronyms appearing in most charts. Students should be cautioned that some agencies use their own "in-house" acronyms that may not appear in guides.
3. Assign students to use a drug guide to investigate their client's prescribed drugs. Assign students to use the guides to look up side effects, dosing for the patient's weight, nursing administration considerations, and compatibility with other prescribed medications.
4. Require the use of clinical calculators to use tools for assessments such as body mass index, pain scales, intravenous rates, and unit conversions. Have students evaluate their use.
5. Assign a Medline literature search of a topic relevant to their client's needs. This helps students develop skills in literature searches and interpreting applicability of findings to clinical situations.
6. Have students develop a brief care plan "on the fly" using their reference tools during the course of a clinical day. Evaluate the quality of their plan, but also have the students evaluate the quality of the reference tools. This assignment can require the use of a nursing diagnosis guide, intervention guide, drug guide, and other tools.
7. Require the use of mobile resources to develop a patient teaching intervention. Have students find peer-reviewed information and images that can be used to assist patients learn about their treatment or condition.

oriented to the software before entering the clinical area so they know its capabilities. Faculty should also discuss with students the appropriate use of these tools and how to wash hands frequently between patient care and use of these devices.

Faculty who use any of these techniques must be well practiced themselves in the use of technology. Students also look to faculty modeling of technology in the clinical setting. Faculty use improves acceptance by staff and reduces students' technologic fears (Secco, Amirault, Doiron-Maillet, & Furlong, 2014).

Health care resources and applications on electronic devices are useful as reference material, for patient teaching, and patient assessment and monitoring. See Box 19-7 for suggestions for using electronic devices in the clinical setting.

Putting It All Together

Teaching in a connected classroom offers the opportunity for using learning technology to best advantage, connecting students with resources, and flipping the classroom. The connected classroom also promotes linkages with clinical practica and promotes learning for application to real-world patient care situations. The connected classroom also provides students an opportunity to investigate and use emerging health care technologies used for health assessment, patient teaching, and evidence-based practice. In the connected classroom, faculty intentionally choose the teaching methods that will enhance learning. For example, "high-tech" is not needed for small-group discussions, debates, or in-class planning of care. Yet all will help students connect with each other and the faculty.

Traditional pedagogy that values memorization over learning for application to patient care will not adequately prepare nursing students for their future practice. Digital technology such as podcasts, ARSs, wikis, and streaming videos may not be directly used in clinical practice but will help students learn in a more active way than previous methods allowed. These tools can be used at little or no cost, but do take preparation to use effectively. When faculty design learning objectives and outcomes that require higher order thinking and application to practice, they will be in a position to choose methods that take advantage of learning technology rather than having technology guide the objectives.

Using mobile technology in the clinical setting is simultaneously a teaching and a practice tool. Solving real-world problems with mobile computing tools helps put students on the path to better practice after graduation. A clear policy on the appropriate use of these tools must be in place before students use the tools clinically. Although clinical agencies may have concerns about privacy violations, faculty can offer reassurance through the use of school and agency privacy policies and the use of appropriate ethical behaviors.

The decision to have a connected classroom is no longer a question of if but of when it will be implemented. The exponential growth of health care information requires students to learn how to locate and use new information. The increasing globalization of health care practice also means a greater need for connections with other health care providers and patients. New technologies will emerge after the publication of this book and faculty need to be ready and able to incorporate them into teaching and clinical practice. All of these factors will lead faculty to find their connections with students, patients, and the world. As Albert Einstein (Frank, 2002, p. 185) noted, "[I do not] carry such information in my mind since it is readily available in books. … The value of a college education is not the learning of many facts but the training of the mind to think."

REFLECTING ON THE EVIDENCE

1. Design an ideal connected classroom. What elements are important to you and your students?
2. Many nursing faculty may not be well versed in the use of technology in the classroom. What would you teach a faculty member about using the technologies?
3. What emerging evidence supports the use of the flipped classroom? What variables are being studied? Must all students be "satisfied" to use this method in connected classroom?
4. There are many health care reference applications for mobile devices. How would you decide which applications to recommend to students?
5. Locate the social media policy at your school. How is it communicated to students? What consequences are in place for students who do not observe the policy? How does this policy relate to other policies at your school that guide ethical, legal, and moral behavior of students and faculty?
6. What new health care or learning technologies are in the news recently? How will they affect your classroom?
7. The use of mobile computers in clinical settings may be in violation of local policies. How would you go about effecting change in those policies?
8. Wearable technologies such as cameras and smartwatches are becoming available. What are the risks and benefits of this technology? How would you integrate these technologies into the connected classroom or clinical setting?

REFERENCES

Abate, K. S. (2013). The effect of podcast lectures on nursing students' knowledge retention and application. *Nursing Education Research, 34*(3), 182–185.

Abel, R., Brown, M., & Suess, J. (2013, September/October). A new architecture for learning. *Educause Review, 88–102.*

Abell, C. H., & Garrett-Wright, D., (2014). E-Books: Nurse faculty use and concerns. *Nursing Education Perspectives, 35*(2), 112–114.

American Association of Colleges of Nursing. (2014). *2013-2014 Salaries of instructional and administrative nursing faculty in baccalaureate and graduate programs in nursing.* Retrieved from, http://www.aacn.nche.edu/media-relations/fact-sheets/nursing-faculty-shortage.

American Nurses Association (ANA). (2015). *Six tips for nurses using social media.* Retrieved from, http://www.nursingworld.org/FunctionalMenuCategories/AboutANA/Social-Media/Social-Networking-Principles-Toolkit/6-Tips-for-Nurses-Using-Social-Media-Poster.pdf.

Amerson, R. (2011). Facebook: A tool for nursing education research. *Journal of Nursing Education Research, 50*(7), 414–416.

Beard, K., & Morote, E. S. (2010). Using podcasts with narrative pedagogy. *Nursing Education Perspectives, 31*(3), 186–187.

Berry, J. (2009). Technology support in nursing education: Clickers in the classroom. *Nursing Education Research, 30*(5), 295–298.

Bull, G. (2013, May). Refresh your flipped classroom with interactive video. *Learning & Leading with Technology, 10–11.*

Button, D., Harrington, A., & Belan, I. (2013). *E-learning and information communication technology (ICT) in nursing education: A review of the literature.* Nurse Education Today. Retrieved from, http://dx.doi.org/10.1016/j.nedt,2013.05.002.

Critz, C. M., & Knight, D. (2013). Using the flipped classroom in graduate nursing education. *Nurse Educator, 38*(5), 210–213.

Dahlstrom, E., Walker, J. D., & Dziuban, C. (2013, September). *ECAR study of undergraduate students and information technology, 2013 (Research Report).* Louisville, CO: EDUCAUSE Center for Analysis and Research. Retrieved from, http://www.educause.edu/ecar.

Doswell, W., Braxter, B., Dabbs, A. D., Nilsen, W., & Klem, M. L. (2013). mHealth: Technology for nursing practice, education, and research. *Journal of Nursing Education and Practice, 3*(10), 99–109.

Doyle, G. J., Garrett, B., & Currie, L. M. (2014). Integrating mobile devices into nursing curricula: Opportunities for implementation using Rogers' Diffusion model. *Nurse Education Today, 34*, 775–782.

Drake, M. A., & Leander, S. A. (2013). Nursing students and Ning: Using social networking to teach public health/community nursing in 11 baccalaureate nursing programs. *Nursing Education Perspectives, 34*(4), 270–272.

Edmonds, M. L. (2013). The use of film in teaching concepts in quantitative inquiry to graduate nursing students. *Journal of Nursing Education, 52*(3), 179–180.

Farrell, M. J., & Rose, L. (2008). Use of mobile handheld computers in clinical nursing education. *Journal of Nursing Education, 47*(1), 13–19.

Frank P. (2002). *Einstein: His life and times.* Boston: Da Capo Press.

George, L. E., Davidson, L. J., Serapiglia, C. P., Barla, S., & Thotakura, A. (2010). Technology in nursing education: A study of PDA use by students. *Journal of Professional Nursing, 26*(6), 371–376.

Glackin, B. C., Rodenhiser, R. W., & Herzog, B. (2014). *A collaborative project assessing the impact of eBooks and mobile devices on student learning.* The Journal of Academic Librarianship. Retrieved from, http://dx.doi.org/10.1016/j.acalib.2014.04.007.

Gonen, A., Sharon, D., Offir, A., & Lev-Ari, L. (2014). How to enhance nursing students' intention to use information technology: The first step before integrating it in the nursing curriculum. *CIN: Computers, Informatics, Nursing, 32*(6), 286–293.

Greenfield, S. (2011). Podcasting: A new tool for student retention? *Journal of Nursing Education, 50*(2), 112–114.

Gregory, L. C., & Lowder, E. (2013). "There's an app for that" Bringing nursing education to the bedside. *Journal of Pediatric Nursing, 28*, 191–192.

Hamdan, N., McKnight, P., McKnight, K., & Arfstrom, K. M. (2013). *The flipped learning model: A white paper based on the literature review titled "A review of flipped learning."* Retrieved from, http://fln.schoolwires.net/cms/lib07/VA01923112/Centricity/Domain/41/WhitePaper_FlippedLearning.pdf.

Hawks, S. J. (2014). The flipped classroom: Now or never? *AANA Journal, 82*(4), 264–269.

Honey, M., & Doherty, I. (2014). Research brief: Using wiki to support student nurses learning discipline specific terminology. *Nursing Praxis in New Zealand, 30*(1), 42–43.

Johnston, A. N. D., Massa, H., & Burne, T. H. J. (2013). Digital lecture recording: A cautionary tale. *Nurse Education in Practice, 13*, 40–47.

June, S., Yaacob, A., & Kheng, Y. K. (2014). Assessing the use of YouTube videos and interactive activities as a critical thinking stimulator for tertiary students: an action research. *International Education Studies, 7*(8), 56.

Kardong-Edgren, S. E., Oermann, M. H., Ha, Y., Tennant, M. N., Snelso, C., Hallmark, E., et al. (2009). Using a wiki in nursing education and research. *International Journal of Nursing Education and Scholarship, 6*(1), 1–10. Article 6.

Kidd, W. (2014). Utilising podcasts for learning and teaching: A review and ways forward for e-learning cultures. *Management in Education, 26*(2), 52–57.

Klein, K., & Kientz, M. (2013). A model for successful use of student response systems. *Nursing Education Perspectives, 34*(5), 334–338.

Lee, S. T., & Dapremont, J. A. (2012). Engaging nursing students through integration of the audience response system. *Nursing Education Perspectives, 33*(1), 55–57.

Marrocco, G. F., Kazer, M. W., & Neal-Boylan, L. (2014). Transformational learning in graduate nurse education through podcasting. *Nursing Education Perspectives, 35*(1), 49–53.

May, O. W., Wedgeworth, M. G., & Bigham, A. B. (2013). Technology in nursing education: YouTube as a teaching strategy. *Journal of Pediatric Nursing, 28*, 408–410.

McDonald, K., & Smith, C. M. (2013). The flipped classroom for professional development: Part I. Benefits and strategies. *Journal of Continuing Education in Nursing, 44*(10), 437–438.

Missildine, K., Fountain, R., Summers, L., & Gosselin, K. (2013). Flipping the classroom to improve student performance and satisfaction. *Journal of Nursing Education, 52*(10), 597–599. http://dx.doi.org/10.3928/01484834-20130910-03.

Morris, A. H., & Faulk, D. R. (2012). *Transformative learning in nursing: A guide for nurse educators.* New York: Springer.

National Council of State Boards of Nursing. (2011). *White Paper: A nurse's guide to the use of social media.* Retrieved from, http://www.ncsbn.org/Social_Media.pdf.

National League for Nursing (NLN). (2015). *A vision for the changing faculty role: Preparing students for the technological world of health care.* Retrieved from, http://www.nln.org/aboutnln/livingdocuments/pdf/nlnvision_8.pdf.

Peck, J. L. (2014). Social media in nursing education: Responsible integration for meaningful use. *Journal of Nursing Education, 53*(3), 164–169.

Revell, S. M. H., & McCurry, M. K. (2010). Engaging millennial learners: Effectiveness of personal response system technology with nursing students in small and large classrooms. *Journal of Nursing Education, 49*(5), 272–275.

Russell, J. S., McWilliams, M., Chasen, L., & Farley, J. (2011). Using clickers for clinical reasoning and problem solving. *Nurse Educator, 36*(1), 13–15.

Schaffhauser, D. (2014, June 4). 3 ways to get faculty up to speed with technology. *Campus Technology, 41*(2), 1–3.

Schlairet, M. C., Green, R., & Benton, M. J. (2014). The flipped classroom: Strategies for an undergraduate nursing course. *Nurse Educator, 39*(6), 321–325.

Schmitt, T. L., Sims-Giddens, S. S., & Booth, R. G. (2012, September 30). Social media use in nursing education. *Online Journal of Issues in Nursing, 17*(3), 2.

Schwartz, T. A. (2014). Flipping the statistics classroom in nursing education. *Journal of Nursing Education, 53*(4), 199–206.

Secco, M. L., Amirault, D., Doiron-Maillet, N., & Furlong, K. (2013). Evaluation of nursing central as an information tool, part I: Student learning. *Nursing Education Perspectives, 34*(6), 416–418.

Secco, M. L., Doiron-Maillet, N., Amirault, D., & Furlong, K. (2014). Evaluation of nursing central as an information tool, part 2: Clinical instruction. *Nursing Education Perspectives, 34*(6), 416–418.

Shellenbarger, T., & Robb, M. (2014). Technology-based strategies for promoting clinical reasoning skills in nursing education. *Nurse Educator, 40*(2), 55–56.

Silverthorn, D. U. (2006). Teaching and learning in the interactive classroom. *Advances in Physiology Education, 30*, 135–140.

Skiba, D. J. (2014a). The connected age and the 2014 Horizon Report. *Nursing Education Perspectives, 35*(2), 131–132.

Skiba, D. J. (2014b). The connected age: Implications for 2014. *Nursing Education Perspectives, 35*(1), 63–64.

Skiba, D. J. (2014c). The connected age: Mobile apps and consumer engagement. *Nursing Education Perspectives, 35*(3), 199–201.

Swan, B. A., Smith, K. A., Frisby, A., Shaffer, K., Hanson-Zalot, M., & Becker, J. (2013). Evaluating tablet technology in an undergraduate nursing program. *Nursing Education Perspectives, 34*(4), 192–193.

Thompson, B. W. (2005). HIPAA guidelines for using PDAs. *Nursing, 35*(11), 24.

Ustun, C., & Cihangiroglu, M. (2012). Health care workers' mobile phones: A potential cause of microbial cross-contamination between hospital and community. *Journal of Occupational and Environmental Hygiene, 9*, 538–542.

Watson, W. R. (2007). An argument for clarity: What are learning management systems, what are they not, and what should they become? *Tech Trends, 51*(2), 28–34.

Watson, J. A., & Pecchioni, L. L. (2011). Digital natives and digital media in the college classroom: Assignment design and impacts on student learning. *Educational Media International, 48*(4), 307–320.

Wilkinson, A., Roberts, J., & While, A. (2013). Nursing students' use of technology enhanced learning: A longitudinal study. *Journal of Nursing Education and Practice, 3*(5), 102–115.

Wittman-Price, R. A., Kennedy, L. D., & Godwin, C. (2012). Use of personal phones by senior nursing students to access health care information during clinical education: Staff nurses' and students' perceptions. *Journal of Nursing Education, 51*(11), 642–646.

20 Teaching and Learning at a Distance

Barbara Manz Friesth, PhD, RN

Technological advances in computers and broadband connectivity continue to open new ways for nursing faculty to connect with their students and deliver media-rich content at a distance. Increasingly, students want to learn in more flexible programs that maximize their time and other life commitments (Urso & Ouzts, 2011). At the same time, higher education programs are recognizing the need to increase student access to distance-accessible programs (Allen & Seaman, 2014). Distance education offers the ability to bring health care practitioners to rural and underserved areas. By educating those who already live in rural areas, there may be a greater likelihood that they will remain and practice in their home towns after completion of their studies (Skillman, Kaplan, Andrilla, Ostergard, & Patterson, 2014).

There is a current faculty shortage in nursing schools, and this trend is expected to worsen in the coming years with advancing faculty age and looming retirements (American Association of Colleges of Nursing [AACN], 2014). Distance education programs offer a means to reduce the faculty shortage and connect specific student learning interests with faculty expertise, despite the distance between the two (Billings, 2010). Distance education delivery systems that encourage innovation and flexibility have the potential for maximizing use of institutional infrastructure, improving access to credit courses, and providing consistency for learning at multiple locations.

Distance education is broadly defined as students receiving instruction in a location other than that of the faculty. This separation of teacher and student could be as close as within the same community or campus or as far away as across states or continents. The options of available delivery systems to implement distant academic courses or continuing education opportunities have become increasingly competitive and are frequently defined by cost, administrator and faculty knowledge, acceptance, and readiness. Additionally, computers, mobile devices, and computer-based communication systems continue to have a positive and dramatic effect on teaching and learning, thus becoming invaluable tools for distance instruction. Faculty must become proficient and comfortable with the use of technology in their practice and as educators (Gerard, Kazer, Babington, & Quell, 2014; Healthcare Information and Management Systems Society, 2011).

Distance education delivery systems are undergoing rapid change. In most cases, technologies have merged with others to form a blend of delivery or are being replaced by new and innovative delivery options. Obsolescence of existing media within the next 5 to 10 years will be commonplace, as the changes in technology continue at a very rapid pace. However, the concepts related to leading, planning, using, supporting, administering, and evaluating student learning in distance education environments remain applicable. The *virtual classroom,* defined for this purpose as the learning environment occurring wherever the student can access information, has become more common as colleges and universities endeavor to offer efficient and effective higher education opportunities to students any place and at any time.

Online education is continuing to grow at a rate that is faster than the overall higher education market in general (Allen & Seaman, 2014). Shachar & Neumann (2010) conducted a metaanalysis of 20 years of research comparing traditional and distance learning modalities and concluded that learning at a distance is at least equivalent to traditional face-to-face courses if not superior. A similar landmark metaanalysis conducted by the United States Department of Education (2009) found similar results overall, and in addition, data to support that blended methods may produce the best outcomes overall. Blended, or hybrid, approaches use a combination of online and face-to-face formats. Recent trend data from undergraduate students reflect a preference for blended learning environments over traditional or online alone (Dahlstrom et al., 2013). Synchronous video technologies offer a way to deliver blended courses to students at a distance, without requiring the time and expense associated with travel to the host site. The use of blended approaches in higher education has increased, and is expected to continue to grow in the coming years (Dahlstrom, 2012; Diaz & Brown, 2010; Fleming, 2013). The technologies available today offer a wide variety in strategies for delivering blended approaches at a distance.

Distance learning tends to capitalize on a constructivist, problem solving approach to learning. Distance learning seems to support Piaget's (2001) position that learning is not just inherent or just experiential in nature, but a combination of both. Constructivism encourages learners to build their own understanding of information, and to apply this information in their own environment (Kala, Isaramalai, & Pohthong, 2010). This constructivist approach is also consistent with an active learning and learner-centered approach as well (Keengwe & Kidd, 2010). Although other instructional media are not excluded from this consideration, computers and networked learning have had a huge effect on the learner's ability to construct and manage his or her own learning environment. Distance learning and computer-based instruction have created a newfound independence for learners.

The variety of options available to support distance instruction continues to increase as technologies improve and the transformation from a teacher-centered focus to a learner-centered focus becomes more prominent (Stanley & Dougherty, 2010). Use of distance learning technologies requires planning and development of materials long before the course begins (Keengwe & Kidd, 2010). State-of-the-art resources for faculty development of instructional materials must be available. Training and support for faculty to develop and use the new technology must be present. In addition, support for students must be provided in the use of the technology. With proper resources for development and support, faculty can deliver distance-accessible programs that meet the educational needs of students enrolled in online courses.

Online course management software, commonly called *learning management systems* (LMS), has had an influence on distance learning. LMSs provide an instructional environment that incorporates a support system for course management. This includes course information and content, announcements, communication for synchronous and asynchronous collaboration, and assessment and evaluation of student learning. The LMS used in conjunction with synchronous and asynchronous strategies opens up the realm of possibilities for connecting students with faculty and peers, and providing media-rich content.

With the shift toward computer-based instruction, the number of courses offered exclusively in the form of face-to-face instruction is decreasing substantially. However, many courses offer a blended, or hybrid, approach with other technologies such as video conferencing, audio conferencing, video streaming, podcasting, and other specialized web-based computer applications to offer a blend of synchronous and asynchronous learning experiences. Some technologies use *synchronous* technologies, or technologies that connect people simultaneously, or at the same time. Other technologies use *asynchronous* approaches, allowing learners to access materials without the constraints of a specific time or place. This chapter covers selected strategies used in educating students who are geographically dispersed and separated from the faculty, and both synchronous and asynchronous approaches. An overview of delivery systems, their advantages and disadvantages, and other pertinent information specific to each medium are also presented in Table 20-1.

Synchronous Technologies

With expected continued growth in the blended format of higher education programs, there is a growing need to use technology to provide face-to-face interactions for students at a distance. Synchronous technologies offer a way to deliver blended courses to students at a distance, without requiring travel to the host site. Synchronous video technologies discussed in this chapter include institutionally based video conferencing systems, institutionally focused web conferencing solutions,

TABLE 20-1 Instructional Delivery Systems

Type	Advantages	Major Disadvantages	Costs Related to Technology
Institutionally based video conferencing systems	• Highest quality audio and video • Easy to use • Multiple sites possible • Students attend classes in groups at their respective sites • Remote sites must have high-speed Internet access but students do not need it in their homes	• Requires hardware at all remote sites • Requires technical support at all remote sites • No ability to provide spontaneous breakout sessions for small group work • Students required to attend at a video conference site and are not able to participate from home	• Expensive, with need for centralized bridge access at the institution level • Hardware units required at host and all remote locations • Support staff at host and remote locations
Institutionally focused web conferencing and cloud based software (two-way)	• Interactive video from multiple participants • Desktop and document sharing with polling capabilities • Ability to have multiple spontaneous breakout groups concurrently for group projects	• Finite limit to number of participants • Video quality decreases with increased number of participants • High-speed Internet required for all participants	• Institutionally purchased software • Cost of computer, web camera, headset with mic, and access to high-speed Internet for both host and recipients • Support for audio and video difficulties
Webinar	• Real-time video over Internet to personal computers • Screen-sharing capabilities • Requires minimum technical assistance for recipients • Numerous participants possible	• One-way video • Response back may be audio or instant message • High-speed Internet required for all participants	• Institutionally purchased software • Cost of computer, web camera, headset with mic, and access to high-speed Internet for host • Recipients require computer and high-speed Internet • Support for audio and video difficulties
Individual or small-group web conferencing	• Very low cost or free software • Easy to install and use	• Limited to one on one or to very small number of interactive video participants	• Proprietary networks require line fees • High demand on network bandwidth • Salaries to provide scheduling and technical support
Audio conferencing	• Learner centered • Low cost • Can be taught from or received at any location that has telephone or high-speed Internet access • High speed internet access for VoIP	• Calls may be joined from remote classrooms or homes • Styles of class presentation may need to be altered • Visual learners and students with hearing limitations may be at a disadvantage	• Long-distance telephone toll charges • Audio conferencing equipment at receive sites, if more than one student is enrolled • Service provider fees • Salaries for site coordinators
Podcast, enhanced podcast, vodcast	• Learner centered • Access anywhere • Real-time and anytime delivery • Engaging across learning styles • Portable • Inexpensive • Fun	• Requires iPod or other mobile device to use in mobile format • Need for faculty to learn new technology • Potential compatibility issues across platforms	• High-speed Internet access • Personal player or computer required • Production staff salaries • Support staff salaries

VoIP, Voice over Internet Protocol.

and one-on-one or small group web conferencing programs. Synchronous audio-only technologies include audio conferencing, over either existing telephone lines or Voice over Internet Protocol (VoIP) systems. VoIP is essentially a telephone connection that uses a computer or hardware and the Internet to digitally transmit the call.

Audio Conferencing

Instruction transmitted over telephone lines is a delivery strategy commonly referred to as *audio conferencing*. A teacher located at the origin site, not necessarily a classroom, interacts with students in one or more receiving sites. Some distance teaching universities and colleges incorporate audio conferencing in a blended manner with other technologies, such as webinars, where additional materials may be presented in a visual manner over the Internet. Existing phone conferencing services may be used for the audio conferences; however, increasingly, VoIP software is used to connect the audio of numerous participants. VoIP software allows one to make phone calls, or conference calls, using software and high-speed Internet, thus eliminating teleconferencing or long-distance charges. Some LMSs have VoIP audio conferencing capabilities built into their software, but freely available software such as Skype and Google Hangouts can be used as well.

If the chosen blend of instruction does not include a visual component, photographs or video of the instructor and students may be shared by electronic or other means at the beginning of the course. In addition, students should be encouraged to identify themselves and their location when they speak during the audio class sessions to facilitate a feeling of classroom community. For the best audio experience, students should be instructed to use a headset with a built-in microphone. Participants not currently speaking should be asked to "mute" their lines to eliminate distractions and extraneous noises during the conference call. Activities that provide opportunity for some student socialization should also be incorporated into early class sessions at the same time that students are provided orientation to use of the technology. Because the teacher is unable to identify nonverbal cues, teaching strategies should include more questioning to determine class understanding of content being addressed. Methods of drawing students into discussion should be planned and appropriately incorporated into classes throughout the course. One common strategy to engage students at remote sites is to call on students on a rotational basis.

Institutionally Based Dedicated Video Conferencing Systems

Many educational institutions, businesses, and health care systems are using dedicated Internet protocol video conferencing systems (such as Polycom or Tandberg) to connect with one or multiple sites. Simultaneous video conferencing of three or more systems, also known as *multipoint video conferencing*, is conducted via use of multipoint control units. These multipoint control units, or bridges, allow video connections from multiple sources and control the throughput of the audio and video to each site. A dedicated video conferencing unit is required at any site wishing to participate in the video conference. One or many participants may be present at any given site. Current state-of-the-art systems employ high-definition cameras, resulting in high-quality video. This high-quality video enables the participants to experience and see details of facial expressions and body language. The cameras can be controlled remotely to zoom in or out and to focus on one or many participants.

Video output from the conference is typically displayed using flat-panel high-definition televisions in the case of very small classrooms or high-definition video projectors in larger classrooms. An important feature of these dedicated video conferencing systems is sophisticated audio handling. The dedicated units use echo cancellation technology, which eliminates problems where the remote parties may hear their own voices speaking back to them over the system (echo) and reverberation or audio feedback. The video output from the conference can be customized to display one or multiple parties on the screen. When using a single-view option of remote sites, the bridge will automatically switch video signals to display the site that is currently speaking. These institutionally based units have the highest quality audio and video available on the market today and are typically very easy to use. Most institutionally based systems also allow remote participants to join using specialized software and their personal computer with camera and microphone.

A high-fidelity version of institutionally based video conferencing is "telepresence." Traditionally telepresence video conferencing uses a combination of life-size, high-definition video technology and special acoustic microphones, speakers, and soundproofing to deliver an experience of near lifelike quality. A recent advancement in telepresence systems involves cameras that use radar and sonar technology to identify who is speaking within a given room, and automatically focuses on the speaker. These automated systems mean that the instructor can focus on teaching, and not have to attend to whether or not the camera is focused on the person currently speaking in the classroom, while still delivering high-quality audio and video for participants at remote sites.

The major advantage to using institutionally based dedicated video conferencing systems is the exceptionally high quality of the video. State of the art systems use high-definition video and enable participants to see facial expressions and body language, which is particularly important in courses that use any role playing or student presentations. The major disadvantage is that managing large groups, or the ability to view large groups of students, can be difficult, and the video connection requires good broadband connectivity by all participants.

Institutionally Focused Web Conferencing and Cloud-Based Solutions

For institutions that are unable to leverage regional and institutionally based video conferencing units where the target students are located, webcasting or web conferencing offers an alternative for distance students. Institutionally focused web conferencing software allows connection of two or more individuals simultaneously. Increasingly these services are being provided by "cloud-based" companies that use the Internet to provide video conferencing solutions to institutions who do not want to maintain or provide the hardware to provide videoconferencing locally. This is an area of rapid growth, with new products and features coming to market often. Examples of such software include Adobe Connect Professional, Web-Ex, GoToMeeting, Wimba Live Classroom, and Zoom. Some web conferencing software requires installation of software on each participant's part, whereas others are strictly web-based applications and require no installation to join. Some of the software solutions are built directly into institutionally deployed LMSs. Each individual who is connecting to the web conference does so via a computer connected to high-speed Internet. Participants may receive audio and video from others, but to share their own video, they must also have a web camera. Web cameras have become standard equipment on newer laptops and many newer computers. To avoid audio feedback problems, participants should be encouraged to use a headphone with a built-in microphone, and to mute their audio when not speaking.

Although it is possible to see all participants who have web cameras, the actual size and quality of the video may vary greatly based on the number of participants and the quality of the bandwidth. The ability to switch between speakers and view multiple participants concurrently varies somewhat across systems.

Most web conferencing software has the ability to share desktops, thus sharing presentations or papers from either the host or participant computers. Many also have polling software and instant messaging available. Web conferences can be recorded and made available for students to view later or for students who miss a particular class session to review at a later date. Some of the systems allow students or faculty to create breakout group areas, allowing for small-group collaboration among participants working on group projects. In addition to using the web conferencing for face-to-face class sessions, office hours may be scheduled using the software, thus enabling a face-to-face interaction for students desiring to take advantage of such support.

Another version of web conferencing is "webinars," which are typically one-way broadcasting of actual video. The actual software used to deliver webinars is the same as that used for web conferencing, and the capabilities of displaying slides and desktop applications are similar. There are several advantages of webinars over interactive two-way video conferences. One advantage is the possible number of participants. Because video is broadcast in only one direction, broadband limitations are generally not affected by multiple participants, and it is possible to have more than 100 participants in any given webinar. Participants may still engage during live sessions, but will do so via polling mechanisms, chat, and audio only. Webinars still require high-speed Internet access, although a web camera is not necessary for participation at remote locations. The obvious disadvantage to webinars is the loss of the face-to-face interaction with the remote sites.

Individual or Small-Group Web Conferencing

Although many institutions may subscribe to professional-level web conferencing software solutions, software also exists for connecting one-on-one or in small groups for no, or very little, charge. Examples of this software include Skype, Microsoft Lync, FaceTime, and Google Hangouts. Most of these web conferencing solutions are offered as a free download with the creation of an account for their service. The software is easy to use and requires a computer with web camera, headphones with microphone, and high-speed Internet access.

Most of these types of software also allow for instant messaging and a "status indicator" to let people know if you are available for web conferencing or messaging. Although not designed to allow multiple video connections at one time, such software is a cost-effective way to enable one-on-one, face-to-face interactions between faculty and students or between small student groups. Such software may be used to facilitate face-to-face tutoring sessions or to bring groups together for project work across geographic locations. Instructors can also use the software to host office hours with students, by posting their availability to students and being available at specified times each week. This software may also be used to bring a guest content expert to your classroom virtually, without the expense and time involved with actual travel. Some of the software allows for desktop sharing but overall the robustness of sharing features is limited compared with institutionally focused web conferencing solutions. Nonetheless, given the inexpensive cost to use these products, these tools offer a valuable way to connect with students.

Support and Strategies for Synchronous Connections

Each synchronous connection medium has identifiable differences specific to the technology but the similarities of required support for planning, and implementing use of the technology in the classroom and online represent the major focus. Virtual classroom teaching requires faculty to carefully plan the best strategies for learning over a distance. Within this overall process, students must be oriented to the technology and clear expectations must be communicated to the learners. Student outcomes can be influenced by both the process and content of learning. Clear and concise orientation is an important step toward improved academic self-concept. A summary of adapted teaching strategies specifically for teaching with synchronous technology is provided in Table 20-2.

TABLE 20-2 Adapting Teaching Strategies for Use with Synchronous Technologies

Rationale for Use in Courses Delivered by Synchronous Technology	Adapted Teaching Strategies
	LECTURE
Provides efficient method of presenting factual information in a short period	• Present key concepts in short mini-lectures (10–15 minutes) or podcasts interspersed with feedback, interaction, questioning, and application opportunities. • Engage learners with key concepts material through self-assessment strategies, reflection, advanced organizers. • Enhance mini-lecture with web- and computer-based materials, and other media such as presentation software, video, and computer graphics. • Coach guest speakers to design interactive presentations, with ample opportunity for question–answer exchanges with learners.
	DISCUSSION
Provides student-centered learning environment Facilitates collaborative learning process Engages learners in active learning Provides opportunity for critical inquiry	• Elicit multiple perspectives, points of view for learners to reflect on, and experiences. • Preassign individuals to give specific reports to enhance discussion. • Call on students frequently; establish a dialogue between learners at various reception sites. • Allow sufficient time for learners to respond to questions and enter the discussion, encouraging all sites to participate. • Ask high-level questions that require students to compare, apply, synthesize, hypothesize, or evaluate. • Repeat and rephrase question while waiting for students to prepare a response. • Encourage participation from learners by effectively using camera to engage in eye contact with learner and focus on those speaking.
	INTERVIEW
Experts or clients bring additional information or viewpoints to the class in an interview format	• Prerecord guest segments with guest "live" for web-based question–answer exchanges or available by telephone. • Moderator should summarize and clarify key points and keep interview timely and on point.

(Continued)

TABLE 20-2 Adapting Teaching Strategies for Use with Synchronous Technologies—cont'd

Rationale for Use in Courses Delivered by Synchronous Technology	Adapted Teaching Strategies
	PANEL DISCUSSION
Facilitates the introduction of a wide-range of informed opinions in an efficient manner	• Learners should be prepared by previous assigned learning activities. • Ensure that panel members understand their role on the panel and what they are to contribute to discussion. Three or four panel members is optimum. Choose panelists with differing viewpoints or areas of expertise. Keep presentations short so all panel members have sufficient time to present their information. Conduct a rehearsal with the panel before class as needed. • Panel members can be geographically dispersed and live or online—but be sure to guide discussion to all panel members. • Moderator's summaries are crucial to identifying important points, and keeping panel members to allotted time so all have an opportunity to speak
	ROLE PLAYING
Encourages simulated decision-making, collaboration, and engagement	• Role playing scenario can be prerecorded and shown during class; consider using groups at different reception sites. • Role playing can be used to follow up a previous assignment such as "What would you do in this situation?" • Prepare learners ahead of time, because there is less spontaneous activity than in a face to face classroom. • Keep role-playing segments short so that students from all sites can react and respond. • Debrief role playing scenario with discussion to emphasize key learning, reflection, feelings, etc.
	LEARNING CIRCLES, DISCUSSION GROUPS, STUDY GROUPS
Facilitates discussion in larger classes Provides opportunity for practical work sessions in a collegial and collaborative environment Encourages participation and active learning, and builds group rapport within the class	• Use technology that supports formation of synchronous or asynchronous groups, divide class into groups of 5 to 10 for discussion purposes. In classes with large groups of students, break the group into smaller groups and ask group to select a "reporter" to present the group work. • Use team-building skills to develop collaborative learning. • Give groups explicit instructions as to the task to be accomplished, such as "develop one question" or "agree on one disadvantage"; keep instructions clear and simple. • Use with problem-based learning and team-based learning scenarios • Have groups report back during videoconference class time.
	QUESTION AND ANSWER
Provides feedback to faculty and learner Stimulates discussion Engages learners in class	• Participants should be encouraged to make note of questions or comments as the class proceeds so they are ready to respond. • Respect for individuals' questions is essential; provide opportunity through asynchronous discussion forums, chat function, live stream, or 800 number to answer questions from individuals who did not have a chance to participate during the class session.
	CASE STUDY/SIMULATION
Helps individuals to weigh and test values, separate fact from opinion, and develop critical thinking skills	• Case studies should be available to learners in advance of class so the learners can review and prepare individual or group responses. • If oral case studies are presented, they can add a change of pace; keep these short (5 to 10 minutes) so that others in the group can assimilate the details. • Incorporate presentation software, video clips, or other media to enhance case study presentation; encourage learners to do the same to enhance their responses to the case study.
	DEBATE
Clarify points and positions Helpful for values clarification and developing critical thinking and communication skills Supports learning in the affective domain	• Plan ahead and give clear directions. • Have groups develop criteria for evaluating presentations. • Be sure learners at all sites can hear points; repeat as needed. • Can preassign positions to be debated to specific groups.
	MULTIMEDIA, GRAPHICS, SLIDES
Provides visual clarity and close-up view of selected material	• Keep graphics simple. • Use "horizontal" or "landscape" aspect. • Use large font size. • Use contrasting background and foreground (blue, gray, and pastel are best as background colors).

As with other instructional delivery strategies, synchronous systems of instruction require marketing, site selection, effective communication, and ongoing course coordination to be managed efficiently. Faculty and administrators must work together closely to ensure that these components of the total educational plan are in place.

Selection of a Synchronous System

The selection of any video conferencing solution for a given institution will vary based on existing resources and the student population. Whether there are already existing regionally based video conferencing units in the locations desired will factor into the decision. Collaborative relationships or rental of remote equipment is also possible in some cases. The regional video conferencing model gives remote students a chance to get to know others geographically close to them, because they come together in remote classrooms. In rural areas or areas with poor broadband access, video conferencing units located at regional hospitals or small-town libraries may be one way to accommodate access to the virtual synchronous classroom, particularly when students do not have access to broadband in their homes.

In areas where students do have access to high-speed Internet, use of a web conferencing solution offers great flexibility for access to the virtual classroom. Many institutions subscribe to a particular product, and use of the institutionally available product will be most cost effective. It is important to note that the quality of the video may not result in the ability to see facial expressions and detail; however, you will have some of the benefits of a face-to-face interaction. When considering web conferencing, one must consider the potential number of students expected at remote sites, and select a product with capabilities to accommodate concurrent anticipated usage. With large numbers of participants, switching to a webinar format may be preferred, although this option must be weighed against the loss of two-way interactive video. One area of considerable growth has been the ability to connect handheld mobile devices such as smartphones and other tablet devices to web conferences. The ability to join mobile devices is significant as research on current students supports that they are likely to own two to three internet-capable devices, including smartphones, tablets, and laptops (Dahlstrom, Walker, & Dzuiban, 2013).

Asynchronous Technologies

Although there is increased growth in use of a variety of synchronous technologies, asynchronous technologies have also grown and become more interactive. Asynchronous technologies do not require the student to be tied in time to a specific time or place, hence offering the greatest flexibility in scheduling and participation in course materials. A variety of audio-only and video-enhanced technologies exist to deliver content and materials to students on their own schedule.

Podcasts

A popular tool for receiving streaming media over the Internet is a podcast. *Podcast* was a term originally derived from Apple's portable music player, the iPod (Podcast, n.d.) and involved the broadcast of audio that could be subscribed to and automatically downloaded to a computer. Now the term *podcast* typically refers to any type of audio programming that can be automatically downloaded to a computer or mobile device. The most common file type for distribution of audio-only podcasts is mp3 files. Students subscribe to a particular podcast with software either in their LMS or other freely available programs to automatically receive the new files.

One popular form of podcasting is to capture live, face-to-face lectures. An easy way for faculty to capture lectures for podcasting is with portable flash-memory audio recorders that record directly in the mp3 format. The recording can be made at a low bit-per-second rate (32 kbps is recommended) that reduces file size without much compromise in audio quality. The use of a lapel microphone will help ensure higher audio quality. Be sure to state the name and date of the class at the beginning to help students know the topic of the audio file. These files require no postrecording processing except for changing the name of the file. Files can be uploaded to a course LMS or even be e-mailed directly to students.

Advantages of this style of podcasting include making content available for additional student review to increase the understanding of difficult concepts and allowing additional note-taking time for items missed during class. An archive of lectures can be created and used for inclement weather dates or in case of faculty illness for future classes. The major disadvantage of this form of podcasting is that it does not foster active learning and that some students may perceive an opportunity to miss class periods. Strategies such as using interactive learning activities in class that build on concepts introduced in the podcast can help discourage this behavior. Another disadvantage of this form of podcasting is that it does not add any additional information to the class.

Another form of podcasting involves replacing lecture time with prerecorded podcasts. Two studies comparing performance on exams after podcasted lectures and face-to-face lectures found no significant differences in the two formats (Abate, 2013; Vogt, Schaffner, Ribar, & Chavez, 2010). Although overall satisfaction with the podcast format was good, the majority of students did not necessarily prefer podcasts to live lectures.

The podcasting of supplementary materials to students is another strategy in the use of podcasting. This allows students to explore topics in greater depth and extend their learning beyond what was received in the classroom. Ideas for podcasting include addressing most common questions from the week, bringing guest lecturers to students, weekly review of top topics, or creating a "precast" of materials prior to class to allow better preparation for in-class periods (Indiana University, Center for Teaching and Learning, 2011). A precast of materials is also a version of a flipped classroom, where traditionally lecture-style content is delivered in advance of other more active learning strategies that are used in learning activities after the podcast (Educause Learning Initiative, 2012).

Enhanced Podcasts

Enhanced podcasts are audio podcasts that include still images that are synced with the audio narration. One common format of an enhanced podcast in education is presentation-style slides with voiceover narration. The slides and audio are synched together, delivered via the distribution feed, and made playable on computers and some mobile devices. The most common file format for enhanced podcasts is the Advanced Audio Coding–encoded audio file. Another popular format is Adobe Presenter, which results in a PDF or Flash-based output file. It is important to note that not all mobile players can play every file format and the capabilities of mobile devices change rapidly. If your institution has a handheld or mobile device requirement, targeting file formats that are most compatible with those mobile devices is important. Computers and laptops are capable of playing any of the file types.

Video Podcasts (Vodcasts)

A video podcast, or *vodcast,* is a podcast that includes video. This video may include enhanced material, such as slides with synced narration, but typically it includes live-action film of the speaker or speakers. Vodcasts may be used to provide content, provide instructions or expectations for assignments, or to clarify content on a routine basis. Courses using instructor-generated video content are touted as a way to increase student engagement (Draus, Curran, & Trempus, 2014) and the social presence of the instructor (Borup, West, & Graham, 2012). One cautionary note on video formats, similar to enhanced podcasts, is that there is less compatibility across devices. For example, Adobe Flash, one of the Internet format standards for *streaming* video, is not playable on any of the Apple mobile devices. A more universally common format for all devices is MPEG4 video, or specifically H.264 codec, used for video compression. HTML5 is another popular video format that is touted to use less power on mobile devices and result in smaller file sizes. All vodcast files tend to be relatively large and therefore careful attention should be given to whether video is a necessary component to the delivery of the material. If video is essential, using shorter clips (less than 5 or 10 minutes) is desired to limit the size of the file download. The size of the playback window can also be reduced to make smaller file sizes for distribution.

Podcast and Vodcast Creation Tools

Simple audio-only files are easy to capture and may be created with a variety of portable recorders. For the most professional results, the use of a soundproof booth and special microphone will result in the best sound quality; however, at a minimum, use of a good microphone in a quiet room will result in much higher quality sound (Indiana University, Center for Teaching and Learning, 2011). Editing of audio files can be done with software such as GarageBand (Mac platform) or Audacity (Mac or PC) that is available for free via the Internet (Foster, Larmore, & Havemann, n.d.). In addition, some universities are making automated podcast systems available in special classrooms to capture live lectures (Marchand, Pearson, & Albon, 2014). This takes the time needed for recording and posting the files out of the individual faculty member's responsibilities and automates the process with technical setup and support ahead of time.

Creation tools for enhanced podcasts include the iLife suite of applications, such as GarageBand, Keynote, and iMovie, on the Mac platform. In addition, a very popular and easy-to-use tool for creation of enhanced podcasts is PowerPoint and Adobe Presenter. Using the Adobe Presenter plug-in within PowerPoint, faculty can create voice-over narrations of their slides and can output the file as streaming video (Flash), a self-contained PDF file, or a movie file. As noted earlier, not all file types are compatible with mobile players, so it is important to target formats that fit the student profile in your institution.

Creation of vodcasts involves cameras to capture the live video, and postproduction software to edit the video. Video may be captured simply by using a smartphone or built-in web cameras, or may be more professionally done with professional video cameras and microphones. Use of professional equipment will result in higher-quality audio and video in the final product. Software needed to edit and process such files includes Adobe Premiere, Adobe Presenter, and iMovie. If extensive editing of video files is required, it is recommended to have support staff that are skilled in the use of such software provide assistance in this area, as learning to use video-editing software with proficiency can be time consuming. Similar to enhanced podcasts, it is important to understand your user group when making vodcasts available and either provide multiple file formats or target those most used by your student group.

Technologies for Distance Education Clinical and Telehealth

Along with the advances and changes in technology that have enabled students to attend courses from a distance, similar technology has allowed for nursing care at a distance (Grady, 2011). *Telehealth* involves the use of electronic communication equipment to share clinical and health-related information (Health Resources Services Administration, 2012). *Telenursing* is the use of these electronic communication devices and equipment to deliver, manage, and coordinate nursing care from a distance (American Telemedicine Association, 2011). Similar technologies that are used to provide care and monitoring to remote locations might also be used in monitoring students at remote sites. Such technologies include video and audio conferencing, computers, and specialized remote monitoring equipment. Students at a distance may use the technology to perform physical assessments, interviews, and interventions at a distance (Klaassen, Schmer, & Skarbek, 2013). Use of the technology can also enable students to gain clinical experiences that may not be geographically located near them (Grady, 2011), as well as enable practice with technology that will likely increase as more health care is delivered in homes (Rutledge, Haney, Bordelon, Renaud, & Fowler, 2014).

Emerging Trends in Distance Education

A recent trend in distance education is massive open online courses (MOOCs) (Bonvillian & Singer, 2013). MOOCs enroll thousands of students in online courses that generally are free (DeSilets & Dickerson, 2013). Although the business models are still emerging on MOOCs, some that have been proposed include offering "badges," which are certificates for verified completion of the course (DeSilets & Dickerson, 2013; Pirani, 2013). Although still in its infancy, the first accredited MOOC-based degree program in a field outside of health care launched in 2014 (Mazoue, 2014), and the notion of MOOCs for credit remains an area with rapid change predicted. See Chapter 21 for further discussion about MOOCs and online education.

Another driving force affecting distance-delivered courses is the mandate for programs that deliver education across state lines to be approved within that state (Poulin & Boeke, n.d.). In 2010 the US Department of Education released its original mandate that programs receive state authorization to deliver programs across state lines. At this writing, the federal mandate calling for state authorization has been vacated, and, although it is expected that it will be reinstated at some future date, state regulations that require authorization for delivery of distance programs are still in place. For institutions that plan to deliver their programs across state lines, a clear understanding of the requirements for obtaining approvals to deliver academic credit programs within the states where students may be served is necessary.

Adapting Teaching for Distance Education

Although there are differences in the technology and intricacies of various distance education delivery systems, there are commonalities that should be considered regardless of the medium used. Primary to teaching through a distance delivery system is the understanding that there must be modifications to the style of teaching and to the materials used (Bower, Dalgarno, Kennedy, Lee, & Kenney, 2014). Planning as a team rather than individually, emphasizing content rather than process, and using a syllabus to cohesively link content are important elements of the distance education planning process. Faculty will take on the role of a facilitator or a guide in distance education (Keengwe & Kidd, 2010). In addition, faculty must ensure that distance-delivered courses include opportunities for active learning, feedback, and interaction with faculty and classmates, as well as creating an environment that respects diversity of learning styles and opinions. Although extensive supports are needed to help faculty in the use of technology, faculty must still possess a baseline in technological capabilities as well as organizational planning.

Needs Assessment

Before a distance education program is initiated, a market analysis of the need for its introduction into the proposed geographic area should be conducted to ensure adequate student enrollment numbers. Nursing education administrators have embraced distance learning because there is perceived need and demand for it. A move forward with the curriculum implies a commitment from the university that students will be able to complete a significant portion, if not all, of the academic or continuing education program through distance instruction. In addition, the target audience needs to be considered in regard to the availability of technology and access to high-speed Internet. Because so many of the current distance technologies rely on high-speed Internet, knowing where potential users have broadband access will dictate to a certain extent the strategies that will be selected. Requiring students to have a minimum level of high-speed Internet connection is one way to ensure that students will be able to use the latest technologies deployed. Following a careful market analysis of the need for the distance course or program, resources for implementing a marketing plan to introduce the course or program in a new geographic area will likely be necessary to ensure adequate registration. Once the program has been initiated, student satisfaction serves as the best method of promoting the program.

Electronic Classroom: The Teacher's View

The classroom remains an essential component of distance education delivery. However, the increasing number of web-based courses and online supplements is changing how the classroom is used for distance instruction. When electronic classrooms are needed to support all or portions of a course, the commitment to technology and the site must be considered as a long-term investment because the cost of equipping the facility will be substantial. A newly designed classroom may comprise complete multimedia systems, including computerized presentation systems and wired and wireless high-speed data networks. Visual presentation can be at the touch of a button from a single touch-panel control module. Camera control, DVR, DVD, Blu-ray DVD, CD, electronic whiteboard, and other computer-based presentation devices are typically integrated into the classroom design for quick and easy access. In addition, portable video conferencing and audiovisual equipment that can be moved to different locations gives flexibility for use in a wide variety of instructional spaces, while still using state-of-the-art technologies.

Although the need for advanced classroom technology is still present, particularly with programs that blend onsite delivery with remote delivery or use of institutionally based video conferencing, increasingly faculty can teach many portions of their content from their offices or even from home. To teach from alternate locations requires that the faculty member still have access to state-of-the-art computers with audio and video capabilities, high-speed Internet access, and technical support. With such supports in place, the faculty member may choose to teach from literally anywhere.

When the opportunity to select a totally new site within a geographic area exists, its location should be considered with respect to its centrality to population, access to public transportation, and relationship to library and computing resources. Most institutions opt to have the origin site located on an existing campus. With the commitment to distance delivery of academic programming, there must also be a financial commitment to infrastructure, including data networks and computing resources for hardware, software, ongoing faculty development and support, and instructional media. Personnel for technical support must also be included in this plan.

Orientation to technology and ongoing development are needed for faculty teaching distance education courses. Faculty must intricately understand the delivery mechanism to give full attention to the learners instead of the technology. Formative development is a desired approach because it improves specific instructional strategies and ensures a strong learning focus. If faculty are given an orientation early in their commitment to teach at a distance, they will have time and opportunity to incorporate innovative tactics into their course design and presentation style and to develop teaching materials appropriate to the technology.

Continuous and formative evaluation during the course of instruction helps ensure that teaching strategies are being implemented appropriately and that learning focus is maintained. Formative evaluation provides opportunities for adjustments and modifications to both teaching and learning so faculty and students can maintain good social presence in the learning environment for the duration of the course.

Electronic Classroom: The Student's View

When distance education technologies that include off-site learning facilities are used, a site coordinator or personnel assigned to assist with technology issues and provide student support is essential to having the program run smoothly. For programs where students attend virtual classrooms from their homes, centralized support systems must be in place to troubleshoot technology at a distance. Students using web conferencing equipment in their homes need to test and practice using such technology prior to the start of the program. Ongoing support during all class sessions is also necessary to ensure that faculty can concentrate on instruction and students can focus on learning, while support personnel assist remote learners with technical problems. Support personnel and time availability can be given to students along with options for contacting them for help via telephone, live chat, or e-mail.

Logistics of ensuring availability of library, computer, and audiovisual resources must be handled by administrative and support staff. Such resources are essential to successful course delivery; however, teaching faculty should not be expected to coordinate the plethora of these other relevant activities. Support efforts to ensure efficient registration; advising; financial aid; locating physical resources; hiring of technicians, site coordinators, or proctors; handling of syllabi and other course materials; obtaining copyright permissions; arranging travel (if a part of the instruction design); and providing other similar services are essential to the success of any distance education delivery program. Support needs will vary depending on the medium being used.

Clinical Site Development

Creating collateral clinical experiences for distance learners can be a challenge for health care educators. It may be necessary to replicate all aspects of clinical practice to meet curriculum mandates for successful skill development and competence. This requires coordination with health care agencies for creation of consistent, high-quality clinical experiences. Site visits may be required to ensure accuracy and calibration with instruction at the main campus. Preceptors and clinical coordinators may be needed to act as mentors to distant students, to ensure adequate skill development, and to support the alliance between programs and agencies.

Clinical observation is required to validate student competence; however the clinical observation may be accomplished using either direct or indirect methods of observation. These methods of observation include simulation, video technologies (synchronous and asynchronous), and computerized simulations (American Association of Colleges of Nursing, 2012). Distance video conferencing technologies can also be implemented to provide for interactive consultation. These technologies, along with other telecommunication systems, make it possible for faculty to work with students remotely, when it has been traditionally done in person. Electronic document transfer, online evaluation instruments, and collaboration over interactive networks have made it feasible to assess student performance at a distance and to guide the student's clinical experience.

Course Enhancements and Resources

Three factors identified as essential for distance instruction include course design, interaction among course participants, and instructor preparation and support (Crawford-Ferre & Wiest, 2012). In a blended approach to distance education, the learning value of the course is enhanced through the use of supplemental media and several adjunct resources that support instructional delivery and student time on task. Electronic document exchanges, e-mail, instant messaging, and audio and video interactions are necessary enhancements. These electronic tools provide faculty and students with increased opportunities for communication throughout the term of instruction. Some institutions have made available toll-free telephone numbers for enrolled students' use to facilitate their communication with faculty, registrar, financial aid advisers, and other home campus support services. Additionally, many institutions are implementing electronic portals for their distance education programs that provide a personalized online interface to all institutional support and educational activities.

Evaluation

First and foremost in evaluation of students is the issue of student authentication and verification that the student enrolled in the program is the one being assessed and evaluated in the course. The Higher Education Opportunity Act of 2008 requires programs that deliver distance-accessible courses to have verification procedures in place to ensure that the student who is admitted to a program and attending a distance accessible course is the same individual (McNabb, 2010). Currently a secure login and pass code are acceptable methods of identification; however, as new technologies for identification of students become available, additional measures may become necessary for verification of student identity (Cummings, 2012).

Ongoing evaluation of student learning provides the best measure of learning success and will provide faculty with information to improve teaching strategies and the use of technology for distance learning. Both formative and summative evaluation of distance education delivery systems should occur. Formative evaluations are extremely important for the success of the online instructor as well as the online student. These evaluations can be used to determine the student understanding of the content as well as instructor effectiveness. Simply asking the student, "What have you liked the most so far in this online class?" or "What have you liked the least so far in this online class?" is an effective way to obtain valuable feedback. Summative evaluations can also be done at the end of the course using a variety of online survey technologies. More in-depth information related to formative and summative evaluation can be found in Chapter 23.

Peer evaluation of the course by other educators familiar with technology and blended learning environments is important. Peer evaluation may occur at the local level by individuals from the school or institution, or nationally through a program such as Quality Matters. Quality Matters is a nationally recognized review process that uses evidence-based standards for online and blended courses, and certifies peer evaluators. These peer evaluators may conduct peer reviews of both online and blended courses, using an evidence-based rubric (Quality Matters, n.d.).

Student and faculty perceptions of the technology and delivery efficacy should be explored, as well as the rate of student success within the course. Reasons for student attrition should be researched and strategies designed to address any negative trends.

Evaluation data should also include the cost of the course to the university or college. Factors considered will include salaries or wages for faculty, technicians, site coordinators, and other support staff; equipment; hardware and software; potential lease fees for facilities and communication systems; travel costs for faculty; mailing or courier charges; and other resources needed for course implementation. All expenditures must be evaluated against the income generated through tuition and provided by other financial support sources.

Summary

Increased opportunities for access to higher education are becoming more readily available for students who live and work in areas remote from a central campus, as well as within a wired or wireless central community. Informational and educational technologies are regularly used to reach undergraduate and graduate nursing students, as well as registered nurses seeking nonacademic continuing education. As technology infrastructures continue to improve and increased research provides greater direction for use of selected instructional paradigms, nurse educators will find additional opportunities to design technology-rich learning environments and curricula to meet the learning needs of students.

Leaders must carefully assess data collected about distance education to set new parameters for future learning. For nursing education, it will be necessary to determine the extent to which distance delivery will be a driving force within the educational process. Will it become the single most important process? Or will it be used predominately to support other more traditional teaching–learning processes? How will it be used to provide opportunities to extend learning to global student audiences? How will distance education influence interprofessional education and other collaborative ways of learning? Can distance delivery be used to forge academic–practice partnerships to facilitate learning? Without a doubt, the advancement of computer-based data networks, innovative instructional design, and creative leadership will provide a solid platform for distance learning environments in the future.

REFLECTING ON THE EVIDENCE

1. Identify issues of concern that could inhibit or significantly delay implementation of one or more instructional distance delivery systems in your institution.
2. How can distance education technologies be used to facilitate innovative teaching and active learning experiences for faculty and a group of geographically dispersed students?
3. How might you adapt your course to be taught through a synchronous video-conferencing distance delivery system? What would be your development needs as a faculty to effectively design and implement the course?
4. Reflect on the cost factor for various approaches to teaching via distance technology. Consider both the origin and the receive sites. How might costs be minimized yet not impede effectiveness of the course delivery?
5. Design an evaluation plan for a selected distance-delivered course that includes formative and summative strategies to evaluate the effectiveness of the course.

REFERENCES

Abate, K. S. (2013). The effect of podcast lectures on nursing students' knowledge retention and application. *Nursing Education Perspectives, 34*(3), 182–185.

Allen, I. E., & Seaman, J. (2014). *Grade change: Tracking online education in the united states.* Retrieved from, http://www.onlinelearningsurvey.com.

American Association of Colleges of Nursing (AACN). (2012). *Criteria for evaluation of nurse practitioner programs.* Retrieved from, http://www.aacn.nche.edu/education-resources/evalcriteria2012.pdf.

American Association of Colleges of Nursing (AACN). (2014, August 18). *Nursing faculty shortage.* (Fact sheet). Retrieved from, http://www.aacn.nche.edu/media-relations/fact-sheets/nursing-faculty-shortage.

American Telemedicine Association. (2011). *Telehealth nursing fact sheet: ATA telehealth SIG.* Retrieved from, http://www.americantelemed.org/docs/default-document-library/fact_sheet_final.pdf?sfvrsn=2.

Billings, D. (2010). Distance education in nursing: 25 years and going strong. *CIN: Computers, Informatics, Nursing, 25*(3), 121–123.

Bonvillian, W., & Singer, S. (2013). The online challenge to higher education. *Issues in Science and Technology.* Retrieved from, http://issues.org/29-4/the-online-challenge-to-higher-education/.

Borup, J., West, R., & Graham, C. (2012). Improving online social presence through asynchronous video. *Internet and Higher Education, 15,* 195–203.

Bower, M., Dalgarno, B., Kennedy, G., Lee, M., & Kenney, J. (2014). *Blended synchronous learning: A handbook for educators.* Retrieved from, http://blendsync.org/handbook.

Crawford-Ferre, H. G., & Wiest, L. R. (2012). Effective online instruction in higher education. *The Quarterly Review of Distance Education, 13*(1), 11–14.

Cummings, J. (2012). *EDUCAUSE Comments: Financial aid fraud and identity verification.* Retrieved from, http://www.educause.edu/blogs/jcummings/educause-comments-financial-aid-fraud-and-identity-verification.

Dahlstrom, E. (2012). *ECAR study of undergraduate students and information technology, 2012.* Retrieved from, http://net.educause.edu/ir/library/pdf/ERS1208/ERS1208.pdf.

Dahlstrom, E., Walker, J., & Dzuiban, C. (2013). *ECAR study of undergraduate students and information technology, 2013.* Retrieved from, https://net.educause.edu/ir/library/pdf/ERS1302/ERS1302.pdf.

DeSilets, L., & Dickerson, P. (2013). A revolutionary journey into learning/education. *The Journal of Continuing Education in Nursing, 44*(1), 8–9.

Diaz, V., & Brown, M. (2010). *Blended learning: A report on the ELI focus session.* Retrieved from, https://net.educause.edu/ir/library/pdf/ELI3023.pdf.

Draus, P., Curran, M., & Trempus, M. (2014). The influence of instructor-generated video content on student satisfaction with and engagement in asynchronous online classes. *MERLOT Journal of Online Learning and Teaching, 10*(2), 240–254.

Educause Learning Initiative. (2012). *7 things you should know about flipped classrooms*. Retrieved from, http://www.educause.edu/library/resources/7-things-you-should-know-about-flipped-classrooms.

Fleming, B. (2013). *Trend to blend: Thoughts from the sloan-C blended learning conference 2013*. Retrieved from, http://www.eduventures.com/2013/07/trend-to-blend-thoughts-from-the-sloan-c-blended-learning-conference-2013/.

Foster, J., Larmore, J., & Havemann, S. (n.d.) The basics of educational podcasting: Enhancing the student learning experience. Retrieved from http://edis.ifas.ufl.edu/pdffiles/MB/MB00400.pdf.

Gerard, S., Kazer, M., Babington, L., & Quell, T. (2014). Past, present, and future trends of master's education in nursing. *Journal of Professional Nursing*, *30*(4), 326–332.

Grady, J. (2011). The virtual clinical practicum: An innovative telehealth model for clinical nursing education. *Nursing Education Perspectives*, *32*(3), 189–194.

Health Resources Services Administration. (2012). *Telehealth*. Retrieved from, http://www.hrsa.gov/ruralhealth/about/telehealth/.

Healthcare Information and Management Systems Society. (2011). *Position statement on transforming nursing practice through technology and informatics*. Retrieved from, http://www.himss.org/files/himssorg/handouts/himssnipositionstatementmonographreport.pdf.

Indiana University, Center for Teaching and Learning. (2011). *Academic podcasting guide*. Retrieved from, http://ctl.iupui.edu/Resources/Instructional-Technology/Academic-Podcasting-Guide.

Kala, S., Isaramalai, S., & Pohthong, A. (2010). Electronic learning and constructivism: A model for nursing education. *Nurse Education Today*, *30*, 61–66.

Keengwe, J., & Kidd, T. (2010). Towards best practices in online learning and teaching in higher education. *MERLOT Journal of Online Learning and Teaching*, *6*(2), 533–541.

Klaassen, J., Schmer, C., & Skarbek, A. (2013). Live health assessment in a virtual class: Eliminating educational burdens for rural distance learners. *Online Journal of Rural Nursing and Health Care*, *13*(2), 6–22.

Marchand, J. P., Pearson, M., & Albon, S. (2014). Student and faculty member perspectives on lecture capture in pharmacy education. *American Journal of Pharmaceutical Education*, *78*(4), 1–7.

Mazoue, J. (2014). *Beyond the MOOC model: Changing educational paradigms. Educause Review online*. Retrieved from, http://www.educause.edu/ero/article/beyond-mooc-model-changing-educational-paradigms.

McNabb, L. (2010). An update on student authentication: Implementation in context. *Continuing Higher Education Review*, *74*, 43–52.

Piaget, J. (2001). *The psychology of intelligence* (M. Piercy & D. E. Berlyne, Trans.) (2nd ed.). New York: Routledge.

Pirani, J. (2013). *A compendium of MOOC perspectives, research, and resources*. Retrieved from, http://www.educause.edu/ero/article/compendium-mooc-perspectives-research-and-resources.

Podcast. (n.d.). Retrieved from, http://en.wikipedia.org/wiki/Podcast.

Poulin, R. & Boeke, M. (n.d.) Retrieved from http://wcet.wiche.edu/advance/state-approval-history.

Quality Matters. (n.d.). Retrieved from https://www.qualitymatters.org.

Rutledge, C., Haney, T., Bordelon, M., Renaud, M., & Fowler, C. (2014). Telehealth: Preparing advanced practice nurses to address healthcare needs in rural and underserved populations. *International Journal of Nursing Education Scholarship*, *11*(1), 1–9.

Shachar, M., & Neumann, Y. (2010). Twenty years of research on the academic performance differences between traditional and distance learning: Summative meta-analysis and trend examination. *MERLOT Journal of Online Learning and Teaching*, *6*(2), 318–334.

Skillman, S., Kaplan, L., Andrilla, C., Ostergard, S., & Patterson, D. (2014). *Support for rural recruitment and practice among U.S. nurse practitioner education programs*. Policy Brief #147, Seattle, WA: WWAMI Rural Health Research Center, University of Washington.

Stanley, M., & Dougherty, J. (2010). A paradigm shift in nursing education: A new model. *Nursing Education Perspectives*, *31*(6), 378–380.

United States Department of Education. (2009). *Evaluation of evidence-based practices in online learning: A meta-analysis and review of online learning studies*. Washington, DC: U.S. Department of Education, Office of Planning, Evaluation and Policy Development, Policy and Program Studies Service. Retrieved from, https://www2.ed.gov/rschstat/eval/tech/evidence-based-practices/finalreport.pdf.

Urso, P., & Ouzts, K. (2011). *Online versus traditional nursing education: Which program meets your needs?*. Retrieved from, http://www.minoritynurse.com/article/online-versus-traditional-nursing-education-which-program-meets-your-needs.

Vogt, M., Schaffner, B., Ribar, A., & Chavez, R. (2010). The impact of podcasting on the learning and satisfaction of undergraduate nursing students. *Nursing Education in Practice*, *10*, 38–42.

Teaching and Learning in Online Learning Communities*

21

Julie McAfooes, MS, RN-BC, CNE, ANEF

Higher education may have reached a tipping point at which the question about how to deliver a course is no longer whether it should be offered online, but whether it should be offered face-to-face. Three fourths of all colleges and universities give students the choice of taking a course online, which increases to more than 90% if examining only 2-year colleges (Parker, Lenhart, & Moore, 2011). *Online learning* is no longer synonymous with *distance education*. The vast majority of institutions offer online courses to their residential students, too. And growing concern for the environment makes online delivery the "green" choice, with a 90% reduction in energy and carbon dioxide emissions because travel is not necessary (Roy, Potter, Yarrow, & Smith, 2005).

Students have embraced online learning. More than 7.1 million students who were enrolled in college in 2013, or 33.5% of the population, had taken at least one course online (Allen & Seaman, 2014). In the same survey, 66% of academic leaders agreed that online education was critical to the long-term success of their institutions, with 77% viewing achievement of learning outcomes equivalent or better with online rather than face-to-face instruction.

English-speaking countries have led the way in international higher education ever since World War II (Marginson, 2014). The West has exploited global developments in communications and information technologies to export online learning across time zones and borders. The result is a one-world approach to science, language, educational policies, and massive open online course (MOOC) offerings that have put higher education within the grasp of a geographically and socioeconomically mobile international community.

The online courses and programs offered today are just as likely to attract students who are living on campus as those who live at a distance. Indeed, even students living on campus may prefer learning from the comfort of their dorm room where they can access course information and work on their assignments when and where it is convenient for them. This increased use of online learning in higher education has occurred for a number of reasons. The learners of today expect ready access to course offerings and flexibility in scheduling to meet their educational needs (Parker & Howland, 2006). The majority of college students use laptops, smartphones, or tablets in class (Parker et al., 2011) and younger students cannot recall a time when computers and the Internet did not exist. A few students are starting to question the value of the faculty in the classroom when they perceive they can search the Internet to learn whatever they need to know (Johnson, 2014). The nursing shortage, improving quality of available technology, and existing evidence that learning outcomes from in-class courses and online courses are similar are other factors that have contributed to the proliferation of online learning (Baldwin & Burns, 2004).

Online learning has a significant presence in nursing education with an ever-expanding number of programs being offered in this mode, especially for those students who are seeking BSN completion and graduate degrees. Providers of continuing education programs also choose online technology to reach larger audiences of health care professionals who appreciate the flexibility and convenience of meeting their educational needs in their own homes. Many nursing faculty are integrating aspects of online learning into courses that are primarily

*The author acknowledges the work of Judith A. Halstead, PhD, RN, FAAN, ANEF, and Diane M. Billings, EdD, RN, FAAN, ANEF, in the previous editions of this chapter.

taught in the classroom in "real time," thus creating blended or hybrid courses that maximize the use of web-based learning resources.

For example, the "flipped classroom" is a pedagogical model that can be delivered in a variety of ways (Critz & Knight, 2013). Flipping involves altering how time in the classroom is spent (Barra, 2014). Students are expected to prepare before the class meeting by accessing online materials including readings, lectures, quizzes, videos, narrated slide presentations, and other media. The flipped classroom has spurred the conversion of face-to-face classes to blended delivery. In some instances, students and faculty may meet entirely online. Interaction is done through social networking instead of meeting face-to-face. Online learning is also facilitating the development of an international learning community within the nursing profession, as nurses from around the world discover they can access educational offerings to meet their learning needs.

Even with the increasing presence of technology in higher education, teaching in online learning communities (OLCs) remains a new experience for many nurse educators. Engaging successfully in online learning requires faculty and students to reconceptualize their roles as teachers and learners in the teaching–learning process. In addition, multiple institutional issues must be considered when the decision is made to implement online education. This chapter defines *online learning*; identifies factors that must be considered in the planning, implementation, and evaluation of online learning; and describes online course design issues. In addition, this chapter discusses the implications of online learning for the teaching–learning process, as well as the development needs for faculty and students. The chapter concludes with evidence of the effectiveness of online teaching and learning.

Online Learning Communities

Online learning uses the Internet paired with various types of software such as learning management systems (LMSs), learning content management systems, learning portals, e-learning platforms, virtual learning environments (VLEs), or course management systems (CMSs) (Wright, Lopes, Montgomerie, Reju, & Schmoller, 2014). These terms are similar but are not identical. The LMS enables the creation of a learning environment in which a community of learners and educators, as well as other content experts such as clinicians and patients, gather for the purposes of teaching and learning (Babenko-Mould, Andrusyszyn, & Goldenberg, 2004; Jafari, McGee, & Carmean, 2006). Online learning takes place in a VLE that is created by an LMS (e.g., Blackboard's Learn, Desire2Learn's Brightspace, Instructure's Canvas, Pearson's Learning Studio, and open-source Moodle). But the LMSs are aging and are, on average, at least 8 years old (Dahlstrom, Brooks, & Bichsel, 2014). Although features abound, faculty and students report an underutilization phenomenon when it comes to engagement and collaboration. This is related to user attitudes that they are ill equipped to use any but the basic features of the LMS. Digital literacy does not necessarily transfer to mastering the LMS.

The demand is increasing for platforms to be adaptable, friendly, customizable, integrated, intuitive, and, of paramount importance, mobile (Dahlstrom et al., 2014). For the most part, the LMS stores content, delivers quizzes, helps distribute assignments, facilitates communication, and publishes grades. Users report they want the LMS to do a better job with instant messaging, video chatting, online tutoring, social networking, grading, accessing multimedia, and alerting them to the need to post and turn in assignments.

The Next Generation of Digital Learning Environments Initiative, funded by the Bill and Melinda Gates Foundation, has been established to identify why higher education is using outdated technology, and how to replace it (Straumsheim, 2014). These VLEs are designed to enhance collaboration and interaction through use of shared workspaces and mobile wireless devices and to provide a full complement of learner support through access to academic advisers, mentors, preceptors, and librarians. The LMSs also typically include assessment and evaluation software such as test generation and administration software, plagiarism detection software, portfolio management software, and online grade books with grade calculation. Additionally, the online learning environment is becoming more integrated with campus services such as the bursar and registrar, thus enabling students to register for courses and receive grades and transcripts (Nelson et al., 2006). The burgeoning number of features and options has led to LMS vendors positioning themselves as solutions providers who will evaluate the customer's needs and propose custom approaches that the vendor will integrate seamlessly into the LMS.

In nursing education, online learning is frequently used to offer individual courses and complete degree programs for academic credit. In clinical settings, online learning may be used to facilitate orientation to clinical practice, meet requirements for mandatory continuing education, and create learning communities to support career development, mentoring, and coaching programs for nurses (Billings et al., 2006; Pullen, 2006). Online learning is a popular means by which nurses participate in lifelong learning and obtain continuing education contact hours.

Educators and learners use the capabilities of online learning in various ways. For example, content may be developed in self-contained *learning modules,* or tutorials. Online learning modules typically contain objectives, learning outcomes, learning activities, and an evaluation component. Because of their self-contained nature, learning modules are flexible and lend themselves to multiple uses. For example, learning modules are useful for providing access to information that can be learned without interaction with faculty or classmates and colleagues. Learning modules can also be used to provide clinical updates, "mandatory" education required in clinical agencies, or background material in preparation for higher-order application in a classroom or clinical setting. Modules are often integrated into classroom or online courses as reusable learning objects (RLOs), predeveloped content with objectives, content, and evaluation that can be used in courses as required or optional learning activities. It is increasingly common for RLOs to accompany textbooks as ancillary teaching materials; they are also available from web-based learning resource repositories such as MERLOT (http://merlot.org).

Online learning can occur in a variety of configurations to support learning in a course. The courses may be designed to be offered fully online, as full-web courses, in which faculty and students do not meet in person. Typically these are courses that include primarily didactic content, but increasingly clinical courses with a preceptor are offered fully online. The preceptor is usually a qualified clinician in the student's geographic region who facilitates application of the course concepts in a clinical setting.

Online courses can also be developed to integrate with face-to-face meetings in classrooms or clinical practice. These blended courses, also referred to as *web-enhanced, web-supported,* or *hybrid* courses, combine the benefits of face-to-face, classroom, or clinical experiences with the OLC (Bonk & Graham, 2005). Here, the educator uses online assignments such as pretests or case studies to assess student knowledge and facilitate learning course concepts before students participate in face-to-face classroom activities. The educator may even decide to deliver a short online video or audio stream on selected course concepts prior to class. Students can receive feedback about their learning before they come to the classroom, and thus faculty and students are better prepared to use classroom time to clarify misunderstood concepts or focus on more complex problems such as those related to developing clinical decision-making skills. Blended courses can use a combination of technologies to meet the needs of students. For example, for those students who are enrolled in the course but live far away from the campus, one-way or two-way web-based video conferencing may be used to "connect" students to the class during the times of on-campus class meetings. The goal of blended learning is to take advantage of faculty expertise, the learning management toolkit, and just-in-time learning to provide learners with opportunities to learn and apply content, practice and receive feedback, think critically, and assume the role of the nurse across all domains of learning. The educator must make well-thought-out decisions as to which experiences should be held in the classroom and which should be held in the OLC. Table 21-1 offers suggestions for blending learning in classroom, clinical, and laboratory settings with an online learning environment.

Interactions in online learning may occur asynchronously or synchronously, depending on the desired nature of the interaction. *Asynchronous* interactions are those that do not depend on time and place. E-mail, threaded discussions in discussion forums, podcasts, and archived video and audio streams are examples of interactions that are asynchronous. Participants involved in an asynchronous interaction can choose to access or respond to the communication at a time that is convenient for them. *Synchronous* interactions are those that occur in real time and require participants to be available at a specific time to participate in the discussions.

TABLE 21-1 Blending Online Teaching with Various Learning Environments

Classroom, Clinical, or Laboratory Learning Environments	Online Learning Environment
Demonstration of psychomotor skills and clinical decision-making skills with simulated or standardized patient scenarios	Assessment and evaluation of student learning through self-testing, practice testing, administration of summative tests Use of simulated and virtual case studies; problem-based learning scenarios Video streams of clinical skills, including students' own return demonstration
Discussion of difficult-to-learn content; clarification of assignments	Discussion forums in which students can lead or manage the application of content without direct guidance from the faculty Peer review of work, where students provide feedback to each other Study guides
Clinical practice (with or without preceptor or faculty)	Reflective learning assignments, such as journaling or follow-up debriefing after simulated or actual clinical experiences Written care plans, concept maps Written assignments requiring synthesis of clinical concepts and experiences
Demonstration of verbal and nonverbal communication skills requiring interpretation and feedback; modeling of professional values and behaviors; evaluation of student presentation style and abilities	Preparation for class by completing mastery test or worksheet Reaction and reflection papers following classroom discussion or laboratory demonstration Personal application of course concepts in response to a focused question Follow-up to in-class assignments
Panel discussions with guest speakers when online presentations are not feasible	Preparation for panel discussion through reading assignments, study guides Reflection on classroom discussion and application of content to own nursing practice Online debates on topic
Clinical practice situations requiring feedback to prevent or reverse an error	Active learning strategies designed to focus on fostering culture of safety and prevention of errors such as root cause analysis, case studies, debate, 1-minute papers, and self-paced learning modules
Administration of high-stakes examinations and psychomotor skills competency validation	Self-evaluation activities; optional learning activities for testing or enhancing learning; remediation learning options

Class meetings using live video conferencing, chat rooms, or webcasts (use of Internet to share information on a desktop through the use of web-based conferencing software) are examples of synchronous interactions. It is also possible to use e-mail or instant messaging in a synchronous fashion, if those involved in the e-mail messaging prearrange the time for sending and responding to the messages. Electronic "office hours" during which the faculty member is available to promptly answer any student e-mails sent during that period is an example of using e-mail in a synchronous fashion.

Regardless of the type of online course the faculty member is teaching, it is important to remember that it is the use of educational practices such as interaction between students and faculty, interaction among classmates, opportunity to receive feedback while learning, and respect for diverse ways of learning that promote interaction, prevent isolation, and ultimately determine students' satisfaction with the learning experience and the attainment of intended outcomes. The remainder of this chapter provides information that will help faculty to successfully plan, implement, and evaluate learning experiences that will promote the development of OLCs.

Institutional Planning for Online Learning

Many issues must be considered when the decision is made to engage in online education. To successfully plan, implement, and evaluate online education, institutions and individual programs must identify how the government and accrediting organizations influence their decisions.

Judith Eaton (2014), the president of the Council for Higher Education, has described the Higher Education Act as where the federal government, colleges and universities, and accreditation meet.

The U.S. Department of Education spends approximately $30 billion a year to subsidize higher education through student aid and institutional grants (Edwards & McCluskey, 2009). Eaton (2014) asserts that the department has been calling into question the effectiveness of accreditation to establish and evaluate quality in educational institutions. The Higher Education Act is one way for the government to assume more control over accreditation, but this may diminish academic freedom, institutional autonomy, and peer review (Eaton, 2014). Others argue that breaking the stranglehold that accreditation has on colleges and universities will free them to explore innovative approaches to teaching and learning, including those delivered online, that would be less likely to achieve accreditation.

Institutions must identify the needed infrastructure for online education, how it will be sustained, and how faculty and student development and support needs will be met. It is common for planning committees consisting of administrators, technology staff, student support personnel, and faculty to be charged with addressing and monitoring these issues. The various perspectives of each of these individuals are important when designing a model for online education that can be sustained within the institution. Policies and procedures specific to online education may need to be developed within the institution.

Before implementing online education, the institution and program need to give some consideration to how offering online courses or programs fits with the mission of the institution. Administrators and faculty should be clear about the forces that are driving the desire to deliver online education. Is the institution or nursing program interested in primarily serving and retaining the current student population, or to extending course or program offerings to a wider target audience, maybe even serving a global market? An understanding of the reasons for engaging in online education will help guide marketing decisions. Before an online course or program is developed, it can be helpful to conduct an environmental scan to gauge the market and identify which other universities are offering online education and the nature of the courses offered online. What niche does the proposed course or program fill that is not being met by another institution? A needs assessment can also be conducted among prospective students to identify the level of interest in enrollment in an online course or program and the reasons for their interest in online education, as well as the level of computer skills and availability of Internet access present within the targeted population. Having this information before an online offering is planned can help ensure that the learners' educational needs will be met.

It is also important to acknowledge that some of the most strategic marketing of online education may need to occur "internally" within the institution (Billings, 2002). Online education is still new to many faculty, students, and administrators. Faculty who are "early adopters" of technology and online education will need to communicate the potential advantages of online learning to faculty who are more skeptical.

Institutions have reported that using benchmark standards helps ensure quality in online courses (Leners, Wilson, & Sitzman, 2007; Little, 2009). To promote the development of quality online education courses and programs, quality indicators and benchmarks have been established by professional organizations and accrediting bodies for institutions to use when planning online programs and courses.

There are numerous regulatory influences on the delivery of online and distant learning. At the federal level, the U.S. Department of Education has state authorization policies that are tied to Title IV funding (Field, 2014). Distance programs must demonstrate compliance with laws in each state in which they operate or their students are not eligible for federal grants and loans.

Most states have established guidelines for the delivery of distance education through the government bodies that regulate higher education, which include state boards of nursing. At times, there is conflict between a state's board of education and board of nursing in terms of what each requires for approval of distance education programs. This can cause confusion for a nursing program that must satisfy both.

There can be wide variation in the regulations among the boards of education and nursing within a state. In addition, there is variation in the regulations among the boards of nursing in the U.S. The National Council of State Boards of Nursing (NCSBN) has examined the regulations for distance education among the boards of nursing and has found inconsistencies in requirements. One example is for faculty who teach clinical and didactic courses (Lowery & Spector, 2014). Some states require that faculty hold licenses only in the home state where the program is located. Others require that faculty be licensed not only in the home state but also in the host states where the students reside and participate in clinical. Sometimes these requirements change depending on whether the course taught is a didactic or clinical course. Other differences pertain to the qualifications, licensing, and monitoring of preceptors. Online programs find that they may be blocked from offering their programs to potential nursing students in a particular state because they cannot satisfy every boards' conflicting requirements.

Boards of nursing are encouraged to consider adopting the Middle States Commission on Higher Education Interregional Guidelines for the Evaluation of Distance Education (Lowery & Spector, 2014).These have already been endorsed by all regional accrediting organizations and organizations that participate in the National Council for State Authorization Reciprocity Agreement. The nationally accepted guidelines reflect institutional, faculty, and curricular themes.

Regulatory guidelines for prelicensure programs have been developed by the NCSBN Distance Learning Education Committee. These include the following:

1. The guidelines for approval should be the same for distance programs as the home state where the program is located.
2. The home state's board of nursing approves the prelicensure program, which includes the distance component.
3. The home state program supervises prelicensure students in the host states.
4. Those who teach clinical experiences to prelicensure students in distance programs must hold a current, active license in the state where the patient is located. Faculty who only teach didactic content need a current, active license in the program's home state.
5. Boards of nursing will report on prelicensure student clinical students in host states.

These best practices, if adopted, help ensure that the innovations made possible by technology to offer nursing programs at a distance are carried out in a manner that maintains quality and safety for patients receiving care from prelicensure nursing students.

Examples of frequently referenced quality indicators include those established by the Online Learning Consortium (2014), formerly known as the Sloan Consortium or Sloan-C. The Online Learning Consortium promotes online learning worldwide through research and development of best practices that are disseminated through various publications and conferences. The Institute for Higher Education Policy (Hunter & Krantz, 2010) is another entity that sets quality indicators and benchmarks. Quality Matters (QM, 2014) is a nonprofit organization that sets national benchmarks for online course design. These organizations identify essential elements that must be addressed to ensure quality in online education: institutional support and commitment; effective course design and teaching–learning principles, faculty development, support, and satisfaction; student support and satisfaction; and outcome evaluation related to learning effectiveness. How each institution decides to address these elements will vary depending on the resources available to the institution and the specific needs of educators and learners.

Accrediting agencies expect that online courses and programs will provide learners with access to learning experiences that achieve the same learning outcomes of traditional "in-class" courses and programs. Online students should receive the same level of support, socialization, and skill development as their counterparts on campus. Faculty need to develop their expertise in using technology for teaching and learning. Everyone must be given adequate technical support. Specific accreditation policies and standards may be written to govern distance and online students such as verification of the identity of the student. The three professional nursing accrediting bodies, the Commission on Collegiate Nursing Education, the Accreditation Commission for Education in Nursing (ACEN), and the Commission for Nursing Education Accreditation (CNEA), have established standards for distance education programs that state the expectation that learner outcomes will be evaluated using appropriate methodology and with the same rigor associated with traditional face-to-face courses (Accreditation Commission for Education in Nursing [ACEN], 2014; American Association of Colleges of Nursing [AACN], 2007; National League for Nursing Commission for Nursing Education Accreditation, 2015). In addition, many institutions have internal approval processes that must be followed to approve a course or program for online delivery before it can be offered to students. Faculty should familiarize themselves with the guidelines that apply to their particular state, institution, and program as they undertake the planning of online learning programs.

A growing challenge for accrediting agencies is their role in evaluating the quality of MOOCs as more colleges and universities explore this avenue for delivering their product (Eaton, 2012).

Institutional Planning and Commitment

At the institutional level, decisions must be made about the institution's commitment to online education in terms of human, fiscal, and physical resources. Organizational and administrative infrastructure, funding sources, technology support services, and student support services are areas that will need to be addressed. For example, who within the institution's organizational structure will provide administrative oversight for the development, implementation, and evaluation of online education? Does the institution already employ the technical and instructional design personnel needed to provide course design and delivery support or will additional positions need to be created and funded? A decision will also need to be made as to which of these services will be centralized within the institution or decentralized to the respective academic units.

How the development, implementation, and evaluation of online courses and programs will be funded is another crucial area in which decisions will need to be made. Although many online nursing programs are initially developed with the use of grant funds, it is important that sustainability of grant-funded initiatives be addressed. It is likely that student technology fees or distance education fees will need to be assessed in addition to tuition fees to sustain online education within the institution. If such technology or distance education fees are collected by the institution, further decisions will need to be made about how the funds will be dispersed across the academic and service units within the institution.

What is the cost of developing an online course? The answer varies. The University of Minnesota (2013) has published its "good, better, best model" for estimating the cost of online course development. It was acknowledged that the ongoing cost of providing each type of course increased according to its complexity and quality. The "good" approach minimizes costs by reusing didactic content already in digital format and using only features already included in the LMS that can meet the instructional goals of the course. The "better" model allowed for some additional instructional methods such as interactive modules. The technological infrastructure would be reused. The "best" model extends the benefits of the instructional approaches to allow for the creation of special media or programming.

Reliable and effective technology support for faculty and students is essential for delivering quality online education. As mentioned previously, a decision will need to be made about which technology support services will be centralized within the institutional structure and which will be decentralized in the individual schools and programs. A combination of centralized and decentralized support may be a more effective support model. Outsourcing support services is another option to be considered, and may be more economically feasible depending on the extent of technology expertise that already exists within the institution. The level and extent of technology support that the institution will provide to faculty and students will also need to be determined (Halstead & Coudret, 2000). Many institutions have found it necessary to provide around-the-clock support services to faculty and students to limit undue frustration and "down time" related to technology issues. Faculty and student satisfaction with online learning is frequently related to their satisfaction with technology support services.

The acquisition and maintenance of the hardware and software necessary to support online education and facilitate access is another area that must receive serious institutional attention. Is the institution's current computer network system and bandwidth capable of providing online access to large numbers of simultaneous users with speed and reliability, or are upgrades required? Do faculty have convenient access to the hardware and software needed to support teaching online? Is there a plan to replace computer hardware and software on a regular schedule in faculty offices and student computer clusters to maintain access to adequate technology resources? Do students have access to broadband Internet services in their geographic region? If not, online courses will have to be developed with these bandwidth constraints in mind and content delivery options that require large amounts of bandwidth, such as video streaming, will need to be minimized or avoided (Richard, Mercer, & Bray, 2005).

It is also important for the institution to make a decision about which LMS software will be used to support the delivery and management of online courses. Selecting an LMS may be the most important software decision that a college or university may make (Wright et al., 2014). The LMS can be the most liked, or most disliked, application at an institution. A selection committee may be formed to set the criteria for evaluation, and the process for determining which LMS to choose.

There are a variety of commercial vendors and LMSs from which to choose. Some of the larger university systems have chosen to design and support their own CMSs. Using an LMS to deliver online courses provides faculty with a relatively easy-to-use, consistent template on which to build their courses. It also provides students with a consistent learning environment with which they can become familiar, transferring this knowledge from course to course. There are advantages and disadvantages associated with each of the various commercial programs available; each institution needs to evaluate the programs to determine which will best meet the needs of the university's faculty and students.

A major decision is whether to select a proprietary, open source, or cloud-based system. Proprietary LMSs are built by professionals, use current technology to remain competitive, offer training, provide technical support, and may come with a warranty. But proprietary systems can be expensive and limit customization options.

Open-source systems such as Moodle and Sakai have a low upfront cost and are built by a collaborative community (Wright et al., 2014). These customizable systems are attractive to faculty who have a troubled history with proprietary systems. But open-source systems may not integrate with existing administrative systems, require more money to operate than anticipated, and lack technical support.

Cloud-based systems are composed of separate cloud-based tools to form a toolbox of web resources, including document sharing, social networking, and media delivery platforms. For example, Facebook serves as a hub for sharing course activities. iTunes U delivers course content. Skype offers face-to-face interaction. YouTube hosts and streams video lectures. Flickr houses photographs. Students and faculty may already be comfortable using these popular tools that are available at little to no cost. But these may be misconceptions. A free application comes with a cost for advanced features that may be necessary to use it for online learning. Users may not be as savvy as assumed, and training may be unavailable. Authentication, which is required by accreditors, is not provided by these tools and other software must be purchased to perform this function. Security and privacy must be safeguarded. Contingency plans should be in place to handle problems that the institution does not control such as poor maintenance, shut downs for repairs, and even ceasing to operate.

The institution will also need to consider the means by which ongoing faculty and student development for teaching and learning with technology will be provided. Faculty development issues that will need to be addressed include intellectual property policies and ownership of any developed online courses; policies related to providing additional compensation and release time, if any, for faculty who design and teach online courses; and the amount and type of resources that will be provided to help facilitate faculty designing online courses and transitioning to online teaching. The institution or program may also wish to consider questions about what the average student enrollment numbers should be in online courses. Student development issues are primarily related to ensuring that students have the technology access and skills needed to participate in online learning and facilitating student transition to online learning.

Adequate institutional planning to address questions similar to those raised in the preceding paragraphs is essential to ensuring the success of any online education efforts. It is also important that an institutional infrastructure be established that allows for such planning efforts to be ongoing and include input from all stakeholders, as constant advancements in educational technology will need to be monitored for the institution to stay current and informed about developing trends in online education.

Faculty Development and Support

The advances in educational technology have changed the way that teaching and learning occurs (Pearsall, Hodson-Carlton, & Flowers, 2012). Faculty who are expert teachers in the classroom may find themselves in the role of a novice when teaching online.

Faculty who are facing the transition from in-class to online teaching need to reconsider their role in the learning process and redesign their pedagogical strategies to facilitate student learning (Ali et al., 2005; Richard et al., 2005; Ryan, Hodson-Carlton, & Ali, 2005; Zsohar & Smith, 2008). A growing number of faculty now teach full-time at a distance from the location of their employer. They seldom, if ever, meet face-to-face with their administrators, colleagues, and students. Although many may find the faculty-at-a-distance nurse educator (FDNE) option to be attractive, it does present challenges (Pearsall et al., 2012). When asked about hiring, acceptance, and success of the FDNE, nurse educators and administrators identified attitudinal barriers as of most concern. Part of faculty development needs to address the perceptions of the FDNE role and how it can promote nursing education excellence through achievement of the National League for Nursing nurse educator competencies.

Faculty development needs encompass the following areas: instructional design and course development, technology management, workload and time management, role reconceptualization, student learner development, student–faculty interactions and socialization, and assessment and evaluation of learner outcomes (Halstead & Coudret, 2000; Lahaie, 2007b; Pearsall et al., 2012).

Before faculty begin any online course development, it is important to assess their knowledge and comfort level regarding conversion of traditional classroom courses into online courses and identify what level of instructional design support will be needed. Developing expertise in online teaching is usually a gradual learning process for faculty and initially may be intimidating even for experienced faculty (Zsohar & Smith, 2008). Scheduling an ongoing series of educational sessions focused on such topics as technology and time management, developing online courses that promote active learning and foster student–faculty interactions, and evaluating learner outcomes throughout the academic year can help faculty acquire the knowledge and skills necessary to successfully design and teach online courses. These topics are covered in more depth later in this chapter.

Faculty Tenure and Promotion

A major issue is how faculty are rewarded for their hard work developing and teaching online courses. New processes are needed to reflect changing needs in workload, promotion, and tenure for online faculty (Kelly, n.d.). The biggest question is whether teaching online requires more or less time when compared with teaching face to face. There is debate about this issue (Van de Vord & Pogue, 2012). The answer is that it depends on the skills of the individual faculty member and the design of the course. For example, one's ability to type on a keyboard is a major factor in the time spent communicating electronically in online discussion, whereas typing proficiency is a negligible consideration for those who are interacting with students in person. Faculty may find that grading hard copies of assignments with red ink is much easier than employing software tools such as comments and tracked changes to provide feedback on electronic submissions.

Preparing teaching materials for an online class has been likened to making a movie. The course is created ahead of time and presented to the students as mostly a finished product. Teaching in the classroom has been compared to performing in a play. There is preplanning, but the delivery is done in real-time before a live audience. Designing, recording, and programming a lesson for online delivery may take considerable time and effort, but once it is finished, it can be shown repeatedly to many students. A stand-up lecture may involve less preparation and more spontaneity, but must be presented in person every time it is taught.

When asked to keep time logs, one aspect of teaching online that stood out as requiring significant amounts of time was grading assignments (Barra, 2014). This may be attributed more to the fact that the subject matter that is typically taught online may not lend itself to objective testing. Instead, evaluation may require that faculty grade papers, projects, and other written assignments that do not lend themselves to quick, computerized evaluation.

Class discussion is another factor to consider. A face-to-face class has a "hard" start and stop and this places limits on how much time the faculty member will interact with the students regardless of class size. But online discussion has no time boundary, and faculty may spend hours responding to students in discussion threads.

Another question about online teaching is whether the devotion to this format reduces productivity in other areas that could affect promotion and tenure (Kelly, n.d.). This influences their portfolios that are submitted for review.

Institutions need to have policies in place but they may vary from department to department. Leadership at the department level influences how online teaching is valued and rewarded. Although the institution may say that online delivery is the way of the future and critical to its success, is this reflected in how the faculty are rewarded who teach online? Are faculty paid extra or given release time to develop an online course? How does authoring a course compare to authoring a book? Faculty who teach face-to-face courses may be resistant to anything that encourages online offerings and may block changes to tenure and promotion policies. The climate and culture of the department is reflected in how receptive its members are to change. The department or program leader plays a pivotal role in setting the direction and explaining the effect of online teaching on workload, promotion, and tenure.

The American Association of University Professors (AAUP) noted in a 2009 report (Committee on Contingency and the Profession, 2009) that almost 70% of faculty members were employed in non-tenure track positions. Although faculty teaching in traditional programs on campus tended to be tenured, faculty teaching online were more likely to be hired on a contingent basis. The report noted that contingent faculty worked for lower wages in teaching-only positions. The AAUP is calling for the organizing of contingent, or adjunct, faculty. The organization argues that contingency is an issue of academic freedom. Also, adjunct faculty who do not view their teaching as their primary source of income still depend on it to maintain their lifestyle. But adjunct faculty may resist organizing because they value the flexibility that the position offers to carve out time for child care or elder care, for example. Part-time online faculty may be a "tough sell" (Kociemba, 2014).

Learner Development and Support

Introducing online education into a program will have a major effect on the delivery of learner support services, especially if the introduction of online education affects more than just a few individual courses. All aspects of the institution's student support services will ultimately be affected and need to be reconsidered to best serve the needs of students who are geographically distant from the campus, as well as those who are on campus (Mills, Fisher, & Stair, 2001; Nelson, 2007). It is a requirement of national higher education accrediting bodies, as well as nursing accrediting bodies, that the academic support services for online students be similar to those available for on-campus students (Baldwin & Burns, 2004). Student support that will need to be reconsidered and redesigned for students who enroll in online programs include academic advising, tutoring, financial aid, library, and bookstore services. Ensuring that all online experiences are accessible to students with disabilities is another important institutional consideration (Nelson, 2007). The admission and registration processes may also need to be restructured so that students who live at a distance will be able to accomplish these tasks without being physically present on campus.

The decision to deliver online education will also result in the need for the institution to make financial decisions regarding tuition costs and any additional student technology or distance education fees. Many universities or colleges automatically charge students on-campus usage fees, such as activity fees and parking fees. Will these fees be waived for students who never come to campus? These decisions and others related to the delivery of student support services will require the consideration and collaboration of numerous departments in the institution so that students will have a quality learning experience.

Faculty should proactively address the development needs of students engaging in online learning. Learners who are new to online learning frequently need some initial guidance in how to manage their time when they are taking online courses. The relatively independent nature of online education requires students to understand that they are assuming responsibility for their own learning to an extent with which they may be unaccustomed (Johnston, 2008). They are moving from the structure of the traditional classroom to a more unstructured learning environment that does not necessarily include the physical, face-to-face presence of faculty and peers and the weekly time commitment to attend class. Some students may assume that an online course will be "easier" than a traditional course, a notion that is usually quickly dismissed after the course begins and they become overwhelmed with the independence that an online course allows them in managing their own time to meet their learning needs. It is easy for students to underestimate the amount of self-direction and self-pacing that is needed to be successful in online learning.

Faculty can help students by clearly identifying expectations for participation and due dates for assignments (Beitz & Snarponis, 2006; Zsohar & Smith, 2008). If weekly online discussion is expected, this should be stated in the course syllabus. During the first two to three weeks of the course, those students who are not participating in the course should be actively sought out. The lack of participation is likely due to technology issues or the inability to be self-directive in learning (Halstead & Coudret, 2000). Reaching out to the student at this critical point in the course may make a difference in whether the student will be successful in completing the course.

Students will also require an orientation to the CMS and any other technology that they may be required to use in their coursework. Although orientation to technology can occur face-to-face or using printed materials, Carruth, Broussard, Waldmeier, Gauthier, and Mixon (2010) developed a 5-day online orientation course for graduate students who lacked sufficient technological skills to be effective learners in their online course. Evaluations indicated that the students had improved technology proficiency and, because attrition for students who did not have the necessary technology skills was reduced, the course is now required. The institution needs to consider how it can provide orientation to technology for distant learners, as well as technology support when students encounter problems.

In addition to an orientation to support services, students who enroll in online programs also need an orientation to the institution, school, and program. The institution needs to consider how best to establish relationships and "create a sense of presence" (Nelson, 2007, p. 188) with students who may attend the institution only from a distance yet will obtain a degree and become alumni. Effective use of websites, social networking, and virtual tours of the campus can help form connections that will lead to satisfactory student–institution relationships. The "Facebook effect" can promote social networking that leads to increased engagement, cultivates classroom community, and stimulates intellectual discourse (Hurt et al., 2012).

Assessment and Evaluation of Online Learning

Faculty and administrators also need to give consideration to how online courses and programs will be assessed and evaluated to determine whether curriculum and program outcomes are being met, as well as for the purpose of continuous quality improvement (Billings, 2000). Effectiveness of online courses and programs can be measured using a variety of methods. As mentioned previously, quality indicators and benchmarks, as well as accreditation standards, provide guidelines for measuring program quality.

For example, QM is a not-for-profit organization that sets a "national benchmark for online course design" (Quality Matters [QM], 2014). Although faculty performance is not assessed, faculty are trained to conduct collegial and collaborative peer reviews to determine if the standards are met in online and blended learning courses. Faculty may become certified peer reviewers by successfully meeting the requirements through online or face-to-face training. Courses that meet the standards may carry the QM certification mark. The standards for the QM rubric encompass:

- Course overview and introduction
- Learning analytics
- Assessment and measurement
- Instructional materials
- Course activities and learner interaction
- Course technology
- Learner support
- Accessibility and usability

A systematic evaluation plan can be established that will foster continuous, ongoing quality improvement efforts in all aspects of program delivery: institutional support, faculty satisfaction, student satisfaction, adequacy of technology and student–faculty support services, and effectiveness in meeting expected learner outcomes, including a comparison to traditional course offerings. Data regarding student enrollment numbers, academic progression, and graduation can be compiled to address retention concerns. Data related to established program outcomes can be collected to demonstrate effectiveness of selected pedagogical strategies (Broome, Halstead, Pesut, Rawl, & Boland, 2011; Hunter & Krantz, 2010). Rubrics can also be established to assist faculty with their own and peer review of their online courses (Blood-Siegfried et al., 2008).

Faculty Role in Online Learning

The faculty member's role as an educator undergoes a change when he or she is teaching online courses (Halstead, 2002). First of all, real-time, face-to-face interaction with students becomes more limited, with many interactions occurring asynchronously. Most important, in online courses the educator is less likely to be the primary source of information for students. Instead, the educator's role becomes one of facilitating students' learning experiences. Students assume more responsibility for identifying their own learning needs and being self-directed in how they choose to meet identified learning outcomes. For some faculty who are new to online teaching, this results in feeling a loss of control over the learning process. Teaching online may require faculty to rethink long-held beliefs about the role of the educator in the teaching–learning process and explore new paradigms of teaching (Shovein, Huston, Fox, & Damazo, 2005).

Becoming a "facilitator" of learning, however, does not lessen the need for the educator or the importance of the educator's role in the learning process. The educator retains responsibility for identifying the expected outcomes of the course, designing learning activities that will promote active student involvement in the learning process and higher-order thinking, and evaluating student performance. Facilitating online discussion is another important role for faculty who are teaching online (Bristol & Kyarsgaard, 2012). Faculty should encourage peer interaction rather than student–instructor conversation. There should be variety in the types of discussion, which may include reflection, critical thinking, and postclinical conferencing. Clear grading rubrics to evaluate discussion provide timely feedback to students, so that they will know whether they are achieving the desired learning outcomes.

Two common concerns of faculty who are engaged in online teaching for the first time are related to how to facilitate and manage asynchronous online discussion and how to manage time most effectively. Faculty have indicated that their workload increases when they engage in online teaching (Ryan et al., 2005). In their comparison of faculty workload in web-based and face-to-face graduate nursing courses, Anderson and Avery (2008) found that, although the amount of faculty teaching time did not increase in a statistically significant manner in online courses, there were differences in the amount of time spent in course preparation and student contact time, with those faculty teaching online courses reporting more time devoted to each of these activities. More research is needed to more fully understand the demands on faculty workload created by online teaching.

Managing Online Discussion

Time management frequently becomes an issue for faculty teaching online courses because of the amount of student communication generated within the course. The communication generated by students in online courses can be overwhelming if the educator has not given some prior thought to how to manage it. Successful management of asynchronous discussion requires the educator to initially identify the purpose of the discussion and to be sure that all students are contributing to the discussion (Halstead, 2002). As the online discussion unfolds, the educator may find it necessary at times to change the direction of the discussion or to correct any factual errors students may have made in their postings. However, faculty usually serve as discussion facilitators (Zsohar & Smith, 2008). It is not desirable to respond to every comment made by students in online discussion; faculty should strive to avoid dominating the conversation, reserving their comments to emphasize or summarize key concepts, praise students and provide feedback as appropriate, and make other similar contributions.

Because online courses promote student flexibility and convenience in learning, students tend to access the course, post comments, and send e-mails to faculty at all hours of the day, 7 days a week. That is why it is essential to implement time management strategies before the course begins. By having a plan in place, faculty can respond to student comments in a timely manner while still retaining a sense of control.

Some strategies for managing online communication that have proven helpful include (1) deciding how quickly to respond to student inquiries (e.g., within 48 hours) and informing students of this time frame so that they will know when to anticipate an answer; (2) establishing individual student electronic file folders in which to retain a record of course communication; (3) using a separate e-mail account or the learning or CMS e-mail option for student communications, so that student e-mail is automatically separated from other professional or personal correspondence; (4) establishing "electronic" office hours to interact with students; and (5) creating and saving standardized responses to the most commonly asked questions that can be quickly accessed and individualized for students. Faculty may also find it helpful to "block out" scheduled amounts of time each week to devote to the online course.

Another means of managing online communication is to have students provide peer feedback to postings in the discussion forums. Students can critique posted assignments, lead and summarize group discussions, and participate in collaborative group learning activities. Students can be responsible for synthesizing and analyzing the responses in the forum, thus providing faculty and classmates from other groups an opportunity to respond to summarized work. Faculty can appoint and rotate student discussion leaders to provide opportunities for all students to experience a leadership role. Not only do these techniques foster timely feedback and reduce sole reliance on the faculty for feedback, but they also promote active learning (Phillips, 2005). These strategies also work to effectively manage discussion in classes that have larger enrollments.

Managing Large Enrollments in Online Courses

Educator shortages, increased student enrollment, and pressures to admit additional students to nursing programs have led to faculty teaching classes with larger enrollments, including traditional online courses. Although there is no evidence to indicate that the quality of teaching and learning is less in larger classes such that students are dissatisfied, faculty are responsible for ensuring quality learning experiences in their courses and need to consider strategies for facilitating learning when course enrollment increases.

What is a large class? The answer to this question depends on the nature of the student (beginner or advanced, graduate or undergraduate); the type of content (simple or complex, easy to learn or difficult to learn, applied in similar or novel circumstances); the experience of the faculty (novice or expert); and the design of the course (first time, in draft form and well designed, tested and revised). Current evidence indicates that, in general, an online class size of 20 can be taught by one faculty member (Colwell & Jenks, 2006). One study revealed no significant difference in student perception of quality in online discussion between small (12 students) and medium (25 students) class size (Bristol & Kyarsgaard, 2012). Some authors have indicated 25 students to be an appropriate enrollment for an online course (Lahaie, 2007b). A few institutions have established a maximum enrollment for online courses because of the increased time commitment for the faculty. Policies regarding class size vary among institutions.

When teaching a traditional online course with large enrollments, faculty must ensure that the course is designed for maximum learning, educational practices are designed to promote learning, and discussion forums are managed to foster higher-order learning. For courses in which enrollment surpasses 15 or so students, it may be more effective to divide the students into smaller discussion groups. These smaller groups encourage interactions among students while allowing faculty to focus on the outcomes of individual and group work.

The amount of time spent providing feedback to and grading students' work increases as class size increases. Faculty can choose teaching and evaluation strategies that promote learning while limiting the faculty time required to respond to nonsignificant issues. Fewer carefully designed assignments that prompt practice and feedback and foster higher order learning are preferable to more assignments that require the faculty or students to process information in lower levels of the cognitive or affective domains. As described earlier, faculty can also create opportunities for feedback that students themselves and their classmates are capable of providing. Faculty can also use "sampling" strategies for grading, whereby faculty read only selected portions of student writing during formative development of written work or read only selected (but varied) portions of care plans, reflection papers, journals, and other written work that is in formative development. Finally, the use of grading rubrics makes expectations clear to students, maximizes the likelihood of success on the assignment, and simplifies the grading process for faculty.

Teaching assistants may be used to help manage the communication generated by larger classes (Parker & Howland, 2006). Depending on the knowledge and preparation of the teaching assistant, teaching assistants can grade papers, facilitate discussion, provide feedback to drafts, answer questions, and assist students with technology problems. Teaching in an online course as a teaching assistant or teaching practicum is one way to prepare nurses and students for future roles as educators.

Despite the potential increase in time demands for faculty who teach online, faculty do experience the same convenience and flexibility in teaching online courses as students enrolled in online courses do. With careful planning, faculty can incorporate their responsibilities for online teaching into their schedules at a time that is most convenient for them. Faculty can remain in contact with their students even when they are traveling and attending professional conferences. Online teaching helps to promote maximum flexibility in balancing the demands of the various aspects of the faculty role: teaching, scholarship, and service.

Adjunct Faculty

Adjunct faculty are a critical part of the nursing education workforce. Programs rely on them to meet clinical, didactic, and online learning instructional needs (Santisteban & Egues, 2014). Part-time faculty may be responsible for the clinical education of nursing students (American Nurses Association (ANA), 2010) or they may teach online courses. These nurse educators are asked to fulfill vacant positions or allow for flexible expansion and contraction of program size (Brannagan & Oriol, 2014).

But adjunct faculty face many challenges. They may have limited exposure to experienced, full-time nurse educators, making opportunities for role modeling scarce. It may be assumed that adjunct faculty arrive armed with the knowledge and expertise to teach nursing students, but they may lack teaching acumen (Santisteban & Egues, 2014).

Not all adjunct faculty lack teaching experience, however. Online faculty have discovered that they can teach for multiple nursing programs at the same time because they are not geographically bound to one area or region, and have no commute time to employment. The online faculty member can log in and teach several courses each day without leaving the keyboard. This flexible workforce can bring a wealth of expertise to multiple programs and to every class they teach, and in turn this can enrich the learning environment of their students.

Adjunct faculty may have less motivation to attend to their teaching responsibilities because of low salaries, conflicts with full-time employment demands, lack of job security, and inadequate support for teaching and scholarship (Brannagan & Oriol, 2014). Overcoming these challenges requires the collaboration of nursing education, nursing practice, and nursing research (Santisteban & Egues, 2014). Exposure to pedagogy and the role of the educator should be part of all nursing education to prepare nurses to understand the intricacies of teaching. Nurse educators in practice settings can provide in-service education about precepting nursing students who affiliate with their facilities. More research needs to be conducted on how to prepare, recruit, and retain adjunct faculty.

Offering nurses in clinical practice an opportunity to try teaching as an adjunct may prompt more to choose an academic career (Robert Wood Johnson Foundation, 2013). Nursing programs need an infrastructure that supports adjunct faculty (American Nurses Association [ANA], 2010).

The Online Adjunct Faculty Mentoring Model recommends pairing a full-time faculty mentor with an adjunct faculty mentee (Brannagan & Oriol, 2014). The adjunct faculty coordinator is responsible for introducing the new educator to the online environment to ensure that they understand the role and job responsibilities. A critical component to successful use of an adjunct or part-time workforce is recruitment. Potential candidates should be screened for their skills in communicating online (e.g., submission of electronic forms). Once employed, the new educator completes a series of online, asynchronous learning modules that mimic teaching in an online course. The mentor and mentee meet via web-conferencing tools to discuss experiences and build rapport. Brannagan and Oriol (2014) point out that not all faculty are naturally inclined to be mentors. Those who show a desire to help new faculty and accept the responsibility undergo orientation and training.

Designing Courses and Learning Activities

Offering a module, course, or academic program fully or partially online provides faculty an opportunity to reconceptualize the way the course or program is designed and sequenced. Evidence for best practices indicates that course design influences how students learn and how well the course influences time on task and productive use of students' learning time (Palloff & Pratt, 2003). Ideally, faculty have access to course design specialists such as instructional designers, graphic artists, and web technicians. Ultimately, however, faculty are responsible for the design and integrity of courses that are moved to the OLC and must be aware of course design basics.

Evaluation of students using methods other than testing has spurred the popularity of grading rubrics. A rubric should not be added as an afterthought when creating an assessment activity but rather it should be integrated during the development process (Dennison, Rosselli, & Dempsey, 2015). If written well, most rubrics can aid in evaluation of both in-class and online assignments with slight modifications (e.g., scholarly papers can be graded with the same rubric; however, the online student submits an electronic file to the LMS rather than turn in a paper version during class).

Nurse educators should develop their online courses according to theories of teaching and learning and instructional design (Bolan, 2003; Hollingsworth, 2002a; O'Neil, Fisher, & Newbold, 2004; Sternberger, 2002). These theories suggest that students learn when they actively engage, interact in a social and applied context, and reflect on their practice. See Chapter 13 for foundational information about theories of teaching and learning, developing courses, and selecting learning experiences.

When developing online courses, faculty first need to consider whether the course, the course content, and the needs of the students can be best met in a fully online course; in synchronous or asynchronous modes; or with a mix of online activities, on-campus meetings in a classroom or laboratory, or clinical practica. At this time, faculty also need to consider what learning or course management tools and online resources are available or need to be acquired to support the pedagogical goals.

Course development should also be guided by frameworks and models that ensure attention to all steps of the teaching–learning process (Sternberger, 2002; Zsohar & Smith, 2008). Course development should also be guided by the use of good practices in education (Bali, 2014; Chickering & Gamson, 1987; Lowery & Spector, 2014), as well as by evidence of best practices (Billings, Skiba, & Connors, 2005; Suen, 2005). These practices include high expectations, active learning, feedback, interaction with faculty, interaction with classmates, time on task, and respect for diverse ways of learning (Table 21-2).

TABLE 21-2 Educational Practices in Online Courses

Educational Practice	Examples in Traditional Online Courses	Examples in MOOCs
High expectations	Communicate learning outcomes and expectations in several places in the course; expect success; online learning is not easier than or less than classroom expectations.	MOOCs may balance the goal of course completion with setting high expectations. If the purpose of the MOOC is to drive enrollment and increase exposure, expectations may be kept low for noncredit courses. This can backfire if students perceive that the courses are of low quality.
Active learning	Use case studies; problem-based learning; discussion; round robin; critical thinking vignettes.	Many MOOCs give quizzes because they lend themselves to auto-grading. Reflective or analytical assignments are other approaches.
Rich, prompt feedback	Create self-graded activities; structure learning activities that require students to produce work for review by self, students, and faculty.	Quizzes that are auto-graded provide prompt feedback. Reflective or analytical assignments are seldom graded unless by peers.
Interaction with faculty	Use online office hours; use course e-mail for individual communications; be available to answer noncourse–related questions; share examples of faculty work; participate in socialization activities.	Most communication is one-way from the faculty to the student through e-mails and announcements. Some courses offer a feedback forum where students may pose questions, and faculty respond in a timely manner.
Interaction with classmates	Use group projects to promote collaborative work; structure communication tools for small group work, learning circles, chats; create opportunities for students to share reflections and experiences; ensure places for public and private communication for class members.	MOOCs are known for encouraging student interaction through discussion forums. Unmoderated forums can lead to dissatisfaction when participants do not follow netiquette rules.
Time on task	Time spent on learning activities should be reasonable; allow sufficient time between assignments; structure online classroom so students are not reading voluminous and nonessential postings and online time is productive and related to course outcomes; create separate "social spaces" as options for participation.	Many MOOCs allow students to choose the level of engagement, and hence the time spent on task.
Respect for diverse ways of learning	Create options for learning and evaluation; present choices for content and learning activities; encourage diverse opinions while creating norms of respect; use reflective journals to assist students to assess their own needs, styles, and values.	There is a potential global audience for a MOOC, which should take into consideration the diverse needs of those from many cultures. Successful MOOCs tend to have translations of media and readings in several languages. Examples are not all U.S.-centric.

MOOC, Massive open online course.

Basic principles of course design are discussed here. However, we suggest that faculty work with an instructional design team when developing courses for the first time.

1. *Start with the learner.* The student is the focal point for designing online courses. Educators must assess student learning styles, learning needs, current knowledge, motivation, and adaptive needs (see Chapter 2). Although not all students prefer learning online or have well-developed self-directed learning skills that are essential to success in an OLC, most students can adapt and draw on strengths and resources that facilitate their learning when online coursework is required. Educators must also understand the current generation of "m-learners," those students who use mobile wireless devices and who are accustomed to multitasking and acquiring and processing information just as they need it and in a context that meets their needs (Alexander, 2004). Faculty should also understand the learner's technology skills and provide learner support and adequate resources, particularly when online courses are offered for the first time.
2. *Define learning outcomes, objectives, and competencies.* Specifying learning outcomes is a curricular process and should be completed within the context of course and curriculum development (see Chapter 10). Outcomes in all domains of learning can be facilitated within online courses, and the course design can accommodate a variety of learning domains and levels within the domains.
3. *Organize content into short, logical units such as lessons or modules.* Courses designed for the classroom are typically planned for the semester and class hour schedule of the institution. With web-based courses, however, there is more flexibility in scheduling, and thus the content can be organized with additional attention to pedagogical principles. Storyboards and course plans facilitate the organization of modules and courses (Hollingsworth, 2002a). Each unit should include an overview, outcomes and objectives, learning activities, readings and assignments, and evaluation (Zsohar & Smith, 2008).
4. *Integrate educational practices.* Educational practices such as those listed in Table 21-2 provide a foundation for developing the course and related learning activities. Mounting evidence indicates that the use of these educational practices enhances outcomes such as learning, socialization, student satisfaction, and transition to practice, as well as a sense of caring and social presence in the course (Billings et al., 2006; Brownrigg, 2005; Burruss, Billings, Brownrigg, Skiba, & Connors, 2009; Diekelmann & Mendias, 2005; Pullen, 2006; Sitzman & Leners, 2006).
5. *Provide students with opportunities to practice and apply course principles in context.* Additionally, learning activities should be designed for the higher levels of the cognitive domain to assist the students in moving from comprehension to synthesis and evaluation and to connect the learning to clinical practice (Benner, Sutphen, Leonard, & Day, 2010).

The course should begin by establishing clear and *high expectations.* These are communicated in the full syllabus. Learning activities should require active learning and participation—interaction with the content, course, classmates, and the teacher. In repeated studies of teaching in courses conducted fully or partially online, findings demonstrate the importance of selecting effective teaching strategies and well-designed learning experiences (Billings, Connors, & Skiba, 2001) to foster active student learning. In general, teaching practices used in the classroom are also effective for promoting discussion and active learning in the online environment. These educational practices (see Table 21-2) have been derived from work by Chickering and Gamson (1987) and adapted for use in the online classroom (Beitz & Snarponis, 2006; Chickering & Ehrmann, 1996; Daroszewski, Kinser, & Lloyd, 2004a; Edwards, Hugo, Cragg, & Peterson, 1999; Phillips, 2005).

A variety of learning activities such as debates, games, concept maps, WebQuests, case studies, questions, treasure hunts, or written work such as papers and reflective journaling and projects engage the student in active learning. Most nursing textbook publishers have created virtual environments and interactive learning activities that accompany the textbook; faculty can integrate these rich resources into the course design to provide students opportunities for active and self-directed learning. Other sources for learning activities include RLOs that are self-contained modules with learning outcomes, learning activities and an assessment component, websites that have developed no-cost learning activities for specific content such as quality and safety (http://www.qsen.org), and consortia that have developed low-cost modules on a variety of topics (Wink, 2009).

Assignments that foster active learning at higher levels are those that promote analysis or critique of a concept. These include concept clarification, case studies, and debates. Identifying a challenging clinical problem or ethical health care issue and having students brainstorm solutions or debate the pros and cons of a given solution to the problem are other examples of higher level discussion techniques that promote discussion and interaction. It is relatively easy for students to identify real-life issues in nursing practice that can be used to generate online discussion. See Box 21-1 for an example of a discussion forum showing the use of a variety of teaching–learning strategies used to promote active learning.

Students must receive *feedback* while they are learning. Feedback in online courses can include acknowledgement, for example, by recognizing that students have submitted work; information, by giving information or direction; and evaluation such as making judgments about students' work and offering information for improvement (Bonnel, 2008). Feedback can come from students themselves, classmates, and the faculty. Bonnel (2008) recommends creating a multitude of opportunities for feedback during the course design stage. These can include use of automated responses and computer-graded practice tests. Self-graded case studies are simple ways for students to check their own progress. Peer review on written work or small study and discussion groups provides students an opportunity to learn from each other. Faculty must provide feedback at every step of the learning process by monitoring student work, correcting errors, and providing examples of expected outcomes. The faculty role also includes developing the students' own capabilities for self-reflection.

BOX 21-1 Discussion Forums

INTRODUCTIONS

Introduce yourself: Tell us where you work, why you are taking this course, and anything else you want us to know about you!

MODULE 1: FOCUS ON THE LEARNER

Post a description of your learners, how you will assess their needs, and what support they need in your web course.

MODULE 2: DEBATE

Question: Should all nursing courses be designed to be offered only on the Internet? Participants with last names A–M will argue the affirmative; participants with last names N–Z will argue the negative. Participant with first last name starting with the letter A, summarize the affirmative; person with first last name starting with the letter Z (or last of alphabet) summarize the negative.

MODULE 3: TREASURE HUNT

In this course, find the various strategies used to inform learners about the course expectations and learning outcomes to be attained. Post your findings and comment on the value of each strategy.

MODULE 4: ROUND ROBIN

Post a response to the question "How can we assist learners in web courses to obtain feedback?"

MODULE 5: CHAT SUMMARY

Summarize the work of your chat room discussion.

MODULE 6: 1-MINUTE PAPER "ONLINE LEARNING COMMUNITIES"

Write a "1-minute paper" describing what helped you become a member of the online learning community in this course.

MODULE 7: MUDDIEST POINT

What is still not clear to you at this point in the course? Post your questions and all (faculty and participants) will try to clear up your muddiness.

STUDENT LOUNGE

This is the place to kick back and relax.

QUESTION OFFICE

Post your questions about the course content, process, or technical aspects here. Answers will be provided within 24 hours.

Interaction is essential in online learning. Students must have opportunities to work with each other, share ideas, collaborate, and work in groups. When students work together there is a sense of social presence and being connected to the course (Brownrigg, 2005). The isolation often attributed to online courses can be overcome by course design that encourages interaction. As noted earlier, faculty, too, must be actively engaged and "present" in the course by responding to students' questions, providing feedback, and establishing a collegial learning environment (Diekelmann & Mendias, 2005). Faculty can demonstrate caring by providing feedback, responding to students in a timely fashion, and conveying a sense of empathy (Sitzman & Leners, 2006). The use of social networking software, web conferencing, and other Web 2.0 tools can be used to facilitate interaction and collaboration.

Online courses must also be designed to respect the diversity of ways that students learn and the diversity of the learners themselves. This occurs by providing options for participating in the course, for ways of learning course material, and for assessing and evaluating learning outcomes. Because of the increasing racial, ethnic, generational, and language diversity of students in nursing schools, faculty must also design courses and communicate expectations for respecting differences of opinion and ways of learning.

1. *Create assessment, evaluation, and grading plans.* The evaluation and grading criteria should be clearly stated. A variety of strategies for evaluation can be adapted for use in online learning environments (see Chapter 23). These include tests, case studies, simulations, journals, debates, discussion, and portfolios. Many classroom assessment techniques (CATs) have been modified as "e-CATs" and are effective for both students and faculty to assess learning (see Chapter 23). Evaluation strategies should be selected to provide formative feedback to students while they are learning and also to evaluate learning outcomes at the end of the module, lesson, or course. The faculty must indicate the grading plans and guidelines to the student at the outset of the course.
2. *Use graphic design principles.* Course design is improved by the use of colors, fonts, and visual images (Hollingsworth, 2002b). The use of colors and fonts must meet design standards and the use of images must not infringe on copyright; faculty are well served by working with design experts. The course designer should integrate media such as videos, audio, and visuals thoughtfully.
3. *Respect copyright laws.* Because of the easy availability of graphics, text, and video media, it is tempting to include many of these resources in online courses. Faculty and instructional designers, however, must work within the guidelines of the U.S. Copyright Act and the Technology, Education and Copyright Harmonization Act (TEACH Act). Reising (2002) advises faculty to be familiar with these laws and consider that copyright works can be used only for educational purposes, for "fair use," and with permission of the copyright holder.

Content Ownership

Technology has made the duplication, distribution, and display of copyrighted material quick and easy. But just because it is possible does not make it legal. Stakeholders including faculty, librarians, and developers need to understand the laws governing the inclusion of copyrighted material in online courses (Baeslack et al., 2013).

There are four types of intellectual property: copyright, trademark, patent, and trade secret. Online courses are influenced the most by copyright law because it covers the rights to duplicate, distribute, derivate, display, and perform content directly, digitally, or through telecommunications (Tillman, 2008). A copyright pertains only to the expression of an idea, such as a video or written work, and not the idea itself. One way to avoid copyright infringement is to transform the presentation of an idea.

Education enjoys a Fair Use Exemption for the reasonable use of copyrighted materials. Four factors are considered when determining whether an exemption applies (Tillman, 2008). Market effect favors an exemption for nonprofit educational institutions because for-profit colleges and universities may be viewed as selling online courses for financial gain.

The Face-to-face Teaching Exemption and TEACH Act allows for nonprofit educational institutions to digitally transmit copyrighted work provided the amount is comparable to that typically displayed in class, and other conditions are met. It is imperative that faculty and students be made aware of copyright laws and violations so that they can be avoided (Tillman, 2008).

A copyright does not mean that a work cannot be inserted into a course. Permission to use copyrighted material may be obtained from the copyright holder. Some agreements will include requirements such as posting the owner's name and copyright status. Others will want payment for the use of the content. Some institutions may be willing to remit a one-time fee, but avoid paying royalties because of the tracking, accounting, and ongoing costs involved.

The "last mile" problem in telecommunications describes the difficulty in hooking up homes and businesses to technology that enables them to connect to the rest of the world. This has been mostly solved for online learners who can visit a local library or workplace and access the Internet when their homes do not have Internet service (Suber, 2008). There is also a "last mile" problem with knowledge that online learners face, but it is not related to technology. Libraries have made the transition from warehouses of print material to distribution centers of electronic information. Online education has been a catalyst for the mass transfer of hard copy, geographically bound books and journals to electronic databases and books. It has never been easier to access research-based evidence from a technological standpoint.

But technology does not eliminate the financial costs that come with toll access to most quality resources. All students, not just those in online classes, need access to resources to research their papers, plan their projects, and locate evidence on which to base their evidence (Suber, 2008). Libraries subscribe to online resources and make them available to enrolled students, but the cost can be considerable.

The federal government has approached this issue by expanding public access, or open access, to the results of federally funded research (Stebbins, 2013). The published results are to be made available to users, without charge, within 1 year of publication in a peer-reviewed journal. The reasoning is that the public pays for the research through their tax dollars. Some argue that this can have a detrimental effect on scholarly publishing because it decreases the amount of money that the publisher can invest in supporting these endeavors.

Online courses combine content developed by faculty, third parties, and educational institutions. Copyright or ownership of the contents depends on contracts and licensing agreements among the parties involved, as well as on laws that govern intellectual property and education use. Traditionally, online courses are offered by the college or university to defined groups of students who have been registered, authenticated, and are affiliated with the institution.

Students in these online courses own the intellectual property that they contribute in the form of papers and discussion posts. An exception may be for a MOOC, which typically includes a disclaimer that submission to the course waives all rights to the content and it may be hosted, displayed, reproduced, modified, distributed, and relicensed (Baeslack et al., 2013). Coursera, edX, and Udacity and others who host MOOCs have created a fourth stakeholder in the issue of who owns the rights to content (Baeslack et al., 2013).

Creating Community

The absence of face-to-face communication in the online community has led to faculty needing to use specific strategies to overcome the sense of distance and create a learning environment in which students feel connected and have a sense of the presence of each member.

At the beginning of each course, the educator can establish a learning community through activities that promote personal student interaction and allow the class to get acquainted with each other as individuals. Sharing pictures, using "icebreaker" activities, and posting brief introductory messages during the first week of the course are just a few examples of some activities that can promote interaction among the students before discussion of course content begins. It is equally important for faculty members to share information about themselves; faculty can use a photograph or a short video introduction to help students learn more about the faculty. Establishing a discussion forum that can be used by students to ask course questions and promote student dialogue without faculty presence can also be helpful in promoting a learning community. Some faculty elect to schedule periodic face-to-face interactions to promote a sense of community, but this is not always possible or even necessary. A learning community can be successfully built online without the participants ever meeting each other.

Caring and Social Presence

Palloff and Pratt (1999) identify six elements that are essential to building communities and promoting interaction: honesty, responsiveness, relevance, respect, openness, and empowerment. For meaningful participation to occur, students must be able to expect that they will receive honest, respectful, constructive feedback and prompt responses from faculty and students. The subject matter and discussion need to be relevant to real life. Respecting students as equal participants in the learning process and empowering them to be self-directed, responsible learners are also important. Finally, students need to feel free to share their thoughts and feelings without fear of retribution in the form of lower grades.

It is also important for faculty to create a sense of caring in the course. In the on-campus classroom, caring is facilitated by expressing concern, being genuine, and the use of facial expressions and body language; different strategies are needed when the classroom is online. Sitzman and Leners (2006), in a small study of students in an online course, asked students to identify the factors that created a caring learning environment. These researchers found that caring occurred when there was frequent feedback, when there was participation and response to postings, and when the faculty member conveyed concern or empathy by asking about the students' welfare. In a subsequent study with a larger sample, Sitzman (2010) further clarified student-preferred caring behaviors and noted that students appreciated clarity in expectations and directions, timeliness in response to postings and e-mails, having faculty who were an empathetic presence, and being fully engaged and available to students. In a replication of the study with graduate students, Leners and Sitzman (2006) found that along with knowing the faculty on a personal level, students also wanted affirmation and encouragement from both classmates and the faculty.

Other researchers refer to the need to create a sense of social presence, an awareness of other persons in the class (Brownrigg, 2005), and to reduce transactional distance, the space of potential misunderstandings between the student and faculty (Patillo, 2007). When students do not feel connected to the members of the class, motivation and engagement decrease (Lahaie, 2007a). Strategies to overcome these barriers include increasing the amount of dialogue, interaction, and collaboration in an online course and establishing small discussion groups. Other strategies are to use web conferencing software (webinars) to facilitate synchronous class meetings; assigning projects that require collaboration and interaction among students; using polling features of the CMS; and increasing the amount of contact students have with faculty through e-mail, communication technologies such as Skype, and, as needed, face-to-face meetings. Emoticons can also be used to convey an affective dimension to the dialogue, although they should be used with caution as they are open to varied interpretation (Lahaie, 2007a).

Social Networking

Another strategy for promoting community in online courses is to use social networking via Web 2.0 tools such as Facebook, YouTube (see Chapter 19), Twitter, wikis, and blogs to facilitate information and media sharing, collaborative work, and professional development. These tools, most of them already a part of students' daily lives, also can be used in the on-campus or online classroom to promote interaction among faculty and students. Suggestions for using these tools for instructional purposes are provided below with the caveat that when used in courses there must be clearly defined instructional purposes and measurable outcomes; communication in the community must be restricted to the members of the online community with safeguards such as passwords; communication must not violate school or university policies or legislation that prohibits public sharing of private information; and there must be an agreement that all members will respect diversity of the opinions shared within the community and observe course norms for appropriate professional behavior.

Social networking sites (for example, Facebook and Twitter) are websites in which members create a profile and add "friends" with whom they wish to share information. Facebook can be used in courses by having students create a Facebook page to introduce themselves to each other, share class notes, and work on class projects; some faculty create a Facebook page for a manikin in the learning resource center and then class announcements and assignments come from the manikin's "Facebook page" (Skiba, 2010). One of the advantages of using Facebook is that many students already have accounts and are accustomed to sharing information in this format. Twitter allows users to send short (140-character) messages ("tweets") to an individual or a group in the social network (Bristol, 2010; Skiba, 2008). The messages are retrieved from an Internet website. Faculty and students can use Twitter to post challenge questions to students, to update assignments, or to share information from a conference. Faculty also use Twitter during a class session to receive responses to questions posed in class.

Blogs promote collaboration and can be used to develop thinking and writing skills (Billings, 2009). A wiki is a single document developed by a group; the software facilitates adding, deleting, and editing members' contributions as well as attaching photographs, video, and audio clips. Wikis can be used for writing group reports or papers, posting the summary of a community assessment, hosting a journal club, or holding "grand rounds" in which each student presents his or her patient and others contribute to the care plan. A blog (web log) is a document composed of sequential postings by members of the learning community. Blogs can be used as reflective journals, with each student posting individual reflections throughout the course. Blogs are also an easy way to elicit comments about a controversial topic, to conduct focus groups, and to share examples of a particular concept.

Professional networking sites (for example LinkedIn) establish interest-focused communities, typically for the purpose of establishing and expanding a list of professional contacts and networking for seeking employment and professional development. Students can use these sites to market themselves and explore employment opportunities.

Clinical Teaching

Although the clinical practice experiences with clients required in nursing cannot be provided online, the tools and strategies that are the strengths of the OLC can be used to support clinical experiences for students and nurses (Babenko-Mould et al., 2004; Billings et al., 2005; DeBourgh, 2001; Lashley, 2005; Vinten & Partridge, 2002). Several types of clinically focused courses lend themselves to being offered in an online environment. For example, Lashley (2005) found that in a physical assessment course students could learn the clinical skills and clinical decision making that were the outcomes for the course. Faculty can use e-mail and chat as well as discussion forums to link students to their instructors, classmates, preceptors, expert nurses, health care professionals, and clients in the broader community of professional practice.

In the clinical teaching environment, the knowledge learned in the didactic course is applied. Here apprenticeship strategies, use of preceptors, and interaction with colleagues facilitate knowledge transfer. For example, Nesler, Hanner, Melburg, and McGowan (2001) found that precepted clinical experiences for students in online courses were important components for professional role socialization, and Billings et al. (2001) found that use of good education practices within the online course correlated highly with socialization and preparation for real-world work. Stewart, Pope, and Hansen (2010) used clinical preceptors in an online program for students seeking an accelerated BSN degree; students who worked with clinical preceptors during five courses reported being well prepared for the real world of nursing practice.

When the clinical courses use preceptors, orientation of the preceptor is imperative and should include information about teaching and evaluating, as well as information about the course and course procedures (Billings et al., 2006; Stewart et al., 2010). In the triad model in which the student, preceptor, and faculty collaborate to promote student learning, the preceptor may be invited to participate in the online course and thus share clinical insights and connect clinical practice to concepts being taught in the online classroom.

The online learning environment has also been used for preconference and postconference discussions associated with a particular clinical experience (Babenko-Mould et al., 2004; Daroszewski, Kinser, & Lloyd, 2004b). For courses in which students are dispersed throughout a range of clinical experiences, the online environment provides an ideal setting for bringing students together to share experiences and apply content to demonstrate attainment of clinical learning outcomes. For example, when directed journaling and reflection were used following a clinical experience in an advanced practice community health course, Daroszewski et al. (2004b) found that students used critical thinking, demonstrated socialization, and had increased understanding of course content. Babenko-Mould et al. (2004) found that students' self-efficacy for nursing competencies improved when they participated in an online computer conference associated with a clinical practicum.

Increasingly, the online learning environment has become a resource environment for students and practicing nurses. Here, links to research findings, evidence for practice, and access to information about drugs and therapeutic interventions provide the basis for informed practice. As students acquire the skills, knowledge, and values of the profession rather than memorize facts, online resources and their access to them by way of mobile devices will become increasingly important.

Evaluating and Grading Learning Outcomes

Evaluation is as important in online courses as it is in the classroom or clinical practice environment. Best practices indicate that evaluation begins with clearly stated and communicated learning outcomes or competencies; provides students with an opportunity to learn and practice the expected behaviors and receive feedback during the learning process; and concludes with judgment or "grading," indicating the degree to which learning has occurred. Special considerations for these evaluation practices as they pertain to the online environment are discussed here.

Timing of Evaluation

Evaluation in online courses, particularly those courses that are fully online, assumes greater significance because of the asynchronous nature of the course and the potential lack of face-to-face communication. Faculty must therefore be deliberate about the timing of the evaluation and thoughtful in choosing evaluation strategies and providing feedback throughout the course.

Formative evaluation occurs during the course and is essential to learning in online courses. Case studies, critical thinking vignettes, and self-tests provide students with opportunities to practice and receive formative evaluation when teaching feedback is included in the test or scenarios. Adapting assessment strategies (see discussion of evaluation strategies in Chapter 23) to the online learning environment is another way to help both students and faculty gauge students' understanding of course concepts. For example, a CAT such as an online "muddiest point" or electronic survey early in the course can help faculty to modify the course or teaching strategies as the course progresses. Taking advantage of the features of an online grade book will help students keep track of their own progress.

Summative evaluation occurs after students have had the opportunity to learn and apply course content. Evaluation strategies that work well in the classroom usually work well in online courses (see discussion of evaluation strategies in Chapter 23). Strategies that are particularly effective include written work, games, debates, discussion, portfolios, electronic poster presentations, and tests (Bloom & Trice, 1997; Reising, 2002; Rossignol & Scollin, 2001).

Evaluation in online courses should take advantage of the course management tools such as discussion forum, e-mail, testing, and portfolio management. Online grade books assist students in tracking their own progress and, to the extent possible, in determining when they are ready for summative or final evaluation such as taking a final examination.

Academic Integrity in Online Courses

Academic integrity must be observed and protected in the online community, as well as in the classroom. Policies may need to be written to include online courses or may need to be adapted to be more inclusive of or specific to the online course. In addition, norms of respect for individuals and their ideas must be observed. All expectations must be communicated to the students in the syllabus.

Recent concern about the reported lapses in academic integrity in higher education has prompted faculty to reconsider how to manage plagiarism and cheating on tests in their on-campus and online classrooms. Plagiarism involves using the work of another without attributing credit to the original author. The electronic environment provides students with easy access to papers and projects from students throughout the world, as well as from students in similar or previous courses within the same school. Faculty have a responsibility to assist students in learning the conventions of citing published work and to be proactive in offsetting the potential for plagiarism. Simple measures include developing an honor code statement, requiring students to submit copies of all cited references, selectively altering assignments each semester, and choosing assignments that can be completed only by using original work such as a care plan for a specific patient. More complicated and expensive measures include purchasing plagiarism detection software that faculty can use to check students' written work for similarities to other student papers or published works.

Cheating on tests offered in the online environment can occur because students may be able to print tests and share them, use textbooks or Internet sites to answer questions, sit together in a computer cluster and assist each other in answering test questions, or have someone else take the test for them (Hart & Morgan, 2009). However, as Hart and Morgan (2010) also point out, in one small study of students in an RN to BSN program, cheating was more prevalent in the on-campus classroom and occurred more frequently among younger students in the traditional classroom. Nonetheless, faculty have responsibility for creating a culture of academic integrity and test security. As in the classroom, methods for ensuring test security can be simple and low cost or they may be complicated and involve additional human and fiscal resources (Reising, 2002). Easy-to-manage security in online tests includes having students log in with a user name and password, using timed tests, adding new questions to each test, giving "open book" tests, and using test software features to scramble test answers or generate alternative versions of examinations. Faculty can also design evaluation and grading plans that use a variety of evaluation methods that do not depend solely on testing. Most faculty ask students to sign academic honesty pledges, and Hart and Morgan (2009) recommend making consequences clear; others find that indicating to the student that it is easy for faculty to track and compare student responses on online examinations is a sufficient deterrent.

More complex measures to prevent or track cheating include tracking Internet protocol addresses for the computers on which students are taking a test, hiring proctors to observe students while taking the test, and purchasing browser security products (Hart & Morgan, 2009). Some faculty have used video cameras to monitor students while they are taking an online test. Students use small cameras on their computers that are monitored by faculty or a proctor. In one study (Mizra & Staples, 2010) researchers found that the experience of being observed on the camera was uncomfortable for the students, and that the students themselves believed it would be easy to cheat because the camera did not view the entire testing area. New advances in proctoring technology use analysis of keystroke rhythms along with web cameras.

Finally, faculty can require students to take the test or skills check-off in a proctored classroom on campus or in the clinical agency. Ultimately, and particularly for high-stakes examinations, faculty are responsible for providing examination security and must take reasonable means to create a secure environment for all students.

Effectiveness and Continuous Quality Improvement

The use of online learning in nursing education continues to increase, particularly as doctorate in nursing practice and PhD programs seek to make their programs distance accessible. There is a growing body of evidence about the effectiveness of online courses and programs and various pedagogical approaches to designing courses and teaching them online. These findings can be used to guide current practice and improve existing courses.

Effectiveness of Online Courses and Programs

Studies of the effectiveness of online courses reveal that student achievement is similar in online courses and in the classroom (Bata-Jones & Avery, 2004; Coose, 2010; Leasure, Davis, & Thievon, 2000; Leners et al., 2007; Little, 2009; Mancuso-Murphy, 2007; Mills, 2007). In different studies, Coose (2010) and Mills (2007) compared achievement of course goals and found student grades to be comparable in online and on-campus courses. Buckley (2003) reported that there were no differences in learning outcomes between a classroom, a web-enhanced, and a web-based nutrition course for undergraduate nursing students. Pullen (2006) found that online learning, when used for continuing professional development, increased learning and knowledge outcomes and that participants also reported improvement in clinical practice.

A metaanalysis of studies by the U. S. Department of Education revealed the level of significance of a number of online approaches (Means, Toyama, Murphy, Bakia, & Jones, 2010): There was no significant difference in the amount that students learned when purely online environments were compared with blended. Multimedia did not enhance online learning. Student control showed slight improvements in online learning. Online quizzing did not lead to better results. Simulation had a mildly positive effect. Reflection showed the most significantly positive gains. The delivery platform played no significant role in the amount of learning.

In other studies, students report satisfaction with online learning (Billings et al., 2001) and favor the online format (Wills & Stommel, 2002). DeBourgh (2003) found that student satisfaction with computer-mediated distance education is most associated with the perceived quality of the instruction and the effectiveness of the instructor. Ali, Hodson-Carlton, and Ryan (2004) found that graduate nursing students were satisfied with the flexibility and convenience of online learning and that timely feedback from faculty was an important indicator of student satisfaction. Doctoral students in a study conducted by Leners et al. (2007) reported satisfaction with the access to the doctoral program and the ability to enroll in a doctoral program while continuing their employment.

Other researchers examined the effectiveness of the educational practices within web courses. For example, Billings et al. (2001) found that the use of active learning strategies and ample opportunity for interaction within the course were correlated with outcomes such as student satisfaction, socialization, and preparation for real-world work. Leners et al. (2007) also found that students believed they were being prepared for professional practice and, because of mentoring in the online course, were becoming socialized. VandeVusee and Hanson (2000) found that faculty could facilitate active learning by carefully structuring the discussion forums that were used to promote outcomes of critical thinking. Billings et al. (2005) found that the educational practices in online courses influenced outcomes, but there were differences between undergraduate and graduate students' perceptions of the educational practices within the course.

Learning analytics study the data trends of student usage to determine patterns (New Media Consortium, 2013). One goal is early identification of at-risk students so that intervention can be taken to increase retention. For example, analytics may reveal that students who spend little time in the course are more likely to drop out. An alert can be sent to the faculty or student advisors prompting them to contact the student to seek ways to increase involvement. Learning analytics may lead to customized displays of information and resources tailored to a particular students. Mobile applications can use analytics to coach productive and successful student behavior.

Continuous Quality Improvement

As with all course development and teaching, faculty must obtain feedback from students and colleagues about their work and use it to continuously improve course quality (Chao, Saj, & Tessier, 2006). Obtaining course evaluations from students is one important way to determine how the course is working for them and to obtain suggestions for improvement (see Chapter 26 for information about course evaluation).

Peer review of web courses is another way to receive feedback about the course design and the effect on student learning (Cobb, Billings, Mays, & Canty-Mitchell, 2001). Peer review may include informal review of the course and teaching by colleagues and integrating suggestions for improvement. Zsohar and Smith (2008) suggest that peer reviewers have experience and expertise teaching online as well as the necessary content expertise and use preestablished criteria for evaluating the course and instruction. Another review method is to invite colleagues outside nursing but with online teaching experience to review the course. More formal review occurs when peers review courses for promotion, tenure, or teaching awards.

Nurse educators should continue to monitor the effectiveness of the use of technology, the educational practices within the OLC, and the outcomes of the courses and educational programs in which online teaching and learning occur. Using the opportunities of new learning environments will continue to challenge assumptions about teaching and learning and in the long run will result in improvement of pedagogical practices.

Summary

Online learning and the use of online courses has become an accepted educational practice in nursing education. Although evidence continues to indicate that online courses are as effective as on-campus courses, the focus of inquiry has shifted to gathering evidence for the best practices for designing full web and blended courses; for using the appropriate mix of classroom and online learning experiences; for using the emerging technologies for maximum effectiveness; and practices for designing, implementing, and evaluating online courses and programs to promote learning for the students who are enrolled in these courses. Nurse educators are leaders on university college campuses in implementing online education and will continue to be in the forefront of identifying the best practices for designing, implementing, and evaluating online courses and programs.

REFLECTING ON EVIDENCE

1. What is the state of the science about teaching and learning in OLCs?
2. What are strategies to promote social presence and caring in online courses?
3. What learning activities can be used in an online course to facilitate socialization to the profession, ethical comportment, and development of the affective domain?
4. When designing (or redesigning) a course, which elements are best offered online? In the classroom? Synchronously or asynchronously?
5. What research questions should be posed to advance the science of teaching and learning in the OLC?
6. What strategies can be used to prevent academic dishonesty in online courses? What are the cost and benefit considerations of these strategies?

REFERENCES

Accreditation Commission for Education in Nursing (ACEN). (2014). *Accreditation manual: Section II policies. ACEN.* Atlanta, GA: Author.

Alexander, B. (2004). Going nomadic: Mobile learning in higher education. *Educause, 39*(5), 29–35.

Ali, N., Hodson-Carlton, K., & Ryan, M. (2004). Students' perception of online learning: Implications for teaching. *Nurse Educator, 29*(3), 111–115.

Ali, N., Hodson-Carlton, K., Ryan, M., Flowers, J., Rose, M. A., & Wayda, V. (2005). Online education: Needs assessment for faculty development. *The Journal of Continuing Education in Nursing, 36*(1), 32–38.

Allen, I. E., & Seaman, J. (2014). *Grade change: Tracking online education in the United States.* Wellesley, MA: Babson Survey Research Group.

American Association of Colleges of Nursing (AACN). (2007). *Alliance for Nursing Accreditation statement on distance education policies. AACN.* Washington, D.C: Author.

American Nurses Association (ANA). (2010). *Cultivating adjunct faculty. NavigateNursing.org.* Retrieved from, http://nursingworld.org/Content/NavigateNursing/AboutNN/Fact-Sheet-adjunct-faculty.pdf.

Anderson, K., & Avery, M. (2008). Faculty teaching time: A comparison of web-based and face-to-face graduate nursing courses. *International Journal of Nursing Education Scholarship, 5*(1). Article 2. Retrieved from, http://www.bepress.com/ijnes/vol5/iss1/art2.

Babenko-Mould, Y., Andrusyszyn, M., & Goldenberg, D. (2004). Effects of computer-based clinical conferencing on nursing students' self-efficacy. *Journal of Nursing Education, 43*(4), 149–155.

Baeslack, W., Crews, K., Hilton, J., Gasaway, L., Gonick, L., Tanner, M., et al. (2013). *Copyright challenges in a MOOC environment.* Educause. Retrieved from, https://net.educause.edu/ir/library/pdf/PUB9014.pdf.

Baldwin, K., & Burns, P. (2004). Development and implementation of an online CNS program. *Clinical Nurse Specialist, 18*(5), 248.s–254.s.

Bali, M. (2014). MOOC pedagogy: Gleaning good practice from existing MOOCs. *Journal of Teaching and Online Learning, 10*(1), 44–55.

Barra, J. M. (2014, July 8). Emerging technologies enhance nursing education. *Standard Examiner.* Retrieved from, http://www.standard.net/Guest-Commentary/2014/07/09/Emerging-technologies-enhance-nursing-education.html.

Bata-Jones, B., & Avery, M. (2004). Teaching pharmacology to graduate nursing students: Evaluation and comparison of web-based and face-to-face methods. *Journal of Nursing Education, 43*(4), 185–189.

Beitz, J., & Snarponis, J. (2006). Strategies for online teaching and learning: Lessons learned. *Nurse Educator, 31*(1), 20–25.

Benner, P., Sutphen, M., Leonard, V., & Day, L. (2010). *Educating nurses.* San Francisco: Jossey-Bass.

Billings, D. (2000). A framework for assessing outcomes and practices in web-based courses in nursing. *Journal of Nursing Education, 39*(2), 60–67.

Billings, D. (2002). Internal marketing. In D. Billings (Ed.), *Conversations in e-learning* (pp. 41–44). Pensacola, FL: Pohl.

Billings, D. (2009). Wikis and blogs: Consider the possibilities for continuing nursing education. *Journal of Continuing Education in Nursing, 40*(12), 534–535.

Billings, D., Connors, H., & Skiba, D. (2001). Benchmarking best practices in web-based nursing courses. *Advances in Nursing Science, 23*(3), 41–52.

Billings, D., Jeffries, P., Daniels, D., Rowles, C., Stone, C., & Stephenson, E. (2006). Developing and using online courses to prepare nurses for employment in critical care. *Journal for Nurses in Staff Development, 22*(2), 1–6.

Billings, D., Skiba, D., & Connors, H. (2005). Best practices in web- based courses: Generational differences across undergraduate and graduate nursing students. *Journal of Professional Nursing, 21*(2), 126–133.

Blood-Siegfried, J., Short, N., Rapp, C., Hill, E., Talbert, S., Skinner, J., et al. (2008). A rubric for improving the quality of online courses. *International Journal of Nursing Education Scholarship*, *5*(1), 1–13.

Bloom, K. C., & Trice, L. B. (1997). The efficacy of individualized computerized testing in nursing education. *Computers in Nursing*, *15*(2), 82–88.

Bolan, C. (2003). Incorporating experiential learning theory into the instructional design of online courses. *Nurse Educator*, *28*(1), 10–14.

Bonk, C., & Graham, C. (2005). *The handbook of blended learning: Global perspectives, local designs*. Indianapolis: Jossey-Bass.

Bonnel, W. (2008). Improving feedback to students in online courses. *Nursing Education Perspectives*, *29*(5), 290–294.

Brannagan, K. B., & Oriol, M. (2014). A model for orientation and mentoring of online adjunct faculty in nursing. *Nursing Education Perspectives*, *34*(6), 128–130.

Bristol, T. (2010). Twitter: Consider the possibilities for continuing education in nursing. *Journal of Continuing Education in Nursing*, *41*(5), 199–200.

Bristol, T., & Kyarsgaard, V. (2012). Asynchronous discussion: A comparison of larger and smaller discussion group size. *Nursing Education Perspectives*, *33*(6), 386–390.

Broome, M., Halstead, J., Pesut, D., Rawl, S., & Boland, D. (2011). Evaluating the outcomes of a distance accessible PhD program. *Journal of Professional Nursing*, *27*(2), 69–77.

Brownrigg, V. (2005). Assessment of web-based learning in nursing: The role of social presence. *Unpublished dissertation*. Denver, CO.: University of Colorado Health Sciences Center.

Buckley, K. M. (2003). Evaluation of classroom-based, web-enhanced, and web-based distance learning nutrition courses for undergraduate nursing. *Journal of Nursing Education*, *42*(8), 367–369.

Burruss, N., Billings, D., Brownrigg, V., Skiba, D., & Connors, H. (2009). Class size as related to the use of technology, educational practices, and outcomes in web-based nursing courses. *Journal of Professional Nursing*, *25*(1), 33–41.

Carruth, A. K., Broussard, P. C., Waldmeier, V. P., Gauthier, D. M., & Mixon, G. (2010). Graduate nursing online orientation course: Transitioning for success. *Journal of Nursing Education*, *49*(12), 687–690.

Chao, T., Saj, T., & Tessier, F. (2006). Establish a quality review for online courses. *Educause Quarterly*, *29*(3), 32–39.

Chickering, A., & Ehrmann, S. (1996). *Implementing the seven principles: Technology as a lever*. Retrieved from, http://www.tltgroup.org/programs/seven.html.

Chickering, A., & Gamson, Z. (1987). *Seven principles of good practice in undergraduate education*. Racine, WI: Johnson Foundation.

Cobb, K., Billings, D., Mays, R., & Canty-Mitchell, J. (2001). Peer review of web-based courses in nursing. *Nurse Educator*, *26*(6), 274–279.

Colwell, J., & Jenks, C. (2006). *The upper limit: The issues for faculty in setting class size in online courses*. Retrieved from, http://www.ipfw.edu/ Committee on Contingency and the Profession. (2009). Tenure and teaching-intensive appointments. American Association of University Professors. Retrieved from, http://www.aaup.org/report/tenure-and-teaching-intensive-appointments.

Coose, C. S. (2010). Distance nursing education in Alaska: A longitudinal study. *Nursing Education Perspectives*, *31*(2), 93–96.

Critz, C. M., & Knight, D. (2013). Using the flipped classroom in graduate nursing education. *Nurse Educator*, *38*(5), 210–213.

Dahlstrom, E., Brooks, D. C., & Bichsel, J. (2014). *The current ecosystem of learning management systems in higher education: Student, faculty and IT perspectives*. Louisville, CO: ECAR.

Daroszewski, E. B., Kinser, A., & Lloyd, S. (2004a). Online, directed journaling in community health advanced practice nursing clinical education. *Journal of Nursing Education*, *43*(4), 175–180.

Daroszewski, E. B., Kinser, A., & Lloyd, S. (2004b). Socratic method and the Internet: Using tiered discussion to facilitate understanding in a graduate nursing theory course. *Nurse Educator*, *29*(5), 189–191.

DeBourgh, G. A. (2001). Using web technology in a clinical nursing course. *Nurse Educator*, *26*(5), 227–233.

DeBourgh, G. A. (2003). Predictors of student satisfaction in distance-delivered graduate nursing courses: What matters most? *Journal of Professional Nursing*, *19*(3), 149–163.

Dennison, R. D., Rosselli, J., & Dempsey, A. (2015). *Evaluation beyond exams in nursing education: Designing assignments and evaluating with rubrics*. New York: Springer.

Diekelmann, N., & Mendias, E. (2005). Being a supportive presence in online courses: Attending to students' online presence with each other. *Journal of Nursing Education*, *44*(9), 393–395.

Eaton, J. (2012). MOOCs and accreditation: Focus on quality of "direct-to-students" education. *Accreditation*, *9*(1). Retrieved from, http://www.chea.org/ia/IA_2012.10.31.html.

Eaton, J. (2014, September 21). *A high-stakes moment: Accreditation, the federal government and reauthorization of the Higher Education Act*. Huffington Post. Retrieved from, http://www.huffingtonpost.com/judith-eaton/a-high-stakes-moment_b_5267419.html.

Edwards, N., Hugo, K., Cragg, B., & Peterson, J. (1999). The integration of problem-based learning strategies in distance education. *Nurse Educator*, *24*(1), 36–41.

Edwards, C., & McCluskey, N. (2009). *Higher education subsidies*. Cato Institute. Retrieved from, http://www.downsizing-government.org/education/higher-education-subsidies.

Field, K. (2014, April 24). Panel is split on distance-education role. Retrieved from, *Chronicle of Higher Education*. http://chronicle.com/article/Panel-Is-Split-on/146171/.

Halstead, J. A. (2002). How will my role change when I teach on the Web? In D. Billings (Ed.), *Conversations in e-learning* (pp. 105–112). Pensacola, FL: Pohl.

Halstead, J. A., & Coudret, N. A. (2000). Implementing web-based instruction in a school of nursing: Implications for faculty and students. *Journal of Professional Nursing*, *16*(5), 273–281.

Hart, L., & Morgan, L. (2009). Strategies for online test security. *Nurse Educator*, *34*(6), 249–253.

Hart, L., & Morgan, L. (2010). Academic integrity in an online registered nurse to baccalaureate in nursing program. *The Journal of Continuing Education in Nursing*, *41*(11), 498–505.

Hollingsworth, C. (2002a). Layout, fonts, colors, graphics. In D. Billings (Ed.), *Conversations in e-learning* (pp. 141–154). Pensacola, FL: Pohl.

Hollingsworth, C. (2002b). Storyboards and course plans. In D. Billings (Ed.), *Conversations in e-learning* (pp. 137–140). Pensacola, FL: Pohl.

Hunter, J., & Krantz, S. (2010). Constructivism in cultural competence. *Journal of Nursing Education*, *49*(4), 207–214.

Hurt, N. E., Moss, G. S., Bradley, C. L., Larson, L. R., Lovelace, M., & Prevost, L. B. (2012). The Facebook effect: College students' perceptions of online discussions in the age of social networking. *International Journal for the Scholarship of Teaching and Learning*, *6*(2). Art. 10.

Institute for Higher Education Policy. (2000). *Quality on the line: Benchmarks for success in Internet-based distance education.* Washington, DC: Author. Retrieved from, http://www.ihep.org/assests/files/publications/m-r/QualityOnTheLine.pdf.

Jafari, A., McGee, P., & Carmean, C. (2006). Managing courses, defining learning. *Educause*, *41*(4), 50–70.

Johnson, B. (2014). *Creating learning environments.* Edutopia. Retrieved from, http://www.edutopia.org/blog/creating-learning-environments-ben-johnson.

Johnston, J. (2008). Effectiveness of online instruction in the radiologic sciences. *Radiologic Technology*, *79*(6), 497–506.

Kelly, R. (n.d.). Faculty promotion and tenure: Eight ways to improve the tenure review process at your institution. *Academic Leader.* Retrieved from, http://uca.edu/idc/files/2011/06/Faculty-Promotion-and-Tenure-Eight-Ways-to-improve-the-Tenure-Review-Process-at-Your-Institution.pdf.

Kociemba, D. (2014). Overcoming the challenges of contingent faculty organizing. *Academe*, *100*(5). Retrieved from, http://www.aaup.org/article/overcoming-challenges-contingent-faculty-organizing#.VY28dLBRHX4.

Lahaie, U. (2007a). Strategies for creating social presence online. *Nurse Educator*, *32*(3), 100–101.

Lahaie, U. (2007b). Web-based instruction: Getting faculty onboard. *Journal of Professional Nursing*, *23*(6), 335–342.

Lashley, M. (2005). Teaching health assessment in the virtual classroom. *Journal of Nursing Education*, *44*(8), 348–350.

Leasure, A. R., Davis, L., & Thievon, S. (2000). Comparison of student outcomes and preferences in a traditional vs. World Wide Web-based baccalaureate nursing research course. *Journal of Nursing Education*, *39*(4), 149–154.

Leners, D. W., & Sitzman, K. (2006). Graduate student perceptions: Feeling the passion of caring online. *Nursing Education Perspectives*, *27*(6), 315–319.

Leners, D., Wilson, V., & Sitzman, K. (2007). Twenty-first century doctoral education: Online with a focus on nursing education. *Nursing Education Perspectives*, *28*(6), 332–336.

Little, B. (2009). Quality assurance for online nursing courses. *Journal of Nursing Education*, *48*(7), 381–387.

Lowery, B., & Spector, N. (2014). Regulatory implications and recommendations for distance education in prelicensure nursing programs. *Journal of Nursing Regulation*, *5*(3), 24–33.

Mancuso-Murphy, J. (2007). Distance education in nursing: An integrated review of online nursing students' experiences with technology-delivered instruction. *Journal of Nursing Education*, *46*(6), 252–260.

Marginson, S. (2014, April 2). Opinion: Why the west's influence on global higher education is waning. Retrieved from *Chronicle of Higher Education.* http://chronicle.com/article/Opinion-Why-the-Wests/145681/.

Means, B., Toyama, Y., Murphy, R., Bakia, M., & Jones, K. (2010). Evaluation of evidence-based practices in online learning: A meta-analysis and review of online learning studies. *Office of Planning, Evaluation and Policy Development.* Washington, D.C.: U. S. Department of Education.

Mills, A. C. (2007). Evaluation of online and on-site options for master's degree and postmaster's certificate programs. *Nurse Educator*, *32*(2), 73–77.

Mills, M., Fisher, C., & Stair, N. (2001). Web-based courses: More than curriculum. *Nursing and Health Care Perspectives*, *22*(5), 235–239.

Mizra, N., & Staples, E. (2010). Webcam as a new invigilation methods: Students' comfort and potential for cheating. *Journal of Nursing Education*, *49*(2), 116–119.

National League for Nursing Commission for Nursing Education Accreditation. Retrieved from, http://www.nln.org/accreditation-services/the-nln-commission-for-nursing-education-accreditation-(cnea).

Nelson, R. (2007). Student support services for distance education students in nursing programs. *Annual Review of Nursing Education, 183–205.*

Nelson, R., Meyers, L., Rizzolo, M. A., Rutar, P., Proto, M., & Newbold, S. (2006). The evolution of educational information systems and nurse faculty roles. *Nursing Education Perspectives*, *27*(5), 247–253.

Nesler, M., Hanner, M. B., Melburg, V., & McGowan, S. (2001). Professional socialization of baccalaureate nursing students: Can students in distance nursing programs become socialized? *Journal of Nursing Education*, *40*(7), 293–302.

New Media Consortium. (2013). *NMC Horizon Report: 2013 higher* (education ed.). Austin, TX: Author.

O'Neil, C., Fisher, C., & Newbold, S. (2004). *Developing an online course: Best practices for nurse educators.* New York: Springer.

Online Learning Consortium (OLC). (2014). *About OLC.* Retrieved from, http://onlinelearningconsortium.org/aboutus.

Palloff, R., & Pratt, K. (1999). *Building learning communities in cyberspace: Effective strategies for the on-line classroom.* San Francisco: Jossey-Bass.

Palloff, R., & Pratt, K. (2003). *The virtual student: A profile and guide to working with online learners.* San Francisco: Jossey-Bass.

Parker, E., & Howland, L. (2006). Strategies to manage the time demands of online teaching. *Nurse Educator*, *31*(6), 270–274.

Parker, K., Lenhart, A., & Moore, K. (2011). *The digital revolution and higher education: College presidents, public differ on value of online learning.* Washington, D.C.: Pew Research Center.

Patillo, R. E. (2007). Decreasing transactional distance in a web-based course. *Nurse Educator*, *32*(3), 109–112.

Pearsall, C., Hodson-Carlton, K., & Flowers, J. C. (2012). Barriers and strategies toward the implementation of a full-time faculty-at-a-distance nurse educator role. *Nursing Education Perspectives*, *33*(6), 399–405.

Phillips, J. (2005). Strategies for active learning in online continuing education. *Journal of Continuing Education in Nursing*, *36*(2), 77–83.

Pullen, D. (2006). An evaluative case study of online learning for healthcare professionals. *Journal of Continuing Education in Nursing*, *37*(5), 225–232.

Quality Matters (QM). (2014). *Quality Matters higher education rubric workbook: Design standards for online and blended courses* (5th ed.). Baltimore: MarylandOnline, Inc.

Reising, D. (2002). Online testing. In D. Billings (Ed.), *Conversations in e-learning* (pp. 213–220). Pensacola, FL: Pohl.

Rhoads, J., & White, C. (2008). Copyright law and distance nursing education. *Nurse Educator, 33*(1), 39–44.

Richard, P., Mercer, Z., & Bray, C. (2005). Transitioning a classroom-based RN-BSN program to the Web. *Nurse Educator, 30*(5), 208–211.

Robert Wood Johnson Foundation. (2013). *Wanted: Young nurse faculty.* RWJF. Retrieved from, http://www.rwjf.org/en/about-rwjf/newsroom/newsroom-content/2013/09/wanted-young-nurse-faculty.html.

Rossignol, M., & Scollin, P. (2001). Piloting use of computerized practice tests. *Computers in Nursing, 18*(2), 72–86.

Roy, R., Potter, S., Yarrow, K., & Smith, M. (2005). *Towards sustainable higher education: Environmental impacts of campus-based and distance higher education systems.* Design Innovation Group, Milton Keynes, UK: Open University.

Ryan, M., Hodson-Carlton, K., & Ali, N. (2005). A model for faculty teaching online: Confirmation of a dimensional matrix. *Journal of Nursing Education, 44*(8), 357–365.

Santisteban, L., & Egues, A. L. (2014). Cultivating adjunct faculty: Strategies beyond orientation. *Nursing Forum, 49*(3), 152–158.

Shovein, J., Huston, C., Fox, S., & Damazo, B. (2005). Challenging traditional teaching and learning paradigms: Online learning and emancipatory teaching. *Nursing Education Perspectives, 26*(6), 340–343.

Sitzman, K. (2010). Student-preferred caring behaviors for online nursing education. *Nursing Education Perspectives, 31*(3), 171–176.

Sitzman, K., & Leners, D. W. (2006). Student perceptions of caring in online baccalaureate education. *Nursing Education Perspectives, 27*(5), 254–259.

Skiba, D. J. (2008). Nursing education 2.0: Twitter & tweets. Can you post a nugget of knowledge in 140 characters or less? *Nursing Education Perspectives, 29*(2), 110–112.

Skiba, D. J. (2010). Nursing education 2.0: Social networking and the WOTY. *Nursing Education Perspectives, 31*(1), 44–46.

Stebbins, M. (2013). *Expanding public access to the results of federally funded research.* Office of Science and Technology Policy. Retrieved from, http://www.whitehouse.gov/blog/2013/02/22/expanding-public-access-results-federally-funded-research.

Sternberger, C. (2002). Embedding a pedagogical model in the design of an online course. *Nurse Educator, 27*(4), 170–173.

Stewart, S., Pope, D., & Hansen, T. S. (2010). Clinical preceptors enhance an online accelerated bachelor's degree to BSN program. *Nurse Educator, 35*(1), 37–40.

Straumsheim, C. (2014, September 23). *Where does the LMS go from here?* Inside Higher Education. Retrieved from, https://www.insidehighered.com/news/2014/09/23/educause-gates-foundation-examine-history-and-future-lms.

Suber, P. (2008). *Open access and the last-mile problem for knowledge.* SPARC Open Access Newsletter. Retrieved from, http://www.sparc.arl.org/resource/open-access-and-last-mile-problem-knowledge.

Suen, L. (2005). Teaching epidemiology using WebCT: Application of the seven principles of good practice. *Journal of Nursing Education, 44*(3), 143–146.

Tillman, J. (2008). *Copyright for higher education: Just because you can does not mean you may!.* Retrieved from, https://www2.masters.edu/Libraries/pdf/Copyright/Copyright%20for%20Higher%20Education.htm.

University of Minnesota. (2013). *Good, better, best model for estimating development of online courses.* Minneapolis: University of Minnesota. Retrieved from, http://digitalcampus.umn.edu/resources/Good-Better-Best-Model.pdf.

Van de Vord, R., & Pogue, K. (2012). Teaching time investment: Does online really take more time than face-to-face? *International Review of Research in Open and Distance Learning, 13*(3). Retrieved from, http://www.editlib.org/p/49702/.

VandeVusee, L., & Hanson, L. (2000). Evaluation of online course discussions. *Computers in Nursing, 18*(4), 181–188.

Vinten, S., & Partridge, R. (2002). E-learning and the clinical practicum. In D. Billings (Ed.), *Conversations in e-learning* (pp. 187–196). Pensacola, FL: Pohl.

Wills, C., & Stommel, M. (2002). Graduate nursing students' precourse and postcourse perceptions and preferences concerning completely web-based courses. *Journal of Nursing Education, 41*(5), 193–201.

Wink, D. (2009). Sources of fully developed course materials on the Web. *Nurse Educator, 34*(4), 143–145.

Wright, C. R., Lopes, V., Montgomerie, T. C., Reju, S. A., & Schmoller, S. (2014). *Selecting a learning management system: Advice from an academic perspective.* Louisville, CO: ECAR.

Zsohar, H., & Smith, J. (2008). Transition from the classroom to the Web: Successful strategies for teaching online. *Nursing Education Perspective, 29*(1), 23–28.

Introduction to the Evaluation Process

22

Mary P. Bourke, PhD, MSN, RN
Barbara A. Ihrke, PhD, RN

Nursing faculty are responsible for evaluating student learning, courses, curricula, and program outcomes, as well as their own teaching practices. They are accountable to students, peers, administrators, employers, and society for the effectiveness of the nursing program. The purpose of this chapter is to present an overview of the process by which nursing faculty can evaluate instructional and program outcomes and report results to stakeholders. The chapter provides an overview of evaluation and delineates a step-by-step evaluation process. Also, this chapter provides information about the use of evaluation models; selection of instruments; data collection procedures; and the means to interpret, report, and use findings. Results can be used to make decisions about improvement in student learning; faculty performance; and course, curriculum, and program quality. This chapter is a link to previous and subsequent chapters that discuss specific evaluation activities and strategies.

Evaluation Defined

Evaluation is a broad term that describes the process of determining value, worth, or quality. In nursing education it is an ongoing process that begins with specifying outcomes and criteria (program outcomes, course outcomes, learning outcomes, promotion, and tenure criteria), providing opportunity to attain the outcomes (participating in instruction and learning activities), receiving information about progress toward attaining the outcomes (skills practice prior to actual clinical performance), and ends with evaluation or a judgment about the extent to which outcomes were attained. A variety of terms are used in describing this process; they are connected, yet distinct. In this book the following terms are used to describe the evaluation process.

Evaluation

Evaluation involves gathering and appraising data or placing a value on data gathered through one or more measurements. Evaluation is a process of making judgments using preestablished criteria that have been communicated to the individual or group prior to their use. In nursing education, faculty evaluate students' learning in cognitive, psychomotor, and affective domains in both classroom and clinical settings; determine the effectiveness of teaching and learning; and judge the outcomes of curricula and academic programs. Evaluation is also a professional activity that educators undertake to reflect on their own performance.

Evaluation may be defined by the time frame in which it is conducted. In *formative evaluation,* the judgment about the performance is conducted while the event being evaluated is occurring. Formative evaluation focuses on determining progress toward purposes, outcomes, learning activities, courses, or curriculum, and provides opportunity for correction and improvement.

Formative evaluation emphasizes the parts instead of the entirety. The aim of formative evaluation is to monitor progress (e.g., in student learning, instituting a new teaching–learning strategy such as simulation, or in curriculum or program development) and make ongoing corrections to ensure the desired end result is attained. For formative evaluation of a program, many schools of nursing use national standardized testing systems. Each semester students take a test that identifies the student's competencies and their placement nationally. This helps to determine student progression through key concepts within the curriculum. Weaknesses within the curriculum can be identified using content-specific testing as the cohorts progress through the nursing program. Thus formative evaluation provides critical data for ongoing changes necessary to improve student outcomes.

One advantage of formative evaluation is that the events are recent, thus guarding accuracy and preventing distortion by time. Another major advantage of formative evaluation is that the results can be used to improve student performance, program of instruction, or learning outcome before the program or course has concluded (Waugh & Gronlund, 2012). Disadvantages of formative evaluation include making judgments before the activity (classroom or clinical performance, nursing program) is completed and not being able to see the results before judgments are made. Formative evaluation can also be intrusive or interrupt the flow of outcomes. There is also a chance for a false sense of security when formative evaluation is positive and the results are not as positive as predicted earlier.

Summative evaluation, on the other hand, refers to data collected at the end of the activity, instruction, course, or program (Waugh & Gronlund, 2012; Story et al., 2010). The focus is on the whole event and emphasizes what is or was and the extent to which objectives and outcomes were met for the purposes of accountability, resource allocation, assignment of grades (students) or merit pay or promotion (faculty), and certification. Therefore summative evaluation is most useful at the end of a learning module or course and for program or course revision. Summative evaluation of learning outcomes in a course usually results in assignment of a final grade.

The advantages of performing an evaluation at the end of the activity are that all work has been completed and the findings of the evaluation show results. The major disadvantage of summative evaluation is that nothing can be done to alter the results.

Assessment

Assessment refers to gathering and using data that are used to improve the factors being evaluated in relation to the specified criteria. Assessment data are used to determine progress and provide guidance toward attaining the desired outcomes. Faculty use assessments to give feedback to student learning, to improve teaching and learning, and to coach and guide students to competency or mastery. Although similar to formative evaluation in that one of the purposes of assessment is to monitor progress, the focus of assessment is on improving teaching and learning. Assessment is an interactive process between students and faculty with the goal of improving learning and teaching. Findings from assessment are diagnostic; the results are used for improvement and are not "graded."

Grading

Grading involves quantifying data from student work and assigning a value. The value is expressed as a "grade," or representation of the value of the student's work. Final grades, grades obtained at the end of the course of study, typically are required in academic programs and are used to communicate to the student, the university, and the public the achievement of the student as determined by the faculty. Grading criteria must be made evident to the student prior to assigning grades. These criteria are published, typically in a syllabus, for both grading of assignments and for calculating a final course grade.

Philosophical Approaches to Evaluation

Conducting an evaluation begins with understanding one's philosophy, or values and beliefs about evaluation. The philosophy will influence how evaluations are conducted, when evaluations are conducted, what methods are used, and how results are interpreted. A philosophy is reflected in attitudes and behavior.

In nursing education, evaluations or judgments are made about performance (students and faculty), program effectiveness (a nursing curriculum or program), instructional media (a textbook, a video), or instruction (course, faculty). Evaluation activities in nursing education are conducted from various perspectives, and these perspectives influence outcomes. Therefore evaluators should be aware of the perspective or orientation as they relate it to the evaluation process.

Several philosophical perspectives tend to influence evaluation. Educators who rely on goals, objectives, and outcomes to guide program, course, or lesson development will likely have a *goals* approach to evaluation. The merits of the activity or program are largely indicated by the success of students meeting those goals or objectives. A *service* orientation toward evaluation emphasizes the student learning process and includes self-evaluation, thus assisting educators to make decisions about learners and the teaching–learning process. Although all evaluation involves judgment, the evaluator with a judgment perspective focuses on establishing the worth or merit of the employee, student, product, or program. Others have a *research* orientation to evaluation and emphasize precision in measurement and statistical analysis to gain a general understanding of why students and programs do or do not succeed. The focus in this perspective is on tools, methods, and designs as they relate to validity and reliability of instruments. Yet another orientation is the *constructivist* view, which emphasizes the values of the stakeholders and builds consensus about what needs to be changed. Although faculty, in their role as evaluators, use a combination of these perspectives, one is likely dominant, and faculty should be aware of the perspective they bring to the evaluation process because their philosophical orientation toward evaluation will guide the evaluation process and influence outcomes. More importantly, results should be used by faculty for course, clinical, and program improvement.

The Evaluation Process

Evaluation is a process that involves the following systematic series of actions:

1. Identifying the purpose of the evaluation
2. Determining when to evaluate
3. Selecting the evaluator
4. Choosing an evaluation design, framework, or model
5. Selecting an evaluation instrument
6. Collecting data
7. Interpreting data
8. Reporting the findings
9. Using the findings
10. Considering the costs of evaluation

The steps can be modified depending on the purpose of the evaluation, what is being evaluated (e.g., students, instruction, program, or system), and the complexity of the units being evaluated.

Identifying the Purpose of the Evaluation

As in the research process, the first step in the evaluation process is to pose various questions that can be answered by evaluation. These questions may be broad and encompassing, as in program evaluation, or focused and specific, as in classroom assessment (Box 22-1). Regardless of the scope of the evaluation, the purpose or reason for conducting an evaluation should be clear to all involved.

BOX 22-1 Purposes of Evaluation

- To facilitate learning—or change behavior of an employee or student
- To diagnose problems—to find learning deficits, ineffective teaching practices, curriculum defects, and so on
- To make decisions—to assign grades, to determine merit raises, to offer promotion or tenure
- To improve products—to revise a textbook, to add content to an independent study module
- To judge effectiveness—to determine whether goals or standards are being met
- To judge cost effectiveness—to determine whether a program is self-supporting

Determining When to Evaluate

The evaluator must also weigh each evaluation event and determine when evaluation is most appropriate. Typically, both formative and summative evaluations are appropriate and lend respective strengths to the evaluation plan.

In determining when to evaluate, the evaluator must also consider the frequency of evaluation. Evaluation can be time consuming, but frequent evaluation is necessary in many situations. Frequent evaluations are important when the learning process is complex and unfamiliar and when it is considered helpful to anticipate potential problems if the risk of failure is high. Finally, important decisions require frequent evaluations (Box 22-2).

BOX 22-2 Situations in Which Frequent Evaluation Is Useful

- Learning is complex.
- Trends are emerging.
- Problems have been identified.
- Problems are anticipated.
- There is a high risk of failure.
- Serious consequences would result from poor performance.
- Major changes have recently been made in curriculum or requirements of a program.

Selecting the Evaluator

An important element in the evaluation process is the evaluator. Selection of an evaluator involves deciding who should be involved in the evaluation process and whether the evaluator should be chosen from the "inside" (internal evaluator) or from the "outside" (external evaluator). Both have merits.

Internal Evaluators

Internal evaluators are those directly involved with the learning, course, or program to be evaluated, such as the students, faculty, or nursing staff. Many individuals (stakeholders) have a vested interest in the evaluation process and could be selected to participate. There are advantages and disadvantages associated with internal evaluators, and often several evaluators are helpful to obtain the most accurate data.

Advantages of using internal evaluators include their familiarity with the context of the evaluation experience with the standards, cost effectiveness, and potential for less obtrusive evaluation. Additionally, the findings of evaluation can be acted on quickly because the results are known immediately.

Disadvantages of using internal evaluators include bias, control of evaluation, and reluctance to share controversial findings. When internal evaluators are chosen and employed, it is important to note their position in the organization and responsibility and reporting lines.

External Evaluators

External evaluators are those not directly involved in the events being evaluated. They are often employed as consultants. State, regional, and national accrediting bodies are other examples of external evaluators. The advantage of using external evaluators is that they do not have a bias, are not involved in organizational politics, may be very experienced in a particular type of evaluation, and do not have a stake in the results. Disadvantages of using external evaluators include expense, unfamiliarity with the context, barriers of time, and potential travel constraints. Because evaluators are so critical to the evaluation process, faculty should select evaluators carefully. Box 22-3 lists questions to ask when selecting an evaluator.

BOX 22-3 Questions to Ask When Selecting an Evaluator

1. What is the evaluator's philosophical orientation?
2. What is the evaluator's experience?
3. What methods or instruments does the evaluator use? Have experience with?
4. What is the evaluator's style?
5. Is the evaluator responsive to the client?
6. Does the evaluator work well with others?
7. Is the evaluator supportive versus critical?
8. What is the evaluator's orientation to evaluation?

Choosing an Evaluation Framework or Model

An evaluation model must be chosen or developed. An evaluation model represents the ways the variables, items, or events to be evaluated are arranged, observed, or manipulated to answer the evaluation question. A model serves to clarify the relationship of the variables to be evaluated and provides a systematic plan or framework for the evaluation.

Using an evaluation model has several advantages. A model makes variables explicit and often reflects a priority about which variables should be evaluated first or most often. A model also gives structure that is visible to all concerned; the relationships of parts are evident. Using an evaluation model helps focus evaluation. It keeps the evaluation efforts on target: those elements that are to be evaluated are included; those not to be evaluated are excluded. Finally, a model can be tested and validated.

Evaluation models for nursing education may be found in the education and nursing literature, may have been adapted from uses in business, or may be developed by nurse educators for a specific use. A model should be selected according to the demands of the evaluation question, the context, and the needs of the stakeholders. Commonly used evaluation models in nursing education are noted here; specific applications of the model are described in relevant chapters.

Program evaluation and accreditation models often have been adopted from higher education. Common models include Chen's theory-driven model, which directs the variables to be measured (Chen, 2004); Stufflebeam's (1971) model, which organizes the variable to be evaluated as context, input, process, and product; and naturalistic models such as those proposed by Lincoln and Guba (1985), which involve the participation of stakeholders in determining consensus about what needs to be changed. (See Chapter 26.)

Adoptions of innovations and change models focus on the extent to which learning or use of a teaching–learning strategy has been integrated into practice. These models can be used to guide change as well as to evaluate process and outcome. Kirkpatrick and Kirkpatrick's (2014) four-level evaluation model evaluates four levels of change: reaction, learning, behavior, and results. The first two levels (reaction and learning) indicate time and resources devoted to teaching and learning, and levels three and four (behavior and results) reveal the lasting outcome of the education. Rogers's (2003) model of adoption of innovations provides a framework for understanding how innovations are diffused through an organization. Adoption of an innovation, such as new curriculum or new teaching strategy, depends on the nature of the innovation, the communications within the organization, the time span, and the social system. Rogers (2003) notes that not all persons involved in the adoption of a change do so at the same time and offers a curve to indicate that there will be a range of adopters from those who are early adopters to those who are later adopters, described as laggards.

Quality assurance or *total quality improvement models* are also used in nursing education. One example is the use of Quality Matters (2014) to evaluate online courses (see Chapter 21). This group has developed benchmarks for online courses with rubrics used to assess standards for the design of online courses. Courses are reviewed by trained reviewers.

Selecting an Evaluation Instrument

After a model has been selected, and the variables to be evaluated and their relationship to each other have been identified, the evaluator then selects evaluation instruments that can be used most easily to obtain the necessary data. The selection of evaluation instruments is determined by the evaluation question and the evaluation model.

Types of Instruments

Many instruments are available for measurement and can be found by doing a literature review. To use a published instrument, faculty must contact the publisher and obtain permission.

Questionnaire

A *questionnaire* is a method in which a person answers questions in writing on a form. The questionnaire is usually self-administered. The person reads the question and then responds as instructed. Questionnaires are cost effective but often lack substance. Questions must be clear, concise, and simple (Polit & Beck, 2013). This type of instrument is often used to measure qualitative variables, such as feelings and attitudes. Questionnaires could be used to measure a student's level of confidence in the clinical setting or to determine students' satisfaction with the nursing program after graduation.

Interview

An *interview* involves direct contact with individuals participating in the evaluation. Exit interviews, for example, are often conducted as a faculty member leaves the school of nursing or as students graduate. Interviews can be used to elicit both qualitative and quantitative data. Interviews can be conducted with an individual or in focus groups. Students or external evaluators may be assigned to collect the data. The interview should be scheduled at a time that is convenient for both the interviewer and the participant.

The interviewer should provide a quiet, private room or office to allow the participant to speak in privacy. A participant may open up more if he or she feels that the conversation will be private and confidential. An objective outline should be created and followed during the interview, and notes should be kept in a file. Great care must be taken to avoid personalizing the information. One negative aspect of interviews is that they are time intensive (Polit & Beck, 2013). Sanders and Sullins (2006) define the guidelines for interviews as follows:

1. Keep the language pitched to the level of the respondent.
2. Clearly explain the purpose of the interview, who has access to the recordings or transcripts, and how it will be kept confidential.
3. Encourage honesty, but let people know they can refuse to answer a question if they choose. Establish rapport by asking easy, impersonal questions first. Avoid long questions.
4. Avoid ambiguous wording. Avoid leading questions.
5. Limit questions to a single idea. Do not assume too much knowledge (Sanders & Sullins, 2006, p. 31).

Rating Scale

A *rating scale* is used to measure an abstract concept on a descriptive continuum. The rating scale is designed to increase objectivity in the evaluation process. Rating scales work well with norm-referenced evaluation, although they are not the best tools to use for this type of evaluation. Grades can easily be assigned to the ratings.

Checklist

A *checklist* is two-dimensional in that the expected behavior or competence is listed on one side and the degree to which this behavior meets the level of expectation is listed on the other side. With a detailed checklist of items and well-defined criteria being measured, the evaluator can easily identify expected behavior or acceptable competence. This type of instrument is useful for formative and summative evaluations. A checklist can be used to evaluate a student's performance of clinical procedures. The steps to be followed can be placed in sequential order and the observer can then check off each action that is taken or not taken.

Attitude Scale

An *attitude scale* measures how the participant (usually a student) feels about a subject at the moment when he or she answers the question. Several popular types of attitude scales are used in nursing education evaluation.

The most popular is the Likert scale. In a Likert scale, several items in the form of statements (10 to 15 statements are recommended) are used to express an opinion on a particular issue. Each item represents a construct of that issue; for example, a particular item may express an opinion about Latino students in nursing when the theme of the survey is diversity. Participants are asked to indicate the degree to which they agree or disagree. Equal numbers of positively and negatively worded items should be used to prevent bias in the responses.

Semantic differential is another scale used to measure attitude. *Bipolar scales* are used to measure the reaction of the participant. Each item on the scale is followed by bipolar adjectives such as good–bad, active–passive, or positive–negative. The number of intervals between each adjective is usually odd so that the middle interval is neutral. A list of five to seven intervals is adequate. Analysis is performed by adding values for each item, which is similar to what is done with the Likert scale (Polit & Beck, 2013).

For analysis of Likert scale data and semantic differential scale data, it is recommended to refrain from treating the data as interval data and to use the Rasch model for analysis. By applying the Rasch model, a more appropriate analysis of the tool and data are accomplished. Typically, Likert data are treated as interval data, although the individual responses are scaled as ordinal. Interval data are assumed. As Bond and Fox (2007) illustrate:

> Five endorsements of the coding of a Likert type scale by a respondent (SD D N A SA) results in a satisfaction score of 25, five times the amount of satisfaction indicated by the respondent who endorses the five SD categories ($5 \times 1 = 5$), or almost exactly twice the satisfaction of someone who endorses two N's and three SD's ($2 \times 3 \times 2 = 12$). Whenever scores are added in this manner, the ratio, or at least the interval nature of the data, is being presumed. That is, the relative value of each response category across all items is treated as being the same, and the unit increases across the rating scale are given equal value.... [T]he data are subsequently analyzed in a rigidly prescriptive and inappropriate statistical way. (p. 67)

The Rasch model treats Likert scale data mathematically more justifiably than the ordered sequence of 1 to 5 "then add them up" approach. Rasch recognizes coding as ordered categories only, in which values of each category are higher than for the previous category but by an unspecified amount. Likert-type scale data need to be regarded as ordinal data, whereas the Rasch model transforms the counts of items into interval scales based on empirical evidence as opposed to an assumption. The empirical evidence is calculated using log transformations of raw data odds and abstraction is accomplished through probabilistic equations.

The Rasch model is "the only model that provides the necessary objectivity for the construction of a scale that is separable from the distribution of the attribute in the persons it measures" (Bond & Fox, 2007, p. 7). The conceptual understanding of the Rasch model is best described as a model created within item response theory. *Item response theory,* as explained by Rudner (2001), uses test scores and specific test item scores based on assumptions concerning the mathematical relationship between abilities or attitudes and item responses. The Rasch model has the ability, through several diagnostic procedures, to diagnose the tool's ability to measure accurately the author's and respondent's intentions. The design of a rating scale has a tremendous influence on the quality of responses provided by the respondents. Diagnostic ability provides a powerful tool for designing, analyzing, and revising attitude scales.

Portfolios

A portfolio is used to provide evidence of program learning outcomes through the accumulation of artifacts collected throughout the program. An artifact is the production of instruction such as an assignment, PowerPoint presentation, concept map, care plan, and so on. A guide for collection of artifacts is provided to students at the start of their program to facilitate successful completion. Portfolios are stored either electronically or in an organized paper version. Often reflections are added to each artifact to show how the artifact met program learning outcomes. Reflections enhance student learning and ensure progress toward meeting program learning outcomes.

Reliability and Validity of Evaluation Instruments Used in Nursing Education

When any instrument is used, its validity and reliability for evaluation should be ensured. Special procedures can be used to determine reliability and validity of instruments used for clinical evaluation, program evaluation, and examinations given to measure classroom achievement. Specific procedures are discussed in appropriate chapters of this book. A general overview of the concepts of validity and reliability are provided here.

Validity

Measurement validity verifies that faculty are in fact collecting and analyzing results they intend to measure. Measurement validity, particularly in the area of educational assessment and evaluation, has attributes of relevance, accuracy, and utility (Prus & Johnson, 1994; Wholey, Haltry, & Newcomer, 2004). *Relevance* of an instrument is achieved when the instrument measures the educational objective as directly as possible. The instrument is *accurate* if it is measuring the educational objective precisely. The instrument has *utility* if it provides formative and summative results that have implications for evaluation and improvement. As a result, valid evaluation instruments have relevance for the local program or curriculum and can provide meaningful results that indicate directions for change (Prus & Johnson, 1994).

Although there are several types of validity, measurement validity is viewed as a single concept. Content-related evidence, criterion-related evidence, and construct-related evidence are considered categories of validity. For interpretation, evidence from all categories is ideal. The validity of an instrument can best be determined when faculty understand the nature of the content and specifications in the evaluation design, the relationship of the instrument to the significant criterion, and the constructs or psychological characteristics being measured by the instrument (Waugh & Gronlund, 2012).

Content-related evidence refers to the extent to which the instrument is representative of the larger domain of the behavior being measured. Content-related evidence is particularly important to establish for clinical evaluation instruments and classroom tests. For example, with classroom tests, the following question is raised: "Does the sample of test questions represent all content described in the course?" In clinical evaluation, the question posed is: "Does the instrument measure attitudes, behaviors, and skills representative of the domain of being a nurse?"

Criterion-related evidence refers to the relationship of a score on one measure (test, clinical performance appraisal) to other external measures. There are two ways to establish criterion-related evidence: concurrent and predictive. *Concurrent evidence* is the correlation of one score with another measure that occurs at the same time. The most common example of concurrent validity is correlation of clinical course grades with didactic course grades. Concurrent validity of the instrument is said to occur, for example, when there is a high correlation between clinical evaluation and examination scores in a class of students. *Predictive study,* on the other hand, is a correlation with measures obtained after completion of an event or intervention, such as a course or lesson. For example, there may be predictive validity between course grades and licensing examination or certification examination scores.

Criterion-related evidence is used to relate the outcomes of one instrument to the outcomes of another. In this sense, it is used to predict success or establish the predictability of one measure with another one. Criterion-related evidence is established by using correlation measures. One example is the correlation between grade point average and scores on licensing or credentialing examinations. When there is a high positive correlation between the grade point average and the examination score, there is said to be criterion-related evidence.

Construct-related evidence is a relationship of one measure (e.g., examination) to other learner variables such as learning style, IQ, clinical competence, or job experience. Construct-related evidence is used to infer the relationship of a test instrument and student traits or qualities to identify what factors might be influencing performance. Examples include the relationship of IQ scores, Scholastic Aptitude Test scores, and other test scores or working for pay as a student nurse and clinical performance.

Reliability

Reliability is the extent to which an instrument (self-report examination, observation schedule, or checklist) is dependable, precise, predictable, and consistent. Pedhazur and Schmelkin (1991) refer to reliability as the degree to which test scores are free from errors of measurement. Reliability answers the question: "Will the same instrument yield the same results with different groups of students or when used by different raters?" According to Newby (1992), "Reliability in testing refers to the idea that tests should be consistent in the way that they measure performance" (p. 253).

Several types of reliability—stability reliability, equivalence reliability, and internal consistency reliability—are relevant to evaluation instruments and achievement examinations. *Stability reliability* of an instrument is the perceived consistency of the instrument over time. An assumption of stability in results is assumed. *Equivalence reliability* entails the degree to which two different forms of an instrument can be used to obtain the same results. For example, when two forms of a test are used, both tests should have the same number of items and the same level of difficulty. The test is given to the group at the same time as the equivalent test is given or the equivalent test is administered at a later date. *Internal consistency reliability* is associated with the extent to which all items on an instrument measure the same variable and with the homogeneity of the items. This reliability is considered only when the instrument is being used to measure a single concept or construct at a time. Because the validity of findings is threatened when an instrument is unreliable, faculty should use measures to ensure instrument reliability.

Collecting Data

The next step of the evaluation process is use of the evaluation instrument to gather data. Although the instrument will determine to some extent what data are collected and how, several other factors should be considered at this time. These include the data collector, the data sources, amount of data, timing of data collection, and informal versus formal data collection.

Data Collector

Consideration must be given to who is collecting the data. For example, the evaluator who gathers the data might be the faculty member evaluating the clinical performance of the students. In other situations, students or research assistants may administer instruments. If the data collectors are not familiar with the data-collecting procedures, they should be oriented to the task. Interrater reliability must be ensured when more than one person is collecting data.

Data Source

Before evaluation, the evaluator must identify sources from which the data will be collected. Will the data be observed (as in clinical evaluation), archival (as when grade point average is obtained from student records), or reported (as obtained from a longitudinal questionnaire of graduates)? At this time in the evaluation process, it is important to determine whether it is possible to have access to records, particularly if permission must be obtained from the participants.

Amount of Data

The amount of data to be collected must also be determined and specified. All data may be collected or a sample may be sufficient, but a decision must be made. For example, in clinical evaluation or classroom testing it is impossible to collect data about each instance of clinical performance or knowledge gained from the classroom experience. In this instance, a sampling procedure is used and guided by the clinical evaluation protocol, blueprint, or plan for the classroom test. It is important to note that the sampling plan must be established at this stage of the evaluation process.

Timing of Data Collection

When is the best time to collect the data? An understanding of the context of evaluation is helpful here. Should the data be collected at the beginning, middle, or end of the activity being evaluated? When gathering data from students, it is important to allow adequate time and to gather data when students are able to give unbiased responses. (For example, course evaluation data collected immediately after test results have been given may not yield the most reflective responses.)

Formal versus Informal Data Collection

Decisions about use of formal and informal data must also be made. Data can be obtained in a formal manner, such as by using a structured evaluation tool. Data can also be collected with informal methods, such as in the form of spontaneous comments made by students. The evaluator must decide whether both formal and informal data will be used in the plan.

Interpreting Data

The interpretation step of the evaluation process involves translating data to answer the evaluation questions established at the beginning of the evaluation process. This involves putting the data in usable form, organizing data for analysis, and interpreting the data against preestablished criteria. When data are interpreted, the context, frame of reference, objectivity, and legal and ethical issues must also be considered.

Frame of Reference

Frame of reference refers to the reference point used for interpretation of data. Two frames of reference are discussed here: norm-referenced interpretation and criterion-referenced interpretation.

Norm-Referenced Interpretation

Norm-referenced interpretation refers to interpreting data in terms of the norms of a group of individuals who are being evaluated. The scores of the group form a basis for comparing each individual with the others. In norm-referenced evaluation, there will always be an individual who has achieved at the highest level, as well as one who has achieved at the lowest level.

Norm-referenced interpretation permits evaluators to compare achievement of students in several ways. Students in the same group can be compared and ranked. Students can be compared with students in another group or class section or with national group norms, as in the case of licensing examinations or nursing specialty certification examinations. Consequently, an *advantage* of norm-referenced interpretation is the ability to make comparisons within groups or with external groups and to use the data for predictive purposes, such as admission criteria. A *disadvantage* of norm-referenced interpretation is the focus on comparison, which may foster a sense of competitiveness among students.

Criterion-Referenced Interpretation

In *criterion-referenced interpretation,* on the other hand, results are judged against preestablished criteria and reflect the degree of criteria attainment. Criterion-referenced interpretation is typically used in competence-based learning models in which the goal is to assist the learner to achieve competence in or mastery of specified learning outcomes. Because students are compared with the outcomes and not each other, all students can achieve competence.

The *advantages* of criterion-referenced interpretation include the following: emphasis on mastery and the potential for all learners to achieve increased learner motivation, sharing and collaboration among students, and ability to give clear progress reports to learners. *Disadvantages* of criterion-referenced interpretation include the inability to compare students with each other or with other groups.

Issues of Objectivity and Subjectivity

The issues of objectivity and subjectivity in evaluation always arise when data are interpreted. Different evaluators can look at the same data yet render different judgments. The differences may be a result of evaluator bias or degrees of difference in objectivity. Studies of performance appraisals in work settings have shown the effects of recency—interpreting findings when other favorable findings have preceded the evaluation (Polit & Beck, 2013). In some ways, faculty need to accept that there is a certain amount of subjectivity in evaluation; after all, this is "evaluation" and not "measurement." However, faculty should recognize subjectivity and the role it may play in interpretation of findings.

Legal Considerations

There may be legal aspects involved in interpretation of findings. Legal consideration is particularly important in the area of student rights. How will the results of evaluations be shared? What data about students can be collected? Does evaluation involve protection of human subjects? Will there be moral or ethical dilemmas in reporting the data? Who is affected by evaluations? How will they respond to the results? What effect will evaluation have on a student, a program, or a curriculum? Accordingly, the evaluator and the audience must be aware of the context of evaluation because these elements can influence how the evaluation is conducted, how results are reported, what will change because of the evaluation, and how due process will be handled. See Chapter 3 for additional discussion of legal aspects of evaluating students' academic and clinical performance.

Reporting the Findings

In this step of the evaluation process, the results of evaluation are communicated to appropriate persons. Factors to consider when findings are reported include when, how, and to whom the findings will be provided.

Who Receives the Findings?

The evaluator must know to whom the data should be reported. Typically, both the persons and group being evaluated and those requesting evaluation receive evaluation reports. Issues of reporting and confidentiality should be established at the outset of evaluation. Confidentiality of the report must be maintained. Only those persons designated to receive the report should do so. The evaluator should then destroy unneeded background information after the report is completed.

In reporting findings, it is also important to consider the recipient of the report. What will the recipient want and need to know? For example, students receiving a test grade are usually prepared only to understand the grade, not the complex methods that were used to determine the grade or the item analysis statistics. Preparing the recipient for the evaluation report may also be helpful if the recipient does not have adequate background information to receive the report.

When to Report Findings

The timing of the report is also crucial. There tends to be a readiness to know the results of evaluation, and if the report of results is delayed, the recipients may lose interest. For example, students prefer having immediate results and can have increased anxiety or lose interest if results are delayed. The timing of the report may also be based on when information is needed, for example, at the end of the semester when grades are to be reported to the registrar.

How to Report Findings

Evaluation reports can take many forms. They may be written or oral, formal or informal. An example of an informal evaluation is talking with the student about his or her performance in a clinical experience, without a structured evaluation. This type of evaluation is far from ideal and leaves the student and the instructor without objective criteria and a sense of fairness. In the event that the student should fail the course, the instructor is not able to defend the decision. In a formal report, statistical analysis of the data will be accessible along with the findings. Specific methods of reporting findings to students, faculty, administrators, and external audiences are discussed in subsequent chapters.

Using the Findings

Evaluation is a mutual effort between the evaluator and the individual, group, or program being evaluated. Although using the findings is the last, and often forgotten, step of the evaluation process, both parties have obligations to use the findings as explained by Sanders and Sullins (2006). It is a waste of valuable resources to conduct an evaluation without follow-up. Target the evaluation results toward uses that will have the most influence on the program. Barrett-Barrick (1993) states that the use of evaluation findings requires purposeful, strategic planning. Four perspective strategies are purpose, people, planning, and packaging. The *purpose* of the evaluation must be identified by faculty and administration. Types of evaluation used in nursing programs include accreditation, criterion-referenced evaluation, decision-focused evaluation, external evaluation, formative evaluation, internal evaluation, outcome evaluation, process evaluation, and summative evaluation. For an evaluation to be successful, the *people* involved in the evaluation should be included in the process. The main strategy in promoting evaluation is *planning* the activities and disseminating the evaluation information. *Packaging* the evaluation report to meet the needs of those who will use the report is a priority. The report should be in a format that is easily understood, and graphs and other visual aids should be used as needed.

Evaluation results can be used in a variety of ways. Common uses in nursing are to assign grades; revise instruction, courses, curricula, or programs; and demonstrate program effectiveness.

Several ways to improve the use of evaluation efforts are as follows:

1. Encourage persons involved in results to be involved in designing the evaluation plan.
2. Involve all concerned in the evaluation process. For example, students can do self-evaluation; faculty can do peer review.
3. Report findings in a timely manner.
4. Make recommendations that are realistic and can be used. For example, when reporting results of a test to a student, the evaluator (teacher) can make recommendations as to how to study for the next test to improve scores. In this way, the report of the results can be useful to the student.
5. Build in time for sharing results. This can be done by having an examination review, an evaluation conference, or a curriculum evaluation workshop.
6. Encourage the recipient to generate alternatives to behavior. For example, the student can make his or her own suggestions about improving test scores. Faculty and staff can establish goals and objectives for course change.
7. Establish trust and be cautious with sensitive findings.
8. Place findings in context. Explain to the recipients what the findings mean and how they can use the results in their own setting.

Considering the Costs of Evaluation

Evaluation can be costly throughout the entire process, and therefore the evaluator and audience must be assured that the cost will match the benefit.

Answers to the following cost-related questions need to be determined at the outset:

- What fees (or faculty time) are associated with evaluation?
- How much time will the evaluator spend in developing tools, administering tools, interpreting data, and reporting results?
- Will undue time be spent on the part of those being evaluated in filling out evaluation tools?
- Will complex evaluation methods involving lengthy evaluation tools or computer time for data analysis contribute to the outcome?
- Will the results of evaluation require changes?
- Will the student fail the course and need to repeat it?
- Will the curriculum require massive revision?

Summary

Evaluation is a means of appraising data or placing a value on data gathered through one or more measurements. The evaluation process involves a systematic series of actions including identification of a clear purpose, the time frame, and the evaluator. Models or frameworks can be used to guide the process, choice of instruments, data collection methods, and reporting procedures. Would a builder construct a house without plans? The same principle applies in evaluation. The framework establishes the guide to the construction of purposeful evaluation. Researching and developing the framework are the most valuable first steps. Selection of the appropriate instruments is integral to success. The instruments should be appropriate for what is being evaluated, easy to use, cost effective, time efficient, valid, and reliable. Results must be interpreted and reported accurately. Finally, after analysis, the findings must be used. To design and implement an evaluation plan and then ignore the results would defeat the purpose of evaluation. It would be analogous to leaving a newly constructed house empty. Box 22-4 presents several websites that provide useful information about the evaluation process.

BOX 22-4 Internet Resources Related to Evaluation

- **www.scup.org/** Society for College and University Planning.
- **http://nces.ed.gov/ipeds/** Integrated Postsecondary Education Data System (IPEDS).
- **http://nces.ed.gov/** "The National Center for Education Statistics (NCES), located within the U.S. Department of Education and the Institute of Education Sciences, is the primary federal entity for collecting and analyzing data related to education."
- **http://nces.ed.gov/NPEC/** "[The National Postsecondary Education Cooperative's] mission is to promote the quality, comparability and utility of postsecondary data and information that support policy development at the federal, state, and institution levels."
- **http://eric.ed.gov/** "The Education Resources Information Center (ERIC), sponsored by the Institute of Education Sciences (IES) of the U.S."
- **www.chea.org/Research/crossroads.asp** *Accreditation at a Crossroads.*
- **www.chea.org/Events/Usefulness/98May/98_05Ewell.asp** *Examining a Brave New World: How Accreditation Might Be Different.*
- **www.chea.org/pdf/HED_Apr1998.pdf#search="Distancelearning"** Distance Learning in Higher Education.
- **www.chea.org/degreemills/default.htm** *The Fundamentals of Accreditation.*
- **www.ion.illinois.edu/resources/tutorials/pedagogy/index.asp** Instructional Strategies for Online Courses.
- **www.umass.edu/oapa/oapa/publications/online_handbooks/program_based.pdf** *PROGRAM-Based Review and Assessment: Tools and Techniques for Program Improvement.*
- **www.managementhelp.org/evaluatn/fnl_eval.htm** Basic Guide to Program Evaluation.
- **http://paws.wcu.edu/gjones/as.assessment_wcu.html** Assessment and evaluation topics.

REFLECTING ON THE EVIDENCE

1. A national nursing accrediting body has notified you that your program is due for reaccreditation in 3 years. What steps must you take to be prepared for the accreditation team? Develop a plan of action to evaluate and document student and program outcomes, and organize the documents obtained.
   a. Based on the best evidence, choose an evaluation model and evaluation tools, develop a method to track outcome evidence, and develop a plan to delegate certain evaluation components.
   b. Develop a timeline and action plan.
   c. Discuss your timeline, action plan, and effect of accreditation with at least two other students.
   d. What are the evaluation obstacles facing your nursing program and what plan do you have to overcome these obstacles?
2. You have been assigned by your program chair to design the evaluation process for your school of nursing. The school of nursing is a baccalaureate program with 160 students, 12 full-time faculty, and 20 adjunct faculty. Your curriculum has not been revised for 10 years and your National Council Licensure Examination pass rate has averaged 70% for 6 years. What model would you choose for evaluation and why?
3. After you have chosen a model in question 2, design a framework to collect data. Address the evaluation process and stakeholders. Also create a theoretical budget for the evaluation process.
4. Your school of nursing has decided to hire an outside evaluator to evaluate the master's degree (nurse practitioner) program. What criteria would you use to hire an outside evaluator? Who will interact with the evaluator? What documents will he or she need to access? What possible outcomes might occur after an evaluation of this sort? Why might an "outside" evaluator be necessary instead of an "inside" evaluator?

REFERENCES

Barrett-Barrick, C. (1993). Promoting the use of program evaluation findings. *Nurse Educator, 18*(1), 10–12.

Bond, T., & Fox, C. (2007). *Applying the Rasch model: Fundamental measurement in the human sciences.* Mahwah, NJ: Lawrence Erlbaum.

Chen, H. T. (2004). A theory-driven evaluation perspective on mixed methods research. *Research in the Schools, 13*(1), 75–83.

Kirkpatrick, J. D., & Kirkpatrick, D. L. (2014). *The Kirkpatrick Four Levels: A fresh look after 55 years—1959–2014.* Retrieved from, www.kirkpatrickpartners.com.

Lincoln, Y. S., & Guba, E. G. (1985). *Naturalistic inquiry*. Beverly Hills, CA: Sage.

Newby, A. C. (1992). *Training evaluation handbook*. San Diego, CA: Pfeiffer.

Pedhazur, E., & Schmelkin, L. (1991). *Measurement, design, and analysis: An integrated approach*. Hillside, NJ: Lawrence Erlbaum.

Polit, D. F., & Beck, C. T. (2013). *Essentials of nursing research: Methods, appraisal, and utilization*. Philadelphia, PA: Lippincott Williams & Wilkins.

Prus, J., & Johnson, R. (1994). A critical review of student assessment options. *New Directions for Community Colleges, 88*, 69–83.

Quality Matters. (2014). *A national benchmark for online course design*. Retrieved from, https://www.qualitymatters.org/.

Rogers, E. M. (2003). *Diffusion of innovations* (5th ed.). New York: Free Press.

Rudner, L. M. (2001). *Item response theory*. Retrieved from, http://echo.edres.org:8080/irt/.

Sanders, J. R., & Sullins, C. D. (2006). *Evaluating school programs*. Thousand Oaks, CA: Corwin Press.

Story, L., Butts, J. B., Bishop, S. B., Green, L., Johnson, K., & Mattison, H. (2010). Innovative strategies for nursing education program evaluation. *Journal of Nursing Education, 49*(6), 351–354.

Stufflebeam, D. L. (Ed.), (1971). *Educational evaluation and decision-making*. Itasia, IL: Peacock.

Waugh, C. K., & Gronlund, N. E. (2012). *Assessment of student achievement* (10th ed.). Columbus, OH: Pearson.

Wholey, J. S., Haltry, H. P., & Newcomer, K. E. (2004). *Handbook of practical program evaluation*. San Francisco: Jossey-Bass.

23 Strategies for Evaluating Learning Outcomes*

Jane M. Kirkpatrick, PhD, RNC-OB, ANEF
Diann A. DeWitt, PhD, RN, CNE

The purpose of this chapter is to discuss uses, advantages, disadvantages, and issues related to a variety of strategies that faculty can use to evaluate student learning. Just as teaching methods are expanding to ensure that nursing education is integrating clinical and classroom instruction (Benner, Sutphen, Leonard, & Day, 2010) to achieve desired student learning outcomes as identified by the American Association of Colleges of Nursing essentials and National League for Nursing competencies, faculty must also expand their use of evaluation strategies to determine if these competencies are attained. Competency in higher order thinking as demonstrated by clinical reasoning, critical thinking, and best nursing practices may need multiple measures to be accurately evaluated. As educators work to develop deep learning and reflective practice, they continue to explore ways that active learning–teaching strategies can be transformed to evaluate the desired learning outcomes.

The chapter includes practical information on a variety of evaluation strategies. Included are ways to select strategies, improve their validity and reliability, and increase the effectiveness of their use.

*This chapter is dedicated to our outstanding colleague and friend, Dr. Lillian Yeager. Dr. Yeager finished her career as Dean for the School of Nursing at Indiana University Southeast following approximately 30 years as an exceptional educator there. It was our pleasure to collaborate with such an outstanding nurse educator and administrator. Lillian had a keen sense of humor and zest for life, both of which aided in her valiant efforts to live life fully in her fight with cancer. She is greatly missed and will long be remembered by many. Thanks for inspiring us, Lillian!

Assessment and Evaluation

Just what is the difference between assessment and evaluation? In many instances it seems that these two terms are interchangeable, but there are distinct differences. *Assessment* involves obtaining information about teaching and learning for the purpose of improvement. Oermann and Gaberson (2014) indicate that "the process of assessment is important to obtain information about student learning, judge performance and determine competence to practice, and arrive at other decisions about students and nurses" (p. 3). The information collected may be quantitative or qualitative depending on how it will be used. The process of assessment requires faculty to make clear the expectations and quality of performance expected and includes the collection, analysis, and interpretation of student work. The information gained from assessment provides evidence about current learning and then is used to promote further learning (Gikandi, Morrow, & Davis, 2011). Normally, assessment is conducted while learning, or the course or program is ongoing and changes and improvements can be made (see Chapters 10 and 22).

Evaluation, on the other hand, occurs at the end of learning, courses, or programs, and suggests that a judgment or decision has been made. Evaluation can be formative or summative. *Formative evaluation* occurs while learning is taking place; opportunity for feedback and improvement is implicit. *Summative evaluation* is more holistic and takes into account all of the aspects that have led to attaining outcomes. Summative evaluation marks the end of the teaching–learning process and leads to a judgment, often expressed as a grade. In clinical disciplines, faculty must evaluate student attainment of course outcomes and defined program competencies to ensure that graduates are prepared for safe practice. The focus of this chapter is on evaluating student achievement.

Selecting Strategies

The strategies discussed in this chapter provide faculty with a variety of techniques to use to assess and evaluate student learning outcomes. Several of the strategies discussed may also be familiar as teaching strategies. The idea of adapting a teaching strategy for use in assessment or evaluation allows students to practice the same process by which they will ultimately be evaluated. Although most strategies can be used for both assessment (formative evaluation) or final evaluation (summative evaluation), some strategies are more appropriate for assessment whereas others are clearly better used to determine final outcomes of learning and assigning grades.

The major reasons for faculty to consider evaluation strategies are so they can better evaluate (1) all the domains of learning (including the affective domain), (2) higher levels of the cognitive domain (e.g., analysis, synthesis), (3) critical thinking and clinical reasoning, and (4) students' preparation for licensing or certification examinations. By providing a more authentic evaluation wherein the student is asked to perform or demonstrate the learning in a way that is as closely related to the ultimate performance required in the real world, the faculty will have richer and deeper evidence of student achievement.

In selecting evaluation strategies, the philosophy of the faculty regarding accountability and responsibility for learning must be considered. Many of the strategies discussed are compatible with active teaching techniques. Critical reflections, short essays, and guided writing assignments encourage students to interact with the material in a different way than if they were learning the material for a multiple-choice test. The major challenges of using these strategies include (1) the time it takes to use the strategy and (2) difficulty in establishing validity and reliability of data-gathering instruments and methods. To avoid some of the pitfalls associated with these strategies, faculty should do the following:

1. Clearly delineate the *purpose* of the evaluation.
2. Consider the *setting* in which the learning and evaluation will take place.
3. Choose the best evaluation *strategy* for the purpose.
4. Determine the *procedure* for the strategy selected.
5. Establish *validity* and *reliability* of the strategy.
6. Assess the overall *effectiveness* of the process.

Purpose

The purpose of evaluation is to ascertain that students have achieved their potential and have acquired the knowledge, skills, and abilities set forth in courses and curricula. The instructional goals and course outcomes and objectives indicate the type of behavior (cognitive, affective, or psychomotor) to be assessed or evaluated. The learning experiences should be designed to have relevance to the students and the evaluation should carry value in the grading system. Finally, the grading criteria should be shared with the students before evaluation occurs.

Setting

Another critical factor to consider is the setting in which the instruction and evaluation will occur. Most faculty are comfortable with evaluation in traditional classroom settings, but a majority of nursing schools are now using some form of computer-based learning support for either completely online instruction or hybrid (blended) instruction. Most of the strategies discussed in this chapter can be used in an online community. For example, a threaded discussion can be used for critiquing or even as a forum for verbal questioning. Concept maps can be developed in an electronic format. Students or faculty can maintain an electronic portfolio representative of student work throughout the course or program. When considering assessment or evaluation strategies in an online environment, the faculty needs to be sure the technology is relevant for the assessment purpose and build in learning time for both students and faculty to become proficient in the use of the technology (Mok, 2012).

The expansion of interprofessional education creates new opportunities to collaborate with educators from other professions. Clearly identified shared competencies (Interprofessional Education Collaborative Expert Panel, 2011) are essential to this process. As with any team teaching effort, consistent application of criteria are essential. Evaluation strategies discussed in this chapter are appropriate for all professions.

Choice of Strategy

When choosing the best strategy for the purpose, faculty must weigh the advantages and disadvantages of each strategy. Faculty should also consider time for preparation, implementation, and grading. Other issues, such as cost, may also be determining factors. Faculty must decide how often to evaluate, who will evaluate, and how the students will be prepared for the evaluation. When selecting an evaluation strategy, it is imperative that students have ample opportunity to practice in the way in which they will be tested.

Procedures

Although procedures for using evaluation strategies vary, any procedure selected must be well planned. The strategy should be pilot tested before it is fully implemented. This process will help prevent unexpected difficulties, and allows for refinement and quality improvements prior to full-scale implementation. It is also important to delineate the responsibilities associated with the methods used. For example, in the case of portfolio evaluation, a decision must be made about whether students or faculty will collect and keep the work. Another area of concern is the environment in which the evaluation will take place. Because of the anxiety and stress associated with the process of being evaluated, faculty must attempt to provide an atmosphere conducive to the process. Appropriately used humor may help place students at ease.

Validity and Reliability

The issues of validity and reliability are critical, especially when the purpose is for evaluation. In Chapter 22, the terms *validity* and *reliability* are defined and described. For the purposes of this chapter, specific examples are given to clarify establishment of validity and reliability when non–multiple choice evaluation methods are used.

In determining validity, faculty must ask whether the technique is appropriate to the purpose and whether it provides useful and meaningful data (Miller, Linn, & Gronlund, 2012). Faculty must consider the fit of the strategy with the identified objectives. In other words, does the strategy measure what it is supposed to measure? For instance, if the objective for an assignment is for the student to demonstrate skill in written communication, evaluating student performance through oral questioning will not provide valid data. Similarly, at the nursing department level, faculty should coordinate strategies with nursing program outcomes such as critical thinking, clinical reasoning, and communication. It is a challenge to develop sound criteria for evaluation that accurately reflect the specified outcomes, objectives, and content. To establish *face validity,* faculty must seek input from colleagues by asking questions such as, "Do these criteria appear to measure the specified objectives?" In addition, obtaining the opinion of other content experts can assist in determining whether there is adequate sampling of the content (*content validity*). These traditional approaches to establishing validity are being replaced by a unitary concept, based on several different categories of evidence (e.g., face-related evidence, content-related evidence). The evidence available to establish validity determines whether validity is considered low, medium, or high (Gikandi et al., 2011; Miller et al., 2012).

Once evaluation criteria are developed, it is essential to establish their reliability or the ability to be dependable in measuring the desired learning outcome (Gikandi et al., 2011). In completing their systematic review of online formative evaluation these authors determined that a reliable evaluation would document and monitor evidence of learning, and incorporate multiple sources of evidence and "explicit clarity of learning goals and shared meaning of rubrics" (p. 2339). A commonly used method for establishing reliability of an evaluation rubric is to have two or more instructors independently rate student performance using the agreed-on criteria for sample work. Ratings are correlated to establish *interrater reliability,* which is expressed as a percentage of agreement between scores. When agreement is less than 70%, faculty should continue to refine the specificity and clarity of each criterion to come to a stronger agreement. An example of using criteria to establish interrater reliability is provided in Box 23-1. It is especially important to establish interrater reliability when multiple faculty are grading the same assignment. Frequently evaluation criteria are placed in rubrics as a way of articulating the grading scale for assessment criteria. Rubrics are defined in greater detail in the section of this chapter on communicating grading expectations.

A multiplicity of evaluation strategies can provide a more complete picture of the student's abilities and therefore contribute to the trustworthiness of the process. It is a serious limitation to rely on a single strategy. Each strategy has limitations and

BOX 23-1 Establishing Interrater Reliability

Develop criteria and apply them to sample work.
Have two or more observers independently rate performance, then correlate.
The formula for % Agreement is as follows:
total # agreements / # of agreements + # of disagreements

Example: Three raters evaluate written communication using the following criteria:

1. Clear expression of ideas
2. Logical flow and organization
3. Correct use of syntax, grammar, American Psychological Association format
4. Incorporation of research findings
   - Item 1: Two agree, one does not
   - Item 2: All three agree
   - Item 3: Two agree, one does not
   - Item 4: All three agree

10 (Total agreements)/10 (Agreements) + 2 (Disagreements) = 10/12 = 0.83 or 83% (>70% is good)

Polit, D. F., & Hungler, B. P. (1999). *Nursing research: Principles and methods* (6th ed.). Philadelphia: Lippincott, p. 416.

issues that can influence the reliability, validity, and appropriateness of the strategy for given student populations. Using multiple strategies provides a more robust and accurate framework for making decisions.

Effectiveness

After the evaluation strategy is implemented, it is essential to determine its overall effectiveness as well as the potential issues that can arise related to the implementation of the strategy. Some questions faculty should ask include: Was the strategy an effective use of resources (e.g., student and faculty time and financial resources)? Was there adequate data to determine if the learning outcome was met? Are there any problems with the implementation of the technique? What revisions are necessary? Would the faculty consider this strategy to be a good choice for future use?

Matching the Evaluation Strategy to the Domain of Learning

Educators must also be mindful of the domain of learning being evaluated (see Chapters 10 and 15). Cognitive learning is typically assessed or evaluated with strategies requiring the students to write, submit portfolios, or complete tests (see Chapter 10). Assessment in the psychomotor domain typically involves simulations and simulated patients and ultimately occurs in clinical practice (see Chapters 18 and 25). Evaluation in the affective domain is particularly important in nursing and is discussed further here.

The taxonomy of the affective domain as applied to nursing has five behavioral categories: (1) receiving, (2) responding, (3) valuing, (4) organization of values, and (5) characterization by a value or value complex (Krathwohl, Bloom, & Mases, 1964). Development of the affective domain is progressive and can be tied to clinical reasoning. Because of the progressive nature of development, formative evaluation (assessment) across the curriculum may be most appropriate, with a summative evaluation at the time of graduation. Many of the evaluation strategies listed in this chapter can be adapted for the affective domain. For example, using the concept of cultural competency, formative and summative evaluation can be planned throughout the curriculum. At the beginning level, students may be expected to become self-aware using exploration of their own cultural and health care practices as well as values. A midprogram outcome could focus on student awareness of the cultural orientation of the patients under their care. At graduation, the expected outcomes (including knowledge, skills, and attitudes) would be to act in a culturally competent manner when providing care to all patients and demonstrate the ability to advocate for an individual patient's unique needs.

Ondrejka (2014) and Olantunji (2014) each discuss the importance of incorporating affective teaching and evaluating affective learning. Olantunji (2014) suggests that colleges and universities tend to overemphasize the cognitive domain with a resultant neglect of the affective domain and proposes that regaining a balance between the cognitive and affective domain during the educational experience would increase the quality of the graduates.

Multiple strategies can be used to evaluate the affective domain. By again considering the example of acquiring cultural competence, faculty might consider using written papers with the purpose of having students identifying their own cultural background or perhaps develop a critical analysis of an interaction in care giving with a patient of another culture. The use of media (e.g., video recording, webpage development, or even a collage) to demonstrate key concepts and values held by a given culture is another method that can be used. These learning activities encourage self-awareness and recognition of the values and value conflicts in areas in which judgments must be made, and can help students appreciate the implications of how respect and caring are communicated in various cultures. The evaluation criteria for these activities must emphasize the desired outcome. For example, if the selected strategy is a written assignment, overemphasis on process (such as writing style) may negate the importance of students' insights and self-awareness.

Other areas within the nursing profession that lend themselves well to evaluation in the affective domain include, but are not limited to, socialization to the roles of the nurse, developing a professional identity, caring for patients who are dying, meeting spirituality needs, and working with sexuality concerns. The Quality and Safety Education for Nurses (QSEN) competencies specifically focus on attitudes as well as knowledge and skills needed by nurses (Cronenwett et al., 2007). QSEN exemplars take a defined concept and list outcomes for the knowledge, skills, and attitudes. For example, an attitudinal competency identified in the category of patient centered care is "Value seeing health care situations 'through patients' eyes'" (http://qsen.org/competencies/pre-licensure-ksas/).

Communicating Grading Expectations

When evaluation strategies are used to collect data for grading purposes, it is imperative that the grading requirements be communicated to the students. Information about grading criteria is typically provided to students in the course syllabus. Other methods such as checklists, guidelines, or grading scales can be used as well. See Box 23-2 for an example of a writing assignment with grading rubric.

Rubrics are rating scales used to determine performance (Stevens & Levi, 2012). Rubrics not only provide exquisite clarity of the grading criteria, they also provide a mechanism to inform students about grading expectations. The two basic types of rubrics are *holistic* and *analytic.* The holistic approach is based on global scoring, often with descriptive information

BOX 23-2 Sample Writing Assignment with Grading Rubric

COLORADO CHRISTIAN UNIVERSITY

COLLEGE OF ADULT AND GRADUATE STUDIES

NUR468A Global Nursing & International Health Care

Final Global Health Paper

PURPOSE OF ASSIGNMENT:

The purpose of this assignment is to provide the student an opportunity to research a current global health issue. In addition, the research and reflections related to this real-life situation will demonstrate knowledge of the key principles explored in this course. Reflections on the cultural perspectives related to this global health issue must also be addressed.

ASSIGNMENT INSTRUCTIONS

Background:

The world has become aware of the Ebola virus crisis in West Africa. It has touched the hearts of many in the United States because of the missionaries who contracted the disease. This paper will be within the context of the Ebola virus outbreak.

Requirements

1. Introduction, including a thesis statement (the purpose or focus of the paper)
2. The body of the paper should clearly explain the topic and include the following:
   a. Overview of the Ebola virus outbreak. Some typical questions might include:
      i. Describe the recent Ebola outbreak.
      ii. What is the disease?
      iii. How does it affect the patients?
      iv. What are the treatment options?
      v. Where is it occurring?
      vi. What effect does it have on that region?
      vii. What is currently being done to contain the virus?
   b. Explain the cultural issues to consider that may affect caring for these patients, families, and communities.
3. The conclusion (a summary of the main points of the paper; no introduction of new ideas)
4. American Psychological Association format (see university writing resources)
5. Be sure to use topic sentences and transitional sentences to enhance the flow of the paper.
6. Three to five pages (not including title page and reference page)

Please follow the scholarly writing rubric and submit through Assignments by the due date.

BOX 23-2 Sample Writing Assignment with Grading Rubric—cont'd

COLORADO CHRISTIAN UNIVERSITY

Division of Nursing and Sciences

Scholarly Paper Grading Rubric

Criteria	Levels of Achievement				Points & Comments
	Poor	Fair	Good	Excellent	
Application of Knowledge: Analysis	0 to 3.5 points Student restates or lists course content.	3.6 to 5 points Student's argument/ perspective is unclear or not cohesive with course material.	5.1 to 5.5 points Student develops a stance/ argument based on themes and/ or connections between course material and references or research.	5.6 to 6.5 points Student provides original perspective, drawing on course content and relevant academic references or research.	
Bloom's Taxonomy	0 to 3.5 points Student shows only basic knowledge of concept (recall/ restate the information).	3.6 to 5 points Student shows comprehension of concept (understand meaning and state in own words).	5.1 to 6 points Student is able to apply, then analyze the concept (use concept in different situation and separate into component parts to understand structure).	6.1 to 7 points Student synthesizes and evaluates the concept (creates new meaning or structure and forms judgments).	
Written Communi- cation: Structure and Transitions	0 to 3.5 points Introduction is not included and/ or there is no clear purpose, subject, or position for the paper.	3.6 to 5 points Introduction does not focus the intention of the paper. The thesis or topic sentence is implied but not specific.	5.1 to 6 points Introduction highlights general subject of paper and includes a thesis to identify a topic, indicating the subject matter the writing is about.	6.1 to 7 points Introduction engages reader and focuses attention on what is to follow. The thesis is interesting, specific, and manageable.	
	0 to 3.5 points Paragraphs with <3 sentences and flow or organization often hard to follow.	3.6 to 5 points Paragraphs with < 3 sentences and/or flow or organization sometimes difficult to follow.	5.1 to 5.5 points Transitions are obvious and/or routine, simply getting the job done.	5.6 to 6.5 points Paragraphs very well developed with logical flow and organization. Minimum of 3 sentences compose each paragraph.	

(Continued)

BOX 23-2 Sample Writing Assignment with Grading Rubric—cont'd

Criteria	Levels of Achievement				Points & Comments
	Poor	Fair	Good	Excellent	
	0 to 3.5 points Transitions not present.	3.6 to 5 points Transitions are choppy/ jarring, and fail to create relationships between paragraphs.	5.1 to 5.5 points Transitions are obvious and/or routine, simply getting the job done.	5.6 to 6.5 points Paragraphs very well developed with logical flow, excellent transitions and organization.	
	0 to 3.5 points Conclusion is not included.	3.6 to 5 points Conclusion is vague and insufficient in summarizing the paper or new ideas appear in the conclusion.	5.1 to 5.5 points Conclusion summarizes the thesis indicating if thesis supported or proved. No new ideas appear in the conclusion.	5.6 to 6.5 points Conclusion examines implications of the thesis and gives the reader a satisfying closure/ summary. No new ideas appear in the conclusion.	
Written Communication: Language, Spelling, and Grammar	0 to 3.5 points Conversational word choice; passive voice only; no variety in sentence structure.	3.6 to 5 points Conversational word choice; limited variety in sentence structure; passive voice is primarily used.	5.1 to 5.5 points Both conversational and academic language used; some variety in sentence structure; active and passive voices are used.	5.6 to 6.5 points Strong, effective academic word choice; variety in sentence structure; active voice is primarily used.	
	0 to 3.5 points Paper contains ≥3 spelling or grammatical errors.	3.6 to 5 points Paper contains 2 spelling or grammatical errors.	5.1 to 5.5 points Paper contains 1 spelling or grammatical error.	5.6 to 6.5 points Paper contains 0 spelling or grammatical errors.	
Use of Evidence: Support, Evidence, and APA Format	0 to 3.5 points Student provides little to no support for statements.	3.6 to 5 points Student attempts to match course materials to assumptions but does not have corresponding references or research for support.	5.1 to 6 points Student's arguments/ perspectives are developed on course content and applicable academic references or research.	6.1 to 7 points Student synthesizes references or research and course content to support their perspective.	
	0 to 3.5 points No connections between argument and references or research made.	3.6 to 5 points Connections between argument and references or research are unclear.	5.1 to 5.5 points Connections between argument and references or research are clear.	5.6 to 6.5 points Connections between argument and references or research are clear and creative.	

BOX 23-2 Sample Writing Assignment with Grading Rubric—cont'd

Criteria	Levels of Achievement				Points & Comments
	Poor	Fair	Good	Excellent	
	0 to 3.5 points Greater than 2 ideas identified that lack in-text citation.	3.6 to 5 points Two ideas identified that lack in-text citation.	5.1 to 6 points One idea identified, which lacks in-text citation.	6.1 to7 points All ideas that are not unique to the student or considered common knowledge are cited in the text of the paper.	
	0 to 3.5 points Use of direct quotes is excessive (≥50%).	3.6 to 5 points Use of direct quotes is moderate (<50%).	5.1 to 5.5 points Use of direct quotes is minimal (<20% of citations).	5.6 to 6.5 points Use of direct quotes is rare (<5% of citations).	
	0 to 3.5 points Less than 50% of sources are from primary sources of evidence from the literature.	3.6 to 5 points Between 50–80% of sources are from primary sources of evidence from the literature.	5.1 to 5.5 points Uses predominantly (>80%) primary sources of evidence from the literature to support arguments and/or claims made in paper.	5.6 to 6.5 points Exclusively uses (>95%) primary sources of evidence from the literature to support arguments and/or claims made in paper.	
	0 to 3.5 points Less than 50% of evidence from the literature used to support arguments and/or claims in paper have been published within the last 5 years or is a classic.	3.6 to 5 points Majority of evidence from the literature (>50%) used to support arguments and/or claims in paper have been published within the last 5 years or is a classic.	5.1 to 6 points Most evidence from the literature (>80–95%) used to support arguments and/or claims in paper have been published within the last 5 years or is a classic.	6.1 to 7 points Almost all evidence from the literature (>95%) used to support arguments and/or claims in paper have been published within the last 5 years or is a classic.	
	0 to 3.5 points Paper contains ≥3 APA formatting errors.	3.6 to 5 points Paper contains 2 APA formatting errors.	5.1 to 5.5 points Paper contains 1 APA formatting error.	5.6 to 6.5 points Paper contains 0 APA formatting errors.	

APA, American Psychological Association.
Adapted from Online Certificate of Advanced Graduate Study (CAGS) Rubric 2014.

for each area based on a numerical scoring system, whereas analytic scoring involves examining each significant characteristic of the written work or portfolio. For example, in evaluation of writing, the organization, ideas, and style may be judged individually according to analytic scoring (Miller et al., 2012). The global method seems more suitable for summative evaluation, whereas the analytic method is useful in providing specific feedback to students for the purpose of performance improvement.

Regardless of the type, rubrics are composed of four parts: (1) a task description (the assignment), (2) a scale, (3) the dimensions of the assignment, and (4) descriptions of each performance level (Stevens & Levi, 2012). The first portion of a rubric contains a clear description of the assignment and should be matched to the learning outcomes of the course. The next part of the rubric is a scale to describe levels of performance. Such a scale may include levels such as "excellent," "competent," and "needs work." The dimensions of the assignment appear in the third part of rubric development where the task is broken down into components. Finally, differentiated descriptions of each performance level are explicitly identified. Rubrics thus provide clarity of expectations to assist students in the successful completion of assignments as well as making grading of these assignments more objective for the faculty. See Box 23-3 for an example of grading rubrics.

BOX 23-3 Examples of Grading Rubrics

"A" GRADE

The final course *synthesis paper* clearly defines a researchable problem; the search strategy provides sufficient relevant data for understanding the problem; the coding sheet is focused and guides the analysis of the data; issues of reliability and validity are identified; the literature is synthesized, rather than reviewed or summarized; the paper concludes with recommendations based on the research synthesis. The paper is written using the IUSON writing guidelines.

Participation in discussions and learning activities integrates course concepts and reflects critical thinking about research synthesis. Participation is thoughtful, respectful, informed, and substantiated. Peer review of the synthesis paper reflects the reviewers' understanding of the synthesis process, provides practical suggestions, and is presented in a collegial manner.

Dissemination of the findings of the research synthesis includes a written *plan for publication* and an oral *presentation* to faculty and classmates. The plan for publication includes thoughtful selection of a journal; draft of a query or cover letter; and, if the paper needs revisions to suit publication guidelines, a statement about revisions needed that matches the journal publication guidelines. The professional presentation is well organized, supported by visual aids (e.g., PowerPoint slides), and uses professional communication style to suit the audience.

"B" GRADE

The final *synthesis paper* clearly defines a researchable problem; the search strategy yields mostly relevant data for understanding the problem; the coding sheet lacks one or more important data or does not reflect the scope of the problem statement; issues of reliability and validity are unclear; the review of literature is primarily synthesis with minimal summary; the paper concludes with mostly appropriate recommendations. The paper is free of major errors in grammar or style.

Participation in discussions and learning activities usually integrates course concepts and reflects critical thinking about research synthesis. Participation is helpful but may not contribute substantially to the focus of the course. Peer review of the synthesis paper does not include relevant aspects of the peer review checklists or overlooks areas in which feedback is needed.

Dissemination of the findings of the research synthesis includes a written *plan for publication* and an oral *presentation* to faculty and classmates. The plan for publication includes appropriate selection of a journal; the drafts of the query or cover letter are generally appropriate to the situation; general revisions are noted but do not consider manuscript guidelines of the journal. The professional presentation is fairly well organized; the visual aids (e.g., PowerPoint slides) enhance the presentation; the presentation is delivered with consideration for the audience.

"C" GRADE

The final *synthesis paper* has an ill-defined problem; the search strategy yields irrelevant or tangential data for understanding the problem; the coding sheet is not well focused or neglects key variables or includes irrelevant variables; issues of reliability and validity are not identified or are ignored; the review is more summary than synthesis; the paper does not include recommendations or includes recommendations that are not drawn from the data. There are substantial errors in grammar or writing style.

Participation in discussions occurs on an irregular basis and is not grounded in course concepts, comments do not reflect critical thinking, and there are breaches of course norms and etiquette. Peer review of the synthesis paper does not provide substantive or helpful feedback to classmates; significant aspects of the peer review checklist are ignored.

Dissemination of the findings of the research synthesis includes a written *plan for publication* and an oral *presentation* to faculty and classmates. There is no plan for publication or the journal selected is not appropriate for the content of the paper; the drafts of the query or cover letters are not clearly written and do not capture attention of the reader; there is not clear understanding of the revisions needed of the paper for the style requirements for the selected journal. The professional presentation is not well organized; visual aids (e.g., PowerPoint slides) or the visuals do not clarify or highlight key points of the presentation; the presentation exceeds time limits or is not suited to the audience. The presenter is unable to answer audience questions, if any, about the material.

IUSON, Indiana University School of Nursing.

The Association of American Colleges and Universities (AAC&U) has developed the Valid Assessment of Learning in Undergraduate Education (VALUE) initiative, a set of standardized rubrics to evaluate multiple skills such as reasoning, critical thinking, and written work across a university or college (Sullivan, 2014). The 16 rubrics are viewed as both an alternative to standardized testing for the evaluation of student learning outcomes and as a way of communicating criteria associated with achievement and student success. These rubrics are not designed for individual grading, but rather for use at the program and university level. The AAC&U is currently building a database in which student work can be deposited and scored using the VALUE rubrics (Sullivan, 2014).

Strategies for Evaluating Learning Outcomes

Nursing faculty have a multitude of available strategies to evaluate student learning. This section identifies several strategies known to be effective in nursing. Table 23-1 provides an overview of these strategies.

Portfolios

Description and Uses

Portfolios at the most basic level are collections of student work. Although the medium most widely used for pen-and-paper portfolios in the past has been some type of binder to contain the data, electronic portfolios, commonly called *e-portfolios,* are more prevalent now (see suggested websites at the end of the chapter for valuable resources). The e-portfolio experience has been shown to be most effective when students have a clear understanding of the technology and have an appreciation for the relevance of using this method of evaluation (Mok, 2012).

Regardless of the format, portfolios are used to obtain a broader sample of student performance (Miller et al., 2012). Portfolios are used for a variety of purposes. They can be used (1) as proof of achievement in a class, (2) as an outcome measure of a program, (3) as a marketing tool for job placement, or (4) for student placement in a program of study.

The purpose of the portfolio needs to be clearly established before work is collected for inclusion. Portfolios for student *assessment* are a collection of student work within the course or program of study that is designed to demonstrate *progress* of the learning. The learning outcomes help in determining the specific materials to be included in the portfolio. Decisions need to be made on whether the portfolio is for formative or summative evaluation or both. The work and assignments to be included, the timing of the collection of the assignments, as well as whether the grading remarks will be included in the portfolio are also decisions that need to be made. *Nonselective portfolios* are collections of all student work for a specified period. The focus of these is more on formative evaluation of student progress. A compilation of certain completed works of students is frequently referred to as a *selective portfolio*. A selective portfolio often contains works that are the best efforts of the student and are usually part of a summative evaluation.

Evaluation of the portfolio may occur during the course or plan of study (formative) or at the end (summative). A comprehensive portfolio may be used to demonstrate the acquisition of competencies during a program of study (Roberts, Shadbolt, Clark, & Simpson, 2014). It is important that clearly established criteria be identified for the assessment, evaluation, or grading of the portfolio. These criteria need to be shared with students at the onset of the process.

Students may be required to *critique* their *progress* as the portfolio develops during the course, clinical placement, or the plan of study. When clearly delineated criteria are used, this exercise engages students in self-assessment and critical reflective skills that more effectively prepare them for real-world practice (Roberts et al., 2014). O'Sullivan et al. (2012) used portfolios in a competency-based medical curriculum and noted that students became very aware of the expected program outcomes as they repeatedly selected the materials to include and completed self-reflections on their progress toward these outcomes.

Portfolios used as an *outcome measure of a program* can include selections of student work acquired throughout the curriculum. Samples of these portfolios can be used to evaluate student progress in an area such as writing skills to provide feedback about the effectiveness of the program (Robertson et al., 2010).

Although liberal arts graduates have used portfolios of their work when seeking employment and

TABLE 23-1 Overview of Assessment Strategies

Technique	Domain/ Assessment Purpose	Possible Applications	Advantages	Disadvantages	Issues
Portfolio (paper and electronic)	High-level cognitive Affective Psychomotor (if video) Formative Summative	Placement in program of study For evidence of progress Outcome measure for individual or program Marketing tool for job placement	Broad sample of student work Documents progress Identifies student strengths and weaknesses Critical thinking with student reflection If e-portfolio is easier to make updates and convenient for online programs	Time for collection and grading Need storage space Not direct observation Limited reliability Additional expenses with electronic portfolios Time needed for learning	Ownership Responsibility for collection Nonselective vs. selective portfolio Are you assessing process or product? Deciding on the format for organizing the portfolio
Role play	Cognitive Affective Psychomotor Formative	Formative feedback for psychomotor skills, communication techniques, problem-solving skills	Active participation of student Stimulates creativity Variables can be controlled Can repeat Provides practice in peer-review skills	Immediate feedback may not be possible Self-consciousness of participant	Takes time to build comfort with technique Need familiarity with material
Reflection	High-level cognitive Affective domain Formative Summative (for trending)	Self-assessment Integration of learning can be demonstrated Appropriate for assessing the higher-level cognitive skills; critical thinking can be assessed	Active student involvement Encourages students to form connections within and between content Assists students to practice self-assessment based on criteria Encourages recognition of learning in students' life experience	Time consuming for both students and faculty Student frustration with lack of clarity of assignment	Grading criteria can be developed jointly Requires a high degree of trust Students will need orientation to this process May want to consider anonymous grading
Paper	High levels of cognitive and affective domains Formative Summative	Critical thinking skills Writing skills Develop arguments Synthesis of ideas	More in-depth information in area of interest A public work to be assessed Writing is the scholarly model for self- expression	Time for both faculty and student Subjectivity in grading Limited sample of ability	Reliability Grading criteria
Essays	High levels of cognitive and affective domains Formative Summative	Critical thinking skills Free-form Demonstrate problem-solving abilities, decision making, and rationale Analysis	Shorter than a paper Assess recall and synthesis at one moment rather than at several times Creativity Easy to construct and administer	Less sample of content and ability Time to write and time to grade	Reliability Grading criteria Clarity of questions Use a test plan to better cover content

TABLE 23-1 Overview of Assessment Strategies—cont'd

Technique	Domain/ Assessment Purpose	Possible Applications	Advantages	Disadvantages	Issues
Oral (verbal) questioning	All ranges of cognitive domain Affective domain Formative Summative	Evidence of thinking process with "why" questions Evidence of verbal skills Defense: determines content mastery and evidence of synthesis	Quick to prepare Inexpensive Opportunity for student to receive immediate corrective feedback Works well for nonlinear ideas	Perceived by students as threatening Bias of evaluator	Must determine the difference between questions for teaching vs. assessment Criteria for assessment should be established before use Can be subjective
Concept mapping	All ranges of cognitive domain Affective Formative	Concepts expressed in a visual way Shows relationships between and among topics	Works well for students who are highly visual in their orientation Computer-based tools available for electronic submissions	Artistic students may have an advantage Can be frustrating to concrete thinkers Time to master electronic format	Reliability Grading criteria must be defined Allow for student creativity
Audio and Video Recording	All ranges of cognitive domain Affective domain Video gives evidence of psychomotor domain Formative Summative	Verbal skills Interviews Group discussion Video captures nonverbal performance	Provides evidence when presence of faculty may be intrusive or when faculty are unable to be present Relatively inexpensive Is a permanent record Evidence can be replayed Works for self-assessment	Limited by mode of recording May be difficult to get quality recording of each group member Requires time to listen Expense and maintenance of equipment	Requires consent Student should be aware of how the recording will be used Must determine whether entire tape or a sampling of the tape will be assessed Confidentiality of patient data is critical
Patient Simulation	Psychomotor High-level Cognitive Affective	Safe practice environment for psychomotor skills Preparation for clinical	Active involvement of students and faculty Team interaction	Expensive Specially trained personnel including faculty Small numbers of active students per scenario Training persons for patient role	Integration into the curriculum Selection of scenarios Opportunity to practice prior to assessment Equipment maintenance Faculty education/ training Personnel needs Efficient scheduling of students
Service learning	Higher levels of cognitive domain Affective domain Formative Summative	Evidence of complex communication and problem-solving skills; teamwork, if group project	Authentic learning and assessment; effect on student, preceptor, and community; student exposure to diverse and/ or underserved populations	Time to coordinate with students, agency personnel; risk that expectations of students and agency for scope of project are not alike	Assessment should include outcomes for student learning, preceptor and agency satisfaction, and impact on targeted community

further study for many years, this approach is now increasing in nursing. In some geographical areas jobs for new graduates are competitive and an outstanding portfolio may assist to secure employment. Karagory and Kirby (2014) have implemented digital badges as an electronic method to demonstrate specific competency acquisition. The digital badge can be linked to the student's electronic resume or portfolio. An employer can open the badge to view samples of the work accomplished by the new graduate. Similarly, a portfolio or dossier may be useful when applying to academic institutions for advanced education. Select BSN completion programs use student portfolios to validate prior learning and experience.

Portfolios are often used in nursing programs for advanced placement of students. The portfolio is a compilation of objective evidence demonstrating expertise and skills acquired through prior learning, practice experience, or both. Guidelines for compiling and assessing such portfolios must be clearly delineated. Examples of documentation that may be included in this type of portfolio include (but are not limited to) a resume, performance evaluation, course syllabi or outlines, and evidence of professional activity.

Similar to student portfolios are those used by faculty; faculty may use portfolios when they are seeking promotion or showing evidence in performance evaluations. Guidelines for construction of such portfolios usually include evidence and assessment of teaching, scholarship, and service, although specific requirements differ among institutions.

Advantages

Portfolios provide a broad sample of student work and can show evidence of progress or accomplishment, especially as they are linked to a program goal or competency. Identification of student strengths and weaknesses allows students to make improvements. Student reflection on the work in a portfolio can stimulate critical thinking and also provide evidence of the developing affective domain. Using portfolios for advanced placement in programs enables students to receive credit for previous experience and reduces repetition of content. The e-portfolio provides increased access by both students and faculty and allows large amounts of data to be gathered, increasing the comprehensiveness of the data. The e-portfolio lends itself well to online courses and programs.

Disadvantages

Although collection of the portfolio papers is not time consuming, the main disadvantage associated with portfolios is the time needed to provide feedback and grades. In addition, it is challenging and takes time for faculty to determine validity and reliability for the established grading criteria or rubrics. If e-portfolios are used, additional resources may be needed, such as the expense for software licensing or online storage costs as well as time for faculty and students to learn the technology.

Issues

Major issues related to student portfolios are ownership of the portfolio, responsibility for collection, fair grading, use of nonselective versus selective portfolios and the format used to organize the portfolio. Both paper and electronic formats are used, although electronic ones are gaining in popularity. When a portfolio is used for classroom or program assessment or evaluation, the faculty must determine the purpose of the portfolio (e.g., to assess writing skill or critical thinking), which works will be collected, who is responsible for maintaining the portfolio, what criteria will be used to assess the collection, the scoring method, and timing of feedback.

When portfolio is used for program assessment purposes, faculty buy-in and adequate faculty development are key (Robertson et al., 2010). These authors emphasize the implications for organizational culture change, the need to clarify faculty role expectations for development and participation in the portfolio review process, institution of reward structures to recognize faculty service provided, and development of tools that adequately reflect the program outcomes that are all necessary for successful implementation of portfolio for program assessment.

Critical Reflection

Description and Uses

The development of self-assessment skills is key to student success and is an essential component of professional development (Benner et al., 2010; Bercher, 2012). The use of reflection is also a technique that can be used in interprofessional education to improve awareness of the mental model individuals apply to a practice experience. Shared mental models are defined as "individually held knowledge structures that help team members function collaboratively in their environments" (McComb & Simpson, 2014, p. 1479). Building shared mental models among members of teams is considered to enhance effectiveness of the team.

Self-monitoring of clinical practice (paying attention to clinical actions while in the moment, purposely examining the effect of one's actions, and using these insights to improve future thinking and practice) should be cultivated by health care professionals (Larkin & Klonoff, 2014). The concept of reflective practice has developed from the work of Schoen (1984) in the early 1980s. Schoen determined two kinds of reflective thinking: The first occurs in the moment and can be characterized by the phrases "thinking on one's feet" or "mindfulness." The second is reflection after the fact. Both of these reflective activities are important for practicing health professionals (Larkin & Klonoff, 2014, p. 56). The purpose of self-reflection is to create a more thoughtful, self-aware, and reflective practitioner who will ultimately contribute to improved quality of care. Reflection generates attribution and judgment about performance that evokes an emotional response. These attributions and emotions can either enhance or decrease students' level of self-efficacy (Bercher, 2012). The use of reflection on experiences as a learning tool promoted self-awareness and supported self-directed learning when nursing students engaged in critical analysis (Tashiro, Shimpuku, Naruse, Matsutani, & Matsutani, 2013).

The use of reflection as a learning activity encourages the students to fully consider a question, an experience, or a thesis, and to process their thoughts. For example, a reflection may focus on preclinical experience exploration of values, postclinical reactions to an experience, or a self-assessment of a component of professional development. The reflection itself may be implemented through a variety of techniques such as short (one- to two-page) papers, progressive journaling, or through oral questioning and discussion with individuals or in groups.

Reflections allow faculty to assess level of understanding and guide students in the awareness of their mental models, and help students expand critical thinking skills, which leads to professional development (Tashiro et al., 2013). Journaling can be a strategy for reflection and can be organized as a preclass (preparing for the class), intraclass (as a result of activities conducted during the class or clinical experience), and postclass (such as a homework reflection where examples may be used to demonstrate understanding of key concepts).

Evaluation of reflection is based on an educational connoisseurship model, in which students become connoisseur critics. According to Eisner (1985), a connoisseur is able to appreciate and distinguish the important from the trivial. Although students may not have enough experience to be true connoisseurs, the faculty member can role model and coach students to develop these skills. Bevis and Watson (1989), in a modification of Eisner's work, identified six levels of critiquing: looking, seeing, perceiving and intuiting, rendering, interpreting meaning, and judging. These steps include identifying an event, viewing it with a focus, interpreting the event on a personal level (complete with value clarification), and discerning the significance of the event. Evaluation criteria can be built around these steps.

Providing feedback to student reflections requires thoughtful responses by faculty. Effective assessment includes feedback about the student's efforts; individualized and clearly expressed comments that focus on the work—not the student as an individual; and concern for the student's learning. Faculty comments should focus on the learning to be obtained from the assignment. Seven components for responding to writing identified by Beach and Marshall (1991) are useful for response and are described in Box 23-4.

Advantages

As a strategy, reflection provides an opportunity to examine critical thinking and values awareness. The process of contemplative learning practices, including completing reflection on experiential learning, serves to reinforce the expected standards (O'Sullivan et al., 2012) and can contribute to deep learning (Kuroda, 2014). Sequential reflections provide evidence of learning over time.

Disadvantages

The use of critical self-reflection for evaluation requires time for both students and faculty. Students may experience initial frustration if the scope of the assignment is not well defined and the skills required for critiquing are not practiced. The process used to grade the critique must be clearly defined. For this type of assignment, the grading may

BOX 23-4 Seven Components for Responding to Writing

1. **Praising:** providing positive reinforcement for students
2. **Describing:** providing "reader-based" feedback about one's own reactions and perceptions of the students' responses that imply judgments of those responses
3. **Diagnosing:** determining the students' own unique knowledge, attitudes, abilities, and needs
4. **Judging:** evaluating the sufficiency, level, depth, completeness, validity, and insightfulness of a student's responses
5. **Predicting and reviewing growth:** predicting potential directions for improving student's responses according to specific criteria and reviewing progress from previous responses
6. **Record keeping:** keeping a record to chart changes across time in student's performance
7. **Recognizing/praising growth:** giving students recognition and praise for demonstrating growth

Excerpt from Beach, R. W., & Marshall, J. D. (1991). *Teaching literature in the secondary school* (pp. 211–212). New York: Harcourt Brace & Company, 1991.

be less focused on form, and more focused on the insights (Pohlman, 2013). Defining the criteria for evaluation and clearly communicating them is essential. For example, Wyss, Freedman, and Siebert (2014) developed a grading rubric for online graduate student discussions, beginning with general directions and criteria. The final rubric was centered on three key attributes and provided clear descriptions of what constituted minimal, basic, and proficient performance. These authors note that student performance improved with the implementation of the rubric.

Issues

Students must be oriented to the elements that are essential to a high-quality reflection. The authors' initial experience with reflection found that students spent the majority of a written reflection assignment describing the event or incident, providing minimal analysis. If the purpose of the reflection activity is to provide evidence of analysis and application, then the assignment needs to be structured for this. A three-part journal framework can accomplish this goal. The first section is for description of the event, the second section requests the student to demonstrate an understanding of the concepts by applying the content from the course to the experience, and the third section asks the student to apply the understanding gained from the analysis to a future professional experience.

Time involved for both students and faculty is an issue. Writing thoughtful reflections requires a time commitment on the part of students. Those who procrastinate may not obtain the benefits of the exercise. For faculty, reading and responding can be a lengthy process. For example, if reflections are assigned in the framework of a sequential journal, faculty must decide whether they are going to read each entry for evaluation purposes or take a sample.

The purpose of the assignment must be clearly established for its full benefits to be realized. Establishing grading criteria before students complete the assignment will convey outcome expectations. Faculty feedback should also be of a critically reflective nature and may be most effective as a formative evaluation. The use of anonymity could be appropriate for grading this kind of assignment, because it can enhance objectivity on the part of the evaluator and minimize student fears that can inhibit honesty and creativity.

In critical reflection, the relationship of the student and faculty changes to shared power in the learning environment. The faculty–student relationship becomes more collegial, and a high level of mutual trust and desire to grow is essential. It is also imperative that the philosophy of the school and faculty support the practice of critical reflection. Students should also know who will view their reflections. If peers will view the reflections (e.g., via threaded discussions, etc.) the amount of self-disclosure students choose to provide may be affected. Confidentiality for the student reflection is an important consideration. If the reflection assignments are kept in an electronic format, password protection adds security.

Papers and Essays

Description and Uses

Papers and assigned essays or essay questions on examinations can be used to demonstrate organizational skills, critical thinking, clinical reasoning, and written communication while encouraging creativity. *Papers* are written reports, whereas *essays* are free-form responses to open-ended questions.

Students are encouraged to be creative in responding to essay questions. Both papers and essays can measure the affective domain, as well as higher levels of the cognitive domain.

Advantages

In-depth information can be obtained through the writing of papers. This helps students clarify their own thinking about topics and learn to write better. Papers are a public work and can be assessed by others in the profession. Writing papers requires students to integrate their ideas with those found in other sources. Similarly, essays are useful for assessing higher-level cognitive skills such as analysis and synthesis.

Using essay questions in a testing environment has the advantage that essay questions are easier to construct than multiple-choice examination questions. It is important to make the essay question clearly understood and focused; providing the grading criteria to students will help them allocate their response time more effectively during the testing session (Davis, 2009). Essay tests can demonstrate the ability of the student to synthesize material they have learned and convey their ideas clearly without the benefit of resources.

Disadvantages

The major disadvantage of papers for both students and faculty is the amount of time involved in writing and grading. Faculty can become distracted from the content of the paper when a student exhibits poor writing skills. As well, faculty feedback may be more focused on supporting the grade assigned even when faculty states their belief that the purpose of feedback is to improve students' skill acquisition (Li & Barnard, 2011). Providing constructive comments can be accomplished through facilitative comments by posting questions versus being authoritative. Davis (2009) suggests using the question, "What do you hope your reader will understand your thesis to be?" instead of a directive statement such as "State your thesis more clearly" (p. 328). Faculty should also avoid the temptation to rewrite the paper while they are grading. An essay test may involve less sampling of the content than a multiple-choice examination.

Issues

Reliability in grading papers is an issue. Reliability can be increased by having clearly established grading criteria and having more than one person grade the paper. This is especially important for papers that receive low or failing grades. Anonymous grading can increase the objectivity of the grader. Faculty should determine the assessment plan based on the purpose of the paper and desired outcomes. For example, if the purpose is to demonstrate critical thinking and creativity, the format of the paper may have less value in the total grade of the paper. Alternatively, if the purpose is for the student to demonstrate scholarly writing, evaluation may emphasize the format and style of writing.

Writing a clear and focused essay question can be a challenge for faculty. The question needs to be stated in such a way that the scope is clear to the students. It is also important to follow a test plan when essay tests are constructed so that the content is adequately sampled. Before grading an essay examination, faculty must establish clear grading criteria. When more than one person is grading, interrater reliability needs to be established. Time required to answer the essay should be determined. Davis (2009) suggests providing approximately twice the amount of time for students to provide their answer in a testing environment as it takes for the faculty member to write out the answer to the essay.

Concept Mapping

Description and Uses

Concept, mind, and *nursing process mapping* are all descriptive terms applied to a strategy in which students express concepts and their relationships in a visual format. This strategy uses a visual means for students to demonstrate how they organize information, understand complex relationships, and integrate theoretical knowledge into practice (Harrison & Gibbons, 2013; George, Geethakrishnan, & D'Souza, 2014). Concept mapping is frequently used as an alternative to traditional nursing care plans as a method for students to demonstrate their understanding of the underpinnings that guide the delivery of nursing care. Multiple problems can be incorporated into a patient-oriented concept map, allowing students to demonstrate the interrelationship of the problems to patient care (Harrison & Gibbons, 2013). Examples of concept mapping are provided in Figures 23-1 and 23-2.

The concepts to be mapped can be provided by the faculty, be generated by the students, or

Example of a Concept Map for Synthesizing Course Concepts in a Graduate Course in Computer Technologies for Nurse Educators

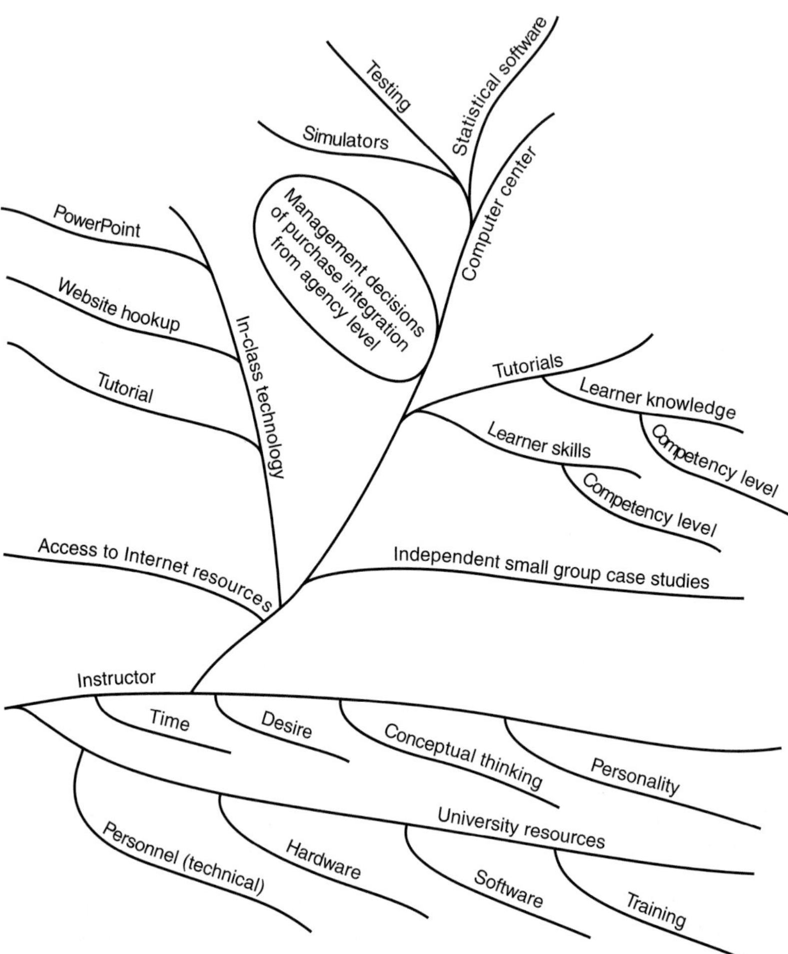

Figure 23-1 Concept map used to assess attainment of major course concepts. Courtesy Mary Beth Riner, Indiana University School of Nursing.

determined by the unique patient care they represent. The structure can be defined or left open to student creativity. A number of computer-based programs are available for constructing concept maps, and are useful for online environments. Using electronic maps allows each piece of the concept map to be hyperlinked to a resource. This application of concept mapping is called a *concept resource map.*

When concept mapping is used for evaluation, the purpose of the assignment drives the criteria. For example, criteria may include such things as a content analysis (the number of items included), the clarity of the organizational structure, accuracy of relationships, and categorization of content. It is possible to have students self-assess or peer assess concept maps as a way of building the professional skills of self-assessment and peer assessment.

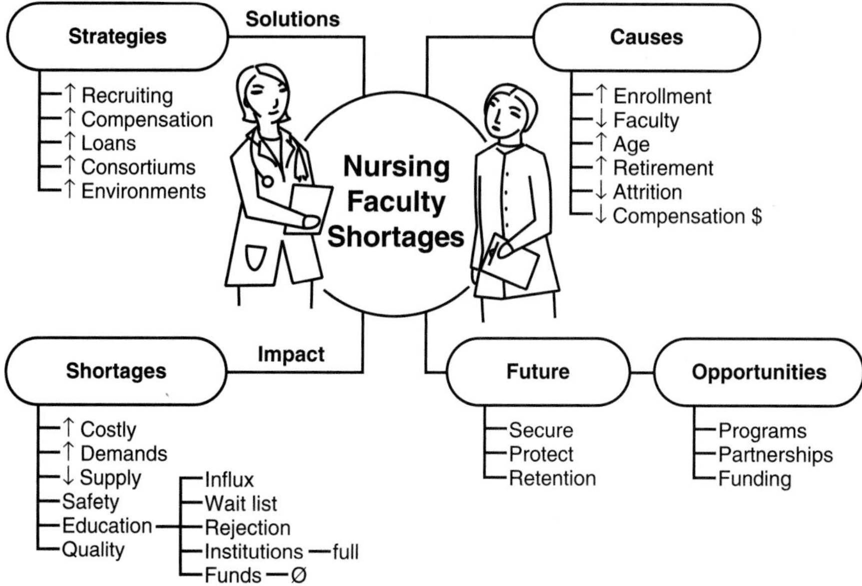

Figure 23-2 Concept map created to analyze the nursing faculty shortages. Courtesy Carolyn Low, RN-BSN graduate from Colorado Christian University.

Advantages

Concept mapping requires students to demonstrate cognitive synthesis skills with a minimum of writing. Mapping also allows faculty to gain insight into the way students assimilate new information and how students are connecting the material. Mapping also lends itself well to assessment, especially in determining the way students view relationships. Having students verbally explain the concept map can add clarity to their understanding of the relationships expressed by the lines on the map.

Disadvantages

The concept map may be large and difficult to follow. It can also be more challenging to interpret the student's intent because only key words and phrases are used. It is possible that the artistic ability and overall appearance of the map, much like handwriting, could influence faculty. For digital concept maps, special software is required. Time required for both students and faculty to learn the program needs to be acknowledged. Time involved in reading and responding to concept maps can be lengthy.

Issues

The faculty must teach students how to successfully create a map and allow them practice in completing maps before using this as an evaluation strategy. By practicing the mapping strategy as an in-class learning experience, the students will have a greater familiarity with the process. This becomes an active learning strategy when small groups work on a concept map during class time and then share their maps with peers. Using the evaluation rubric to provide peer feedback not only provides the students an opportunity to practice feedback, it familiarizes them with the expectations of the assignment. Special software can improve the capabilities of concept mapping in an electronic environment. Software to support concept mapping can add a learning curve for students. Regardless of the method used to construct the map, a limitation of mapping is the challenge of uncovering the rationale for the relationship of ideas. One way of addressing this limitation is to use the map as the focus for a faculty–student conference.

The grading of the exercise can easily become subjective unless clear criteria for grading are established. These criteria should be defined for the students before submission of their work. Faculty need to establish the validity and reliability of their tools for this strategy.

Oral Questioning

Description and Uses

In the quest to assess the student's ability to think critically and develop clinical reasoning skills, faculty have historically used oral questioning. At the graduate level, oral questioning is used for the defense of the dissertation and thesis. In this process, the student must demonstrate a working knowledge of the discipline and the ability to express arguments orally. The answers to these questions demonstrate the knowledge, skills, and attitudes held by the student. For health professions, the use of oral questioning during clinical learning is designed to elicit assessment at all levels of the cognitive domain and affective domain and to provide evidence of critical thinking. Questions can solicit only factual information or ask for comparisons, priorities, and rationale. During a questioning session, students can be asked to elaborate and justify their responses. Questioning as an assessment technique can be sequenced to move the student from a basic level (factual information) to a higher cognitive level (clarifying relationships). A high degree of trust and sense of collaboration for learning growth in the relationship of faculty and learner is a key for success in this method. Subsequent assessment can demonstrate the effect of this formative feedback process (Al Wahbi, 2014). For examples of how Bloom's Taxonomy can be used to generate questions, see Box 23-5.

BOX 23-5 Examples of Questions to Assess the Cognitive Domain

REMEMBER

Define __________.
List the five principles for __________.
Based on your assignment, what do you recall about __________?

UNDERSTAND

Explain the meaning of __________.
Tell me in your own words what is meant by __________.
Which of the examples demonstrates __________?

APPLY

What is a new example of __________?
How could __________ be used to __________?
Show how this information could be graphed.

ANALYZE

What are the implications of __________?
What is the meaning of __________?
What are the key components of __________?

EVALUATE

Explain the effectiveness of this approach.
Which solution would you choose? Justify your opinion.
What are the consequences of __________?

CREATE

What are some possible solutions to the problem of __________?
From this information, create your own model of __________.
Suppose you could __________. How would you approach __________?

Adapted from Hansen, C. (1994). Questioning techniques for the active classroom, and King, A. Inquiry as a tool in critical thinking. In D. F. Halpern (Ed.), *Changing college classrooms: New teaching and learning strategies for an increasingly complex world* (pp. 13–38, 93–106). San Francisco: Jossey-Bass.
Cognitive taxonomy dimensions based on Krathwohl (2002). A revision of Bloom's taxonomy: an overview. *Theory into Practice, 41*(4), 212–218.

Advantages

Oral questioning is inexpensive, requires no special equipment, and can be quickly developed by faculty. During oral questioning, it is possible to give immediate feedback to the student, which makes this an excellent option for formative assessment.

Disadvantages

Students may feel highly stressed by the experience. As well, not all faculty are skilled in providing feedback. Al Wahbi (2014) found that as many as 40% of clinical faculty overestimated their proficiency in providing feedback and could benefit from specific training in feedback practices. The lack of established interrater reliability is also a concern when using oral exams (Rahman, 2011).

Unless the session is recorded, there is no permanent record of it. The evaluator may be biased by a variety of factors during the assessment. For example, if the student performs well at the beginning of the session and the performance deteriorates as the session progresses, the earlier performance may be biased by what occurred subsequently. It is imperative that the criteria for assessment be fully developed before the questioning session.

Issues

Using questions for evaluation must be distinguished from using questions to encourage active student learning. Avoid leading or loaded questions. Consider giving students a minute to write down an answer. This can minimize the stress of a questioning session. It is important for faculty to avoid interrupting the student as an answer is being given. Oral feedback from the teacher to the student, especially when correcting the student, needs to have as its primary focus the purpose of improving future performance. That makes this technique most suited as an assessment strategy. Not all faculty are well trained in this technique. The criteria for evaluation must be established before the session with the student. Because of the lack of a permanent record of the interaction, risk of subjectivity is greater in this kind of assessment.

Audio and Video Recording

Description and Uses

Audio recording can be used to evaluate communication skills, group process, clinical caregiving simulations, and interviewing skills. Audio recording allows the evaluator to focus on verbal communication without other distracters. Video recording captures a more complete essence of the competencies being evaluated. For example, evaluation of psychomotor skills as well as aspects of clinical reasoning can be demonstrated in the video capture. Faculty must determine at the outset if audio and video recording is used as an assessment to provide feedback to students for performance improvement or if their performance is being evaluated and graded.

Using a video camera to record student performance can be a means of evaluating several performance parameters. Video of student performance is useful for evaluation communication skills because it picks up the student's actual words and inflections, as well as body language. The live-action feature of the video recording also provides evidence of the sequencing of student actions in hands-on skill performance. This method works well for skill validation and is very useful for students to self-assess their performance using a rubric. The video capture has been long used for debriefing after simulations. Basic video recording equipment has become fairly inexpensive; cameras are included as part of many cell phones, tablets, and computers. Comprehensive audio-video capture equipment specifically designed to link with high-fidelity simulation can be very expensive.

Advantages

Obtaining audio recording equipment is relatively inexpensive. Most digital cameras, cell phones, tablets, and computers have video recording capabilities and are fairly inexpensive. In the case of audio recording, the presence of the microphone may be less threatening to the student than use of a video camera or direct faculty observation. Video recording works well for evaluation of mastery, particularly with psychomotor skills. These techniques allow students to practice and record their skills in private, listen to or view and critique their own performance, and even rerecord the procedure until they are satisfied with the performance prior to submitting for a grade.

This strategy affords flexibility in scheduling for both students and faculty. Faculty can conduct a secondary analysis of the recording if necessary. With both audio and video recording, faculty can assess student performance with patients without being intrusive in the dynamic of the student–patient relationship.

Disadvantages

It can be difficult to distinguish individual voices in a group of participants when listening to an audio recording. One suggestion is to have each group member state his or her name at the beginning of the recording so that voices can be identified. In addition, communication has both verbal and nonverbal components. Thus one limitation of audio recording as a strategy is that only the verbal components of the skill can be evaluated.

A certain level of competence is required in knowing how to position video equipment correctly to secure quality visual and audio recording. The skill of the cameraperson and the camera angle can affect the quality of the recording. It may be necessary to use small microphones to adequately secure the audio components. More expensive options are commonly found in high-fidelity simulation rooms where video cameras may be mounted in multiple sites throughout the room and inputs from each camera are synchronized in a control room. Extra technical personnel are usually needed to maintain the equipment. If patients are involved, their consent is required. Requirements of the Health Insurance Portability and Accountability Act of 1996 (HIPAA) privacy rules are of concern whenever there is digital data from patients; therefore protocols should be in place to maintain security. Students should be educated about the uses of the recordings, especially the issues surrounding confidentiality of the materials, and sign agreements indicating their understanding.

The experience of being recorded can cause stress to some students who may feel self-conscious about being "on camera." However, in some cases, the stress level may be lower than that experienced with direct observation by the faculty member. If patients are also being video recorded, explanations of expectations should be provided as well as consent obtained before the recording begins. Evaluators need good observational skills.

Issues

The protocol for scoring must be determined before this strategy is instituted. Students need an opportunity to practice with the strategy before it is used in the assignment of a grade. A decision needs to be made about whether the entire recording or a sampling will be used for evaluation. Confidentiality is an issue, as well as the need to obtain consent from all individuals who are included in the recording. HIPAA guidelines are required for digital patient data.

Role Play

Description and Uses

In role play, the learner portrays a specific individual and is generally given much freedom to act out that role spontaneously. Role play is particularly appropriate for objectives related to developing interpersonal relationships with patients, peers, and other health care providers (Oermann & Gaberson, 2014). The role-playing process provides a live sample of human behavior that serves as a vehicle for students to (1) explore feelings; (2) gain insight into their abilities, values, and perceptions; (3) develop their problem-solving skills and attitudes; and (4) explore subject matter in different ways.

The time for role play can vary according to the time available and the complexity of the role-play situation. The student is informed of the concept or role to be performed and given time to be creative in its presentation. The content, and not the performance ability, should be assessed. The content and process can be assessed for use of communication techniques. Role reversal is used in situations in which the purpose is to change attitudes. This facilitates an understanding of opposing beliefs. On termination of the role play, the student observers analyze what occurred, what feelings were generated, what insights were gained, why things happened as they did, and how the situation is related to reality.

Advantages

Situations can be structured or prepared as open-ended responses. After students critique the role play, the process can be repeated. Role play affords the opportunity for students to practice peer review. This technique actively involves the students and fosters creativity.

Disadvantages

Role play can be awkward for the faculty and student if it is not practiced before the time of assessment or evaluation. Immediate feedback is difficult to provide if many groups are performing at the same time.

Issues

Using role play as a teaching mode before its use in evaluation assists students and faculty to become familiar with the technique and material. All that could happen cannot be anticipated. Students need to be informed in advance about the use of this technique for assessment. It may take time and experience to build comfort with this technique.

Patient Simulation

Description and Uses

Simulation is the creation of a representation or model of a real-life situation (adapted from http://sb.thefreedictionary.com/simulate). In nursing, simulations are used to provide a safe practice environment for student learning, assessment, and evaluation (Jeffries, 2012). The continuum of simulation ranges from role playing to high-fidelity, computer-supported simulation that uses the most up-to-date mannequins and computer-driven equipment to closely replicate real-life situations.

Use of standardized patients (individuals who are trained to act as patients) is another form of role playing used to evaluate student performance in simulations. Faced with limited clinical resources, both standardized patients and high-fidelity simulations are being widely adopted in nursing education programs. The National Council of State Boards of Nursing study on simulation has demonstrated that undergraduate students can experience up to 50% of clinical instruction via simulation (Hayden, Smiley, Alexander, Kardong-Edgren, & Jeffries, 2014), and when used as clinical instruction, faculty also need to consider the most appropriate way to assess and evaluate clinical learning outcomes and determine when simulation is best used for assessment including feedback for improvement or for evaluation and grading. (See Chapter 18.)

Advantages

Standardized patients and low-fidelity and high-fidelity simulation provide safe environments to assess and evaluate skills that are essential for quality nursing practice. Low-fidelity simulations can allow the opportunity for students to practice psychomotor skills in a more authentic environment. For example, instead of setting up individual stations where students validate their ability to perform procedures, a more authentic simulation involves new orders on a given patient that requires performance of the skills in the context of patient care. The combination of video recording with simulation provides opportunities for debriefing with students. Faculty must carefully consider if these situations are appropriate for evaluation, or are best used to help students learn.

In addition to assessing individual skill performance and demonstration of higher order thinking skills, simulations allow for assessment of team and interprofessional interaction. High-fidelity simulations have been used with students of various disciplines to improve communications and teamwork across disciplines. Students and faculty alike find the simulated patient care environment interesting and stimulating. Again, faculty must be thoughtful in their decision to use simulations for grading and evaluation in these situations.

Disadvantages

The main disadvantage of using high-fidelity simulations for evaluation is the time and expense involved. While equipment cost is decreasing, it remains rather high for the initial purchase. Another disadvantage is that simulations can only accommodate a small number of active participants at a given time. Similarly, disadvantages of using standardized patients include the training required, the expense involved, and increased faculty workload for evaluation.

Issues

Major issues related to using simulation as an evaluation strategy include but are not limited to selection of scenarios, opportunity for practice prior to evaluation, maintenance of equipment, faculty education and training, personnel needs, and efficient scheduling of students. The format of the scenario for evaluation should match the format used for practice. There is a need for ample opportunity for student practice prior to evaluation. This assists the students to become more comfortable with the simulated environment before they receive a grade (even if it is satisfactory or unsatisfactory). *Creating reliable and valid instruments* for evaluation and ensuring interrater reliability for their use is another issue.

How to efficiently schedule students for evaluation must be addressed as simulations only accommodate a small number of active participants. It is necessary to work out the mechanics of scheduling students whether simulations are used as a teaching, assessment, or evaluation strategy. If collaborative partnerships have been developed between practice and academia for shared simulation equipment and space, then scheduling issues may be more complicated.

Service Learning

Description and Uses

Many college campuses have embraced service learning either as the framework for a course or a component within a course. According to the definition provided in The National and Community Service Trust Act of 1990 (1999), service learning should meet community needs, foster civic responsibilities, and be structured in a way that supports the students' educational goals and provides the opportunity for students to reflect on the experience. A service learning project can take multiple forms. It can be designed as an individual project where one student works on a project that meets a need for an agency (e.g., developing an in-service for a nursing unit on a given topic) or it may be a group project wherein several students work together (e.g., develop and carry out a health fair for senior citizens at a community center). The ability to effectively work as a member of a team is a common outcome associated with service learning (Foli, Braswell, Kirkpatrick, & Lim, 2014). Using assessment strategies such as an appreciative inquiry reflection at the midpoint of the project can be useful in addressing challenges with the group (Kirkpatrick & Braswell, 2010). Timing of this assessment midway through the project allows readjustments in group processes and helps with self-awareness. Typically a final group presentation or report is completed and submitted for evaluation and grading.

Advantages

A service learning project has relevance for the students because the learning experience is authentic and based in a real-world situation. It also is meaningful to those who benefit from the projects these students complete. Seating the learning in the context of reality exposes students to situations they may encounter after graduation, and allows them the opportunity to find their way while still having the support of faculty. Service learning can contribute to positive visibility for the school when contributions provided by the service learning projects meet needs of the community. As well, service learning projects provide students the opportunity to better understand needs of individuals and communities.

Disadvantages

Time for faculty to manage service learning projects can be viewed as a disadvantage because out-of-class time is required to meet with the agencies, arrange the experiences, and follow up regularly with students and agencies. It takes care to be sure that the expectations of the agency are in concert with the expectations of the faculty for the learning requirements and that evaluation criteria align with both sets of expectations. Faculty may need to help students clarify and resolve conflicts with agencies and within groups. There is also a risk that the student group may fall short of the expectation of the agency and the reputation of the school could be jeopardized in the community.

Issues

The ultimate question becomes how to evaluate the learning that takes place. Again, the faculty must focus on the desired learning outcomes. For example, if the primary purpose is to help students learn to work in teams, evaluation strategies that emphasize growth in self-awareness, communications, and conflict resolution are appropriate. A variety of strategies may be used. It is fairly common to have reflections or papers as a means to consider the outcomes. Group work or teamwork can be triangulated by looking at individual and group reports as well as observation by the faculty and the agency staff. In some cases, students may be asked to provide peer review. Evaluation should address the measurable effect of the experience on the student, the agency, the preceptor, and the community served. Organizing, supervising, and evaluating service learning activities requires time from the faculty to develop, nurture, and maintain relationships with the community partner.

Summary

There are many strategies to effectively evaluate learning outcomes in both the classroom and clinical setting. Using more than one strategy will more fully demonstrate student outcome achievement. When using any evaluation strategy, students should have the opportunity to practice before the activity is used for grading. The strategies addressed in this chapter include portfolios, reflections, papers, essays and essay tests, concept mapping, oral questioning, audio and video recordings, simulations, role play, and service learning. To select the best strategy, faculty members must consider the purpose and setting; the time required for preparation, implementation, and grading; the cost; and the advantages and disadvantages of each strategy. Although it requires time, energy, and persistence to plan evaluation of student achievement of learning outcomes, the effort ultimately benefits students and the patients they are preparing to serve.

Faculty who implement evaluation strategies will continue to increase the evidence base for best practices and contribute to the scholarship of teaching. The findings from the use of assessment and evaluation strategies can be used for a variety of purposes. The most obvious is to provide feedback to the learner and to revise instruction and learning activities. Evidence of critical thinking, clinical reasoning, and therapeutic communication are a part of the systematic program assessment plan. In addition, assessment and evaluation data are also helpful for the individual faculty as evidence of teaching excellence. As nursing education meets current challenges, the refinement of assessment and evaluation strategies will continue to expand in tandem with the development of teaching strategies, thereby contributing to the ever-increasing quality of education for nurses of the future.

REFLECTING ON THE EVIDENCE

1. Select a course or program outcome and determine an assessment strategy for that outcome by applying the six steps discussed in the chapter.
2. Compare two different assessment strategies and discuss application in the classroom or clinical setting.
3. Identify ways to enhance the reliability and validity of assessment strategies presented in the chapter. Construct a grading rubric for an assessment or evaluation strategy to be used to assess learning outcomes in a course.

REFERENCES

Al Wahbi, A. (2014). The need for faculty training programs in effective feedback provision. *Advances in Medical Education and Practice, 5*, 263–268.

Beach, R., & Marshall, J. (1991). *Teaching literature in the secondary school*. San Diego: Harcourt.

Benner, P., Sutphen, M., Leonard, V., & Day, L. (2010). *Educating nurses: A call for radical transformation*. San Francisco: Jossey-Bass.

Bercher, D. (2012). Self-monitoring tools and student academic success: When perception matches reality. *Journal of College Science Teaching, 41*(5), 26–32.

Bevis, O. M., & Watson, J. (1989). *Toward a caring curriculum: A new pedagogy for nursing*. New York: National League for Nursing.

Brookhart, S. M., & Nitko, A. J. (2014). *Educational assessment of students* (7th ed.). Upper Saddle River, NJ: Pearson Education.

Cronenwett, L., Sherwood, G., Barnsteiner, J., Disch, J., Johnson, J., Mitchell, P., et al. (2007). Quality and safety education for nurses. *Nursing Outlook, 55*(3), 122–131. http://dx.doi.org/10.1016/j.outlook.2007.02.006.

Davis, B. G. (2009). *Tools for teaching* (2nd ed.). San Francisco: Jossey-Bass.

Eisner, E. (1985). *The educational imagination* (2nd ed.). Macmillan: New York.

Foli, K., Braswell, M., Kirkpatrick, J., & Lim, E. (2014). Development of leadership behaviors in undergraduate nursing students: A service-learning approach. *Nursing Education Perspectives, 35*(2), 76–82.

George, A., Geethakrishnan, R., & D'Souza, T. (2014). Concept mapping: a child health nursing practical exercise. *Holistic Nursing Practice, 28*(1), 43–47.

Gikandi, J. W., Morrow, D., & Davis, N. E. (2011). Online formative assessment in higher education: A review of the literature. *Computers and Education, 57*(4), 2333–2351. http://dx.doi.org/10.1016/j.compedu.2011.06.004.

Harrison, S., & Gibbons, C. (2013). Nursing student perceptions of concept maps: From theory to practice. *Nursing Education Perspectives, 34*(6), 395–399.

Hayden, J. K., Smiley, R. A., Alexander, M., Kardong-Edgren, S., & Jeffries, P. R. (2014). The NCSBN national simulation study: A longitudinal, randomized, controlled study replacing clinical hours with simulation in prelicensure nursing education. *Journal of Nursing Regulation, 5*(2), S3–S64.

Interprofessional Education Collaborative Expert Panel. (2011). *Core competencies for interprofessional collaborative practice: Report of an expert panel*. Washington, D.C.: Interprofessional Education Collaborative. Retrieved from: http://www.aacn.nche.edu/education-resources/IPECReport.pdf.

Jeffries, P. (2012). *Simulation in nursing education: From conceptualization to evaluation*. New York: National League for Nursing.

Karagory, P., & Kirby, K. (2014, November 20–22). *Digital badges in nursing education: An innovative tool to showcase student knowledge, skills, and competencies (poster)*. Baltimore, MD: AACN Baccalaureate conference.

Kirkpatrick, J., & Braswell, M. (2010). Service-learning. In L. Caputi (Ed.), (2nd ed.) *Teaching nursing: The art and science. vol. 2*. (pp. 879–899). Glen Ellyn, IL: College of DuPage Press.

Krathwohl, D. (2002). A revision of Bloom's taxonomy: An overview. *Theory Into Practice, 41*(4), 212–218.

Krathwohl, D. R., Bloom, B. S., & Mases, B. (1964). Taxonomy of educational objectives. *Handbook II, affective domain*. New York: David McKay (pp. 66–91).

Kuroda, A. (2014). Contemplative education approaches to teacher preparation program. *Procedia-Social and Behavioral Sciences, 116*(21), 1400–1404. http://dx.doi.org/10.1016/j.sbspro.2014.01.405.

Larkin, K. T., & Klonoff, E. A. (2014). *Specialty competencies in clinical health psychology*. New York: Oxford University Press.

Li, J., & Barnard, R. (2011). Academic tutors' beliefs about and practices of giving feedback on students' written assignments: A New Zealand case study. *Assessing Writing, 16*(2), 137–148.

McComb, S., & Simpson, V. (2014). The concept of shared mental models in healthcare collaboration. Shared mental models. *Journal of Advanced Nursing, 70*(7), 1479–1488.

Miller, M. D., Linn, R. L., & Gronlund, N. E. (2012). *Measurement and assessment in teaching* (11th ed.). Upper Saddle River, NJ: Prentice-Hall.

Mok, J. (2012). As a student I do think that the learning effectiveness of electronic portfolios depends, to quite a large extent, on the attitude of students!. *The Electronic Journal of e-Learning, 10*(4), 407–416. Retrieved from www.ejel.org.

O'Sullivan, A. J., Harris, P., Hughes, C. S., Toohey, S. M., Balasooriya, C., Velan, G., et al. (2012). Linking assessment to undergraduate student capabilities through portfolio examination. *Assessment & Evaluation in Higher Education, 37*(3), 379–391.

Oermann, M., & Gaberson, K. (2014). *Evaluation and testing in nursing education* (4th Ed.). New York: Springer.

Olantunji, M. O. (2014). The affective domain of assessment in colleges and universities: Issues and implications. *International Journal of Progressive Education, 10*(1), 101–116.

Ondrejka, D. (2014). *Affective teaching in nursing: Connecting to feelings, values and inner awareness*. New York: Springer.

Pohlman, S. (2013). Reading Ella: Using literary patients to enhance nursing students' reflective thinking in the classroom. *International Journal of Nursing Education Scholarship, 10*(1), 283–291.

Rahman, G. (2011). Appropriateness of using oral examination as an assessment method in medical or dental education. *Journal of Education and Ethics in Dentistry, 1*(2), 46.

Roberts, C., Shadbolt, N., Clark, T., & Simpson, P. (2014). The reliability and validity of a portfolio designed as a programmatic assessment of performance in an integrated clinical placement. *BMC Medical Education, 14*, 197. http://dx.doi.org/10.1186/1472-6920-14-197.

Robertson, J., Rossetti, J., Peters, B., Coyner, S., Koren, M., Hertz, J., et al. (2010). Portfolio assessment: One school of nursing's experience. In L. Caputi (Ed.), (2nd ed.)*Teaching nursing: The art and science. vol. 2*. (pp. 525–558). Glen Ellyn, IL: College of DuPage Press.

Schoen, D. (1984). *The reflective practitioner: how professionals think in action*. New York: Basic Books.

Stevens, D. D., & Levi, A. J. (2012). *Introduction to rubrics: An assessment tool to save grading time, convey effective feedback and promote students learning*. Sterling, VA: Stylus.

Sullivan, D. F. (2014). *It's time to get serious about the right kind of assessment: A message for presidents*. Retrieved from https://www.aacu.org/value/right-kind-of-assessment.

Tashiro, J., Shimpuku, Y., Naruse, K., Matsutani, M., & Matsutani, M. (2013). Concept analysis of reflection in nursing professional development. *Japan Journal of Nursing Science, 10*(2), 170–179. http://dx.doi.org/10.1111/j.1742-7924.2012.00222.x.

The National and Community Service Trust Act of 1990. (December 17, 1999). *P. L. 106-170*. Retrieved from http://www.nationalservice.gov/pdf/cncs_statute.pdf.

Wyss, V. L., Freedman, D., & Siebert, C. J. (2014). The development of a discussion rubric for online courses: Standardizing expectations of graduate students in online scholarly discussions. *TechTrends, 58*(2), 99–107.

E-PORTFOLIO WEB RESOURCES

http://ddp.alverno.edu/.
http://www.wix.com/.

CONCEPT MAP WEB RESOURCES

http://www.socialresearchmethods.net/mapping/mapping.htm.
https://library.usu.edu/instruct/tutorials/cm/CMinstruction2.htm.

SERVICE LEARNING WEB RESOURCES

http://www.compact.org/initiatives/service-learning/.
http://www.compact.org/disciplines/reflection/structuring/.
http://citl.indiana.edu/programs/serviceLearning/ResourcesforService-Learning.php.
http://www.purdue.edu/cie/learning/servicelearning/faculty/courses.html.

CLASSROOM ASSESSMENT TECHNIQUES

http://cft.vanderbilt.edu/guides-sub-pages/cats/.
http://www.cmu.edu/teaching/assessment/assesslearning/CATs.html.

Developing and Using Classroom Tests: Multiple-Choice and Alternative Format Test Items*

24

Diane M. Billings, EdD, RN, FAAN, ANEF

Using test questions, either written by the faculty or selected from a test bank (and revised as needed) is one more strategy that nurse educators can use to assess student attainment of learning outcomes. Although developing classroom tests seems like a relatively straightforward task, it is, in fact, an involved process. The purpose of this chapter is to offer a step-by-step approach to planning, developing, administering, analyzing, and revising classroom tests. Understanding these steps will not only assist faculty to develop their own fair, reliable, and valid tests, but will also provide information for judging the quality of test items used on standardized tests and preparing tests from commercially developed test banks.

Planning the Test

Developing or using a test that is valid (representative) and reliable (consistent) requires much thought and planning (Tarrant & Ware, 2012). During the planning stage faculty must make thoughtful and informed decisions about the test design, administration, and use of the test results. These decisions must be based on evidence, follow best practices, and be made *before* the test is administered and graded. This section discusses determining the purpose of the test, understanding criterion-referenced versus norm-referenced tests, developing a table of specifications, choosing item types, writing structured response test items, and improving the reliability and validity of a test.

*The author acknowledges the work of Lori Rasmussen, MSN, RN; Diana J. Speck, MSN, RN; and Prudence Twigg, MSN, RN, in the previous editions of the chapter.

Purpose of the Test

Tests in nursing education are given for a variety of reasons and faculty must first determine how the test will be used. If using an already developed test, it will also be important to understand the validity and reliability and other metrics of the test because test results have significant consequences for evaluating learning as well as determining students' admission, progression and graduation.

Tests Used to Determine Admission, Progression, and Graduation

One of the first tests nursing students may encounter are those used for admission. Although there are a variety of standardized college admissions tests such as the Scholastic Aptitude Test (SAT) and the Graduate Record Exam (GRE), many schools of nursing now use a battery of tests specifically designed to test basic academic skills of nursing students. Standardized tests are also used, particularly in prelicensure nursing programs, to monitor students' progress throughout the program, and as an exit exam at the end of the program that may be used to determine if the student graduates (Santo, Frander, & Hawkins, 2013). Because the decisions made based on these tests have serious consequences for the applicant or the student admitted and progressing through the program, these tests are referred to as *high-stakes* tests (Sullivan, 2014).

When administering high-stakes tests to make decisions about admission, progression, and graduation, the National League for Nursing (2010) recommends faculty make thoughtful decisions and understand how the test was developed, what constructs the test measures, the validity and reliability of the test, the readability of the test items, and the presence of linguistic or cultural bias. If the test will be used for predicting success on a licensing examination, faculty must know how those data are determined and for which population of students. When using commercially developed high-stakes tests, faculty must also consider the ethical and legal aspects of using these tests as well as the cultural and socioeconomic diversity of the students who will be taking the tests (Santo et al., 2013). For example, faculty must consider the implications for students when standardized tests are used to determine progression or graduation for students who have paid tuition, demonstrated attainment of learning on teacher-made tests, and demonstrated requisite knowledge, skills, and attitudes in clinical practice.

Tests Used to Determine Readiness or Placement or as Advance Organizers

If the test is to be given *before* instruction, as a pretest, the test may be used to determine readiness (the grasp of prerequisite skills needed to be successful) or placement (the level of mastery of instructional objectives). Administering a test that is similar to a unit or final exam can also serve as an "advance organizer" to alert students to significant content that should be learned and will be subsequently tested (Carey, 2014).

Tests Used to Improve Learning (Practice Tests)

During instruction, the test may be used as a *formative* evaluation of learning or as a diagnostic tool to identify learning problems. With the wide availability of test banks, such as those that accompany textbooks, and the ease of creating tests in a test-authoring component of a learning management system, faculty can also use tests as a way for students to practice and assess their own learning.

Tests Used to Determine Grades

As measures of learning outcomes, tests provide summative evaluation of learning on which grading decisions may be based. See Table 24-1 for a summary of test measures based on timing of administration.

Tests may serve a variety of additional functions. For example, testing may provide the structure (e.g., deadlines) that some students need to direct their learning activities or faculty may use testing as one means of evaluating teaching effectiveness by measuring the outcomes of student learning.

TABLE 24-1 Test Measures Based on Timing of Administration

Timing	Type of Test	Measure
Before	Readiness	Prerequisite skills
	Placement	Previous learning
During	Formative	Learning progress
	Diagnostic	Learning problems
After	Summative	Terminal performance

Types of Tests

Criterion-Referenced Tests

Criterion-referenced tests are those that are constructed and interpreted according to a specific set of learning outcomes (McDonald, 2013). This type of test is useful for measuring mastery of subject matter. An absolute standard of performance is set for grading purposes. Typically, nurse educators tend to use criterion-referenced tests because the goal of nursing education is for all students to attain mastery of the content. For example, criterion-referenced tests are frequently used to ensure safety in areas such as drug dosage calculation, in which the absolute standard of performance may be set as high as 100%, regardless of the performance of other students.

Norm-Referenced Tests

Norm-referenced tests are those that are constructed and interpreted to provide a relative ranking of students (McDonald, 2013). This type of test is useful for measuring differential performance among students. A relative standard of performance is used for grading purposes. Standardized tests such as the SAT and GRE are examples of norm-referenced tests.

Table of Specifications

The purpose of developing a table of specifications (test map, test grid, test plan, test blueprint) is to ensure that the test serves its intended purpose by representatively sampling the intended learning outcomes and instructional content. The first step in developing a table of specifications is to define the specific learning outcomes to be measured. Specific learning outcomes, which are derived from more general instructional outcomes (e.g., course and unit objectives), specify tasks that students should be able to perform on completion of instruction (Miller, Linn, & Gronlund, 2012).

Bloom's taxonomy (Bloom, Englehart, Furst, Hill, & Krathwhol, 1956) has been used as a guide for developing and leveling general instructional and specific learning outcomes. Although the cognitive components of the affective and psychomotor domains can be evaluated with structured choice tests, tests have most often been used to determine achievement of outcomes in the six levels of Bloom's cognitive domain (Table 24-2). Anderson and Krathwohl (2001) have revised Bloom's taxonomy, defining knowledge dimensions and cognitive processes. The knowledge dimensions are factual, conceptual, procedural, and metacognitive. The cognitive processes are remembering, understanding, applying, analyzing, evaluating, and creating (Table 24-3). Any of the six cognitive processes may be applied to the various dimensions of knowledge. The licensing exams offered by the National Council of State Boards of Nursing (NCSBN) use Anderson and Krathwohl's (2001) taxonomy.

TABLE 24-2 Bloom's Taxonomy with Action Verbs for the Cognitive Levels

Cognitive Level	Action Verbs
Remembering	Define, identify, list
Understanding	Describe, explain, summarize
Applying	Apply, demonstrate, use
Analyzing	Compare, contrast, differentiate
Evaluating	Critique, evaluate, judge
Creating	Construct, develop, formulate

TABLE 24-3 Anderson and Krathwohl's Taxonomy with Action Verbs for the Cognitive Processes

Cognitive Processes	Action Verbs
Remember	Retrieve, recognize, recall
Understand	Interpret, classify, summarize, infer, compare, explain, exemplify
Apply	Execute, implement
Analyze	Differentiate, organize, attribute
Evaluate	Check, critique
Create	Generate, plan, produce, reorganize

TABLE 24-4 Content Outline and Relative Teaching Time

	Content	Teaching Time (%)	No. of Items/ Section*
I.	Antipsychotic agents	25	10
II.	Antianxiety agents	25	10
III.	Antidepressant agents	25	10
IV.	Antimanic agents	12.5	5
V.	Antiparkinson agents	12.5	5
Totals		100	40

*Percentage of teaching time × Total no. of items = No. of items/section.

Additional attention is being given to those cognitive processing skills used by nurses, such as critical thinking, clinical judgment, and clinical decision making (Wendt & Harmes, 2009b). Test items should address these processes as well, and a mixture of cognitive processes should be evaluated at each stage of instruction, placing an increasing emphasis (or weight) on higher-level skills. This is vital because higher-level skills are more likely to result in retention and transfer of knowledge. In addition, this will assist in preparing students for the licensing and certification examinations that test primarily at the levels of application and analysis.

The second step in developing a table of specifications involves determining the instructional content to be evaluated and the weight to be assigned to each area. This can be accomplished by developing a content outline and using the amount of time spent teaching the material as an indicator for weighting (Table 24-4).

Finally, a two-way grid is developed, with content areas being listed down the left side and learning outcomes being listed across the top of the grid (Table 24-5). Each cell is assigned a number of questions according to the weighting of content and cognitive processes of learning outcomes.

Some faculty prefer to use a three-way table of specifications. With a three-way grid, the five steps of the nursing process are listed on the left side, outcomes are listed across the top, and the number of items or specific content areas is listed within each cell. Weighting of the steps of the nursing process again depends on the level of instruction. For example, early in the instructional process, assessment and diagnosis might carry the most weight,

TABLE 24-5 Two-Way Table of Specifications

Outcomes* (Content†)	Apply (20%)	Analyze (40%)	Evaluate (40%)	Totals
Antipsychotic agents (25%)	2	4	4	10
Antianxiety agents (25%)	2	4	4	10
Antidepressant agents (25%)	2	4	4	10
Antimanic agents (12.5%)	1	2	2	5
Antiparkinson agents (12.5%)	1	2	2	5
Totals	8	16	16	40

*Arbitrarily determined by level of instruction.
†Percent determined by teaching time.

whereas all stages may be tested equally by the end of instruction. Tables 24-6 and 24-7 are examples of three-way tables of specifications.

Alternatively, a table of specifications can be created by using the test plan of the current licensure or certification examination (National Council of State Boards of Nursing, 2014). When developing a test plan based on these examinations, the faculty must also be using these test plans with appropriate learning outcomes and teaching–learning strategies.

Other Considerations in the Planning Stage

Selecting Item Types

Several types of items can be used to test attainment of learning outcomes. Items may be selection-type, providing a set of responses from which to choose, or supply-type, a constructed response type requiring the student to provide an answer. Common selection-type items include true–false, matching, ordered-response, and multiple-choice questions. Supply-type items include fill-in-the-blank (usually requiring an absolute answer derived from a mathematical calculation), short-answer, multiple-response, hotspot, and essay questions (Wendt & Kenny, 2009).

The primary reason for choosing one type of item over another can be determined by answering the question: "Which type of item most directly measures the intended learning outcome?" Both selection-type and supply-type questions can be developed for all levels of the cognitive domain (Su, Osisek, Montgomery, & Pellar, 2009) and to test critical thinking, problem solving, and clinical decision-making skills. Other factors may also influence the item-type selection. For example, a large class size may prohibit the use of supply-type items because of the time required for grading.

TABLE 24-6 Three-Way Table of Specifications: Number of Items per Cell

Outcomes* (Content†)	Apply (20%)	Analyze (40%)	Evaluate (40%)	Totals
Assessment (40%)	6	6	4	16
Diagnosis (10%)	1	3	—	4
Planning (10%)	1	2	1	4
Intervention (20%)	—	2	6	8
Evaluation (20%)	—	3	5	8
Totals	8	16	16	40

*Arbitrarily determined by level of instruction.
†Percent determined by teaching time.

TABLE 24-7 Three-Way Table of Specifications: Content to Be Tested per Cell*

Outcomes* (Content†)	Remember (20%)	Understand (40%)	Apply (40%)	Totals
Assessment (40%)	P, A, A, D, D, M	P, P, A, D, M, PA	P, A, D, PA	16
Diagnosis (10%)	P	A, D, M	—	4
Planning (10%)	PA	A, D	P	4
Intervention (20%)	—	P, A	P, A, A, D, M, PA	8
Evaluation (20%)	—	P, PA, D	P, A, D, D, M	8
Totals	8	16	16	40

A, Antianxiety agents; *D*, antidepressant agents; *M*, antimanic agents; *P*, antipsychotic agents; *PA*, antiparkinson agents.
*No. of each type of content item determined by teaching time.
†Percent determined by teaching time.

In addition to multiple-choice items with one correct answer, licensing exams use alternative-format questions, which include fill-in-the-blank questions, multiple-response questions, drag-and-drop or ordered-response questions, and picture or graphic questions, as well as questions that use audio files; using video clips in test questions is under consideration (Wendt & Harmes, 2009b). Current information on the examination format can be obtained at the website for the NCSBN (www.ncsbn.org).

Selecting Item Difficulty

Determining the item difficulty, the percentage of the number of students who answered the question correctly, primarily depends on the purpose and type of the test. If the purpose of the test is to evaluate learning to assign a grade, the test should be moderately difficult and distinguish the students who have learned the content from those who have not. If the test is a criterion-referenced test, difficulty should match the level of the learning that reflects the skills to be mastered. For some questions, therefore, the item may be an "easy" item. Norm-referenced tests involve eliminating easy items and using average-difficulty items to maximize the differences among students.

Determining Number of Items

Determining the number of items to include on a test depends on the number of learning outcomes to be evaluated. Although test reliability increases with the number of test items, the number of test items is limited by many practical constraints. For example, more selection-type items than supply-type items can be answered in a given period. Similarly, items that require higher-level thinking skills take more time to answer than those that require lower-level skills.

A general guide for planning is to allow 1 minute for each moderately difficult multiple-choice item. For tests with greater difficulty and longer questions such as multiple-response type questions, the time allocation may need to be longer, approximately 1.5 minutes per question. Faculty should also consider the numbers of culturally and linguistically diverse students in the class and create a supportive test taking environment by allowing sufficient time for all students to process the question and respond to the answer options (Fuller, 2013).

Writing Test Items

Understanding the Structure of Multiple-Choice and Alternative-Format Test Questions

Writing most types of test items used by nurse educators involves creating a *scenario*, a description of a nursing care situation that requires problem-solving, making judgments and clinical decisions; a *stem*, or question; and a set of *answers*, or options, one or more of which are correct and others that are incorrect (*distractors*). See Box 24-1 for general guidelines for writing test items.

Writing Multiple-Choice and Alternative-Format Test Items

The most common types of questions used by nursing faculty are multiple-choice and alternative-format questions. Alternative-format questions include chart and exhibit, short-answer and

BOX 24-1 Guidelines for Writing Test Questions

SCENARIO

1. Present a single, realistic clinical encounter that requires the student to solve a problem or make clinical judgments or decisions.
2. Include relevant and irrelevant data to test students' ability to differentiate significant data, but at the same time avoid unnecessary information or excessive descriptive information.
3. Specify age, gender, ethnicity, or race only when essential to answering the question.
4. Do not use names for clients.

STEM

1. Poses the question; can be a complete or an incomplete sentence; can ask for priorities such as what the nurse should do first.
2. Should be clear enough to answer without looking at the options.
3. Write the stem in a precise manner. If it is too complex, the student will spend too much time trying to decipher it.
4. State the stem in a positive rather than a negative manner. Highlight (underline, italicize, or use bold font for) key words such as *not, never, first,* and *next*.
5. Use action verbs that are consistent with the cognitive process being measured. The cognitive level of the question must match with the learning outcome it is being used to evaluate.
6. Avoid clue words in the stem.
7. Keep as much information in the stem to avoid repeating it in the options.
8. Write the stem using active voice.
9. Use precise terms and measurements; avoid words such as *frequently, often,* and *some.*

ANSWERS AND OPTIONS

1. Keep all options grammatically consistent with the stem to avoid giving clues to the correct option.
2. Arrange the options in either alphabetical or numerical order.
3. Keep the options the same length.
4. Make all the options reasonable and homogenous.
5. Use only one best answer on which all authorities would agree.
6. Avoid the use of "all of the above" or "none of the above." Students can often guess the correct answer with only partial knowledge. Multiple response type questions can be used to evaluate students' ability to cluster data.
7. All options must be plausible.

fill-in-the-blank, hotspot (rollover), drag and drop or ordered response, graphic and graphic response, audio, video, and multiple choice. Multiple-choice and alternative-format items are used on licensing exams. Multiple-choice questions are typically used on certification exams. The definitions, advantages, disadvantages, guidelines for writing, and an example of each of these types of test items follow.

Multiple-Choice Items

A multiple-choice item consists of a scenario, which provides data about a client situation; a stem, which can be a question or an incomplete statement; and options (answers), one of which is correct and three of which are incorrect (distractors). Multiple-choice items, when carefully constructed, can measure critical thinking and higher levels of the cognitive domain (McDonald, 2013; Su et al., 2009).

Advantages

Multiple-choice items allow the faculty to sample a large amount of content in a single test. Test items can be scored easily and objectively. Scores on multiple-choice tests are less influenced by guessing than are scores on true–false tests. These items are versatile because they can measure learning of several levels of cognitive processes.

Disadvantages

Writing good items with plausible distractors can be time consuming. This item type takes more time for the student to read and understand. These items may discriminate against the creative, verbal student. Scores can be affected by students' reading ability and the instructor's writing style. This item type can raise the score of the student who can recognize rather than produce the correct answer.

Example

An older adult is admitted to the hospital because of severe diarrhea. The client is thirsty and skin turgor is poor. The blood pressure is 92/64 and pulse is

100. The serum sodium ($Na+$) level is 165 mmol/L. The nurse should develop a plan to:
1. Protect the skin from friction.
2. Increase fluids.
3. Prevent excoriation of the rectal area.
4. Place the client on "falls alert."

Multiple-Response Items

A multiple-response item, like a multiple-choice item, has a scenario, stem, and options; however, there are more than four options (usually five or six) and the options are written so that two or more of the responses are correct. Students are instructed to choose all correct responses ("select all that apply") to receive credit for the question.

Advantages

Multiple-response items allow for several correct answers and require students to cluster correct responses. There is less opportunity for choosing options by process of elimination than with standard multiple-choice items. The use of multiple-response items avoids using "all of the above" as an option.

Disadvantages

Multiple-response items require more options (usually five or six) and thus more distractors than standard multiple-choice items. Scoring, particularly by computer, may be more difficult.

Example

The nurse implements a medication safety teaching plan for an older adult. Which statements by the patient indicate that the teaching has been effective? "I will" (Select all that apply.)
1. throw away any medications I am no longer using."
2. have my prescriptions filled at different pharmacies to get the best price."
3. tell my physician about any nonprescription medications I am taking."
4. crush any medications that I have difficulty swallowing."
5. take all of my medications with food to avoid stomach upset."
6. report possible side effects of my medications to my physician."

Chart and Exhibit Questions

These questions, an example of interpretive questions, assess the test-taker's ability to seek and use data presented on a client's chart or health record. The data will be presented from one or more chart "tabs": prescriptions, history and physical, laboratory results, miscellaneous reports, imaging results, flow sheets, intake and output, medication administration record, progress notes, and vital signs. When the test is administered by computer, the test-taker will be required to search in a way that simulates search through a client's chart or computerized patient record. The question may be similar to a multiple-choice question with four responses, with one correct response, or a multiple-response question with more than four options that asks the test taker to "select all that apply."

Advantages

Chart and exhibit questions test the ability to consider which data are needed for client care and to test in higher levels of cognitive domain. These questions require test-takers to use data for clinical decision making and use them to interpret a set of data, for example, trend data on a vital signs record. These questions also simulate obtaining data from a client's chart; test-takers can be timed to ascertain whether they know what data to obtain and where on a chart to find it.

Disadvantages

Chart and exhibit questions are time consuming to develop. Chart and exhibit questions may require duplicating chart forms to develop the test questions.

Example

A parent has brought a 4-month-old to the immunization clinic. The nurse is reviewing the immunization record on the progress notes (see table).

Progress Notes	
11/1/2015	1-month well-child visit; administered HepB #1
12/3/2015	2-month well-child visit; administered DTaP #1, IPV #1

The infant will receive which immunization(s) at this visit? (Select all that apply.)
1. DTaP #3
2. HepB #2
3. IPV #2
4. MMR #1
5. Varicella

Fill-in-the-Blank Questions

The short-answer or fill-in-the-blank item requires the student to produce an answer (Miller et al., 2012). The question can have a scenario and a stem, but the "answer" is constructed by the student. This item type is used when the instructor wants the student to recall or calculate the answer (fill in the blank). The student could also be asked to visually represent the answer, for example, "Calculate a drug dosage, then mark the answer on a picture of a syringe." When fill-in-the blank questions are used on the licensing exam, the test-taker provides one answer that can be noted to be either correct or incorrect, and typically includes calculation of intake and output, drug dose, or drip rate for intravenous infusions.

Advantages

This item type reduces guessing. This item type works well for math problems because it requires the student to work out the answer. A broad range of material can be tested.

Disadvantages

It is difficult to phrase the question so there is only one correct answer. Scoring can be time consuming because the student may supply an answer the instructor had not considered. The student's spelling can make it difficult to score.

Example

The nurse is to give morphine elixir, 4 mg, sublingually. The drug available is morphine, 20 mg/mL. How much should the nurse give? (Round to the nearest tenth.)

______________________________ mg

Hotspot (Rollover) Questions

Hotspot questions ask the test-taker to locate a specific "spot" on a chart or figure. Hotspot questions use a scenario, a stem and directions to identify a particular "spot" on a diagram or illustration. When the questions are developed to be administered in paper-and-pencil formats the faculty can develop and number four options and place four "spots" on the figure (one correct, three incorrect spots) and ask the test-taker to identify the number of the correct "spot." Hotspot questions are more effectively developed for computer-administered examinations in which the test-taker can use the mouse to roll over the correct spot on the chart or figure.

Advantages

Hotspot questions provide an easy way to test understanding and application of anatomic knowledge. They offer an effective way to test understanding of physical assessment techniques. They can be used to test procedures and nursing skills with correct or incorrect positioning.

Disadvantages

Hotspot questions are most effective in computer applications where a mouse can be used to roll over to identify the hotspot. Hotspot questions may be more difficult to develop because of the need to have an illustration as a reference point.

Example

A client has not voided for 10 hours. Identify the anatomic area where the nurse should assess for bladder distension.

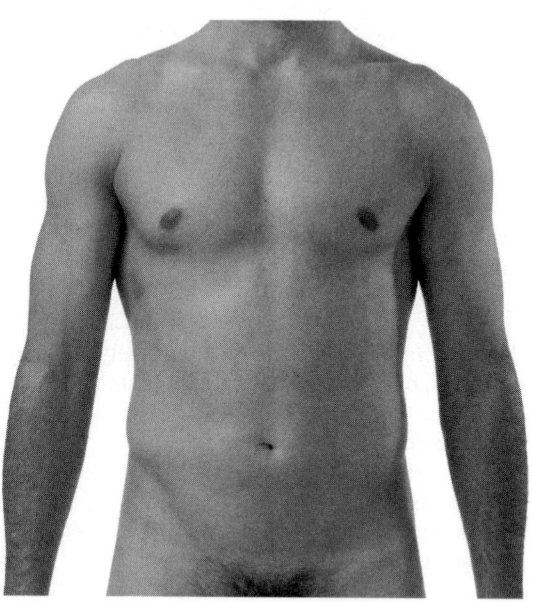

Figure from Wilson, S. F., & Giddens, J. F. (2011). *Health assessment for nursing practice* (5th ed.). St. Louis, MO: Mosby.

Drag-and-Drop and Ordered-Response Questions

Ordered-response questions require the test-taker to place information in a specified order. For example, questions can be developed to ask the test-taker to put steps of a procedure in order or, given a set of clients, to determine priorities for nursing care. These items have a scenario and a stem, and the options, all of which are correct, must be placed in the correct order. On the licensing examination, candidates drag each response in the left column and drop it into the correct order in the right column.

Advantages

Ordered-response questions evaluate test-takers' understanding of the order for steps of a procedure or how to set priorities for a client or groups of clients. They are relatively easy to develop. When writing for paper-and-pencil tests, the order can be "scrambled" and the item writer can pose four or more possible sequences.

Disadvantages

Ordering all of the steps or priorities may be confusing. Steps, sequences, and priorities may be controversial or context-specific; thus the item needs to be structured such that experts will agree on the correct order, correct answer, and rationale.

Example

A client begins to have a seizure. The nurse should do which actions in order from first to last?

1. Note the time.
2. Notify the physician.
3. Protect the client from injury.
4. Obtain a history of events prior to the seizure.

Graphic Items

Graphic items use photographs or illustrations in the question or in the answer options (graphic response). This type of question has a scenario, stem, and options. The test-taker responds to details in the graphic to answer the question, or chooses the answer by selecting the correct answer from four different graphics.

Advantages

Graphic items test assessment and evaluation skills, and clinical decision making.

Disadvantages

Graphic items require use of art; expense could be involved to obtain images of incorrect responses. They may be time consuming to develop.

Example

The nurse is evaluating a client who has just been instructed on how to walk with crutches. The nurse should instruct the client (see figure) to:

1. Lean forward 30 degrees.
2. Pad the tops of the crutches.
3. Keep the arms on the rungs of the crutches as shown.
4. Lower the head to watch for objects on the floor.

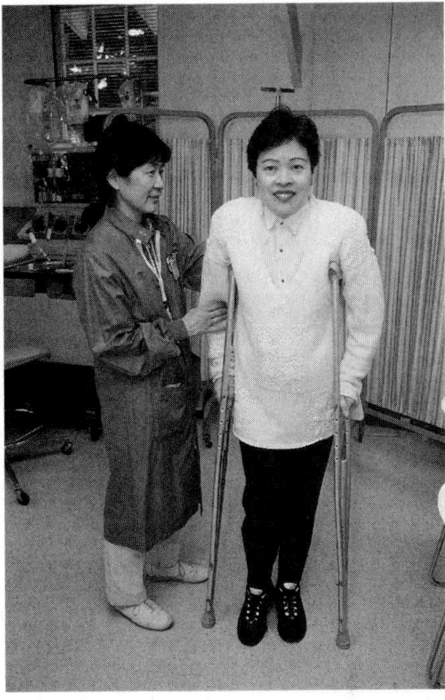

From Ignatavicius D. D., Workman L. M. (2013). *Medical-surgical nursing: Patient-centered collaborative care* (7th ed.). Philadelphia: W. B. Saunders Company.

Audio and Video Items

In audio and video items, an audio or video clip is used as a stimulus in a part of the question or answer. Audio and video items use a scenario, stem, and answers. The audio or video clip is included in the scenario; the student clicks on the icon that brings up the audio file. The National Council Licensure Examination–Registered Nurse (NCLEX-RN) exam currently uses audio item types and has considered the use of video item types (Wendt & Harmes, 2009a, 2009b).

Advantages

Audio and video items test students' ability to identify sounds or respond to video information and make a clinical judgment based on information provided in the audio or video file. Test questions can be written at higher levels of the cognitive domain and require students to synthesize data from the scenario and the data provided in the audio or video file. These questions test competencies that may be difficult to assess with other test item formats.

Disadvantages

Audio and video items can be administered only in a computer-managed environment that supports access to the audio and video files. Finding access to no-cost or low-cost files may be difficult; purchase of files may be necessary as copyright protections must be observed.

Example

The nurse is assessing the breath sounds of a client who is hospitalized with bacterial pneumonia. Click here to listen to the breath sounds. *[The sounds are coarse crackles.]* The nurse should do which first? *[Note: The correct answer depends on the test-taker correctly identifying the breath sound and selecting the appropriate nursing action.]*

1. Have the client take a deep breath and cough to expectorate retained secretions.
2. Encourage the client to drink one glass of fluids every hour.
3. Check the blood levels of the antibiotic the client is receiving.
4. Tell the client the breath sounds are clear and to continue the deep-breathing exercises.

Avoiding Potential Bias in Test Items

Students of equal ability should have an equal probability of correctly answering a test item. If systematic differences in responses to an item exist among members of particular groups, independent of total scores, then the item may be biased. Bosher (2003) classifies potential areas of bias in test items in four categories of bias: testwise flaws, irrelevant difficulty, linguistic bias, and cultural bias.

Testwise flaws are those errors in items that provide cues to the correct answer within the item or test itself. These flaws potentially provide an unfair advantage to students with more test-taking experience or training and to native English speakers who can more easily recognize grammatical and other cues.

Items with *irrelevant difficulty* may be missed for reasons related more to format than to content. This type of bias can occur from writing, unclear stems, providing superfluous information, or using negative phrasing.

Linguistic complexity, grammatical errors, and inconsistent word use also may result in biased items. *Linguistic modification* involves writing short and clearly understood questions (Abedi, 2014). Faculty can reduce the reading load of test items by eliminating irrelevant information, using simple words, and short sentences. Faculty also should avoid using idioms or "slang" that may only be understood by certain groups of students. Faculty can also reduce linguistic load in test questions by using the present tense and active voice.

Faculty must also guard against *cultural bias* when constructing test items (Hicks, 2011). These items depend on culturally specific knowledge and should not be used unless cultural practices *per se* are the domain of the question. The guidelines for writing items are designed to avoid bias.

Ensuring Readability of Test Items

Test items must be written at the level of reading comprehension of the test-taker. Readability refers to the semantic and syntactic complexity of the test item. There are several tests of readability such as the Lexile Framework, Fry, and the Flesch–Kincaid readability tests. Word processing software also have simplified versions of readability tests. If interested, faculty can obtain a rough estimate of readability of their tests using one of these programs. The National Council of State Boards of Nursing (NCSBN) uses grade reading levels linked to the Lexile scale to determine readability of their licensing exam (O'Neill, 2004). The readability level for the Practical Nurse exam does not exceed eighth grade reading level; the reading level for the Registered Nurse exam should not exceed a tenth grade reading level

If the test is to be administered by a computer, the faculty and instructional designer must also consider the perceptual readability, which includes elements such as the screen position, screen color, and font size. Most colleges and universities follow Americans with Disability Act guidelines for readability of computer screens. The NCSBN assumes that the candidate can read text presented on a computer screen. Candidates who do have difficulty with reading computer screens and have a documented disability can request an accommodation from their state board of nursing.

Editing Test Items

After test items have been developed, it is necessary to edit them and make any needed corrections. At this stage, peer review of the questions is helpful for refining the questions, ensuring accuracy and readability, reviewing the test items for fairness and cultural sensitivity, and eliminating grammatical errors. Appropriate peers include those with the content knowledge to check for errors and those with editorial skills to edit for clarity and language usage. When using peers to review the test times, provide sufficient time for a thoughtful review.

Editing can be done in a question or checklist format. Questions to consider when editing a test include the following:

1. Are items stated in a precise manner? Are the items written using short, simple, direct sentences?
2. Do items match the table of specifications?
3. Is there one best answer for each item (except for multiple-response items)?
4. Does each item stand alone?
5. Are sentence construction and punctuation correct?
6. Have stereotyping, prejudices, and biases been eliminated?
7. Have "slang" or words with several meanings been eliminated?
8. Does the question eliminate gender bias, such as referring to the nurse as "she"?
9. Has the use of humor been avoided?
10. Has extraneous information been deleted?
11. Has a colleague reviewed the test?
12. Is the placement of correct options varied so there is no obvious pattern?
13. Is the terminology used on the test the same as has been used in the classroom and in reading assignments?
14. Does the layout of the test on the page facilitate easy reading of the question? Is there sufficient "white space"? Is the entire question on the same page (no page breaks within in the scenario, stem, and options).

Using Test Banks and Test-Authoring Systems

Faculty should attempt to create a large pool of questions from which the items for a specific test can be drawn. Although it is time consuming to amass a large number of questions, the effort is rewarded by being able to administer different versions of the test or to generate a "makeup" test for students who were not able to take the test at a regularly scheduled time. Having the test items available in a word-processing file makes revision of the test easier. All test files should be secured in password-protected areas of a file server.

Many textbook publishers provide test items free of charge to faculty adopting their texts. Often these test items are written to test specific knowledge presented in the various chapters of the textbook, are written at lower levels of the cognitive domain, or contain item writing flaws (Masters et al., 2001), and do not test critical thinking or clinical judgment skills (Clifton & Schriner, 2010). If using these test items, faculty must review them for fit with their learning outcomes and test specifications or blueprints. Faculty can revise questions from test banks to test at higher cognitive levels and to meet the needs of a particular course.

The task of creating test items can be simplified by using computerized test development software that typically is included as a component of a learning management system (see Chapter 21). This software can facilitate test development by creating a collection of test items (test bank) from which faculty can select appropriate questions according to the test blueprint. Alternative forms of tests can also be generated because the item pool can be large enough so that questions can be selected randomly. Some test-authoring software can be used for online testing in a computer classroom or on the Internet, thus simplifying the test administration process.

Assembling a Test

Once the items are written and edited, they must be assembled into a test. This step includes arranging the items, writing test directions, reproducing the test, and administering the test.

Arranging Items within the Test

Unless using test-administration software in which items will be randomly generated, faculty can next determine how the test items should be arranged on the test. For the purposes of enhancing thought tracking, increasing student confidence, and preventing students from becoming anxious about early items, the following guidelines are suggested:

1. Group similar item types together (e.g., all true–false items).
2. Place items within each group in ascending order of difficulty.
3. Place item types in ascending order of difficulty (e.g., true–false items first, essay items last).
4. Begin the test with an easy question.

Writing Test Directions

Test directions should be self-explanatory and include the following information:

1. *Purpose of the test:* This may not need to be included if it has been addressed earlier in the instructional process.
2. *Time allotted to complete the test:* This information allows the students to pace themselves when responding to items.
3. *Basis for responding:* This provides the student with information necessary to choose the appropriate response (e.g., choose only one answer; matching options can be used more than once).
4. *Recording answers:* Answers may be recorded in a variety of ways to expedite grading (e.g., recording answers on a computer sheet using a No. 2 pencil, marking an X through the correct answer on a separate answer sheet for stencil grading, marking answers directly on the test booklet in the left column).
5. *Guessing:* Encouraging students to answer all questions prevents the inflation of scores of bolder students as a result of guessing.
6. *Value/points assigned to items:* This information allows the student to effectively plan the use of his or her time.
7. *Academic honesty policy:* Some faculty cite the policy or remind students of the policy. Faculty may also ask the student to sign that they are complying with the policy.

Reproducing the Test (Paper and Pencil Tests)

When preparing the test in a paper and pencil format, the test should be easy to read and follow. Use standard font and type size; observe guidelines for page layout and use of white space. Space items evenly. Number items consecutively. Keep an item's stem and options on the same page. Place introductory material (e.g., graph or chart) before an item (and make sure it reproduces clearly). Keep matching lists on the same page. Proofread the test after it is compiled but before it is duplicated. Print on one side only.

Administering and Maintaining Security of Tests

Maintaining an Appropriate Physical Test-taking Environment

The physical environment should be conducive to the task. In a classroom, this includes adequate lighting, a comfortable temperature, sufficient workspace, and minimal interruptions. To reduce student anxiety, the faculty member should maintain a positive, nonthreatening attitude and avoid unnecessary conversation before and during the test. Faculty should avoid giving unintentional hints to individual students who ask for clarification of questions during the test.

When administering the test in an online environment, faculty must determine if the test will be administered in a proctored testing center in the school of nursing or on the campus or if the test will be administered to students on their own computer and during a specified period. The student should have a comfortable chair, desk, and computer, as well as sufficient space.

Maintaining a Secure Test Environment

In recent years, maintaining a secure test environment and ensuring academic honesty has become a challenge (DiBartolo & Walsh, 2010; Klocko, 2014). Some suggestions for preventing cheating on tests administered in the classroom include the following:

1. Maintain test security (e.g., lock up copies of the test). Number tests and make sure all copies of tests are returned to the instructor before students leave the classroom.
2. Modify tests from one semester to another.
3. State the consequences of cheating early in the instructional process and inform students of academic honesty policies at the time of testing.
4. Have students sign an honor pledge that has been written on the test (or precedes an online test) that the work during the test is their own.

5. Require that book bags, cell phones, and items of clothing such as hats in which "cheat sheets" can be stored be brought to the front of the room.
6. Proctor students consistently throughout testing; depending on class size, additional proctors may be necessary. Have a clear plan about how proctors are to manage cheating when it is observed or suspected.
7. Designate special seating arrangements (e.g., have an empty chair between students; have students sit in an assigned order).
8. Use alternative versions of the test.
9. Use alternative answer forms (e.g., listing responses down the page, listing responses across the page).

See Chapter 21 for information about maintaining security for online tests. See Chapter 3 for general issues relating to academic honesty.

Accommodations for Test Taking

Students with disabilities or circumstances that require special consideration may request accommodations for test taking (see also Chapter 4). Considerations may be given for the following reasons: allowing extra time for taking the test, needing additional or extra time for rest breaks, requiring adaptations for using a computer such as reading a computer screen (need for increased font size or color change) or for use of a trackball mouse, having hearing or other auditory disabilities, having visual or eyesight difficulties (such as requiring a Braille, large print), requiring a quiet space with limited distractions, having a reader to read or record test-taker responses, needing a sign language interpreter, or having a medical device in the room.

At a college or university, the policies for accommodations for classroom tests are established by the faculty and made public. Students must have documented need for accommodations on file with the office that deals with Americans with Disabilities Act compliance (see Chapter 4) and follow established procedures for implementing the request for accommodation for taking a test. For other tests, such as licensing exams or certification exams the policies are set by the test administration service (state board of nursing in the case of the PN or RN licensing exam) and the test-taker must make the request in writing and have a letter from an appropriate health professional confirming the diagnosis or disability. Approval or disapproval of these requests can be determined based on the effect the disability has on the candidates' ability to practice nursing in the state.

Analyzing Test Results

Once the test has been administered and scored, faculty should review the results using concepts of measurement and data analysis. On the basis of these findings, faculty assign grades. Faculty at most schools of nursing have access to test scoring services that calculate test statistics and provide item analysis. Although there may be a fee associated with the service, the data provided by test scoring services are helpful, particularly for the first few times the test is used. Faculty should seek the assistance of these services and the consultation that can be obtained at testing centers.

Concepts of Measurement

A variety of metrics are used to determine the effectiveness of a test. These include validity, reliability, and measures of central tendency.

Validity

The concept of validity refers to the appropriateness, meaningfulness, and usefulness of inferences made from test scores. Validity is the judgment made about a test's ability to measure what it is intended to measure. This judgment is based on three categories of evidence: content-related, criterion-related, and construct-related.

Content-related patterns of evidence should show that the test adequately samples relevant content. In nursing education, the relevant content is defined by nurse educators, the course, and the profession. Some examples of content-related evidence of validity are correspondence of the test content with the following:

1. The table of specifications
2. Professional judgments of peers
3. Core material as defined by professional organizations
4. Standards of care as defined by agencies and professional organizations

Criterion-related patterns of evidence should show that the test adequately measures performance, either concurrently or predictively. The performance must be compared with some criterion variable. Nurse educators may use performance on the licensing examination (NCLEX-RN or NCLEX-PN) as the criterion variable (pass or fail).

Construct-related patterns of evidence should show a relationship between test performance and some "quality" to be measured. This is a broad category of evidence that must include specifics about the test (from the content and criterion categories) in addition to a description of the quality or construct being measured.

Some of the factors that may adversely affect test validity are unclear directions, inconsistent or inadequate sampling from the table of specifications, poorly written test items, and subjective scoring (McDonald, 2013). Careful preparation of the test can improve test validity. (See Box 24-2.)

Reliability

Reliability refers to the ability of a test to provide dependable and consistent scores. A judgment about reliability can be made based on the extent to which two similar measures agree. Reliability is a necessary but not sufficient condition for validity. However, reliability may be high even with no validity. Nurse educators look for evidence to judge tests as both reliable and valid.

Among the factors that may adversely affect test reliability are insufficient length and insufficient group variability. For the purpose of increasing reliability, a minimum test length of 25 multiple-choice questions with an item difficulty sufficient to ensure heterogeneous performance of the group is sufficient for classroom testing.

Reliability could be measured by giving the same test to the same group and noting the correspondence (test-retest method) or by giving "equivalent" tests to the same group. Both of these methods have major disadvantages for classroom testing and are not generally used by nurse educators. Reliability can be measured with a single test administration by using either the split-half or internal consistency method. The split-half method separately scores responses to odd and even questions and then compares the "odd-question" score to the "even-question" score. The internal consistency of a test can be calculated by using one of the Kuder-Richardson formulas (McDonald, 2013). Many computer grading programs supply a test reliability coefficient as part of the results (Figure 24-1).

Reliability is measured on a scale of 0 to 1.00. A reliability coefficient of 1.00 represents 100% correspondence between two tests or measures. Many standardized tests have reliability coefficients of 0.9 or higher. Good test reliability is greater than 0.80; acceptable test reliability is 0.70 to 0.80; poor test reliability is less than 0.70 (Tarrant & Ware, 2012). For the test results shown in Figure 24-1, the reliability coefficient is 0.844, indicating good internal consistency of the test. Measures of test reliability are based on the assumption that all students had adequate time to answer all questions and that all test items are of about the same difficulty. Because the reliability coefficient functions better when the variability of scores is maximized, tests administered to smaller groups of students (N) may have lower reliability coefficients. See Box 24-3.

BOX 24-2 Improving Test Validity

- Use a table of specifications (blueprint).
- Develop test items based on common nursing practice.
- Base test items on standards of care.
- Develop test items using evidence for best nursing care practices.
- Obtain peer review of blueprint and test questions from a clinical content expert.

Test Statistics

Various test statistics can be calculated, generated by test-authoring software, or reported from computer scoring services (see Figure 24-1). These statistics help faculty interpret test results and provide data for item revision. Test grading software typically provides students' raw and percentage scores, individual student reports, and test statistics such as central tendencies and test reliability indices as well as item analysis data.

Raw Score

The raw score is the number of test questions answered correctly. Raw scores are the most accurate test scores but yield limited information. A frequency distribution can be used to arrange raw scores to create class intervals. If tests are scored by computer, a frequency polygon is likely. The percentage score compares the raw score with the maximum possible score.

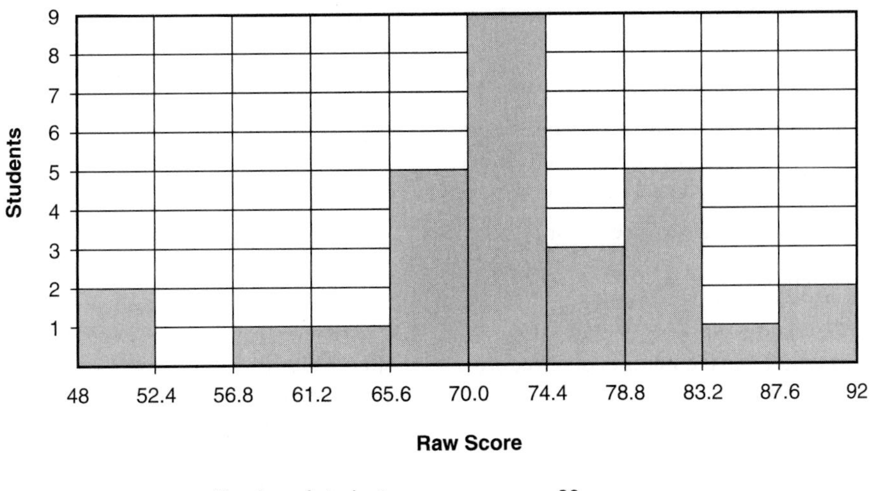

Number of students	29
Number of items	100
Maximum point value	100
Highest score	92 (92.0%)
Lowest score	48 (48.0%)
Median	73
Mean	72.690
Standard deviation	9.813
Test reliability	0.844
Standard error of measurement	3.872

Figure 24-1 Sample test statistics report from a computer test scoring program.

> ### *BOX 24-3* Improving Test Reliability
>
> - Increase number of test items.
> - Improve discrimination levels.
> - Increase number of test takers (less than 25 decreases reliability).
> - Increase variability of scores (mastery tests have low variability).

$$\text{Percent score} = \text{Raw score}(x) / \text{maximum possible score}$$

Central Tendency

Central tendency is a descriptive statistic for a set of scores. Measures of central tendency include the mean, median, and mode. The mean (or average) has the advantage of ease of calculation. The mean is calculated as the sum of all scores divided by the total number of scores.

$$\text{Mean}(m) = \text{Sum of all scores}(x\text{'s}) / \text{Number of scores}(N)$$

The median divides the scores in the middle (i.e., 50% of scores fall below the median and 50% of cores are above the median). The median is a better measure of central tendency than the mean if the scores are not normally distributed.

Variability

Variability refers to the dispersion of scores and is thus a measure of group heterogeneity. Variability of scores affects other statistics. For example, low variability (homogeneity of scores) will tend to lower reliability coefficients such as the Kuder-Richardson coefficient (Lyman, 1997). Relative grading scales are most meaningful when they are applied to a wide range of scores. Mastery tests, by design, may show little variability. As groups of students progress in a nursing program, there may be less variability in scores because of attrition of students (failure or withdrawal from the program).

Range

The range is the simplest measure of variability and is calculated by subtracting the lowest score from the highest score. Thus:

$$\text{Range} = \text{Highest score} - \text{Lowest score}$$

Standard Deviation

The standard deviation (SD) of scores is the best measure of variability. Most computer scoring programs provide the SD of the scores with the results. Calculators with statistical functions can also be used to figure the SD. For more information on formulas and methods for calculating the SD, consult a statistics text. The SD is just the average distance of scores from the mean. In Figure 26-1, the SD is given as 9.8. The SD can be used in making interpretations from the normal curve (Lyman, 1997).

Normal Curve

The normal curve is a theoretical distribution of scores that is bell shaped and symmetrical. The mean, median, and mode are the same score on a normal curve. Also, for a normal curve, 68% of scores will fall within ±1 SD of the mean and 95% of scores will fall within ±2 SDs of the mean. This distribution may be used in assigning grades.

Standard Error of Measurement

The standard error of measurement is an estimate of how much the observed score is likely to differ from the "true" score. That is, the student's "true" score most likely lies between the observed score plus or minus the standard error.

$$\text{True score} = \text{Observed score} \pm \text{Error}$$

The standard error of measurement is calculated by using the SD and the test reliability. Many computer scoring programs calculate the standard error of measurement. Some faculty members give students the benefit of the doubt and add the standard error to each raw score before they assign grades.

Standardized Scores

Standardized scores allow for ease of comparison between individual scores and sets of scores. The z score converts a raw score into units of SD on a normal curve. The z score can be calculated as follows:

$$x = \frac{x - m}{SD}$$

where x = observed score, m = mean, and SD = standard deviation. For example, for a raw score of 34:

$$z = \frac{34 - 36.8}{6.6} = -0.42$$

Thus a raw score of 34 falls approximately 0.5 SD below the mean.

Because z scores are expressed by using decimals and both positive and negative values, many faculty prefer to use t scores instead. The z score can be used to calculate the t score. Converting raw scores to t scores has the following advantages:

1. The mean of the distribution is set at 50.
2. The SD from the mean is set at 10.
3. t scores can be manipulated mathematically for grading purposes.

$$t = 10z + 50$$

For example, the z score of –.42 would be transformed as follows:

$$t = 10(-0.42) + 50 = 45.8$$

Conducting the Item Analysis

Classic test theory is used for this discussion of item analysis and the discrimination index. Classic test theory and related inferences assume a norm-referenced measure. For a critique of classic test theory and an explanation of the newer item response theories, see *Developing and Validating Multiple-Choice Test Items* (Haladyna, 2004). Item response theories depend on large samples and thus are of limited application to classroom tests.

Item analysis assists faculty in determining whether test items have separated the learners from the nonlearners (discrimination). Many computer scoring programs supply item statistics.

Item Difficulty

The item difficulty index (P value) is simply the percentage correct for the group answering the item. The upper limit of item difficulty is 1.00, meaning that 100% of students answered the question correctly. The lower limit of item difficulty depends on the number of possible responses and is the probability of guessing the correct answer. For example, for a question with four options, $P = 0.25$ is the lower limit or probability of guessing. An item difficulty index of greater than 0.80 indicates low difficulty; an index of 0.30 to 0.80 indicated medium difficulty, and less than 0.30 indicates high difficulty (Tarrant & Ware, 2012). McDonald (2013) recommends keeping the *P* values of the items in the range of 0.70 to 0.80 to help ensure that questions separate learners from nonlearners (a good discrimination index). Clifton and Schriner (2010) recommend using 0.50 as a quick reference point, with low limits at 0.30 and high limits at 0.80. Some items may be slightly easier or more difficult, however, and faculty can determine the range of difficulty that is appropriate for their students and tests.

Item Discrimination

Item discrimination, the item discrimination index, refers to the way an item differentiates students who know the content from those who do not. Discrimination can be measured as a point biserial correlation. The point biserial correlation compares each student's item performance with each student's overall test performance. If a question discriminates well, the point biserial correlation will be highly positive for the correct answer and negative for the distractors. This indicates that the "learners," or the students who knew the content, answered the question correctly and the "nonlearners" chose distractors. An index of greater than 0.40 indicates excellent discrimination; an index of 0.30 to 0.39 indicates good discrimination; an index of 0.15 to 0.29 is satisfactory; an index of less than 0.15 indicates low discrimination; and an index of 0 indicates that there is no discrimination (Tarrant & Ware, 2012). Haladyna (2004) cautions that if the item difficulty index is either too high or too low, the discrimination index is attenuated. The discrimination index is maximized when the item difficulty is moderate ($P = 0.5$). Ultimately, test reliability depends on item discrimination. Inclusion of mastery level material on a norm-referenced test tends to lower test reliability because that item tends to be answered correctly by many students and will thus be a poor discriminator.

Distractor Evaluation

In addition to the evaluation of the correct answer to an item for a positive point biserial correlation, each distractor should be individually evaluated. Effective distractors should appeal to the nonlearner, as indicated by negative point biserial correlation values. Distractors with a point biserial correlation of zero indicate that students did not select them and that they may need to be revised or replaced with a more plausible option to appeal to students who do not understand the content. Distractors that were not selected increase the chances that a student could have obtained the correct answer by guessing. One way to develop appealing distractors is to periodically ask open-ended questions to determine the most common errors in thinking. Distractors for questions with numerical answers may need to be worked out by following the most typical mistakes that students make.

Revising Test Items

Developing a valid and reliable test is an ongoing process. It is helpful to revise the test immediately after administering it while faculty can recall items and student responses to them. Item revision should be conducted after item analysis. One way to analyze items for revision is to use a test item analysis form (Figure 24-2). The result of item analysis for each question is entered in the form. Those items falling outside of the "ideal" range should be considered for revision. Items to be revised should include those with the following statistical characteristics:

1. Items with *P* values that are too high or too low (around 0.5 is ideal)
2. Correct answers with low positive or negative point biserial values (>0.30 is ideal)
3. Distractors with highly positive point biserial values (negative values are ideal)

Other considerations for revising test items include those questions that were scored incorrectly, items not written clearly or noted by students who did not understand the question because of linguistic or cultural bias, or were not matched with the teaching–learning process of having clear learning outcomes, clarity of instruction, and opportunity for practice with feedback.

Test 2
Date 3/08

P (Item Difficulty) / D (Item Discrimination)		>.50	.40–.49	.30–.39	.20–.29	.10–.19	.01–.09	Negative	Total
Very difficult	P = 50% or less								
Difficult	P = 51%–69%	20	10	4	2, 18, 26				6
Average	P = 70%–80%	3, 5, 25, 27	9, 14, 19, 24	12, 16, 17, 23, 29					13
Easy	P = 81%–100%			6, 8, 11, 15, 21, 28	1, 7, 13, 22, 30				11
Total number of items		5	5	12	8				

$\bar{X}$ 75
KR .75
SD 3.7
SEM 2.8

Figure 24-2 Sample test item analysis form for a 30-item test.

Assigning Grades

Grades provide both feedback and motivation for students. In the academic setting, assignment of grades may be guided by the institution grading policy or scale. Many computer software programs are available to assist faculty with assigning grades accurately and efficiently. The two basic methods for assignment are the absolute and the relative ("curved") scales (described in the following sections). Principles of good grading include the following (McDonald, 2013):

1. Informing students of the specific grading criteria at the beginning of the course (stated explicitly in the syllabus)
2. Basing the grades on learning outcomes (not factors such as attendance or effort)
3. Gathering sufficient data (amount and variety) for the assignment of a valid grade
4. Recording data collected for grading purposes quantitatively (e.g., 89%, not B+)
5. Applying the grading system equitably to all students
6. Keeping grades confidential
7. Using statistically sound principles for assigning grades

Absolute Scale

An absolute grading scale rates performance relative to a standard (McDonald, 2013). The student's earned points are compared with the total possible points and are expressed as a percentage earned. The standard should be included in the syllabus at the beginning of the course. Theoretically, all students could receive an A (or an F) with this scale. In reality, the dispersion of the grades depends on the difficulty of the tests. See Table 24-8 for an example of an absolute grading scale.

Relative Scale

A relative grading scale rates students according to their ranking within the group. To assign grades in this system, faculty record scores in order, from high to low. Grades may then be assigned by using a variety of techniques. One method is to assign the grades according to natural "breaks" in the distribution. This method has the disadvantage of being subjective. A better method of assigning grades

TABLE 24-8 Sample Absolute Grading Scale

Percentage Correct	Assigned Grade
90–100	A
80–89	B
70–79	C
60–69	D
<60	F

based on a relative scale is to use the test statistics to create a "curve":

1. Decide whether to use the mean or the median as the best measure of central tendency. If the mean and median are approximately the same, use the mean. If the distribution is skewed, use the median.
2. Determine the SD. The C grade will be set as the mean plus or minus one half of the SD (encompassing 40% of the scores). See Table 24-9 for an example of a relative grading scale.

Table 24-10 shows a comparison of the grades assigned to the raw scores with the absolute and relative grading scales described.

Relative grading scales may also be developed by using linear scores such as z scores or t scores (see the section on standardized test scores for directions for calculating these scores). t scores are more commonly used for grading purposes because there are no negative values in this system. The mean score becomes a t score of 50. The z score and t score are figured for each raw score. The faculty member decides what grade to assign to the ranges of t scores. Assuming a normal curve, a t score of 50 would be assigned a grade of C. Computer grading programs that calculate grades according to absolute or relative scales are available. Many experts in assessment and grading do not recommend the use of relative grading scales (Haladyna, 2004; McDonald, 2013).

TABLE 24-9 Sample Relative Grading Scale

Grade	Calculation	Example	Range
A	> Upper B	>45.5	>45.5
B	Upper C + 1 SD	40.5 + 5	40.6–45.5
C	Mean ± 0.5 SD	38 ± 2.5	35.5–40.5
D	Lower C – 1 SD	35.5 – 5	30.5–35.4
F	< Lower D	<30.5	<30.5

TABLE 24-10 Comparison of Grades Assigned by Three Methods

Raw Score	Percent Score	Grade (Absolute)	Grade (Relative)
49	98	A	A
45(2)	90	A	B
42(2)	84	B	B
40	80	B	C
39(3)	78	C	C
38(4)	76	C	C
37	74	C	C
35(2)	70	C	D
34(3)	68	D	D
33	66	D	D
30	60	D	F
28	56	F	F

Grading Standards, Grade Inflation, and Grade Indexing

Periodically, faculty, administrators, boards of trustees, or consumers raise questions about the relative meaning of grades and potential or actual grade "inflation." Some possible causes for grade inflation are improved academic readiness of admitted students; student retention programs; competency-based assessments; competitive admission standards; a student population of older, mature, and career-directed students; and pass–fail grading systems.

Grade indexing involves indicating how many students in a given course or section of a course received grades that equaled or exceeded the grade of a given student. This index may appear on the student's transcript.

Nursing faculty as a whole should review grading policies and practices on a regular basis. A consistent philosophy about grading and fair and equitable grading practices communicates concern to the students and competence to nursing's varied publics. Faculty must also continually strive to administer valid and reliable tests that measure students' attainment of course and program competencies.

Summary

Although developing, administering, and analyzing classroom tests may seem like a monumental task, the step-by-step approach presented in this chapter can be used as a guide to simplify this process. By following these guidelines, faculty can create written tests that can be used as effective measures of outcomes in the classroom. Assigning grades is the last step in this process.

REFLECTING ON THE EVIDENCE

1. Compare the six cognitive domains of Bloom (1956) and the six cognitive processes of Anderson and Krathwohl (2001). Notice the relative positioning of evaluation and synthesis and creation in the two taxonomies. What is the evidence for creation as a higher-level cognitive process than evaluation in the newer taxonomy? Hint: Think about the structure of a good literature review.
2. Evaluate an instructor-developed test (your own or another instructor's). What is the evidence for the construct, content, or criterion validity of the test? If such evidence does not exist, how would you go about establishing the evidence for validity?
3. Search the literature for an article about item response theory and an article about classic test theory. Compare the assumptions and usefulness of the two theories. Note: This question is most appropriate for the reader with a strong statistical background or interest.
4. Are you using commercially prepared "high-stakes" tests? What are the advantages and disadvantages for using these tests? Support your response with evidence.
5. Following the administration of an exam, students tell you that several students were observed cheating. What will you do? How will you respond to the students who reported the incident? What measures can you take to prevent cheating incidents during the next test?
6. The students in your class ask you to "curve" the grades on a classroom test. Write a short explanation of this practice, based on the evidence, in terms understandable to an undergraduate (i.e., what you would tell the students). Take and defend a position on whether you would or would not agree to "curving" the grades.

REFERENCES

Abedi, J. (2014). *Linguistic modification, part I: Language factors in the assessment of English language learners: The theory and principles underlying the linguistic modification approach.* Retrieved from, http://www.ncela.us/files/uploads/11/abedi_sato.pdf.

Anderson, L. W., & Krathwohl, D. R. (2001). *A taxonomy for learning, teaching, and assessing: A revision of Bloom's taxonomy of educational objectives.* New York: Longman.

Bloom, B. S., Englehart, M. D., Furst, E. J., Hill, W. H., & Krathwhol, D. R. (1956). *Taxonomy of educational objectives: The classification of educational goals. Handbook 1: Cognitive domain.* New York: Longman.

Bosher, S. (2003). Barriers to creating a more culturally diverse nursing profession: Linguistic bias in multiple-choice nursing exams. *Nursing Education Perspectives, 24*(1), 25–34.

Carey, B. (2014). *Why flunking exams is actually a good thing,* Retrieved from, http://www.nytimes.com/2014/09/07/magazine/why-flunking-exams-is-actually-a-good-thing.html?smprod=nytcore-ipad&smid=nytcore-ipad-share.

Clifton, S. L., & Schriner, C. L. (2010). Assessing the quality of multiple-choice test items. *Nurse Educator, 35*(1), 12–16.

DiBartolo, M. C., & Walsh, C. M. (2010). Desperate times call for desperate measures: Where are we in addressing academic dishonesty? *Journal of Nursing Education, 49*(10), 543–544.

Fuller, B. (2013). Evidence-based instructional strategies, facilitating linguistically diverse nursing student learning. *Nurse Educator, 38*(3), 118–121.

Haladyna, T. M. (2004). *Developing and validating multiple-choice test items* (3rd ed.). Mahwah, NJ: Lawrence Erlbaum.

Hicks, N. (2011). Guidelines for identifying and revising culturally biased multiple-choice nursing examination items. *Nurse Educator, 36*(6), 266–270.

Klocko, M. (2014). Academic dishonesty in schools of nursing: A literature review. *Journal of Nursing Education, 53*(3), 121–125.

Lyman, H. B. (1997). *Test scores and what they mean* (6th ed.). Boston, MA: Allyn & Bacon.

Masters, J. C., Hulsmeyer, B. S., Pike, M. E., Leichty, K., Miller, M. T., & Verst, A. L. (2001). Assessment of multiple-choice questions in selected test banks accompanying text books used in nursing education. *Journal of Nursing Education, 40*(1), 25–32.

McDonald, M. E. (2013). *The nurse educators' guide to assessing learning outcomes.* Sudbury, MA: Jones & Bartlett.

Miller, M. P., Linn, R. L., & Gronlund, N. E. (2012). *Measurement and assessment in teaching* (9th ed.). Upper Saddle River, NJ: Pearson Education.

National Council of State Boards of Nursing. (2014). *A test plan for the National Council Licensure Examination for registered nurses.* Retrieved from, http://www.ncsbn.org.

National League for Nursing. (2010). *High stakes testing.* Retrieved from, http://www.nln.org/aboutnln/reflection_dialogue/refl_dial_7.htm.

O'Neill, T. (2004). *Readability of NCLEX exams. NCLEX, psychometric technical brief.* Volume 1, Chicago: National Council of State Boards of Nursing.

Santo, L., Frander, E., & Hawkins, A. (2013). The use of standardized exit examinations in baccalaureate nursing education. *Nurse Educator, 38*(2), 81–84.

Su, W. M., Osisek, P. J., Montgomery, C., & Pellar, S. (2009). Designing multiple-choice test items at higher cognitive levels. *Nurse Educator, 34*(5), 223–227.

Sullivan, D. (2014). A concept analysis of "high stakes testing." *Nurse Educator, 39*(2), 72–76.

Tarrant, M., & Ware, J. (2012). A framework for improving the quality of multiple-choice assessments. *Nurse Educator, 37*(3), 98–104.

Wendt, A., & Harmes, J. C. (2009a). Developing and evaluating innovative items for the NCLEX, part 2, item characteristics and cognitive processing. *Nurse Educator, 34*(3), 109–113.

Wendt, A., & Harmes, J. C. (2009b). Evaluating innovative items for the NCLEX, part I, usability and pilot testing. *Nurse Educator, 34*(2), 56–59.

Wendt, A., & Kenny, L. E. (2009). Alternate item types: Continuing the quest for authentic testing. *Journal of Nursing Education, 48*(3), 150–156.

25 Clinical Performance Evaluation*

Wanda Bonnel, PhD, RN, APRN, ANEF

In times of of profound change in health care, evaluating students' attainment of clinical knowledge, skills, and abilities remains constant. From patient safety to student confidence as clinicians, conducting careful clinical performance evaluations for each student is essential. As students and health care teams come together to establish a culture of safety and quality patient care, using best practices in evaluation of clinical performance is imperative. Providing fair and reasonable clinical evaluation is one of the most important and challenging aspects of the faculty role. Faculty must discern whether students can think critically within the clinical setting, maintain a professional demeanor, interact appropriately with patients, prioritize problems, have basic knowledge of clinical procedures, and complete care procedures correctly. All the while, faculty need to minimize student anxiety within the complex health care setting so that student clinical performance and not extraneous factors, such as anxiety or fatigue, are being observed.

Evaluation of clinical performance provides data from which faculty can judge the extent to which students have acquired specified learning outcomes. This chapter discusses general issues in evaluating clinical performance, clinical evaluation methods and tools, and the clinical evaluation process.

General Issues in Evaluating Clinical Performance

When clinical performance is evaluated, students' skills are judged as they relate to an established standard of patient care. Acceptable clinical performance involves behavior, knowledge, and attitudes that students gradually develop in a variety of settings. A review of literature about clinical evaluation has identified challenges in obtaining this full picture. For example, the concept of clinical judgment, or evaluating students' thinking and problem solving ability, is consistently noted as both important and challenging. In a survey of clinical faculty, researchers found that, although clinical faculty are intent on gaining a holistic student evaluation, much time is spent on task completion and observing task skills (Ironside, McNelis, & Ebright, 2014). The literature also describes the need for models to evaluate clinical judgment and problem solving. Tanner (2006) describes a model of clinical judgment, incorporating components such as student reflection in action and reflection on action. The critical decision model, adapted to incorporate both observation and questioning, related to students' clinical situation awareness, cues for action, and pattern recognition has also been described (McNelis, Ironside, Zvonar, & Ebright, 2014). Incorporating additional evaluation approaches, such as writing, active learning cases, and simulation, discussed in later sections, can help gain a comprehensive evaluation.

The ultimate outcome for clinical performance evaluation is safe, quality patient care. Clinical performance evaluation provides information to the student about performance and provides data that may be used for individual student development, assigning grades, and making decisions about the curriculum. Students have the right to a reliable and valid evaluation that assesses achievement of competencies required to take on the role of the novice nurse. Box 25-1 provides some "quick tips" to be considered at the beginning of the evaluation process.

*The author acknowledges the work of Dorothy A. Gomez, MSN, RN; Stacy Lobodzinski, MSN, RN; and Cora D. Hartwell West, MSN, RN, in the previous editions of the chapter.

BOX 25-1 Quick Tips for Clinical Evaluation

- Define clearly both knowledge and skills that students will need to demonstrate.
- Use multiple sources of data for evaluation.
- Be reasonable and consistent in evaluation of all students.
- Use formative mini-evaluations and suggest minor, easy corrections at the time they are needed.
- Present feedback and evaluation in nonjudgmental language, confining comments to a student's behavior.
- Provide evaluation "sandwiches," commenting first on a strength, then on a weakness, then on a strength of the student's behavior.
- Carry an anecdotal record or mobile device equivalent for each student, maintaining privacy of data.
- Make specific notes, focusing on specific details of a student's behavior.
- Document student patterns of behavior over time through compilation of records.
- Invite students to complete self-assessments and summarize what they have learned.
- Help students prioritize learning needs and turn feedback into constructive challenges with specific goals for each day.

Good practice includes multidimensional evaluation with diverse evaluation methods completed over time, seeking student growth and progress. All evaluation should respect students' dignity and self-esteem. In addition to the concepts of assessment and evaluation, grading is considered part of a systems approach that includes integrating evaluation as the final component of learning (Walvoord, Anderson, & Angelo, 2010). Before assessing and evaluating clinical performance, faculty must consider several issues. These issues include who will be participants in the evaluation, evaluation timing, and evaluation access and privacy.

Using the Team: Participants in Evaluation

Faculty

Clinical evaluation is complex. Although faculty have primary responsibility for the student clinical evaluation, gaining multiple individuals' perspectives or a team approach enhances the evaluation as designated others contribute. Faculty are knowledgeable about the purpose of the evaluation and the objectives that will be used to judge each student's performance. This clarity of purpose provides direction for selection of evaluation tools and processes. Initial faculty challenges in completing clinical evaluations include factors such as faculty value systems, the number of students supervised, and reasonable clinical opportunities for students. Faculty need to be aware of their own value systems to avoid biasing the evaluation process. When faculty are supervising a group of students in the delivery of safe and appropriate nursing care, faculty can only sample student behaviors. Limited sampling of behaviors or individual biases may result in an inaccurate or unfair clinical evaluation. Because of these limitations, faculty use a variety of evaluation methods to capture the broader picture of student competence. Faculty strive to identify equitable assignments and can consider evaluation input from other sources with potential adjunct evaluators, including students, nursing staff and preceptors, peer evaluators, and patients.

Students

Completion of self-assessments by students provides not only data, as part of the evaluation process, but also a learning experience for the students (Bonnel, 2008). Student self-evaluation provides a starting point for reviewing, comparing, and discussing evaluative data with faculty. Initial student involvement in self-assessment tends to facilitate student behavior changes and provides a positive environment for learning and improvement. Participation in their own evaluation also empowers students to make choices and identify their strengths. Self-assessments are further discussed later in this chapter as a component of self-evaluation and self-reflection.

Nursing Staff and Preceptors

New models for clinical education, including dedicated units with entire patient care staff engaged in educating students, dedicated preceptors, and academies to support clinical teaching, emphasize the need to focus on engaging preceptors as part of the clinical evaluation team. Nursing staff and other designated preceptors often provide input to the evaluation process and tend to provide data from an informed perspective as a result of collaboration with students. Even with newer clinical evaluation models, these team members often have limited experience with clinical evaluation. The nursing literature indicates that clinical preceptors consistently report wanting more knowledge about conducting clinical evaluation and giving feedback. There is also a need for addressing the issue of faculty and preceptor interrater reliability. Preceptors indicate the need for faculty support, especially when students are unprepared for clinical (Dahlke, Baumbusch, Affleck, & Kwon, 2012; McClure & Black, 2013).

Nursing staff should understand their role in student evaluation, with staff expectations in the evaluation process clearly articulated. This includes determining whether staff feedback should be provided directly to the student only or shared with faculty as well. One of the disadvantages of including nursing personnel in the evaluation process is that expectations in the clinical area may differ from course performance objectives. Sharing course objectives, expectations of students, and clinical evaluation forms with staff promotes an evaluation partnership. Although evaluation is time consuming for busy nurses, this may be part of a nurse's career development or joint appointment responsibilities.

Preceptors have a specified role in modeling and facilitating clinical education for students, especially for advanced nursing students. Typically preceptors serve a more formal role in evaluation, such as an adjunct faculty role, and provide evaluative data as part of a faculty team. If staff nurses and nurse preceptors provide data for the evaluation process, they should be oriented to the nursing school's evaluation plan. Roles should be clarified, indicating whether staff will be asked to provide occasional comments, to report only incidents or concerns, or to complete a specific evaluation form. Hrobsky and Kersbergen (2002) describe the use of a clinical map to assist preceptors in identifying student strengths and weaknesses. Seldomridge and Walsh (2006) note the importance of adequately preparing adjunct evaluators for their role, teaching these individuals to provide good feedback with tools such as rubrics to promote consistency and specifying clinical activities to evaluate.

Peer Evaluators

Peer evaluation can help students develop collaborative skills, build communication abilities, and promote professional responsibility. Students have described value in peer review roles, but also indicate the need for faculty support and clear guidelines for peer review (Burgess, Roberts, Black, & Mellis, 2013). As some debate the appropriateness of having student peers act as evaluators in the clinical setting, student peers should only evaluate competencies and assignments that they are prepared to judge. A potential disadvantage is that peers may be biased in providing only favorable information about student colleagues or may have unrealistic expectations of their student colleagues. Providing students with this peer evaluation opportunity and then appropriately weighting the contribution can be a reasonable practice (Boehm & Bonnel, 2010). Peer review, an important component of team and group work, includes learning to share thoughtful, objective critique against standards such as rubrics. Providing student peers opportunities to critique and give feedback to each other can also be a team learning opportunity. Faculty can help students appreciate the importance of peer review, use basic rubrics, and practice professional peer communication (Institute of Medicine, 2014).

Patients

Patients provide data from the product consumer viewpoint. Patient satisfaction is considered an important marker in quality health care and can be considered as part of student evaluation. Judgments about student performance are made from patients' personal experiences and data should be weighted for their value. Patients often have positive comments to make about their students, which can be positive for the students to hear. Particularly as health care moves to incorporate patients into stronger team member roles, their perceptions of student care can add value.

Evaluation Timing: Formative and Summative Evaluation

Faculty must consider the appropriate timing of evaluation and student feedback. Formative evaluation focuses on the process of student development during the clinical activity, whereas summative evaluation comes at the conclusion of a specified clinical activity to determine student accomplishment. Formative evaluation can assist in diagnosing student problems and learning needs. Appropriate feedback enables students to learn from their mistakes and allows for growth and improvement in behavior. Summative evaluation attests to competency attainment or meeting of designated objectives. Each of these concepts has unique contributions to the evaluation process, which is discussed further in Chapter 22.

All parties involved in the clinical performance evaluation should be aware of evaluation time frames at the outset. Timely feedback to students from faculty, both ongoing and formally scheduled, decreases the risk of unexpected evaluation results. Ongoing formative evaluations keep students and faculty aware of the progress toward attainment of learning outcomes and promote opportunities for goal setting. This early intervention by a faculty member may provide needed direction for improvement and prevent a student from receiving an unsatisfactory evaluation in clinical performance.

Access to Evaluation Data and Privacy Considerations

There are both ethical and legal issues relevant to privacy of evaluation data that can affect the student, faculty, and institution. Before conducting clinical evaluations, the educator must determine who will have access to data. In most cases, detailed evaluative data are shared only between the faculty member and the individual student. Program policy should identify who additionally may have access to the evaluation and how evaluative information will be stored and for how long. Evaluative data should be stored in a secure area. As designated by the Family Educational Rights and Privacy Act, students 18 years of age or older or in postsecondary schools have the right to inspect records maintained by a school (U.S. Department of Education, 2013). A school's program materials such as catalogues and handbooks can be tools to ensure the creation of reasonable and prudent policies that are in compliance with legal and accrediting guidelines. Additionally anecdotal notes, text-based summaries of student performance, should be objectively written as they have potential to be subpoenaed in legal proceedings. Privacy of written anecdotal notes and computer documents or mobile device notes also need to be maintained. Inadequate security of this information could lead to a breach of student privacy.

The need to protect patient privacy can also become an issue, particularly when evaluating students' use of electronic health records. Although protecting health information privacy for patients, the Health Insurance Portability and Accountability Act may create challenges for faculty and students in accessing written clinical data. Because electronic health records are an important component of student learning, faculty need to be familiar with the guidelines and procedures that clinical agencies have developed for students and faculty to access needed patient care documents. Ongoing discussions about students' electronic record use and its role in evaluation are important to future clinicians (Niederhauser, Schoessler, Gubrud-Howe, Magnussen, & Codier, 2012). If clinical access to electronic health records is limited, another way to evaluate the student's ability is to provide simulations using those commercial products designed to teach about the electronic health record. Additional legal considerations are discussed in Chapter 3.

Clinical Evaluation Methods and Tools

Many methods and tools are used to measure learning in the clinical setting. A variety of approaches should be incorporated in clinical evaluation, including cognitive, psychomotor, and affective considerations as well as cultural competence and ethical decision making (Gaberson, Oermann, & Shellenberger, 2014). Additionally, educators cannot ignore the social connotations of grading, including the effect that evaluation has on the learning process and student motivation (Walvoord et al., 2010).

The goal of evaluation is an objective report about the quality of the clinical performance. Faculty need to be aware that potential exists for evaluation of students' clinical performance to be subjective and inconsistent. Even with "objective" instruments based on measurable and observable behavior, subjectivity can still be introduced into a tool that is viewed as objective. Faculty should be sensitive to the forces that contribute to the subjective side of evaluation as they strive for fairness and consistency (Oermann & Gaberson, 2014).

Fair and reasonable evaluation of students in clinical settings requires use of appropriate evaluation tools that are ideally efficient for faculty to use. In a synthesis of the literature, Krautscheid, Moceri, Stragnell, Manthey, and Neal (2014) summarized that much variability exists in clinical evaluation tools. Although common agreements were found that tools needed to include criterion-based, clear standards and be consistent with program objectives and mission, common challenges were identified to include evaluator bias, subjectivity, and misinterpretation of guidelines. The authors summarized that the best tools are reliable clinical tools that guide in determining how well students meet objectives, verify their competency as safe practitioners, and allow opportunities for formative and summative feedback.

Any evaluation instrument used to measure clinical learning and performance should have criteria that are consistent with course objectives and the teaching institution's purpose and philosophy. Attention to student clinical progress, not only across semesters but across a program, can be considered with similar, consistent evaluation processes and tools that progress across the program (Bonnel & Smith, 2010).

Faculty teams should be engaged in ongoing discussions about the tools they choose to use and their purposes. Ongoing orientation and practice with the tools and ratings is recommended (Krautscheid et al., 2014). Faculty must make decisions about using these instruments according to their purpose for clinical evaluation.

Primary strategies for the evaluation of clinical practice include (1) observation, (2) written communication, (3) oral communication, (4) simulation, and (5) self-evaluation. Because clinical practice is complex, a combination of methods used over time is indicated and helps support a fair and reasonable evaluation. See Table 25-1 for a summary of common strategies and clinical evaluation tools by category. These are also discussed in the following paragraphs.

TABLE 25-1 Sample Evaluation Strategies and Tools by Category

Observation	Anecdotal notes Checklists Rating scales Videotapes
Written	Charting and progress notes Concept maps Care plans Process recordings Written tests Web-based strategies
Oral	Student interviews and case presentation Clinical conferences
Simulations	Interactive multimedia patient simulators Role play and clinical scenarios Standardized patient examinations
Self-evaluation	Clinical portfolios Journals and logs

Evaluation Strategies: Observation

Observation is the method used most frequently in clinical performance evaluation. Student performance is compared to clinical competency expectations as designated in course objectives. Faculty observe and analyze the performance, provide feedback on the observation, and determine whether further instruction is needed. A large national survey specific to faculty clinical evaluation and grading practices confirmed the predominance of observation in clinical evaluation (Oermann, Yarbrough, Saewert, Ard, & Charasika, 2009). Authors noted that continuing issues in clinical evaluation include wide variability in clinical environments, increasingly complex patients, and more diverse students.

Real-time observation and delayed video observation are both considered in this discussion. Advantages of observation include the potential for direct visualization and confirmation of student performance, but observation can also be challenging. Sample factors that can interfere with observations include lack of specificity of the particular behaviors to be observed; an inadequate sampling of behaviors from which to draw conclusions about a student's performance; and the evaluator's own influences and perceptions, which can affect judgment of the observed performance (Oermann & Gaberson, 2014).

Faculty should seek tools and strategies that support a fair and reasonable evaluation. The more structured observational tools are typically easy to complete and useful in focusing on specified behavior. Although structured observation tools can help increase objectivity, faculty judgment is still required in interpretation of the listed behaviors. Problems with reliability are introduced when item descriptors are given different meanings by different evaluators. Faculty training can help minimize this problem.

Tracking Clinical Observation Evaluation Data

An abundance of information must be tracked in clinical observation. Faculty can benefit from systems to help document and organize this information. Faculty can carry copies of evaluation tools and anecdotal records or can consider the use of mobile devices to help facilitate retrieval and use of clinical evaluation records. A variety of strategies exist for using mobile devices in the clinical setting (Lehman, 2003). Privacy in mobile device records is also needed.

Common methods for documenting observed behaviors during clinical practice vary in the amount of structure. Examples include anecdotal notes, checklists, rating scales and rubrics, and videotapes.

Anecdotal Notes

Anecdotal or progress notes are objective written descriptions of observed student performance or behaviors. The format for these can vary from loosely structured "plus–minus" observation notes to structured lists of observations in relation to specified clinical objectives. Serving as part of formative evaluation, as student performance records are documented over time, a pattern is established. This record or pattern of information pertaining to the student and specific clinical behaviors helps document the student's performance pattern for both summative evaluation and recall during student–faculty conference sessions. The importance of determining which clinical incidents to assess and the need to identify both positive and negative student behaviors is noted (Hall, Daly, & Madigan, 2010; Liberto, Roncher, & Shellenbarger, 1999).

Checklists

Checklists are lists of items or performance indicators requiring dichotomous responses such as satisfactory–unsatisfactory or pass–fail (Table 25-2).

TABLE 25-2 Example of Checklist Items and Format

Professional Domain	Midterm			Final	
	Satisfactory	**Unsatisfactory**	**Not Observed**	**Satisfactory**	**Unsatisfactory**
Practices within legal boundaries according to standards.					
Uses professional nursing standards to provide patient safety.					
Follows nursing procedures and institutional policy in delivery of patient care.					
Displays professional behaviors with staff, peers, instructors, and patient systems.					
Demonstrates ethical principles of respect for person and confidentiality.					
Participates appropriately in clinical conferences.					
Reports on time; follows procedures for absenteeism.					

Gronlund (2005) describes a checklist as an inventory of measurable performance dimensions or products with a place to record a simple "yes" or "no" judgment. These short, easy-to-complete tools are frequently used for evaluating clinical performance. Checklists, such as nursing skills check-off lists, are useful for evaluation of specific, well-defined behaviors and are commonly used in the clinical simulated laboratory setting. Rating scales and rubrics, described in the following paragraph, provide more detail than checklists concerning the quality of a student's performance.

Rating Scales and Rubrics

Rating scales incorporate qualitative and quantitative judgments regarding the learner's performance in the clinical setting (Box 25-2). A list of clinical behaviors or competencies is rated on a numerical scale such as a 5-point or 7-point scale with descriptors. These descriptors take the form of abstract labels (such as A, B, C, D, and E or 5, 4, 3, 2, and 1), frequency labels (e.g., *always, usually, frequently, sometimes,* and *never*), or qualitative labels (e.g., *superior, above average, average,* and *below average*). A rating scale provides the instructor with a convenient form on which to record judgments indicating the degree of student performance. This differs from a checklist in that it allows for more discrimination in judging behaviors as compared with dichotomous "yes" and "no" options. Rubrics, considered a type of rating scale, help convey clinically related assignment expectations to students (Suskie, 2009). They provide clear direction for graders and promote reliability among multiple graders. They can support accurate, consistent, and unbiased ratings. The detail provided in a rubric grid allows faculty to provide rapid and informative feedback to students without extensive writing (Walvoord et al., 2010). Typical parts to a rubric include the task or assignment description and some type of scale, breakdown of assignment parts, and descriptor of each performance level (Stevens & Levi, 2005). Serving as a scoring guide, rubrics help focus all on expectations for best practices in completing skills and improve communications. Rubric examples exist for providing detailed feedback for clinical-related assignments such as written clinical plans and conference participation. A web search by topic of interest, such as team communication, can provide samples for review. Skill-based rubrics can provide students direction in their skill practice and learning. Students can use these tools for self-assessments and participate in peer assessments to promote learning. These tools can be distributed to students, as well as be completed by faculty, and tracked or monitored over time (Bonnel & Smith, 2010).

BOX 25-2 Example of Rating Scale Items and Format

Instructions: On a scale of 1 to 5, rate each of the following student behaviors:

(Rating Code: 1 = marginal; 2 = fair; 3 = satisfactory; 4 = good; 5 = excellent; NA = not applicable)

___ 1 Serves as patient caregiver (independence when providing patient care, timely completion of all patient care).

___ 2 Functions in the role of team member.

___ 3 Uses correct procedure when performing nursing interventions.

___ 4 Relates self-evaluation to clinical learning objectives.

___ 5 Displays positive behavior when given feedback.

Videos as Source of Observational Data

Another method of recording observations of a student's clinical performance is through videos. Often completed in a simulated setting, videos can be used to record and evaluate specific performance behaviors relevant to diverse clinical settings. Advantages associated with videos include their valuable start, stop, and replay capabilities, which allow an observation to be reviewed numerous times. Videos can promote self-evaluation, allowing students to see themselves and evaluate their performance more objectively. Videos also give teachers and students the opportunity to review the performance and provide feedback in determining whether further practice is indicated. Use of videos can contribute to the learning and growth of an entire clinical group when knowledge and feedback are shared. Videos are particularly popular for simulation debriefing as well as evaluation in distance learning situations. Videos can also be used with rating scales, rubrics, checklists, or anecdotal records to organize and report behaviors observed on the videos.

Additionally, an approach to involving students as observers in evaluation is to engage them in observing and evaluating online clinical videos such as the National Institutes of Health (NIH) Stroke Scale training. In this example, video cases were developed based on needed competencies for appropriate use of the Stroke Scale. Students complete testing specific to these competencies as they refer to the online video cases (NIH Stroke Scale, n.d.). This approach allows students to participate in a type of standardized testing. There may be additional opportunities for students to observe videos as components of clinical evaluation, for example critique of online videos developed by faculty or others.

Evaluation Strategies: Student Written Communication

Use of written communication, whether paper-based or electronic, enables the faculty to evaluate clinical performance through assessing students' abilities to translate what they have learned to the written word. Review of student nursing care plans or written notes allows faculty to evaluate students' abilities to communicate with other care providers. Through writing assignments, students can clarify and organize their thoughts. Additionally, writing can reinforce new knowledge and expand thinking on a topic. Reflective writing assignments, appropriately designed, can help faculty see students move from telling or describing data to translating information to knowledge (Wear, Zarconi, Garden, & Jones, 2012). Faculty evaluation focuses on the quality of the content and student ability to communicate information and ideas in written form. The rater can determine the student's perspectives and gain insight into the "why" of the student's behavior. A scoring tool such as a rubric with specified objectives for a designated assignment can promote consistency and efficiency in grading specified assignments (Stevens & Levi, 2005). Written data help support faculty clinical observations.

Patient Progress Notes and Electronic Health Record Documentation

The use of electronic text-based communication in the changing health care system is increasing, and being able to write cogent nursing and clinical progress notes is an important clinical skill. Reviewing student documentation provides faculty with an opportunity to evaluate students' ability to process and record relevant data. Students' skill in using health care terminology and documentation practices can be examined and critical thinking processes can be demonstrated in these notes (Higuchi & Donald, 2002). With the focus on electronic records as a tool in patient safety, orienting students to these tools and evaluating students' skill in this area is essential (Bonnel & Smith, 2010). In some clinical practice settings, there may be limited student access to electronic health records or unfamiliar electronic systems, but faculty can use clinical lab settings and simulations to first engage students in learning to use electronic health records and then evaluating their documentation using case studies. Developing ongoing strategies with clinical agency partners may be needed to continue evaluation of students' electronic documentation abilities as they advance in clinical patient care.

Concept Maps

Concept maps are another tool for evaluating students' ability to document thinking processes and allow students to create a diagram of patient needs and nursing responses, including relationships among concepts. These tools can help students visualize and organize patient-specific data relevant to diagnostic work and nursing and medical diagnoses. Concept maps can serve as worksheets for students and serve as organizing tools for documentation (Schuster, 2000). Faculty can evaluate students' understanding of concepts and relationships among relevant concepts and assist in clarifying students' misconceptions. These tools also provide faculty with opportunity to complete a quick review of students' thinking patterns and determine further learning needs before students perform patient care (Castellino & Schuster, 2002; King & Shell, 2002; Vacek, 2009). Some authors suggest that in today's complex health care world, concept maps may better represent care processes than more traditional linear models of documentation (Kern, Bush, & McCleish, 2006). Concept maps, further discussed in Chapter 23, can provide a useful tool in evaluating students' abilities to synthesize concepts in care of specific patients.

Nursing Care Plans

Nursing care plans allow faculty to evaluate students' ability to determine and prioritize care needs according to understanding and interpretation of individual patients' health care problems. Historically, nursing care plans have been used by students to document clinical thinking processes, but some argue that the availability of numerous standardized care plans has minimized the critical thinking component. Some programs report replacing detailed clinical care plans with concept maps or clinical journals and logs. Mueller, Johnston, and Bligh (2001) describe a strategy for modifying care plans and combining them with concept maps to help students clarify the interrelationship of patient problems.

Process Recordings

Process recordings are used to evaluate the interpersonal skills of students within the clinical setting. This form of evaluation requires students to write down their patient–nurse interactions and self-evaluate the communication skills they used. A type of self-reflection, process recordings provide a form of student self-evaluation that allows students to analyze their own interactive behavior, enabling them to better identify the strengths and weaknesses of their interpersonal communication (Sigma Theta Tau International, 2005). This approach to evaluation has traditionally been used in communication courses and in psychiatric nursing. Additional note has been made of process recording benefits for students working with hospice patients (Hayes, 2005).

Written or Electronic Testing Formats

Written testing is frequently used to assess students' basic knowledge for problem solving and decision making in clinical practice. Various test formats (true–false, multiple choice, matching, short answer, essay) can be incorporated into preclinical or postclinical conferences to gauge students' understanding of specific concepts. (See Chapter 24 for information about writing test questions).

Web-Based Strategies

Written evaluation formats can also include web-based clinical evaluation formats. For example, faculty can implement post-clinical conferences or lead clinical case discussions within online learning management systems (Johnson & Flagler, 2013). Within online learning systems, students can submit electronic clinical logs to document patterns of ages and diagnoses of patients seen. Opportunities exist for faculty to provide rapid feedback to students on written clinical papers, threaded discussion boards, or e-journals. Although not limited to students at a distance, web-based strategies are especially popular for clinical evaluation of students in geographically diverse settings. They may be useful as well for clinical conferences and student evaluation in community health courses with clinical coursework in diverse community settings.

Evaluation Strategies: Oral Communication Methods

Communication and information sharing are common nursing tasks and important nursing skills. Oral communication strategies such as student interviews, case presentations, and clinical conferences provide evaluative opportunities. These can be used to assess the student's ability to verbalize ideas and thoughts clearly. In addition, these strategies allow faculty to assess a student's critical thinking skills and pose questions to elicit more complex forms of thinking. Evaluation strategies identified as verbal communication methods are described in the following paragraphs.

Student Interviews and Case Presentation

In simple interview format, faculty ask questions and students respond. These question-and-answer sessions provide faculty with the opportunity to probe for more detail from students and clarify misconceptions. Faculty can focus on asking "higher-order" questions, moving beyond just factual recall, to better promote student critical thinking (Boswell, 2006). Student case presentations, such as "bullet-point" summaries of patient problems and care strategies, assist students in developing concise presentation skills. Faculty can provide feedback to students and obtain evaluative information about students' thoughts and approaches for patient care.

Clinical Conferences

Clinical conferences provide opportunities for students to integrate theory and practice in terms of their own clinical experiences. Questions, reflections, and discussion within conferences encourage critical thinking and allow for peer feedback. Debriefing of clinical experiences, similar to the debriefing of simulations, provides students with opportunity to reflect and further cement learning. As students debrief, they gain opportunity to assess what happened during their clinical care, compare this to accepted criteria, and consider how well they did. Conferences provide an opportunity for faculty to gauge students' abilities to analyze data and critique plans. The multiple student participants in clinical conferences enable faculty to evaluate more than one student at a time. Asking students to engage in goal setting for further learning is another important component of clinical conference debriefing (Bonnel & Smith, 2010).

Interprofessional conferences are another form of clinical conference in which the process of problem solving and decision making is a collaborative effort of the group. Involving multiple health care disciplines, evaluation is concerned with the student's active participation within the group and abilities to present ideas clearly in terms of the care plan for the patient. Increased focus on interprofessional education makes this an important time to address student abilities to clearly communicate and collaborate in problem solving with team members (Institute of Medicine, 2014). Students may find a degree of risk involved with sharing their knowledge and being evaluated critically by other disciplines.

Evaluation Strategies: Clinical Simulations

Simulations can range from simple case role plays to interactions with complex electronic manikins. Through simulations an instructor can identify specific clinical objectives to be demonstrated and focus on student cognitive and psychomotor behaviors defined for the case. Simulations help to create a safe environment for student learning. Benefits of simulations include skill validation in a standardized setting with no risk to actual patients (Harder, 2010; Jeffries, 2012).

With the changing health care setting, students will likely not have opportunities to care for all types of patients in the various clinical settings for which they will be responsible after graduation. Teaching pattern recognition with case studies and scenarios in safe, structured learning environments is becoming an increasingly important strategy. Sample approaches to simulations include technology-based patient simulations, role play and clinical scenarios, and standardized patient examinations.

Technology-Based Patient Simulations

Rapidly advancing technologies provide additional opportunities for clinical evaluation, including virtual case-based simulations and high-fidelity simulations. Virtual case-based simulations, with similarities to high-fidelity simulation, include web-based avatars in online simulated settings. Avatars, a type of on-screen representation of students, placed in virtual health care settings provide a semirealistic learning experience for students to assume nursing roles, interact with a virtual patient, and make care decisions (Robert Wood Johnson Foundation, 2014). Through the use of interactive multimedia, these nursing case studies can be presented in a safe setting without clinical environmental distractions or the risk involved in student clinical decision making

High-fidelity patient simulations involve more traditional clinical lab-supported activities around a patient being simulated by technology. Benefits include that student skills may be demonstrated efficiently and that students have multiple opportunities for practice in a safe environment. Novice nursing students reported gaining comfort and confidence for clinical care when using high-fidelity patient simulation as a learning tool (Bremner, Aduddell, Bennett, & VanGeest, 2006; Jeffries, 2012).

Research findings regarding high-fidelity simulations as both teaching and evaluation tools are becoming increasingly available. Meyer, Connors, Hou, and Gajewski (2011), for example, studied benefits of simulation on students' traditional clinical performance using direct performance measures and comparison groups. They found that students completing simulations prior to scheduled hospital clinical experience attained higher performance measures more quickly than the control group and maintained high performance levels. A model can be used to guide simulation development for both teaching–learning and testing purposes (Jeffries, 2005). Faculty should clarify for students whether a simulation activity is formative (for teaching purposes) or summative (for outcomes evaluation).

Debriefing and feedback to students, as formative evaluation, are considered to be critical elements in the teaching–learning process with high-fidelity patient simulation (Henneman & Cunningham, 2005; Issenberg, McGaghie, Petrusa, Gordon, & Scalese, 2005; Waznonis, 2014). These debriefing sessions provide opportunity for students to gain insight into their performance and consider opportunities for improvement. High-fidelity patient simulators as mechanisms to document student competencies are taking on increasing importance in today's health care settings. Further discussion of simulations as a form of clinical evaluation can be found in Chapter 18.

Role Play and Clinical Scenarios

Role play provides an opportunity for students to try out new behaviors, simulating aspects of nursing care in relation to clinical practice. As students implement the roles called for in specified case guidelines (or scripts for role plays), they gain opportunities to practice competent nurse interactions and behaviors. Students practice interpersonal communication skills and gain opportunity to observe, evaluate, and provide feedback to each other.

Additionally, clinical scenarios created with audio or video clips provide students with the opportunity to review an approach to a clinical scenario and actively learn while faculty facilitate the procedure (Dearman, 2003). Students can respond to audiovisual scenarios orally or in writing. The potential for diverse, varied cases promotes relevance to a majority of nursing arenas and can be used as evaluation in a variety of settings. An advantage that these methods offer is a readily available means of judging specific clinical practices without having to wait for a similar opportunity to arise in the clinical setting. Clinical scenarios can be economically beneficial in the educational setting with large groups of students. Additionally, many of these clinical scenarios have the potential to be used in online settings.

Standardized Patient Examinations

Standardized patient examinations, sometimes referred to as *objective structured clinical examinations* (OSCEs), are another way to evaluate competencies in clinical education. These OSCEs can be described as actors or "pretend patients" in a created environment designed to simulate actual clinical conditions A simulation center, modeled as an authentic clinical environment with standardized patients, can provide a safe setting in which to observe and document student competencies.

Standardized patients can provide feedback to students and help ensure competence before students begin practice in the complex "real" world. Potential exists for multiple evaluators to observe and test students in the performance of numerous skills during brief examination periods. The OSCE process, considered an acceptable and powerful approach in clinical performance evaluation, allows rapid feedback to students about identified clinical deficits. Many programs use the OSCE as a learning tool with formative feedback. If the OSCE is used as high-stakes testing, then building in a remediation plan should be considered (McWilliam & Botwinski, 2010). Specific approaches for implementing standardized patients into clinical evaluation across a curriculum have been described; students have reported learning and satisfaction with the standardized patient experience (Ebbert & Connors, 2004; Gibbons et al., 2002).

Evaluation Strategies: Self-Reflection and Self-Evaluation

Reflecting on one's practice has been described as an integral component of clinical learning (Freshwater, Taylor, & Sherwood, 2010). Reflection, considered to be an introspective process with self-observation of one's thoughts and feelings, provides opportunity to consider and make sense of experiences; it can both instruct and help evaluate the learners' progression. Potential outcomes of reflection include new perspective on experience, change in behavior, readiness for application, and commitment to action (Sherwood & Horton-Deutsch, 2012).

Self-evaluation and self-reflection are related concepts. In self-evaluation students complete criteria-based assessments using self-reflection. Self-evaluation against a standard has been noted as a critical tool for assisting students to gain lifelong learning skills (Fink, 2013). In self-evaluation, students describe and make qualitative judgments about specified experiences, helping balance the quantitative nature of evaluation with qualitative data. Self-evaluation against a rubric or standard can be a significant student learning tool, helping students examine their progress, identify their strengths and weaknesses, and set goals for improvement in the areas indicated. It can also help faculty better understand student attitudes and values as well as thinking processes (Suskie, 2009).

Self-reflection provides students with an opportunity to think about what they have learned and promotes becoming reflective clinicians. Clinical reasoning depends on both cognitive and metacognitive (thinking about one's thinking) skill development (Kuiper & Pesut, 2004). There are different ways to incorporate reflection into clinical practice, including preactivity, during activity, and postactivity. As faculty consider reflection as an important tool for clinical evaluation, continued focus is needed on being precise and thoughtful about approaches, including purposes and the key elements students are being asked to reflect on (Wear et al., 2012). Box 25-3 provides sample reflective prompts.

A potential disadvantage of self-evaluation is that students may not be honest about their level of self-understanding in an effort to protect

BOX 25-3 Sample Reflective Prompts for Clinical Learning

The following are sample written prompts to encourage student reflection and provide faculty opportunity for considering affective and cognitive learning.

PRECLINICAL ACTIVITY

- Why are you here?
- What are your learning goals?
- What concepts and competencies do you hope to attain?
- What is your commitment to engage in learning opportunities?

DURING CLINICAL PATIENT CARE

(Questions to consider during care, and then summarize following your clinical experience.)

- What stands out for you in this situation?
- What are you concerned about in this situation?
- What assumptions are you making? What else could it be?
- What do you already know that can help you in this situation?
- What clinical decisions will you make?
- What action will you take?
- What response do you anticipate if you do that?

POSTCLINICAL ACTIVITY

- What did you learn?
- How has this been helpful to you?
- Did your plans for the patient/family/community work out as planned?
- What could you have done differently?
- What next? How will you use this information?

Adapted from Sherwood and Horton-Deutsch (2012).

themselves against potential criticism (Walker & Dewar, 2000). The ability to critically reflect on individual performance may be influenced by the maturity and self-esteem of the student. Students are more likely to share summaries and reflections with faculty if a foundation of trust has been established. If self-evaluation begins at the onset of the students' clinical experience, students can benefit from examining their ongoing progress. Through the teacher–student interaction process, observations and perceptions can be shared, student strengths and weaknesses can be discussed, and self-evaluation strategies can be improved. Student–teacher relationships can become stronger and more constructive as students progress.

Portfolios

Portfolios provide students opportunity to assemble evidence that documents different types of learning, providing opportunity for a holistic approach to evaluation (Kaplan, Silver, LaVaque-Manty, & Meizlish, 2013). Described as collections of evidence prepared by students, they provide a collage or album of student learning rather than a one-time snapshot. Portfolios allow integration of a number of assessments and can help provide progressive documentation of specified clinical learning outcomes (see Chapter 23). Reflective portfolios are designed to help students consider their progress in clinical learning and also help faculty understand students' clinical learning processes. Faculty can provide portfolio guidelines that help students organize their portfolio components and incorporate reflective summaries (Suskie, 2009). Portfolios can help students learn strategies for documenting clinical competencies as a part of lifelong learning. Evidence exists that when portfolios are well implemented, they prove practical and effective in helping students take learning responsibility and supporting their professional development (Tochel et al., 2009).

Journals and Logs

Journals and logs are, in essence, written dialogues between the self and the designated reader. These written dialogues provide opportunity for students to share values and critical thinking abilities. Journals give students the opportunity to record their clinical experiences and review their progress. This enables students to recall areas of needed improvement and allows them to work on problems and clinical performance weaknesses. The concepts of *clinical logs* and *journals* are sometimes used synonymously, but clinical logs can vary in the amount of detail, ranging from a listing of types of patients and noted student care roles to a more detailed log with a reflection on each patient care experience. A guided reflection, such as reflective prompts based on a clinical judgment model, provides clear direction for helping students communicate about their clinical thinking (Lasater & Nielsen, 2009). Other criteria for written reflections are noted to include description of an event, student's reaction to the event, perceived value of the learning event, learning that occurred, and student's future plans (Blake, 2005). Students have described more active learning and thinking about their actions and processes with use of a detailed reflective clinical log.

Faculty should provide specific guidelines as to the amount of detail required in clinical journals or logs and provide clear guidelines as to how (or if) journals or logs will be graded (Kennison & Misselwitz, 2002). If self-reflective materials such as journals are to be graded, concepts such as student depth of thought, making connections between theory and practice, and relating beliefs and behaviors may be developed as an evaluation rubric. Faculty feedback about student self-reflections provides opportunity for further dialogue on learning experiences (Murphy, 2005). Self-reflection and self-evaluation can become part of the process for lifelong, self-directed learning.

Clinical Evaluation Process

Before the evaluation process begins, faculty and students need a clear understanding of the outcomes to be attained at the culmination of the experience. Clinical evaluation is a systematic process that can be considered as having three consecutive phases: (1) preparation, (2) clinical activity phase, and (3) final data interpretation and feedback. A listing of sample tasks within each phase and the roles faculty will assume during each phase are provided in Box 25-4. Additional discussion of selected points in each phase follows.

BOX 25-4 Roles of Faculty Evaluator during the Evaluation Process

PHASE I: PREPARATION

Determine objectives and competencies. Identify evaluation methods and tools. Choose clinical site.

Orient students to the evaluation plan. Focus on objectivity in evaluation.

PHASE II: CLINICAL ACTIVITY

Orient students and staff to the student role. Provide students clinical opportunities. Ensure patient safety.

Observe and collect evaluation data from multiple perspectives. Provide student feedback to enhance learning.

Document findings and maintain privacy of records. Contract with students regarding any deficiencies.

PHASE III: FINAL DATA INTERPRETATION AND PRESENTATION

Interpret data in fair, reasonable, and consistent manner. Assign grade.

Provide summative evaluation conference (ensure privacy and respect confidentiality).

Evaluate experience.

Preparation Phase

Choosing the Clinical Setting and Patient Assignment as Part of the Evaluation Process

Faculty are responsible for providing each student with ample opportunities to achieve course objectives and must give careful attention to choosing a clinical site that will give students these opportunities. Especially when traditional clinical settings will be the evaluation site, advance planning is needed. Even in the ideal clinical setting, daily variability exists in terms of patients, providers, and the activity level of the unit, which can complicate evaluation. In addition to unit assignments, specific patient clinical assignments should also be considered as part of a fair evaluation. This includes both the types of patients assigned to students and the duration of clinical assignments.

Teaching and learning in a natural setting provide unique challenges for both students and faculty. Negotiating the balance between student independence and supervision is complex. Faculty must provide adequate supervision to ensure safe delivery of care with the welfare and the safety of patients as the first priority. Before the clinical experience begins, the faculty must develop criteria for what is considered unsafe or inappropriate behavior and what consequences will occur if such behavior is observed. Communication between faculty and students before the clinical experience begins is essential, including orientation to the grading process (Walvoord et al., 2010).

The faculty must be prepared to remove a student from the clinical setting if the student is not adequately prepared to provide safe nursing care; students have the right to know the standard used for safe practice and evaluation. Students should also be given an orientation to the clinical facility and to the policies and procedures that will apply to the clinical experience. Unit orientations, as well as orientation to evaluation methods, are important in decreasing the anxiety that can hamper student clinical performance.

Students and faculty are essentially visitors in an established system, and the status of student comfort and support in the clinical environment should be considered in evaluation as well. Chan (2002) noted the importance of a positive clinical learning environment for student learning; students should have opportunity to share with faculty their evaluation of the clinical setting. A sample form for student evaluation of a clinical setting is provided in Box 25-5.

Determining the Standards and Evaluation Tools

Faculty have the responsibility for choosing the appropriate methods and tools for evaluation of the learners' clinical performance. Specific evaluation instruments chosen will be the means of documenting and communicating judgments made about student performance. These tools should document performance expectations relevant to course objectives and be practical and time efficient.

The concepts of interrater reliability (whether results can be replicated by other raters) and content validity (whether a tool measures what is desired) at minimum should be considered in selection of a specific clinical evaluation instrument. More discussion of reliability, interrater reliability, and validity is provided in Chapter 23.

Inconsistencies in evaluation can result if each course coordinator develops course tools independently. Wiles and Bishop (2001) recommend that faculty work in groups to determine or develop tools that reflect the increasing complexity of competencies required as students progress from program beginners to graduating seniors and to promote consistency from course to course.

Clinical Activity Phase

In both obtaining and analyzing clinical evaluation data, faculty need to make professional judgments about the performance of students, being aware of the subjective nature of evaluation. To prevent

BOX 25-5 Student Evaluation of Clinical Setting

Name of Agency
Specific Unit

DIRECTIONS

Print the name of the instructor and the name of the agency, the specific unit where you had your clinical experience, and the days of the week you were assigned.

Please respond to the following statements with the rating that best describes your opinion.

A. Strongly Agree
B. Agree
C. Disagree
D. Strongly Disagree

Please qualify any rating of C or D with comments or suggestions. The agency personnel have asked that you make comments because this is the only way they can make improvements or know what is positive. Your ratings and written comments will be used to determine clinical placement for future students and may be shared with individuals in the setting but only in summary form.

APPLICATION OF COURSE MATERIAL

1. The staff facilitated my ability to meet clinical objectives.
2. I was able to meet the objectives of this course in this setting.

POPULATION/PATIENTS

3. Patients presented clinical problems appropriate to the objectives for this course.
4. Culturally diverse patients (e.g., cultural, social, economic) were available in the setting.

HEALTH PROFESSIONALS

5. Nurse managers, staff nurses, and support staff were accepting of students and student learning.
6. Nurse managers, staff nurses, and support staff were available to me to answer questions and provide assistance.
7. The nursing staff were positive role models.
8. Nurses demonstrated professional relationships with other health care professionals.

PHYSICAL ENVIRONMENT

9. The setting was conducive to working with patients and other health care team members.
10. Space was available for conferences with faculty and other students.

OVERALL IMPRESSION OF SETTING

11. I have a positive impression of the quality of care provided in this setting.
12. I would recommend this setting for future students taking this course.
13. Add statements specific to the clinical setting not already covered.

How could your clinical experience have been improved in this clinical setting?

Please use the back of this sheet to make comments and suggestions.

Adapted with permission from a form used by University of Kansas School of Nursing.

biased judgments, faculty need to be aware of the factors that can influence decision making and must actively use strategies to prevent biases.

Strategies that can help support trustworthiness of the clinical evaluation data include the following:

- Have specified objectives or competencies on which to base the evaluation.
- Use multiple strategies and combined methods of evaluation for compiling data.
- Include both qualitative and quantitative measures.
- Determine a practical sampling plan and evaluate it over time.
- Provide clear scoring directions for tools to promote consistency between raters in collection and interpretation of data.
- Train faculty in use of specific clinical evaluation tools and approaches for consistency and fairness in grading.
- Be aware of common errors such as the halo effect (assuming that positive behaviors in one evaluated competency will be similar in others).
- Incorporate teacher self-assessment of values, beliefs, or biases that might affect the evaluation process (Oermann & Gaberson, 2014).

Final Data Interpretation and Presentation Phase

Clinical Evaluation Conference

The findings of the clinical evaluation are usually shared with the student individually at the end of the clinical experience or course. No surprises should be presented at this time. The timely feedback of the earlier formative evaluation should provide students with information sufficient to prepare them for this evaluation. A student's self-evaluation is often submitted before the evaluation conference and discussed at this time.

Evaluation results are commonly reported in both written and oral forms. Often, the primary evaluation tool is presented to show student improvement and specifically recall incidents. The faculty should clarify initially that the purpose of the conference is to provide information on the student's clinical performance. The results should be explained, giving specific incidents in which the student had difficulties, excelled, performed adequately, or improved. In addition, the faculty member needs to assist the student in establishing ongoing learning goals. Finally, the faculty member needs to summarize the conference and end on a positive note.

The environment in which the evaluation conference takes place should be comfortable for the student, and privacy should be maintained. An hour during which the student is responsible for patient care or directly after a tiring clinical experience is not the most conducive time for a conference. An appointment during office hours away from the clinical site provides a more comfortable and private setting for students to listen to constructive criticism or encouraging comments.

Student Response

The student's response to the faculty evaluation can vary. Typically a student perceives the results as fair if his or her own appraisal is congruent with that of the faculty. A student self-evaluation submitted before the conference helps faculty gain insight into student perceptions and can give faculty time to prepare a response. However, the best way to ensure congruent results is for faculty to provide the student with a sufficient number of formative evaluations and time to reflect on his or her own performance. Faculty need to be sensitive to the student's needs, emphasizing the student's strengths as well as weaknesses and encouraging goals and aspirations.

Working with Students with Questionable Performance

Supporting At-Risk Students

Developing a positive learning environment is a basic step in promoting positive, supportive student learning relationships. Students have a right to expect respect. Pointing out areas in which students need to improve and specific ways to achieve clinical goals promotes a positive learning environment and minimizes potential legal risks.

Scanlan (2001) discusses the importance of clarifying definitions of safe and unsafe clinical practices and having clear policies and guidelines for working with "problem" students. Minimum patient safety competencies can be observed, checked off, and documented in the learning lab. School policies can indicate minimum safety competencies that need to be achieved in the learning laboratory before a student moves into the actual clinical setting. Students' behaviors that put patients at safety risk also typically put students at risk for failing. The need exists for further discussions about the culture of safety, which includes discussing and learning from mistakes, rather than being punitive (Tanicala, Barbara, Scheffer, & Roberts, 2011).

Zuzelo (2000) summarizes the following key points, which, although relevant to all evaluations, have particular merit in evaluating a student with questionable clinical performance behaviors.

- Ensure that the criteria for student success (i.e., the written course objectives or competency statements) are clear to all parties.
- If a student is at risk, objectively document a pattern of marginal or failing behavior.
- Report poor performance to students as formative evaluation and provide students with opportunities for remedial work.
- Use strategies such as clinical probation for supporting the at-risk student. Student clinical contracts can be used to document these plans for improvement. The written student contract should clarify student and faculty expectations and what student behaviors need to occur for passing status to be achieved.
- Follow written procedure from school handbooks.

Anecdotal records should be written objectively and used to document a pattern of behaviors. Failing behaviors need to be identified in writing and a contract for corrections should be signed by the faculty member and the student (Osinski, 2003). An annotated record of each counseling session and student evaluation should be signed by both the student and the faculty member and maintained by the faculty member.

Unsatisfactory Performance

Faculty often feel challenged in assigning failing grades, including emotional responses when students fail and anxiety as to whether their evaluations were correct. Poorman and Mastorovich's (2014) study, relating to these concerns, found faculty worried about limited evaluation experience and the subjective nature of judgments about data. In addition to ongoing faculty preparation, study implications included the need for faculty to help students better understand and prepare for evaluations; they also included the need for all team members to focus on caring and professional relationships.

Boley and Whitney (2003) note that when a student is given a failing grade, faculty must be aware of the standards to meet, grades must not be "arbitrary or capricious," and faculty must be able to explain how grades are determined related to the program and course objectives. When a fair judgment is made that a student's performance is unsatisfactory or failing, strategies should be used to avert interpersonal or legal problems. The need to have clear program policies, a clear chain of command for communicating problems (prospectively) and team support was reiterated (Poorman & Mastorovich, 2014).

Once the decision is made, communication with the student is essential. Documentation from formative evaluation conferences and student contracts can provide support for this decision. Published school policies and procedures should be followed, including documentation that decisions were made carefully and deliberately. Support from the university or college is essential when performance is determined to be unsatisfactory, and the administration should be notified of impending problems early in the grading process.

Final evaluations that result in unsatisfactory or failing performance require special tact and concern. Faculty need to share specific findings that resulted in a student not meeting the expected clinical objectives. Student contracts not fulfilled need to be identified. Students need time to process the information and should not feel rushed. Faculty need to listen attentively, with a strong show of concern and support, to the student's perceptions. The student may need time to reflect and return for another conference after adjusting to the facts.

Student Reactions to receiving a failing grade

The student who has received a failing grade may react in a variety of ways. Caring faculty will recognize these behaviors and provide empathetic support. Students may respond with denial, providing their own perception of how a specified incident did or did not occur and offering excuses. Faculty need to steer the conversation to the student's not meeting the clinical course objectives and provide support for the student's emotional needs. A student may attempt to bargain for a passing grade.

Faculty need to stand firm and focus on the evaluation results. Faculty can be prepared to provide information about any program options that are available to students who fail a clinical course. As the reality of the loss is recognized, the student may respond with despair, confusion, lack of motivation, indecision, and tears. Faculty should provide support, listen attentively, and generally convey caring behaviors; in some cases faculty may also need to recommend professional counseling. The student may come to terms with the outcome and begin to make plans for the future. Assistance from the faculty in considering further options is often sought by the student. How well the student adapts to the final evaluation typically depends on how well he or she has been prepared for the results.

The student may respond with anger. The student may become demanding or accusing and may have the potential to become violent. In this case, faculty need to take steps to ensure their own safety and that of the student. Faculty should not take the anger personally but provide guidance about feelings and focus on the anger as a part of loss. Thomas (2003) has recommended handling anger with a "professional deep breath."

Additionally, an established grievance policy should be available. Both students and faculty share responsibility for knowing about and appropriately employing such a policy. Students have a right to respond appropriately to grievances. See Chapter 3 for further discussion of legal issues.

Dismissing an Unsafe Student from Clinical Practice

Faculty must immediately address student behaviors that are unsafe for patient care such as lack of preparation, violence, and substance abuse. Pierce (2001) notes the importance of a broad and thorough policy that allows for safe and appropriate actions to protect both the patient and the student. School policies and procedures need to be followed. Clear policies help prevent arbitrary or capricious responses to an incident. O'Connor (2014) summarizes key points related to the student who is unsafe to care for patients, noting that safety of the patient is the first priority in removing a student, but that faculty have an obligation to ensure that all students are returned to an area of safety as well. The student unprepared to care for an assigned clinical patient should be sent to the library or laboratory to prepare. Student orientation to clinical practice should include a review of relevant policies and clarification of professional student behaviors.

Evaluation of the Evaluation

After the final student conference, the student and faculty need to evaluate the entire experience as a whole. The clinical site is evaluated on how well it met the learning and practice needs of the students. Was the philosophy of the staff congruent with that of the faculty and students? Were the students given the opportunity to meet all objectives? As these questions are answered, the preparation phase for evaluation begins again. A continuous quality improvement process for clinical evaluation should be considered, with attention given to structure (appropriate evaluation tools with appropriate clinical environment and patient care opportunities), process (appropriate plans for sampling and evaluating clinical behaviors and for sharing feedback and results of evaluation), and outcome (satisfactory evaluative outcomes indicating safe, competent graduates). Ongoing questioning of evaluation practices, including new approaches that further incorporate students' perspectives is recommended (Rankin, Malinsky, Tate, & Elena, 2010).

Summary

Clinical evaluation is important to both patients' safety and students' skills and confidence. Especially in times of changing clinical contexts, best practices include multidimensional evaluation with diverse evaluation methods completed over time, seeking student growth and progress. Advances in technology are promoting new opportunities for clinical performance evaluation. Clinical performance evaluation provides students with a means for critical reflection on their future nursing roles. An appropriate evaluation process sets the stage for productive assessment of student learning.

REFLECTING ON THE EVIDENCE

1. How do you currently provide formative feedback to students? What strategies do you use to challenge students to self-reflect and set further learning goals? How do these strategies contribute to active learning and critical thinking?
2. How can selected methods described in this chapter be incorporated into documentation of students' clinical competency? For example, how can students' written assignments best be used to contribute to clinical evaluation? What other approaches that you read about will you incorporate into your evaluation practices?
3. What is your current process for completing a clinical evaluation? In what ways do you incorporate multiple clinical indicators into evaluation (e.g., data from interview, observation, and document review)? How do you then synthesize these diverse pieces of clinical evaluation data? How will you evaluate the success of these approaches?
4. What are the benefits of anecdotal records and rubrics in the clinical evaluation documentation process? How does your faculty team currently use these tools? Are there ways you could expand or improve the use of these tools? How will you determine whether these approaches improve your efficiency and effectiveness in clinical evaluation?
5. What is your current process for using technologies in clinical evaluation? For example, what ways are best practices used with high-fidelity patient simulators as part of clinical evaluation? How are high-fidelity patient simulators incorporated into your clinical evaluations? What models do you use to guide your work? What processes are most efficient and effective? What research supports these practices?

REFERENCES

Blake, T. (2005). Journaling: An active learning technique. *International Journal of Nursing Education Scholarship, 2*(1) Article 7.

Boehm, H., & Bonnel, W. (2010). The use of peer review in nursing education and clinical practice. *Journal for Nurses in Staff Development, 26*(3), 108–115.

Boley, P., & Whitney, K. (2003). Grade disputes: Considerations for nursing faculty. *Journal of Nursing Education, 42*(5), 198–203.

Bonnel, W. (2008). Improving feedback to students in online courses. *Nursing Education Perspectives, 29*(5), 290–294.

Bonnel, W., & Smith, K. (2010). *Teaching technologies in nursing and the health professions*. New York: Springer.

Boswell, C. (2006). The art of questioning: Improving critical thinking. In M. Oermann & K. Heinrich (Eds.), *Annual review of nursing education innovations in curriculum, teaching, and student and faculty development, 4* (pp. 291–304). New York: Springer.

Bremner, M., Aduddell, K., Bennett, D., & VanGeest, J. (2006). The use of human patient simulators: Best practices with novice nursing students. *Nurse Educator, 31*(4), 170–174.

Burgess, A., Roberts, C., Black, K., & Mellis, C. (2013). Senior medical student perceived ability and experience in giving peer feedback in formative long case examinations. *BMC Medical Education, 13*(79), 1–5.

Caldwell, L. M., & Tenofsky, L. (1996). Clinical failure or clinical folly? A second opinion on student performance. *Nursing and Health Care Perspectives, 17*(1), 22–25.

Castellino, A., & Schuster, P. (2002). Evaluation of outcomes in nursing students using clinical concept map care plans. *Nurse Educator, 27*(4), 149–150.

Chan, D. (2002). Development of the clinical learning environment inventory. *Journal of Nursing Education, 41*(2), 69–75.

Dahlke, S., Baumbusch, J., Affleck, F., & Kwon, J. (2012). The clinical instructor role in nursing education: A structured literature review. *Journal of Nursing Education, 51*(12), 692–696.

Dearman, C. N. (2003). Using clinical scenarios in nursing. In M. Oermann & K. Heinrich (Eds.), *Annual review of nursing education* (pp. 341–356). New York: Springer.

Ebbert, D., & Connors, H. (2004). Standardized patient experiences: Evaluation of clinical performance and nurse practitioner student satisfaction. *Nursing Education Perspectives, 25*(1), 12–15.

Fink, L. D. (2013). *Creating significant learning experiences: An integrated approach to designing college courses* (2nd ed.). San Francisco: Jossey-Bass.

Freshwater, D., Taylor, B., & Sherwood, G. (2010). *International textbook of reflective practice in nursing*. Indianapolis: Sigma Theta Tau International.

Gaberson, K. B., Oermann, M. H., & Shellenberger, T. (2014). *Clinical teaching strategies in nursing* (4th ed.). New York: Springer.

Gibbons, S. W., Adamo, G., Padden, D., Ricciardi, R., Graziano, M., & Levine, E. (2002). Clinical evaluation in advanced practice nursing education: Using standardized patients in health assessment. *Journal of Nursing Education, 41*(5), 215–221.

Gronlund, N. (2005). *How to make achievement tests and assessments* (8th ed.). Needham Heights, MA: Allyn & Bacon.

Hall, M., Daly, B., & Madigan, E. (2010). Use of anecdotal notes by clinical nursing faculty: A descriptive study. *Journal of Nursing Education, 49*(3), 156–159.

Harder, B. N. (2010). Use of simulation in teaching and learning in health sciences: A systematic review. *Journal of Nursing Education, 49*(1), 23–28.

Hayes, A. (2005). A mental health nursing clinical experience with hospice patients. *Nurse Educator, 30*(2), 85–88.

Henneman, E., & Cunningham, H. (2005). Using clinical simulation to teach patient safety in an acute/critical care nursing course. *Nurse Educator, 30*(4), 172–177.

Higuchi, K. A., & Donald, J. G. (2002). Thinking processes used by nurses in clinical decision making. *Journal of Nursing Education, 41*(4), 145–153.

Hrobsky, P. E., & Kersbergen, A. L. (2002). Preceptors' perceptions of clinical performance failure. *Journal of Nursing Education, 41*(12), 550–553.

Institute of Medicine. (2014). *Assessing health professional education: Workshop summary*. Washington, DC: The National Academies Press.

Ironside, P., McNelis, A., & Ebright, P. (2014). Clinical education in nursing: Rethinking learning in practice settings. *Nursing Outlook, 62*(3), 185–191.

Issenberg, S., McGaghie, W., Petrusa, E., Gordon, D., & Scalese, R. (2005). Features and uses of high-fidelity medical simulations that lead to effective learning: A best evidence medical education systematic review. *Medical Teacher, 27*(1), 10–28.

Jeffries, P. (2005). A framework for designing, implementing, and evaluating simulations used as teaching strategies in nursing. *Nursing Education Perspectives, 26*(2), 96–103.

Jeffries, P. (2012). *Simulation in nursing education: From conceptualization to evaluation*. Philadelphia: Lippincott Williams & Wilkins.

Johnson, G., & Flagler, S. (2013). Web-based unfolding cases: A strategy to enhance and evaluate clinical reasoning skills. *Journal of Nursing Education, 52*(10), 589–592.

Kaplan, M., Silver, N., LaVaque-Manty, D., & Meizlish, D. (2013). *Using reflection and metacognition to improve student learning: Across the disciplines, across the academy*. Sterling, VA: Stylus Books.

Kennison, M. M., & Misselwitz, S. (2002). Evaluating reflective writing for appropriateness, fairness, and consistency. *Nursing Education Perspectives, 23*(5), 238–242.

Kern, C. S., Bush, K. L., & McCleish, J. M. (2006). Mind-mapped care plans: Integrating an innovative educational tool as an alternative to traditional care plans. *Journal of Nursing Education, 45*(4), 112–119.

King, M., & Shell, R. (2002). Teaching and evaluating critical thinking with concept maps. *Nurse Educator, 27*(5), 213–216.

Krautscheid, L., Moceri, J., Stragnell, S., Manthey, L., & Neal, T. (2014). A descriptive study of a clinical evaluation tool and process: student and faculty perspectives. *Journal of Nursing Education, 53*(3), S30–S33.

Kuiper, R., & Pesut, D. (2004). Promoting cognitive and metacognitive reflective reasoning skills in nursing practice: Self-regulated learning theory. *Journal of Advanced Nursing, 45*(4), 381–391.

Lasater, K., & Nielsen, A. (2009). Reflective journaling for clinical judgment development and evaluation. *Journal of Nursing Education, 48*(1), 40–44.

Lehman, K. (2003). Clinical nursing instructors' use of handheld computers for student recordkeeping and evaluation. *Journal of Nursing Education, 42*(1), 41–42.

Liberto, T., Roncher, M., & Shellenbarger, T. (1999). Anecdotal notes: Effective clinical evaluation and record keeping. *Nurse Educator, 24*(6), 15–18.

McClure, E., & Black, L. (2013). The role of the clinical preceptor: An integrative literature review. *Journal of Nursing Education, 52*(6), 335–341.

McNelis, A., Ironside, P., Zvonar, S., & Ebright, P. (2014). Advancing the science of research in nursing education: Contributions of the critical decision method. *Journal of Nursing Education, 53*(2), 61–64.

McWilliam, P., & Botwinski, C. (2010). Developing a successful nursing objective structured clinical examination. *Journal of Nursing Education, 49*(1), 36–41.

Meyer, M., Connors, H., Hou, Q., & Gajewski, B. (2011). The effect of simulation on clinical performance: A junior nursing student clinical comparison study. *Simulation in Healthcare: The Journal of the Society for Simulation in Healthcare, 6*(5), 269–277.

Mueller, A., Johnston, M., & Bligh, D. (2001). Mind-mapped care plans: A remarkable alternative to traditional nursing care plans. *Nurse Educator, 26*(2), 75–80.

Murphy, J. I. (2005). How to learn, not what to learn: Three strategies that foster lifelong learning in the clinical setting. In M. Oermann & K. Heinrich (Eds.), *Annual review of nursing education strategies for teaching, assessment, and program planning* (pp. 37–58). New York: Springer.

National Institutes of Health (NIH) Stroke Scale (NIHSS) training—Online or mobile. (n.d.). American Heart Association. Retrieved from, http://www.strokeassociation.com.

Niederhauser, V., Schoessler, M., Gubrud-Howe, P., Magnussen, L., & Codier, E. (2012). Creating innovative models of clinical nursing education. *Journal of Nursing Education, 51*(11), 603–608.

O'Connor, A. B. (2014). *Clinical instruction and evaluation* (3rd ed.). Boston: Jones & Bartlett.

Oermann, M. H., & Gaberson, K. (2014). *Evaluation and testing in nursing education* (4th ed.). New York: Springer.

Oermann, M. H., Yarbrough, S. S., Saewert, K. J., Ard, N., & Charasika, M. E. (2009). Clinical evaluation and grading practices in schools of nursing: National survey findings Part II. *Nursing Education Perspectives, 30*(6), 352–357.

Osinski, K. (2003). Due process rights of nursing students in cases of misconduct. *Journal of Nursing Education, 42*(2), 55–58.

Pierce, C. S. (2001). Implications of chemically impaired students in clinical settings. *Journal of Nursing Education, 40*(9), 422–425.

Poorman, S., & Mastorovich, M. (2014). Teacher stories of blame when assigning a failing grade. *International Journal of Education Scholarship, 16*(11). article 1.

Rankin, J. M., Malinsky, L., Tate, B., & Elena, L. (2010). Contesting our taken-for-granted understanding of student evaluation: Insights from a team of institutional ethnographers. *Journal of Nursing Education, 49*(6), 333–339.

Robert Wood Johnson Foundation. (2014). Simulation and virtual reality. *Charting Nursing's Future, 23*, 1–8. Retrieved from, http://www.rwjf.org/content/dam/farm/reports/issue_briefs/2014/rwjf415763.

Scanlan, J. M. (2001). Learning clinical teaching: Is it magic? *Nursing and Health Care Perspectives, 22*(5), 240–246.

Schuster, P. (2000). Concept mapping: Reducing clinical care plan paperwork and increasing learning. *Nurse Educator, 25*(2), 76–81.

Seldomridge, L., & Walsh, C. (2006). Evaluating student performance in undergraduate preceptorships. *Journal of Nursing Education, 45*(5), 169–177.

Sherwood, G., & Horton-Deutsch, S. (2012). *Reflective practice: Transforming education and improving outcomes*. Indianapolis: Sigma Theta Tau.

Sigma Theta Tau International. (2005). *Resource Paper on The Scholarship of Reflective Practice*. Author, Retrieved from, http://www.nursingsociety.org/aboutus/PositionPapers/Documents/resource:reflective.pdf.

Stevens, D., & Levi, A. (2005). *Introduction to rubrics: An assessment tool to save grading time, convey effective feedback and promote student learning*. Sterling, VA: Stylus.

Suskie, L. (2009). *Assessing student learning: A common sense guide* (2nd ed.). San Francisco: Anker.

Tanicala, M., Barbara, K., Scheffer, B., & Roberts, M. (2011). Defining pass/fail nursing student clinical behaviors phase I: Moving toward a culture of safety. *Nursing Education Perspectives*, *32*(3), 155–161.

Tanner, C. A. (2006). Thinking like a nurse: A research-based model of clinical judgment in nursing. *Journal of Nursing Education*, *45*(6), 204–211.

Thomas, S. P. (2003). Handling anger in the teacher–student relationship. *Nursing Education Perspectives*, *24*(1), 17–24.

Tochel, C., Haig, A., Hesketh, A., Cadzow, A., Beggs, K., Colthart, I., et al. (2009). The effectiveness of portfolios for post-graduate assessment and education: BEME Guide No 12. *Medical Teacher*, *31*(4), 279–281.

U.S. Department of Education. (2013). *The Family Educational Rights and Privacy Act. Uninterrupted Scholars Act Amendment*. Retrieved from, http://www.ed.gov/.

Vacek, J. (2009). Using a conceptual approach with concept mapping to promote critical thinking. *Journal of Nursing Education*, *48*(1), 45–48.

Walker, E., & Dewar, B. (2000). Moving on from interpretivism: An argument for constructivist evaluation. *Journal of Advanced Nursing*, *32*(3), 713–720.

Walvoord, B., Anderson, V., & Angelo, T. A. (2010). *Effective grading: A tool for learning and assessment*. San Francisco: Jossey-Bass.

Waznonis, A. R. (2014). Methods and evaluations for simulation debriefing in nursing education. *Journal of Nursing Education*, *53*(8), 459–465.

Wear, D., Zarconi, J., Garden, R., & Jones, T. (2012). Reflection in/and writing: Pedagogy and practice in medical education. *Academic Medicine*, *87*(5), 603–609.

Wiles, L., & Bishop, J. (2001). Clinical performance appraisal: Renewing graded clinical experiences. *Journal of Nursing Education*, *40*(1), 37–39.

Zuzelo, P. R. (2000). Clinical issues, clinical probation: Supporting the at-risk student. *Nurse Educator*, *25*(5), 216–218.

Systematic Program Evaluation

26

Peggy Ellis, PhD, RN, FNP-BC

Program evaluation is a systematic assessment and analysis of all components of an academic program through the application of evaluation approaches, techniques, and knowledge to improve the effectiveness of the program in reaching the program goals. A program evaluation plan is a document that serves as the blueprint for the evaluation of a specific program. The evaluation plan describes the goal, methods used, frequency, and the individual or group responsible for each component of the evaluation along with the expected results or the desired goals of each component. The purpose of this chapter is to provide information on why and how to conduct comprehensive evaluation of nursing education programs. Background information about program evaluation and its benefits is followed by a description of the processes of conducting a program evaluation.

Purposes and Benefits of Program Evaluation

The purpose of a comprehensive, systematic evaluation of a program is to determine the extent to which all activities for an academic program meet the established desired goals or outcomes. Program evaluation is conducted for all levels of educational programs from licensed practical or vocational nurse to doctor of nursing practice and doctor of nursing philosophy (PhD) to determine the effectiveness of the program and make improvements in the program. Program evaluation may be developmental, designed to provide direction for the development and implementation of a program, or outcome-oriented, designed to judge the merit of the total program being evaluated. It also evaluates what was planned, what was implemented, and what students experienced to identify discrepancies (Merritt, Blake, McIntyre, & Packer, 2012). The more advanced a program is in its implementation, the more complex the program evaluation. Specific purposes of program evaluation are as follows:

1. To determine how various elements of the program interact and influence program effectiveness
2. To determine the extent to which the mission, goals, and outcomes of the program are realized
3. To determine whether the program has been implemented as planned
4. To provide a rationale for decision making that leads to improved program effectiveness
5. To identify what resources and how those resources can be used most efficiently to improve program quality and effectiveness

Relationship of Program Evaluation to Accreditation

Accrediting bodies exert considerable influence over nursing programs. Accrediting bodies including the state board of nursing, professional nursing organizations, and regional accrediting bodies for universities are involved in ensuring that standards are met and quality maintained (see Chapter 27). Nursing programs have historically depended on accreditation processes to guide program evaluation efforts. Some nursing programs do not fully engage in program evaluation until preparation of the self-study for an accreditation site visit has begun. To fulfill its purposes, program evaluation must be a continuous activity. Program evaluation built solely around accreditation criteria may lack examination of some important elements or understanding of the relationship between elements that influence program success. However, more nursing programs are using accreditation criteria as the framework for building an evaluation plan. Although the use of only accreditation criteria may not consider some elements of what might influence program effectiveness, building the assessment indicators identified by these bodies into the evaluation process ensures ongoing attention to state and national standards of excellence.

Historical Perspective

The earliest approaches to educational program evaluation were based on Ralph Tyler's (1949) behavioral objective model. Tyler's behavioral objective model was a simple, linear approach that began with defining learning objectives, developing measuring tools, and then measuring student performance to determine whether objectives had been met. Because evaluation occurred at the end of the learning experience, Tyler's approach was primarily summative. Formative evaluation, which includes testing and revising curriculum components during the development and implementation of educational programs, became popular during the 1960s and continued into the 1970s.

Outcomes assessment became the focus of educational evaluation in the 1980s. In 1984 the National Institute of Education Study Group on the Conditions of Excellence in American Postsecondary Education endorsed outcomes assessment as an essential strategy for improving the quality of education in postsecondary institutions (Ewell, 1985). By the mid-1980s the regional accrediting agencies began mandating outcomes assessment in their accreditation criteria (Ewell, 1985). By the early 1990s the National League for Nursing Accrediting Commission (NLNAC) added assessment of learning outcomes to its accreditation criteria. The Commission on Collegiate Nursing Education (CCNE) also included outcomes assessment in its initial accreditation standards, first published in 1997, as has the NLN Commission for Nursing Education Accreditation (NLN CNEA). The United States Department of Education also emphasizes outcomes, particularly outcomes pertaining to progress and graduation rates. In the past decade most of the nursing literature related to program evaluation has focused on specific elements of program evaluation, rather than on comprehensive evaluation.

Program Evaluation Models

Evaluation Models

Models provide an organizing or systematic approach to overall program evaluation. Table 26-1 provides a summary related to evaluation models and frameworks used in the past. Although it may be helpful to use a specific model to increase the effectiveness and efficiency of the program evaluation, most are no longer commonly used in nursing education. Many of these models are complex and difficult to apply. A study by Sauter (2000) found that most baccalaureate nursing education programs do not use a theory-driven approach to evaluation but instead are influenced by professional accrediting bodies. Currently, most schools continue to use nursing accreditation criteria as a framework to develop an evaluation plan that is systematic and comprehensive.

In all evaluation models, a commonality is the cycle of defining what is to be evaluated, how the evaluation will be conducted, a report of the findings, and recommendations for subsequent revisions. It is always important to repeat the cycle to ensure continual improvement. Figure 26-1 depicts this cycle.

Regardless of the model or theory used, program evaluation is needed to make decisions about the program, the curriculum, and the improvements needed to offer high quality programs. The evaluation plan can be divided into areas so that all aspects of the program are examined and analyzed for program decisions. Although the evaluation plan is important to the continued process, the use of assessment data to guide change involves the commitment of faculty to collect and examine the data and decide what and how to make improvements based on that data.

The Program Evaluation Plan

The program evaluation plan provides a road map for organizing and tracking evaluation activities. The plan is a systematic and written document that contains the evaluation framework, activities for gathering and analyzing data, responsible parties, time frames, accreditation criteria and standards, and the means for using information for program decisions. The program evaluation plan provides the mechanism for maintaining continuous evaluation of program effectiveness.

TABLE 26-1 Evaluation Models

Models provide an organizing or systematic approach to overall program evaluation. It may be helpful to use a specific model to increase the effectiveness and efficiency of the program evaluation. Nursing faculty often do not subscribe to one model of evaluation more than others. However, the following models are commonly found in nursing program evaluation.

SCRIVEN'S GOAL-FREE EVALUATION MODEL

Scriven's model was developed in the 1960s. It provides a broad perspective of evaluation and introduced the ideas of "formative" and "summative" evaluation. The model suggests that the evaluation of goals is unnecessary. The model measures outcomes or the actual effects of the program against the identified needs. Processes, procedures, outcomes, and unanticipated effects, both positive and negative, are examined. Scriven encourages the use of an outside, objective evaluator to avoid bias. The outside evaluator is used to learn about the program and its results with no knowledge of the goals of the program. This method encourages an assessment of both intended and unintended outcomes, as well as a broad range of outcomes (Scriven, 1991).

STAKE'S COUNTENANCE MODEL

Stake's model was introduced in the 1960s and describes three components: antecedents, transactions, and outcomes. *Antecedents* refer to things that existed before the instruction occurred such as an individual's readiness and ability to learn. The transaction phase includes the instructional methods and processes involved in the teaching. Outcomes are the products that result from the antecedents and transactions. It was introduced in 1967 and emphasizes description and judgment. This model takes into account the stakeholders such as students and teachings, the educational experiences, and the outcomes (Stravropoulou & Strouboukі, 2014).

TYLER'S BEHAVIORAL OBJECTIVE MODEL

Tyler's Behavioral Objective Model was developed in the 1930s and is based on what the faculty would like students to achieve at the end of a course or program, or the determination of the objectives. The model also asks what experiences are needed to reach the objectives, how the experiences can be organized, and how faculty can determine whether the objectives have been met. The educational objectives should be derived from the assessment of society, the learners, and the subject-matter to be mastered. The experiences are prescribed by the faculty. However, Tyler recognized that those experiences are not totally under the control of faculty; they are influenced by the perceptions, interests, and previous experiences of the student. The defined objectives are then used as a benchmark against which it can be determined whether the student learned what was intended (Lunenburg, 2011).

STUFFELBEAM'S CIPP MODEL

Stuffelbeam's model originated in the late 1960s and is used as a guide for formative and summative evaluations. The CIPP model is a systems model with the acronym representing *context evaluation, input evaluation, process evaluation,* and *product evaluation.* Context evaluation looks at the context of the program being evaluated. During this stage the evaluator looks at needs, problems, assets, and opportunities. This information is used to define goals, priorities, and desired outcomes. Input evaluation identifies a potential plan for achievement of the goals, and examines what might be used to implement that plan. During this stage, alternative approaches are considered along with possible action plans and staffing plans. The budget needed to meet the needs and achieve the goals is identified and resources are allocated through grants or other mechanisms available. Process evaluation involves the implementation of the plan or instructional strategies, and the judgment of program performance and interpretation of outcomes. Product evaluation is the assessment of the outcomes and the determination of whether the targeted outcomes were met. Going through this process will help answer the questions of whether the plan is succeeding or has succeeded, and what needs to be done or changed in order to reach the proposed goals. This model emphasizes improvement and corrections for problems within a program (Stufflebeam, 2003).

DEMING'S CONTINUOUS QUALITY IMPROVEMENT MODEL

The CQI process was developed by W. Edwards Deming in the 1950s. This evaluation model is seen as a continuous process that is embedded in the culture of the school and its day-to-day work. It should be seen as a natural part of everyday routine. It is described as consisting of four phases: plan, do, study, and act. These phases represent a continuous cycle of activities. *Plan* includes the development of goals and objectives to identify the desired outcomes of the program. Data collection is the *do* phase. The analysis or *study* of data occurs to determine if the program is performing as planned or where and how the program needs improvement or change to reach the intended outcomes. *Act* involves making the changes indicated in the analysis. Then the cycle starts all over so that a continuous process of plan, collect data, analyze, and make changes can occur (Brown & Marshall, 2008).

In all models, a commonality is the cycle of defining where you are headed, how you will get there, an analysis of whether you got there or what is the result, and what you should do next. It is always important to then redo the cycle so that you are continually evaluating and improving. Figure 26-1 depicts this cycle.

CHEN'S THEORY-DRIVEN MODEL

Chen's model was introduced in 1980 and provides a framework that identifies the elements of the program, provides the rationale for interventions, and describes the causal linkages between the elements, interventions, and outcomes. Chen's theory calls for the study of the design and conceptualization of an intervention, its implementation, and its utility, then using models to guide the formulation of questions and data gathering in order to discover the cause of intended and unintended outcomes (Chen, 1990).

CIPP, Context, input, process, and product; *CQI,* continuous quality improvement.

Define or review outcomes and quality. Establish objectives/outcomes/ benchmarks: What do you expect to accomplish? How do you plan to accomplish the outcomes? How do you know when your outcomes are met?
Design strategies for implementing the proposed plan. Collect data to determine if outcomes have been met.
Analyze the data you have collected. Were the outcomes and benchmarks accomplished? Why or why not?
Where are the gaps according to the data? Where do changes need to occur to improve and/or maintain quality? Implement changes.
Quality program built on a vision and mission

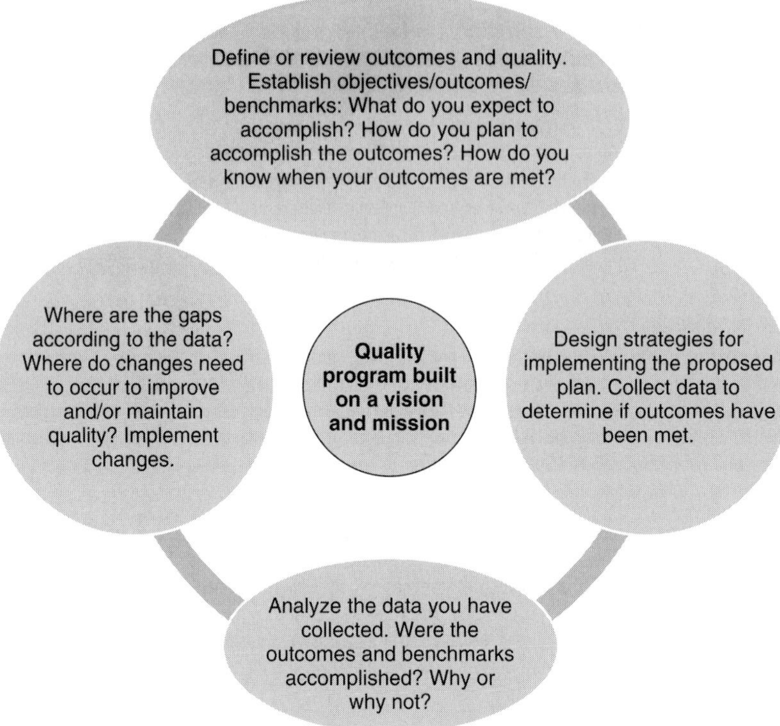

Figure 26-1 Evaluation cycle.

Accrediting agencies require a systematic evaluation plan. Some may mention specific components that are needed in the plan. Accrediting agency guidelines may be good to reference as the evaluation plan is developed.

Table 26-2 provides a sample evaluation plan for mission and goal evaluation applied to a nursing education program. This sample demonstrates how all elements of the program evaluation plan may be articulated, including the program's theoretical elements, assessment activities, responsible parties, time frames, and related accreditation criteria. There are a variety of approaches to the evaluation plan. This example illustrates the important components of the plan. For the remaining evaluation components presented in this chapter, only examples of theoretical elements and methods for gathering and analyzing assessment data related to the review of expected and actual outcomes are provided. The theoretical elements and assessment strategies that are suggested here are not all-inclusive but may assist nursing faculty in further development of their own program theory and program evaluation plan.

Mission and Goal Evaluation

Program evaluation must begin by determining that the appropriate mission, philosophy, program goals, and expected outcomes have been defined. The mission and goals need to be examined for agreement with the university mission and goals. The expectations of both internal and external stakeholders must be considered. Internal stakeholders may include administrators, faculty, students, and university governing boards. External stakeholders may include religious organizations for private schools with religious affiliations, regional accrediting bodies, national discipline-specific accrediting bodies, state education commissions and boards of nursing, the legislature, the community, and professional organizations. There should be congruency between the expectations of stakeholders and the program's mission, philosophy, goals, and outcomes. For private institutions with

TABLE 26-2 Nursing Program Comprehensive Evaluation Plan

CCNE Element	Responsibility for Collection and Review	Timeline	Evidence Resources	Expected Outcomes
Standard 1: The mission, goals, and expected program outcomes are congruent with those of the parent institution, reflect professional nursing standards and guidelines, and consider the needs and expectations of the community of interest. Policies of the parent institution and nursing program clearly support the program's mission, goals, and expected outcomes. The faculty and students of the program are involved in the governance of the program and in the ongoing efforts to improve program quality.				
Key Element 1-A: The mission, goals, and expected program outcomes are congruent with those of the parent institution and consistent with relevant professional nursing standards and guidelines for the preparation of nursing professionals.	Dean and Faculty	Every 5 years in spring semester or as needed. (2013, 2018, 2023, etc.)	1. Comparison of university mission, and goals with School of Nursing mission, goals, and outcomes 2. Comparison of mission and goals with AACN Essentials and other standards as defined	1. There is congruency between the School of Nursing, Professional Standards, and the University's mission, goals and standards.
Key Element 1-B: The mission, goals, and expected student outcomes are reviewed periodically and revised, as appropriate, to reflect professional nursing standards and guidelines and the needs and expectations of the community of interest.	Dean and Faculty	Every 5 years in spring or as needed. (2013, 2018, 2023, etc.)	1. Comparison of expected student outcomes with professional standards and community needs 2. Demonstrated in faculty meeting minutes 3. Executive Advisory Board minutes Student Advisory Board minutes	1. Professional nursing standards and community needs and expectations are reflected in School of Nursing minutes and actions.
Key Element 1-C: Expected faculty outcomes are clearly identified by the nursing unit, are written and communicated to the faculty, and are congruent with institutional expectations.	Dean and Faculty	Every year in the fall	1. List of faculty accomplishments 2. Faculty performance expectations as written in the LU Faculty Guidebook 3. Faculty yearly evaluations	1. Faculty performance correlates with expectations listed in the LU Faculty Guidebook. 2. Faculty evaluations reflect expected outcomes
CCNE Element	**Responsibility for Collection**	**Timeline**	**Evidence**	**Expected Outcomes**
Key Element 1-D: Faculty and students participate in program governance.	Dean and Faculty Student Advisory Council	Every year in spring	1. Minutes from faculty meetings 2. Reports in faculty meetings about university-level committees 3. University Faculty Guidebook 4. University Faculty Council Bylaws 5. Faculty membership on Faculty Council Committees 6. Student Advisory Council Minutes 7. LU and SONAHS Student Handbooks 8. Faculty Council Bylaws	1. Faculty meeting attendance demonstrates that 100% are active in School of Nursing governance. 2. Faculty serve on at least one university- level committee. 3. Minutes from Student Advisory Council and Faculty Meetings reflect that student and faculty input is solicited and considered.

(Continued)

TABLE 26-2 Nursing Program Comprehensive Evaluation Plan—cont'd

CCNE Element	Responsibility for Collection and Review	Timeline	Evidence Resources	Expected Outcomes
Key Element 1-E: Documents and publications are accurate. A process is used to notify constituents about changes in documents and publications.	Dean and Faculty	Every year in summer and ongoing as needed	1. Documents and publications (i.e. Student Handbook, University Catalog, Recruitment materials, website, etc.) are reviewed annually for accuracy and completeness and revised as needed. 2. A process is in place for notifying constituents about changes.	1. All documents are accurate. 2. A documented process exists and is followed for notification of changes.
Key Element 1-F: Academic policies of the parent institution and the nursing program are congruent and support achievement of the mission, goals, and expected student outcomes. These policies are fair and equitable, published and accessible, and reviewed and revised as necessary to foster program improvement.	Dean and Faculty	Every year in summer	1. Table showing congruence of university policies and School of Nursing policies as well as the mission, goals, and expected student outcomes 2. LU catalog and LU Student Handbook online and in print form. 3. SONAHS Student Handbooks and syllabi	1. There is congruence between university policies and School of Nursing policies as well as the mission, goals, and expected student outcomes. 2. Policies are fair, equitable, and published.

Standard 2: The parent institution demonstrates ongoing commitment to and support for the nursing program. The institution makes resources available to enable the program to achieve its mission, goals, and expected outcomes. The faculty, as a resource of the program, enable the achievement of the mission, goals, and expected program outcomes.

CCNE Element	Responsibility for Collection and Review	Timeline	Evidence	Expected Outcomes
Key Element 2-A: Fiscal and physical resources are sufficient to enable the program to fulfill its mission, goals, and expected outcomes. Adequacy of resources is reviewed periodically and resources are modified as needed.	Dean, Program Directors, Faculty, and Staff	Every year in fall and as needed	1. Strategic plan 2. Faculty state that physical resources are adequate. 3. Resources are reviewed in faculty meetings and adequacy is discussed. 4. Faculty communicate needs for resources through dean as evident in meeting minutes reflecting discussion of resource needs.	1. Resources are adequate to meet program needs and enable fulfillment of mission and expected outcomes. 2. Faculty report they are provided an opportunity for input. 3. Classroom space provides room for all classes, as evidenced by room schedule 4. Ongoing fiscal requests reflect faculty input.
Key Element 2-B: Academic support services are sufficient to ensure quality and are evaluated on a regular basis to meet program and student needs.	Dean, Program Directions, Faculty, Dean's Forum, and Student Advisory Council	Every year in summer	1. University survey of academic support services 2. List of support services available in the University Student Handbook and on the University website 3. Student Community Website 4. Student Advisory Council minutes	1. EBI demonstrates 5 out of possible 7 on questions related to support services 2. Information on support services is accurate and up-to-date.

TABLE 26-2 Nursing Program Comprehensive Evaluation Plan—cont'd

CCNE Element	Responsibility for Collection and Review	Timeline	Evidence Resources	Expected Outcomes
			5. Dean's Forum minutes 6. Faculty meeting minutes reflect discussion of academic support services.	
Key Element 2-C: The chief nurse administrator: is an RN; holds a graduate degree in nursing; holds a doctoral degree if the nursing unit offers a graduate program in nursing; is academically and experientially qualified to accomplish the mission, goals, and expected program outcomes; is vested with the administrative authority to accomplish the mission, goals, and expected program outcomes; and provides effective leadership to the nursing unit in achieving its mission, goals, and expected program outcomes.	Dean and Vice President for Academic Affairs	Every five years (2017, 2022, 2027)	1. Chief nurse administrator's (Dean's) vita. 2. Dean job description 3. Performance review of Dean	1. Dean holds RN licensure, a graduate degree in nursing and a doctoral degree in nursing or a related field. 2. Job description demonstrates administrative authority.
Key Element 2-D: Faculty are: sufficient in number to accomplish the mission, goals, and expected program outcomes; academically prepared for the areas in which they teach; and experientially prepared for the areas in which they teach.	Dean and Program Directors	Every year	1. Teaching schedule 2. Enrollment report 3. Faculty vitas compared to teaching assignments 4. Faculty performance standards	1. Faculty/student ratio is 1:10 or less for appropriate clinical experiences and 1:20 or less in the classroom. 2. 70% of faculty are doctorally prepared or in candidacy. 3. Faculty vitas are current and faculty expertise is reflected in teaching assignments.
Key Element 2-E: Preceptors, when used by the program as an extension of faculty, are academically and experientially qualified for their role in assisting in the achievement of the mission, goals, and expected student outcomes.	Dean and Program Directors	Each semester	1. Preceptor vitas 2. Preceptor evaluations completed by faculty and students 3. Preceptor qualifications	1. All preceptors are academically and experientially qualified. 2. 100% of preceptors meet the established criteria. 3. Action plans on preceptor evaluations. 4. EBI evaluation of preceptors demonstrates 5 out of 7 rating.

(Continued)

TABLE 26-2 Nursing Program Comprehensive Evaluation Plan—cont'd

CCNE Element	Responsibility for Collection and Review	Timeline	Evidence Resources	Expected Outcomes
Key Element II-F: The parent institution and program provide and support an environment that encourages faculty teaching, scholarship, service, and practice in keeping with the mission, goals, and expected faculty outcomes.	Dean and Vice President of Academic Affairs	Every Year	1. Description of faculty expectations in Faculty Guidebook 2. Faculty vitas and monthly accomplishment reports. 3. Faculty report of support 4. IT annual "wish list	1. Faculty perform activities in all aspects of the faculty role. They state they feel supported. 2. 100% of faculty participate in professional development opportunities annually. 3. 100% of faculty have individual offices with computers and necessary equipment. 4. Classrooms and labs are available and well equipped.

Standard 3: The curriculum is developed in accordance with the program's mission, goals, and expected student outcomes. The curriculum reflects professional nursing standards and guidelines and the needs and expectations of the community of interest. Teaching–learning practices are congruent with expected student outcomes. The environment for teaching–learning fosters achievement of expected student outcomes.

CCNE Element	Responsibility for Collection & Review	Timeline	Evidence	Expected Outcome
Key Element 3-A: The curriculum is developed, implemented, and revised to reflect clear statements of expected student outcomes that are congruent with the program's mission and goals, and with the roles for which the program is preparing its graduates.	Dean, Program Directors, and Faculty	Every five years (2015, 2020, 2025) or at the development of a new program.	1. Comparison of mission and goals with the expected student outcomes. 2. Copies of course syllabi and materials 3. Student handbook 4. Course proposal forms	1. Expected student outcomes are congruent with the program's mission and goals.
Key Element 3-B: Curricula are developed, implemented, and revised to reflect relevant professional nursing standards and guidelines, which are clearly evident within the curriculum and within the expected student outcomes (individual and aggregate).	Dean, Program Directors, and Faculty	Every five years (2015, 2020, 2025) or more often if needed	1. Comparison of identified professional nursing standards and guidelines with the curriculum and expected student outcomes 2. Copies of course materials that provide evidence standards and guidelines 3. Course proposal forms	1. Curriculum and expected student outcomes are congruent with identified professional nursing standards.
Key Element 3-C: The curriculum is logically structured to achieve expected student outcomes	Dean, Program Directors, and Faculty	Every five years	1. Full and part time sequenced plans of studies 2. Review of course content and placement 3. Course syllabi 4. DARS report	1. Curriculum is logically structured. Pre- and co-requisites listed for courses to ensure progression of knowledge and skills.

TABLE 26-2 Nursing Program Comprehensive Evaluation Plan—cont'd

CCNE Element	Responsibility for Collection and Review	Timeline	Evidence Resources	Expected Outcomes
Key Element 3-D: Teaching–learning practices and environments support the achievement of expected student outcomes.	Program Directors and Faculty	Each semester	1. Review of teaching practices in syllabi 2. Student assignment grades 3. Student course evaluations	1. Students achieve expected outcomes as evidenced by satisfactory grades and portfolio review. 2. Students evaluate teaching strategies and environments highly on course evaluations.
Key Element 3-E: The curriculum includes planned clinical practice experiences that enable students to integrate new knowledge and demonstrate attainment of program outcomes; and are evaluated by faculty.	Program Directors and Faculty	Each semester	1. Review clinical experiences and related objectives 2. Review variety of clinical contracts 3. Review student clinical evaluations 4. Established clinical site criteria for each clinical course	1. Students achieve expected outcomes as evidenced by clinical project or assignment include portfolio review. 2. Clinical sites meet criteria established for each clinical course.
Key Element 3-F: The curriculum and teaching-learning practices consider the needs and expectations of the identified community of interest.	Dean, Program Directors, and Faculty	Each semester	1. Course evaluations 2. Preceptor input 3. Employer evaluations 4. Executive Advisory Committee minutes 5. Faculty meeting minutes	1. Course evaluations demonstrate 3.5 on a 5-point scale or 3 on a 4-point scale. 2. Programmatic feedback reflecting needs and expectations of the community of interest.
Key Element 3-G: Individual student performance is evaluated by the faculty and reflects achievement of expected student outcomes. Evaluation policies and procedures for individual student performance are defined and consistently applied.	Program Directors and Faculty	Each semester	1. Course syllabi 2. Course grades and evaluation measures 3. LU and SONAHS Student Handbooks 4. LU and SONAHS Grading policies 5. Signed Student Handbook Acknowledgement Form	1. Evaluation procedures defined in the syllabus are consistent with LU and SONAHS stated policies. 2. Students understand evaluation policies and procedures and know where to find them. 3. 100% of students have signed the Student Handbook Acknowledgement Form.
Key Element III-H: Curriculum and teaching–learning practices are evaluated at regularly scheduled intervals to foster ongoing improvement.	Dean, Program Directors, and Faculty	Every year in spring	1. Course and clinical evaluations 2. Faculty meeting minutes 3. Student Advisory Council minutes	1. Faculty meeting minutes reflect responses to evaluation data.
Standard 4: The program is effective in fulfilling its mission and goals as evidenced by achieving expected program outcomes. Program outcomes include student outcomes, faculty outcomes, and other outcomes identified by the program. Data on program effectiveness are used to foster ongoing program improvement.				

(Continued)

TABLE 26-2 Nursing Program Comprehensive Evaluation Plan—cont'd

CCNE Element	Responsibility for Collection	Timeline	Evidence	Expected Outcome
Key Element 4-A: A systematic process is used to determine program effectiveness.	Dean and Faculty	Reviewed every five years (2014, 2019, 2024)	A written, systematic plan is in place	1. The systematic plan is fully implemented
Key Element 4–B: Program completion rates demonstrate program effectiveness.	Dean, Program Directors, and Faculty	Every year in June	1. Numbers of students completing the RN to BSN program within 4 years of enrolling in the first nursing course	1. Expected graduation rate is 70%.
Key Element 4-C: Licensure and certification pass rates demonstrate program effectiveness as appropriate.	Dean and Faculty	Every year in May	1. Alumni survey results	1. Of those attempting certification within 3 years postbaccalaureate, 80% will pass (certification is not required).
Key Element 4-D: Employment rates demonstrate program effectiveness.	Dean and Faculty	Every year in June	1. Exit survey 2. Alumni survey results	1. Graduates will be 70% employed within 1 year of graduation.
Key Element 4-E: Program outcomes demonstrate program effectiveness.	Dean and Faculty	Every year in June	1. Portfolios 2. Student grades in all courses 3. Alumni survey 4. Employer satisfaction with graduates 5. Capstone project	1. Graduates demonstrate that all programs outcomes have been met. 2. EBI demonstrates 5 out of 7 in overall alumni satisfaction. 3. Employers report in focus groups satisfaction with graduates.
Key Element 4-F: Faculty outcomes, individually and in the aggregate, demonstrate program effectiveness.	Dean and Faculty	Every year in spring	1. Faculty self-evaluations 2. Faculty evaluations by dean 3. Monthly and annual reports to Provost on faculty achievement 4. Digital measures 5. Course evaluation of faculty	1. Faculty course/teaching evaluations demonstrate a minimum of 3.5 on a 5-point scale or 3 on a 4-point scale. 2. 100% of faculty participate in university, professional, or community service yearly.
Key Element 4-G: The program defines and reviews formal complaints according to established policies.	Dean and Faculty	Every year in June	1. Written formal complaints and written outcomes 2. LU and SONAHS Student Handbooks	1. Policies are in place and followed for review of formal complaints. 2. Minutes of meetings where formal review of concerns and conflicts have occurred.
Key element 4-H: Data analysis is used to foster ongoing program improvement.	Dean and Faculty	Every year in June	1. Faculty meeting minutes demonstrating data analysis and response	1. Data are used to foster improvement.

AACN, American Association of Colleges of Nursing; *BSN,* bachelor of science in nursing; *CCNE,* Commission on Collegiate Nursing Education; *DARS,* Degree Audit Reporting System; *EBI,* Educational Benchmarking, Inc.;

religious affiliations, some perspectives may be prescribed and must be included in mission, philosophy, goals, or outcomes.

The mission of the nursing department or school should be congruent with the university's mission. Incongruence could indicate that the university would not be supportive of the nursing program. Comparison of key phrases in the department's mission with key phrases in the university's mission may be done to assess congruency between mission statements. The identification of gaps between the two mission statements provides information about areas where attention is needed. The assessment should be performed periodically and whenever changes are made to either mission statement.

The evaluation plan should be designed for use in all program levels including doctoral level. Although existing accrediting bodies do not evaluate PhD programs in nursing, use of an evaluation plan for assessing quality is an important aspect of program quality improvement. Quality indicators are identified and accessible online for use in evaluation of PhD nursing programs.

There should be consensus among the faculty regarding the nursing school or department's mission and philosophy. A modified Delphi approach to determine the level of agreement among the faculty for each statement in the mission and philosophy is a useful strategy. The Delphi approach is useful for both the development and the evaluation of belief statements (philosophy). It gathers individual viewpoints and visions to reach a consensus. This approach allows for participants to be in multiple locations and can be done without the need for frequent face-to-face dialogue in a manner that protects the anonymity of participants. In this method, questionnaires that list proposition statements about each of the content elements of the belief statement are distributed. A common breakdown of Delphi responses is a five-point range from "strongly agree" to "strongly disagree" so that respondents can indicate their level of support for each proposition. Respondents are provided with feedback about the responses after the first round of questionnaire distribution, and a second round may occur to determine the intensity of agreement or disagreement with the group median responses (Aguilar, Stupans, Scutter, & King, 2013). After several rounds with interim reports and analyses, it is usually possible to identify areas of consensus, areas of disagreement so strong that further discourse is unlikely to lead to consensus, and areas in which further discussion is warranted. In the evaluation of an established belief statement, the same process will provide data about which propositions continue to be supported, which no longer garner support, and which need to be openly debated (Aguilar et al., 2013). The result provides a consensus list of propositions that either supports the belief statement as it is or suggests areas for revision. Chapter 7 provides further information on the development of mission and philosophy.

All accrediting bodies have expectations related to mission, philosophy, program goals, and expected outcomes. Clear statements of mission, philosophy, and program outcomes are expected. For example, the required outcomes in the accreditation criteria for baccalaureate and higher degree programs for the Accreditation Commission for Education in Nursing (ACEN), National League for Nursing Commission for Nursing Education Accreditation (NLN CNEA), and CCNE include outcomes such as graduation rates, job placement rates, licensure and certification pass rates, and program satisfaction (American Association of Colleges of Nursing, 2013; Commission on Collegiate Nursing Education [CCNE], 2013; NLN CNEA, 2015). Expectations exist regarding congruency of the program's mission, goals, and outcomes with those of the parent institution, professional nursing standards and guidelines, and the needs of the community of interest.

Professional organization guidelines and standards may be considered in the program mission, philosophy, and goals. They may include but are not limited to the American Nurses Association (ANA), the American Association of Colleges of Nursing (AACN), the National League for Nursing (NLN), and the National Organization of Nurse Practitioner Faculties. Other nursing organizations may be included as appropriate and as desired by the program faculty. Program goals and outcomes should be congruent with the chosen and required nursing organization standards and guidelines. Standards and guidelines that are often used include ANA's Standards of Practice (American Nurses Association, 2010), the Criteria for Evaluation of Nurse Practitioner Programs (National Organization of Nurse Practitioner Faculties, 2012), the Institute of Medicine (IOM) Report (2011) and Quality and Safety Education for Nurses (Cronenwett, Sherwood, & Gelmon, 2009).

Other important external stakeholders to consider in the development of the mission and goals include local constituencies, such as health care agencies, that provide clinical learning experiences or employ graduates of the program. A survey of current and potential employers of graduates will help faculty to determine the knowledge and skill requirements of the marketplace and satisfaction with the program's graduates. Many nursing programs establish advisory committees to provide additional information and selected focus groups to add richness to the information. This information is used to ensure that program goals and outcomes are appropriate, to address marketplace needs, and to provide input for curriculum planning. They are also used to develop evaluation questions and tools for determining whether market needs are being met.

The mission and program goals should be clearly and publicly stated. Nursing schools that offer several different nursing programs will need to clearly articulate the purpose and program goals of each of the programs offered. Public announcement of the mission and program goals should be available through the Internet and in printed program brochures and catalogues. Box 26-1 lists the theoretical elements for mission and goal evaluation.

BOX 26-1 Elements for Mission and Goal Evaluation

- The mission of the nursing school or department is congruent with that of the university.
- There is consensus among the faculty regarding the mission and philosophy.
- There is congruency between the nursing mission, philosophy, conceptual framework, goals, and outcomes for each program.
- There is congruency with professional nursing standards and guidelines as identified by the nursing program.
- Expectations of the accrediting and approval bodies are known and considered in the program's mission, goals, philosophy, and outcomes.
- The Nursing Program Advisory Committee has meaningful input into program goals and outcomes.
- Documents and publications accurately reflect the mission and goals.

Curriculum Evaluation

One of the most critical elements of program effectiveness is curriculum design. Curriculum design is an organizing framework that arranges the curriculum elements into a logical order for learning. Curriculum design provides direction to both the content of the program and the teaching and learning processes involved in program implementation. Curriculum content involves both discipline-specific knowledge and the liberal arts foundation. Before the curriculum design can be developed, faculty must first determine their definition of the discipline of knowledge so that they may select courses that will best serve the students to prepare to practice. Faculty must determine what ways of knowing, or methods of inquiry, are characteristic of the discipline and what skills the discipline demands. Program goals and outcome statements provide a guide for the development of the curriculum. The curriculum design and content should be congruent with the nursing program philosophy. The philosophy should define the concepts of person, health, nursing, and education. Those definitions provide some guidance for what should be in the curriculum and how it should be organized. The program goals link the mission and faculty belief statements (philosophy) to the curriculum design, teaching and learning methods, and outcomes. Consequently, the evaluation of the curriculum builds on the evaluation of mission and goals. More information on curriculum design can be found in Chapter 6.

Evaluation of Curriculum Organization

Curriculum must be appropriately organized to move learners along a continuum from program entry to program completion. The principle of vertical organization or scaffolding guides both the planning and the evaluation of the curriculum. Vertical organization or scaffolding provides the rationale for the sequencing or building of curricular content elements (Brown, Bourke-Taylor, & Williams, 2012). For example, nursing faculty often use depth and complexity as sequencing guides; that is, given content areas may occur in subsequent levels of the curriculum at a level of greater depth, breadth, and complexity. Faculty may also use a simple to complex model where the curriculum begins with what the faculty defines as simpler concepts and builds to more complex concepts. In evaluation of the curriculum, faculty must assess for increasing depth and complexity to determine whether the sequencing was useful to learning and progressed to the desired outcomes. Determination of whether course and level objectives demonstrate sequential learning across the curriculum during each semester can be used as a test of vertical organization. The analysis can be performed using Bloom's (1956) Taxonomy as a guide for determining whether objectives follow a path of increasing complexity. Bloom's Taxonomy was adapted to demonstrate the levels of learning and relate those levels to verbs. Figure 26-2 is an example of Bloom's Taxonomy and Learning Wheel.

The concept of sequencing related to the vertical organization helps guide the curriculum structure so that new information and experiences are not presented until existing knowledge has been assimilated. In other words, what prior knowledge must be present to provide a link for new knowledge in

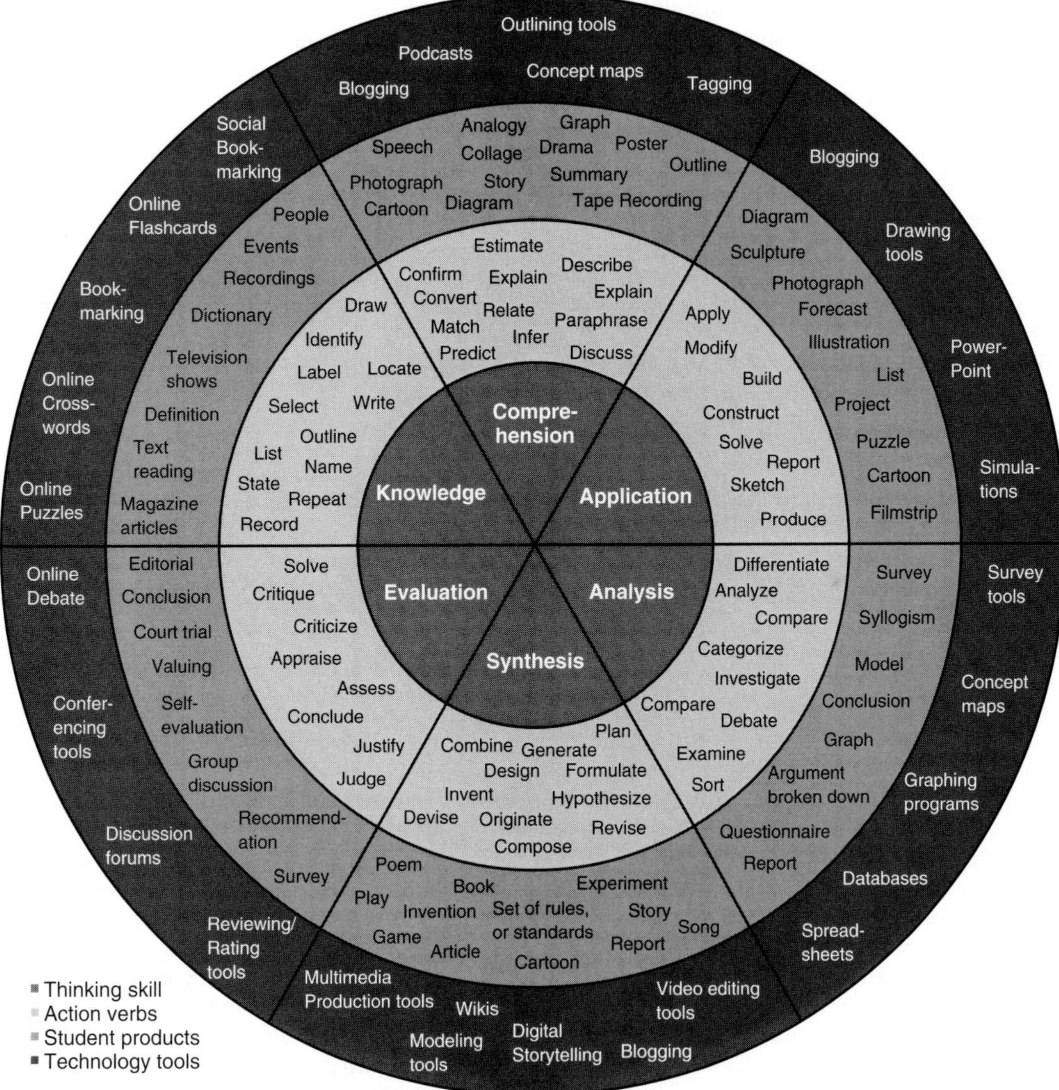

Figure 26-2 Bloom's Taxonomy and the Levels of Learning Wheel. Graphic created by Emily Hixson, Janet Buckenmeyer, and Heather Zamojski, 2011. Reprinted with permission of authors.

long-term memory? Often faculty believe everything needs to be learned at once. Of course this is not possible. An appropriate question is: "What entry skills and knowledge does the student need as a condition of subsequent knowledge and experiences?" How faculty answer this question will determine curriculum design and implementation. The evaluation question would address the extent to which students have the entry-level skills needed to progress sequentially in the curriculum. This is a critical question in light of the changing profile of students entering college-level programs. It is often difficult to determine which prerequisite skills should be required for entry and which should be acquired concurrently. Computer skills are a good example. Students enter programs with varying ability in using computers. It is necessary to determine the prerequisite skills needed and the sequence in which advanced skills should be acquired during the program of learning.

The principle of linear congruence, sometimes called *horizontal organization* or *alignment* assists faculty in determining the concurrent nature of courses during each semester or year level (Brown et al., 2012). This alignment means that the same concepts are built in more depth in each course.

The principle of internal consistency is important to the evaluation of the curriculum. The curriculum design is a carefully conceived plan that takes its shape from what its creators believe about people and their education as defined in the program philosophy. The intellectual test of a curriculum design is the extent to which the elements fit together. Four elements should be congruent: course objectives and outcomes, content taught, teaching and learning strategies, and assessments (Willett, Marshall, Broudo, & Clarke, 2007). Evaluation efforts should include examination of the extent to which the objectives and outcomes are linked to the mission and belief statements. Program objectives should be tracked to level and course objectives. One method of assessing internal consistency is through the use of a curriculum matrix or map (Willett et al., 2007). The curriculum map is a visual representation that lists all nursing courses and shows the placement of major concepts flowing from the program philosophy and conceptual framework. It also demonstrates the relationship of the learning outcomes to the curriculum. Curriculum mapping provides a broad picture of the curriculum and its components. This allows you to see where topics are taught and whether there are gaps or redundancies, as well as inconsistencies.

Some nursing programs use a specific conceptual framework that identifies essential program "threads" and provides further direction to curriculum development and implementation. Congruency between program threads, program goals, course objectives, and course content will also need to be assessed. Further information on curriculum development and curriculum frameworks can be found in Chapter 6.

Course Evaluation

Individual courses are reviewed to determine whether they have met the tests of internal consistency, linear congruence, and vertical organization. A triangulation approach to course evaluation is useful. This approach uses data from three sources—faculty, students, and materials review—to identify strengths and areas for change. Each course is evaluated to determine whether content elements, learning activities, assessment measures, and learner outcomes are consistent with the objectives of the course and the obligations of the course in terms of its placement in the total curriculum.

Faculty should clearly articulate the sequential levels of each expected ability to determine what teaching and learning strategies are needed to move the student to progressive levels of ability and to establish the criteria for determining that each stage of development has been achieved. This need is important in relation not only to abilities or competencies specific to the discipline or major but also to the transferable skills acquired in the general education component of the curriculum (Merritt et al., 2012). Some faculty achieve this by creating content maps for each major thread or pervasive strand in the curriculum with related knowledge and skill elements. The content maps chart the responsibility of each course in facilitating student progression to the expected program outcome. The maps also provide a guide for the evaluation of whether the elements were incorporated as planned and not repeated unnecessarily.

Many tools are available to help with evaluation of teaching–learning strategies. Content and curriculum mapping, as discussed under "Curriculum Evaluation" earlier in this chapter, is useful to determine content evaluation and course consistency. The meeting of course outcomes is also essential to course evaluation.

Evaluation of Support Courses and the Liberal Education Foundation

Liberal education is fundamental to professional education. Expected outcomes for the liberal arts component of professional programs have received much attention in recent years (Association of American Colleges and Universities, 2002). Expected outcomes for today's college students include effective communication skills; the use of quantitative and qualitative data in solving problems; and the ability to evaluate various types of information, work effectively within complex systems, manage change, and demonstrate judgment in the use of knowledge. In addition, students should demonstrate a commitment to civic engagement, an understanding of various cultures and global issues, and the ability to apply ethical reasoning. The goals of the liberal arts curriculum should be congruent with the university mission. Nursing faculty should work collaboratively with faculty across disciplines to ensure that the general education curriculum supports the expectations of a twenty-first-century liberal education.

Evaluation questions about general education courses should address the extent to which the courses selected enable student learning and contribute to the expected outcomes. They should also be examined for sequencing to ensure that the support courses are appropriately placed to ground and complement the major and enrich the data mix for the organization and use of knowledge in practice. To develop evaluation questions related to the general education courses, faculty must first articulate what the rationale is for each course, what the expected outcomes are from the courses, and how the courses support the major to provide a broad, liberal education. When the expectations are clear, it is easier to select the measures needed to determine whether expectations have been met. Evaluation of the outcomes of the general education courses will be discussed in the section on outcomes.

External accrediting agencies also have expectations about liberal education. The ACEN, NLN CNEA, and the CCNE state that a liberal arts education provides a strong foundation for nursing. A liberal arts foundation enhances the knowledge and practice of a nurse (American Association of Colleges of Nursing, 2013; NLN CNEA, 2015; Commission on Collegiate Nursing Education [CCNE], 2013). Box 26-2 provides a summary of the elements associated with curriculum evaluation.

BOX 26-2 Elements of Curriculum Evaluation

- Course and level objectives demonstrate sequential learning across the curriculum that builds in depth and breadth (vertical organization).
- Course objectives are congruent with level objectives, which are congruent with the program goals (internal consistency).
- Course sequencing is defined with appropriate rationale for prerequisites and co-requisites so that concepts build in depth (horizontal organization).
- Course content (coursework and clinical experiences) provides graduates with the knowledge and skills needed to fulfill course and level objectives, the program's goals, and defined competencies.
- Support courses enhance learning experiences and provide a foundation in the arts, sciences, and humanities.

Evaluation of Teaching Effectiveness

Evaluation of teaching effectiveness involves assessment of teaching strategies (including instructional materials), assessment of methods used to evaluate student performance, and assessment of student learning. Teaching strategies are effective when students are actively engaged, when strategies assist students to achieve course objectives, and when strategies provide opportunities for students to use prior knowledge in building new knowledge. Teaching effectiveness improves when teaching strategies are modified on the basis of evaluation data. See Chapter 15 for information on designing teaching strategies and student learning activities.

To demonstrate and document teaching effectiveness, faculty need multiple evaluation methods (Johnson & Ryan, 2000). Evaluation methods may include student feedback about teaching effectiveness obtained through course evaluations and focus group discussions, feedback provided through peer review, formal testing of teaching strategies, and assessment of student learning.

Student Evaluation of Teaching Strategies

The institution or nursing department may develop course evaluations to obtain student feedback on teaching effectiveness. The advantage of internally developed evaluations is that they can be customized to the program. The primary disadvantage of internally developed tools is that they may lack reliability and validity. Standardized evaluation tools, such as those found in Individual Development and Educational Assessment (IDEA), offered by the Individual Development and Educational Assessment Center at Kansas State University, and the National Survey of Student Engagement, offered by the Indiana University School of Education Center for Postsecondary Research and Planning, have documented reliability and validity and provide opportunities to compare results among and between academic programs, departments, schools with the institutional score, and a national benchmark.

Focus groups have been used extensively in marketing and social research, and have the potential to serve as powerful tools for program evaluation (Wilson, Morreale, Waineo, & Balon, 2013). A focus group discussion with students can provide a qualitative assessment of teaching effectiveness. Focus groups provide an opportunity to obtain insights and to hear student perspectives that may not be discovered through formal course evaluations. The focus group leader should be an impartial individual with the skill to conduct the session. The leader should clearly state the purpose of the session, ensure confidentiality, provide clear guidelines about the type of information being sought, and explain how information will be used. Group leaders should solicit opinions from all participants, record all comments, and produce a formal report (Nestel et al., 2012). The reliability and validity of information obtained from a focus group discussion is enhanced when the approach is conducted as research with a purposeful design and careful choice of participants. However, the danger is that students may not be willing to share negative aspects of the course or faculty because of the fear of the information not being confidential. It is important to develop a rapport between the focus group members and the interviewers so that there is mutual trust and respect.

Peer Review of Teaching Strategies

Peer and colleague review may provide information on teaching effectiveness through classroom observation and assessment of course materials. In this context, a peer is defined as another faculty member within the same discipline with expertise in the field, and a colleague is an individual outside of the discipline with expertise in the art and science of teaching. Peer review can serve to promote quality improvement of teaching effectiveness and as documentation for performance review. Before peer review is implemented, there is a need to be clear about what data will be gathered, who will have access to the data, and for what purposes they will be used. Faculty and administrators, as stakeholders in the endeavor, should collaborate to establish the norms and standards. Data from peer review may be used prescriptively to assist faculty in developing and improving teaching skills. At some point, peer review data may be needed for performance review and administrative decision making. Some schools require both classroom visits and opportunities to observe master teachers for all new faculty and periodic classroom visits for all faculty thereafter. In some schools the observation of teaching is voluntary. The age of the classroom as the private domain of the teacher is disappearing rapidly, and both accountability and the opportunity to demonstrate the scholarship of teaching are causing colleges and universities to require increased documentation of teaching as a routine part of the evaluation process.

Although classroom observation has been used as a technique for the peer review of teaching for a number of years, the reliability and validity of this method has been suspect. The validity and reliability of classroom observation as an evaluation tool is increased by (1) including multiple visits and multiple, unbiased visitors; (2) establishing clear criteria in advance of the observation; (3) ensuring that participants agree about the appropriateness and fairness of the assessment instruments and the process; and (4) preparing faculty to conduct observations (Danielson, 2012; Rui & Feldman, 2012). Before classroom teaching visits are made, the students should be advised of the visit and should be assured that they are not the focus of the observation. Peer reviewers should meet with the faculty member before the visit and review the goals of the session, what has preceded and what will follow the session, planned teaching methods, assignments made for the session, and an indication of how this class fits into the total program. This provides a clear image for the visitors and establishes a beginning rapport. Some faculty have particular goals for growth that can be shared at this time as areas for careful observation and comment. Finally, a postvisit interview should be conducted to review the observation and to identify strengths and areas for growth. This may include consultation regarding strategies for growth with the scheduling of a return visit at a later date. Many visitors interview the students briefly after the visit to determine their reaction to the class and to ascertain whether this was a typical class rather than a special, staged event. Unless there is a designated visiting team, the faculty member to be visited is usually able to make selections or at least suggestions about the visitors who will make the observation. Peer visits to clinical teaching sessions should follow the same general approach as classroom visits, although specific criteria for observation will be established to meet the unique attributes of clinical teaching and learning. An additional requirement is that the visitor be familiar with clinical practice expectations in the area to be visited.

Evaluation of Teaching and Learning Materials

The review of teaching and learning materials is another element of evaluation of teaching effectiveness that may be conducted through peer review. Materials commonly included for review are the course syllabus, textbooks and reading lists, teaching plans, teaching or learning aids, assignments, and outcome measures. In all cases, the materials are reviewed for congruence with the course objectives, appropriateness to the level of the learner, content scope and depth, clarity, organization, and evidence of usefulness in advancing students toward the goals of the course.

The syllabus is reviewed to determine whether expectations are clear and methods of evaluation are detailed. It is especially important that students understand what is required to "pass" the course. Grading scales and weighting of each of the evaluation methods used in the course should be explained.

In the review of textbooks for their appropriateness for a given course, multiple elements may be considered. The readability of a text relates to the extent to which the reading demands of the textbook match the reading abilities of the students. This assumes that the faculty member has a profile of student reading scores from preadmission testing. Readability of a textbook is usually based on measures of word difficulty and sentence complexity. Other issues of concern include the use of visual aids; cultural and sexual biases; scope and depth of content coverage; and size, cost, and accuracy of the data contained within the text (Sellers & Haag, 1993). Another factor of importance is the analysis of the textbook. This element relates to the organization and presentation of material in a logical manner that increases the likelihood of the reader's understanding of the content and ability to apply the content to practice. A review should determine the ratio of important and unimportant material and the extent to which important concepts are articulated, clarified, and exemplified. Do the authors relate intervening ideas to the main thesis of a chapter and clarify the relationships between and among central concepts? The ease with which information can be located in the index is important so that students can use the book as a reference. Because of the high cost of textbooks, it is useful to consider whether the textbook will be a good reference for other classes in the curriculum. A review of a textbook must also include consideration of whether the content has supported student learning. When student papers or other creative products are used for evaluation purposes, it is common to review a sample of these papers or products that the teacher has judged to be weak, average, and above average to provide a clearer view of expectations and how the students have met those expectations. This review provides an opportunity to demonstrate student outcomes. If a faculty member wants to retain copies of student papers and creative works to demonstrate outcomes, he or she should obtain informed consent from the students. Accrediting bodies often wish to see samples of student work, and faculty may use them to demonstrate learning outcomes for purposes of their own evaluation. Each student's identity should be protected and consent should be obtained.

The review of teaching and learning aids depends on the organization and use of these materials. The organization may be highly structured in that all are expected to use certain materials in certain situations or sequences, or materials may be resources available to faculty and students for use at their discretion according to the outcomes they wish to achieve. Students may be expected to search for and locate materials, to create materials to facilitate their learning, or simply to use the materials provided in a prescribed manner. The emphasis will determine whether evaluation questions related to materials are based on variety, creativity, and availability or whether the materials have been used as intended. Regardless of the overall emphasis, teaching and learning materials should be evaluated for efficiency and cost-effectiveness. Efficiency can be evaluated by determining whether the time demands and effort required to use the materials are worth the outcomes achieved. Cost-effectiveness can be determined by considering whether the costs of the materials justify the outcomes.

Formal Measures for Evaluating Teaching Strategies

Formal, objective measures of teaching strategies may include experimental or quasiexperimental designs, with randomization of subjects and control of treatments. For example, a teacher may establish a control group and a treatment group to try different teaching techniques and to evaluate outcomes to prove or disprove a predetermined hypotheses. This technique is often used when there are multiple sections of a given course, although it can be accomplished within a section. A common method is to use the traditional strategy with the control group and the new strategy with the experimental group. A common examination or other assessment measure is used with both groups. Analysis may include checking for a significant difference in the scores of the two groups, as well as checking areas in which the most questions were missed for congruence or no congruence between the two groups.

A weakness of some of these efforts is that they are context bound and not generalizable. A strength of these testing strategies is the provision of feedback of value to evaluation questions within a given curriculum.

Another measure for evaluating teaching strategies is to have faculty complete a course report. The course report provides a record of the types of instructional methods used, the rationale for choosing these methods, and results of changes to these methods. Course reports can be reviewed annually through a peer review process or by program administrators. See Box 26-3 for a sample of a didactic course report for the evaluation of teaching strategies and Box 26-4 for a sample of a clinical course report for the evaluation of teaching strategies.

Assessment of Student Learning

It is unacceptable to claim that teaching strategies are effective unless there is evidence that links the teaching transaction with student learning. Assessment within the classroom provides evidence for interim outcome evaluation. Interim evaluation refers to outcomes of specific learning episodes, course outcomes, or level outcomes as opposed to outcomes assessed at the conclusion of the program of learning. Glennon (2006) notes that outcomes relate directly to professional practice and differentiates this from objectives that relate to instruction. Course grades are often subjective and insufficient. Therefore real outcomes are needed not only to assist students in learning better but also to aid faculty in better assessing student learning. (Glennon, 2006).

Both formal and informal methods may be used in the classroom to assess student progress and to evaluate the effectiveness of teaching strategies. Chapters 23, 24, and 25 cover these methods in detail. Informal classroom assessment is useful to

---

BOX 26-3 Example: Course Report for a Didactic Course

PROGRAM EVALUATION PLAN: TEACHING STRATEGIES EVALUATION

The Program Evaluation Plan asks the following questions about teaching strategies and curriculum evaluation: (1) "Are we doing what we meant to do?" (2) "Are we doing the right things right?" This part of the program evaluation plan examines (a) teaching strategies, (b) the ability of chosen teaching strategies to accomplish course objectives, (c) opportunities to expand students' knowledge base, and (d) evaluation of student performance.

TEACHING STRATEGIES

1. Teaching strategies facilitate achieving course objectives.
2. Rationale can be identified for all major teaching strategies.
3. Teaching strategies provide opportunities to use prior knowledge in building new knowledge.
4. Teaching strategies are modified based on evaluation data.

List each course objective.

1. List the teaching strategies for each objective.
2. Identify the rationale for each strategy.
3. Identify how prior knowledge is used in building new knowledge. Examples of strategies include textbooks, assignments, presentations, homework, supplemental assigned readings, lectures, discussions in class or in online discussion forums, audiovisuals, group activities, guest speakers, web-based/web-supported courses, other.
4. Describe the effectiveness of each strategy. Include student comments where appropriate. What will be changed the next time you teach this course?

BOX 26-4 Example: Course Report for a Clinical Course

PROGRAM EVALUATION PLAN: TEACHING STRATEGIES EVALUATION

1. Teaching strategies facilitate achieving clinical objectives.
2. Rationale can be identified for all major teaching strategies.
3. Teaching strategies provide opportunities to use prior knowledge in building new knowledge.
4. Teaching strategies are modified based on evaluation data.

List each course objective.

1. List the teaching strategies used for each objective.
2. Indicate the rationale for each strategy.
3. Identify how prior knowledge is used in building new knowledge. Examples of strategies include daily data sheets, journaling, nursing process papers/care plans, instructor skill demonstration (lab or clinical), student return demonstration (lab), direct observation of skill performance and nursing care given, questioning, observational experiences, planned teaching projects, post conferences, role play activities, case studies, computer-based activities/study modules, math competency testing, skills testing in lab, purposeful teaching assignments, and other.
4. Describe the effectiveness of each strategy. Include student comments where appropriate. What will be changed the next time you teach this course?

the teacher for determining how well students are learning. Data from the assessment can be used by the teacher in making changes to improve student learning. This form of classroom assessment is often not graded and is anonymous to get honest feedback. However, faculty also use more formal classroom assessments that are graded to get a feel for the quality of the teaching and determine how well the students are learning,

Students can use the formative assessment to set their own academic goals, compare how hard they have worked or methods used for studying with what they have learned, and to help them prepare for future assessments (Reig, 2007).

The use of formalized external testing in prelicensure programs is another option that assists in the evaluation of student learning. For example, several commercial testing products provide both content mastery and comprehensive predictor examinations that provide indicators of student learning. These assessments provide questions similar to those that students will experience on the licensure examination and provide faculty with feedback that indicates need for improvement in specific content areas. Faculty can then provide focused review of content in which students' scores were low. Tracking student scores in individual nursing courses also can be insightful in revising course content as well as curricula to improve student learning outcomes.

Evaluation of individual student performance must be effectively communicated to students. Documentation should provide evidence that evaluation leads to improvement in performance. This is especially important in clinical evaluation. Clinical evaluation tools should be congruent with course and program objectives. They should be designed to provide students with clear information about expectations. The evaluation tool should clearly demonstrate the student's performance as well as the appropriate feedback provided regarding their performance and how it can be improved. The tools should also include information about how students responded to the feedback and how behavior changed.

Evaluating Student Performance Measures

In addition to documenting that teaching methods are effective, methods of evaluating student performance must be valid and reliable. Multiple-choice examinations are a common, cost-effective, and time-efficient method of testing knowledge acquisition both as students progress in a course and at the conclusion of the course and program. This format provides rapid, quantitative data for individual assessment and aggregate data for centralized evaluation. Other methods of evaluation are discussed in Chapters 23, 24, and 25.

Box 26-5 provides a summary of the elements associated with evaluation of teaching effectiveness. Box 26-6 provides an example of a course report related to student performance.

Evaluating Student Admission, Progression, and Graduation Policies and Procedures

The evaluation of admission, progression, and graduation (APG) policies and procedures begins with an examination of whether a sufficient number of qualified students are enrolled. Academic

BOX 26.5 Evaluation of Teaching Effectiveness

- Students are satisfied with teaching strategies.
- Teaching strategies are modified based on evaluation data.
- Teaching strategies facilitate achieving course objectives.
- Teaching materials are effective and efficient.
- Evaluation of individual student performance is communicated to students and leads to improvement in performance.
- Methods of evaluating student performance are valid.

and demographic profiles of prospective students are important to consider. A first consideration is the mission and goals of the institution and school or department. If diversity is a goal, the selection of students will be different than in schools where high selectivity is a goal. State and private schools may differ in the types of students they wish to attract. Trends in health care provide an important database for defining student enrollment goals. For example, health care reform has opened the market for nurse practitioners to the extent that many schools of nursing have targeted this population. Once a determination of the nature of the student to be recruited has been made, the methods

BOX 26-6 Example: Course Report—Theory

PROGRAM EVALUATION PLAN: TEACHING STRATEGIES EVALUATION

Evaluation of Student Performance

1. Methods of evaluating student performance are valid and consistently applied.

Course Evaluation of Student Performance

Exams	Data	Describe the effectiveness of these methods. Include student comments where appropriate.	What will be changed the next time you teach this course?
How do you use item analysis to improve your tests?	List range of KR 20 values on unit exams, excluding the final exam. Range Fall Spring Summer (The KR20 has a normal range between 0.00 and 1.00 with higher numbers indicating higher internal consistency. You should not expect a score higher than 0.80 [commercially available tests will approach 0.95]).	Comment on reliability of your tests, difficulty level of the tests, and the ability of questions to discriminate between high/low achievers.	
What percent of the course grade is the final exam/assignment? (specify which)	Fall ________% Spring ________% Summer ________% ________exam ________assignment		
Is the final exam/assignment comprehensive?	Fall ________ yes ________ no Spring ________ yes ________ no Summer ________ yes ________ no		

BOX 26-6 Example: Course Report—Theory—cont'd

Course Evaluation of Student Performance

How many students (number and percent of class) did **not** achieve an average exam score of 80%, but passed the course based on written assignments, homework, and/or student presentations?	Fall	________ ________ %
	Spring	________ ________ %
	Summer	________ ________ %

Other Methods of Evaluation

What other methods of evaluation are used in this course?	________ Written assignments ________ Student presentations ________ Homework ________ Blackboard discussion ________ Quizzes ________ Other (List ___)
Rubrics are used for all other graded work (yes or no). If no, what is used to determine validity and assure consistent application?	yes no (explain)
Grading policies from the Dept. of Nursing Policy Manual are followed in this course (yes or no). If no, describe what and why.	yes no (explain)

External measures of student performance (ATI):

			What did you learn from test analysis data provided by ATI?	What (and why) will be changed the next time you teach this course?
Identify ATI Content Mastery test given in this course.				
What was the total number of students that took the Content Mastery Exam?	Fall Spring	________ ________		
What number and percent of class achieved the benchmark on the test? (Proficiency Level 2 and above)	Fall Spring	________ % ________ %		

ATI, Assessment Technologies Institute.

of recruitment require attention. Marketing methods and materials should be reviewed in terms of access to catchment targets, clarity of the message delivered, and results of the effort. An entry inquiry as to the source of the student's information about the school is one way to determine the extent to which marketing materials influenced application decisions.

Admission policies should be clearly defined and support program goals. They should be reliable and valid with a goal of preventing unnecessary attrition while graduating students who are well qualified and who will ultimately pass licensing or certification exams. Student profiles are an important way to track trends in the characteristics of students admitted to programs of learning. Many colleges and universities require entrance examinations related to basic skills, including standardized examinations such as the Scholastic Aptitude Test or discipline-specific tests and institutional examinations in mathematics, English, and reading skills. Grade inflation in both secondary and postsecondary schools has rendered transcript review a difficult measure of student ability. Breckenridge, Wolf, and Roszkowski (2012), found a variety of factors contributed to success in prelicensure students and identified a variety of risk factors. In addition to factors such as GPA, SAT, and grades in science courses, other factors such as income at poverty level and having English as a second language were even more important to academic success and passing the licensing exam. A relationship between scores on the Test of Essential Academic Skills from Assessment Technologies Institute is also predictive of success (Newton, Smith, Moore, & Magnan, 2007). It may be helpful to use an overall profile of criteria to guide the selection of students with attributes suited to the challenges of current health care delivery systems and who more closely match the diversity of the populations they serve.

Admission policies should be checked for discriminatory elements. One must sort those educational discriminators that ensure a fit between the student and the program of learning, and those that are clearly discriminatory from the perspective of social justice. For example, it is appropriate to require that students complete any remediation before admission to the program so they will have the basic skills necessary for success, especially if diversity is a goal. It is not appropriate and it is illegal to exclude students on the basis of gender, sexual orientation, religion, race, or ethnic origin.

Many states are increasing high school requirements with a concurrent shift in college entrance requirements. Individuals who perform evaluation reviews must keep abreast of these changes to maintain congruence and to determine what remediation programs may be needed for students who graduated from high school before the increased requirements were established. Plans must be in place to ensure communication of the changes in a timely fashion. Some programs find it useful to complete correlation studies to determine the relationship of admission criteria to such outcome measures as program completion or success on licensing or certification examinations after graduation. Although this approach does not measure the potential success of those not admitted, it may provide data about criteria that seem to have little relationship to success indicators.

Progression must be fair and justifiable, support program goals, and be congruent with institutional standards. For example, are there conditions for progression related to grade point average at the end of each semester? If a student must drop out of school for any reason, what are the conditions and standards for return? Are they realistic? Are they known to the students? Do they apply equally to all students with exceptions made only in cases that are clearly exceptional?

Records of student satisfaction and formal complaints should be used as part of the process of the student dimension evaluation. An academic appeals process should be in place for students who wish to challenge rulings, and students should know about the process and how to access it. Some form of due process should be in writing and in operation for the review of disputes regarding course grades or progression decisions. Whether these are discipline specific or campus specific is a function of the size and complexity of the institution. An annual review of appeals and the decisions regarding those appeals provides important information for making revisions to policies and processes that are in place or are needed. All stakeholders should participate in appeals reviews. Most programs have an appeals committee composed of both students and faculty with channels to administrative review.

An internal method of review is to survey or interview students who leave the program. An obvious data set is information about why students are leaving. Common reasons include academic difficulties or academic dismissal, financial problems, role conflicts, family pressure, military service, and health issues. An examination of the underlying reasons for leaving often suggests alternatives for intervention that reduces the attrition rate. These alternatives may relate to student services or specific program issues.

Some programs also gather data about antecedent events that may have influenced the potential to complete the program. The extent of data gathered depends on the goals of the review. Data that can be gathered from the student record are not included on the student survey. With the student's permission, data obtained from the record may include preentrance test scores, grade point average, progression point at the time of withdrawal, specific course grades, and any history of withdrawals and returns. These data are extensive but can be used to develop a profile of the student who does not complete a program in an attempt to identify elements within the control of the school for potential intervention strategies. Including a control group of students who completed the program in the study gives more meaning to the findings by identifying success indicators and allowing for determination of significant differences between the two groups. Box 26-7 provides a summary of the elements associated with evaluation of APG policies and procedures.

Evaluation of the Faculty

There must be a sufficient number of qualified faculty to accomplish the mission, philosophy, and expected outcomes of the program. The nature of the program, the expectations of the parent institution, the number of students, and the requirements of accrediting bodies influence the desired number and qualifications of faculty. Qualifications of faculty may be measured from several perspectives: credentials, diversity, and professional experience.

> **BOX 26-7** Evaluation of Admission, Progression, and Graduation Policies and Procedures
>
> - An adequate number of qualified students are recruited to maintain program viability.
> - Admission policies are clearly defined, published, and support program goals.
> - Progression policies are fair and justifiable, published, and support program goals.
> - Records of student satisfaction and formal complaints are used as part of the process of ongoing improvement.
> - Possible reasons for attrition are evaluated and addressed.

Qualifications of Faculty

Faculty should possess credentials appropriate to their teaching assignment, to the program levels in which they teach, and to the service and scholarship mission of the school. Faculty members' professional experience, education, and specialty certification should be congruent with their teaching assignments. Evaluation of the level of degree preparation of nursing faculty is related to the program level in which they teach. A master's degree in nursing is the minimum expectation for teaching in associate or baccalaureate degree programs. A doctorate in nursing or a terminal degree in a related field with a master's degree in nursing is the expectation for teaching in graduate programs. Many nursing schools also strive to have faculty with terminal degrees teaching in prelicensure nursing programs. The nursing profession has been challenged to meet these expectations because of the lack of nurses with terminal degrees. The AACN 2013 Annual Report stated that only 47.9% of nursing faculty are doctorally prepared. This report also identified that approximately 88% of unfilled nursing faculty positions are still seeking candidates with doctoral degrees in nursing or a related field (American Association of Colleges of Nursing, 2014). To address the shortage of nurses with terminal degrees, some nursing schools may provide additional incentives and support to faculty with master's degrees to assist them in pursuing their doctorates. In this situation, care must be taken to avoid "inbreeding," which may result in a disproportionate number of faculty with degrees from the same institution. Representation of a wide variety of educational institutions in the faculty profile demonstrates a commitment to diversity of ideas and openness to creative differences. "Inbreeding" of faculty may perpetuate the status quo.

Evaluation of faculty qualifications should also include the profile of faculty related to rank, classifications for tenure or non–tenure track appointments, and the balance of full-time and part-time positions. Assessment of the number and proportion of faculty for each level of rank provides a measure of faculty experience and expertise in their teaching role. If few faculty members within the school have achieved higher ranks, such as associate or full professor, there may be a lack of senior-level faculty or an inequity in nursing promotions compared with other academic units. In some universities, there are multiple categories of faculty, including non–tenure-track lecturers and clinical instructors, tenure-track faculty, and scientist tracks (see Chapter 1). In some universities, only tenure-track faculty may participate in the governance of the larger institution. Standing committees within both the school and the university may have criteria for rank and tenure as a condition of membership. A goal of full participation in governance issues at the university level can be compromised or enabled by the number of faculty eligible to participate. On the other hand, a faculty composed largely of tenured members could be a barrier to the recruitment of a more diverse faculty or a goal of increasing the number of faculty members with specific areas of expertise. The balance of full-time and part-time faculty is also of concern in ensuring adequate involvement in governance, meeting needs for academic advising, curriculum development, and program evaluation.

Setting goals for faculty qualifications allows the nursing school to measure progress in achieving those goals. Once the goals for qualified faculty have been identified, the faculty profile can be evaluated or analyzed in terms of those goals. Factors that may be interfering with the achievement of the goals will also need analysis. It is essential to track the profile of faculty who are within 5 to 10 years of retirement and to examine reasons for faculty turnover. Control of the faculty profile is influenced not only by recruitment goals but also by faculty retention factors.

A factor related to both recruitment and retention of qualified faculty is the salary structure. If a goal of the school of nursing is to support quality programs and to achieve national stature, salaries must be competitive to attract the mix of faculty that promotes excellence. There are multiple sources for comparison of salaries. Internally, it is important to demonstrate that faculty salaries in the school are congruent with those in the larger institution for comparable rank and productivity. External data are available from such sources as the AACN, the NLN, the American Association of University Professors, and regional groups such as the Big Ten universities. AACN provides salary information for full-time administrative and instructional nursing faculty, including mean and median salaries by rank and degree, and by region of the country (American Association of Colleges of Nursing, 2014). The College and University Professional Association for Human Resources conducts an annual survey of faculty salaries for public and private institutions offering baccalaureate and higher degrees. The National Faculty Salary Survey for Four-Year Institutions provides salary data by discipline and rank (College and University Professional Association for Human Resources, 2014). The results of this survey are available online. In addition, customized reports that sort data by variables such as region of the country, size of the institution's operating budget, and religious affiliation for private schools can be requested. Customized reports may provide a more accurate comparison in determining how faculty salaries compare with peer institutions. Some nursing schools may be able to obtain salary information by networking with a select cohort of peer institutions that agree to share data.

Faculty Development

Faculty development begins with orientation to the university or college, school, and department or division. In this orientation, faculty begin the process of socialization into the academy. They are introduced to the mission and goals of the institution and school at each level represented in the structure. Expectations are reviewed and any documents that will reinforce and guide movement toward those expectations are shared. For example, new faculty are usually given the institutional handbook that contains general policies and teaching, service, and research expectations. Support systems and personnel available to maintain them are introduced and a tour of the physical plant is conducted. More specific orientation occurs at each level. In addition to faculty development offerings at the campus and institutional levels, the school or department may offer a series of open and planned sessions for new and continuing faculty. The focus of the sessions may be related to common concerns, concerns identified through a needs analysis, or issues related to changes in the school. For example, many schools are offering regular sessions on the use of new technology as it is acquired. It may be necessary to offer faculty development related to policy changes, curriculum changes, or any other new development in the school or institution.

Once orientation is completed, faculty should receive support for professional development. Universities may have an office of research to assist faculty in research efforts or may have teaching centers or technology experts to assist faculty in their teaching role. Use of travel monies and planning that encourages faculty to attend conferences, seminars, and research colloquia are important parts of development and should be implemented and tracked as a part of the evaluation effort.

An increasing number of schools are developing mentoring programs that may provide generalist mentoring or specific mentoring in research and teaching. Mentoring is a multidimensional activity that consists of highly individualized dyadic processes and relationships. The ideal mentor is dedicated to helping the mentee develop in both a personal and professional way. The attributes of the mentor include: credibility, trustworthiness, generosity, and the possession of qualities that the mentee wants to emulate (Carey & Weissman, 2010), the mentor and mentee develop a reciprocal relationship in which there is a knowledge differential between participants, and a relationship effect beyond the mentor relationship. Mentors listen, affirm, counsel, encourage, seek input, and help the novice develop status and career direction. Whatever the view of the mentor, the role needs to be clear to the mentor and mentee and allow for individualization. In large schools, the assignment of a mentor may occur at the department level. In smaller schools, the assignment is often the responsibility of a central administrator or a school committee of faculty. It is common for a senior faculty member to be assigned as a mentor for a period of 1 year, with continuing assignment based on individual need or the development plan. Each member of the mentoring dyad should evaluate the nature and effectiveness of the mentoring relationship at the end of the year or at regular intervals if the relationship extends beyond the year. The role of the mentor may vary by institution, but common functions include advice and counsel, review of course materials, observation of instruction, assistance in processing evaluation data, modeling master teaching, encouragement, and coaching.

Those who provide mentoring for research often assist the faculty member in accessing support systems on campus identifying funding sources, and developing a research focus. The mentor can also serve as a resource as the mentee progresses in meeting promotion and tenure expectations. The purpose of the relationship is generally consultative and constructive; however, some schools may prefer a more directed, prescriptive approach, especially with new faculty. In an effort to create safety and opportunity for faculty development, the mentor does not become an evaluator.

Finally, larger schools may have their own department of continuing education. In those schools, one expectation of that department may be to participate in faculty development. Through continuing education, a department may offer a series of workshops related to teaching strategies, test construction, evaluation, or other issues of concern to faculty in general. These are usually open to others as well to create a more diverse mix of participants and to provide fiscal support to the department. Some continuing education departments assist faculty in hosting conferences related to their areas of expertise and cosponsor research colloquia or other events that serve faculty in their professional development and provide an opportunity for faculty to share their professional expertise as presenters.

Faculty Scholarship

Faculty achievements in scholarly activity should support program effectiveness. Many schools use Boyer's (1990) model of scholarship as a basis for evaluating faculty scholarship. Knowledge development (the scholarship of discovery) and the scholarship of teaching are essential to the academy, and are an expectation for all faculty (see Chapter 1). Those who select research as their area of excellence will be measured against criteria established within the school or division. Those criteria will need to withstand the scrutiny of peer review both within and beyond the discipline. The volume of research and publications is less important than the quality of the effort. Some committees ask faculty to select two or three of their best research studies and best publications for review rather than submitting the entire body of work for review. This highlights the focus on quality. An additional expectation is that evidence of both external peer review and review by one's department chairperson be included in the work submitted for review. Selection of one's works for publication or presentation is evidence of its value to the reviewers. Where publications appear may also be of importance. Articles in refereed journals and journals held in high esteem in the discipline are considered evidence of quality review. Before publication, it is important to know the standards of the given institution. For example, some schools give greater weight to articles in refereed journals or to entire books as compared with chapters in a book. Sole authorship versus joint authorship or placement in the listing of authors may be weighted as well. Invited works are often considered evidence of their value. Some institutions also consider invited creative works such as radio or television productions, videotapes, musical scores, and choreography evidence of scholarship or excellence. Receipt of major awards and other forms of recognition as a leader in one's field provides compelling evidence of quality.

Funding for research, scholarly work, and special projects is widely accepted as evidence of scholarship. Weighting may be assigned on the basis of the source of the monies. Internal funding may not be weighted as heavily as external funding. External funding may be weighted as well. For example, funding from major foundations or federal programs may receive a more favorable review than several small grants from lesser known sources. Whether one is the principal investigator or a participant may be weighted in the review process. A growing value is attached to applied research that has meaning for a wider audience. Keys to the consideration of any scholarly endeavor are evidence of analysis and synthesis in studies grounded in theory, rather than simple descriptive studies. Variations occur according to the mission of the institution so that each school must determine criteria within the context of that mission. In the final analysis, scholarly works are best judged by one's intellectual peers.

The scholarship of application is demonstrated through professional practice and service. Practice as professional service is an area of emphasis in some institutions, whereas in other institutions faculty believe it is not valued as highly as research. Again, evidence exists that more and more institutions are attempting to develop criteria to reflect scholarly service and to grant that service the recognition it merits. A common standard of evidence of scholarly clinical practice and clinical competence is national certification in one's field, especially for those faculty who wish to seek recognition and promotion in the clinical track. With some variation based on institutional mission, the focus on service is its connection to the faculty member's professional expertise. Internally, faculty may demonstrate service through participation and leadership in committees and projects within the department or division and, more broadly, at the campus or institutional level. Committees that affect decision making for innovative enterprises or improvement and policy development demonstrate thoughtful participation. Administrative appointments are generally accepted as evidence of professional service within the institution.

Beyond the institution, faculty may demonstrate service through practice and participation in professional, civic, and governmental organizations relevant to their expertise in a manner that reflects the application of knowledge and the extension and renewal of the discovery element of scholarship. Examples include providing technical assistance to an agency and analysis of public policy for governmental agencies or private organizations. Joint appointments or contracts with practice agencies that call on professional expertise are other examples. Certainly, faculty-run clinics are a strong example of such service. Some institutions place applied research in this category of review.

In addition to the listing and description of activities in the area of service, faculty are expected to have documented evidence of the merit or worth of that service. In this area as well, letters from external sources and awards based on service are evidence of merit. Within the institution there is a need for more systematic feedback to those who provide valuable service. Often faculty receive perfunctory notes of thanks for service that do little to define the value of that service. A practice of thanking those who serve with comments about the special expertise provided and outcomes achieved as a result of that service is a valuable form of evidence.

The scholarship of integration is demonstrated through interdisciplinary research, interpreting research findings, and bringing new insight to the field of study. Presentations to the lay public that serve to advance public knowledge of discipline-related issues, development of new and creative teaching materials and modes of delivery, and professional presentations and publications are examples of integrative scholarship. The scholarship of integration may be evaluated by determining whether the activity reveals new knowledge, illuminates integrative themes, or demonstrates creative insight (Boyer, 1990).

It is not possible for a given faculty member to excel in all areas subject to review within the institution. The Boyer (1990) model attempts to respond to a need to look at scholarship differently and to provide multiple ways for faculty to demonstrate worthy productivity. Research and publication are important elements of the academy and are critical to comprehensive and research universities. Limiting the focus of faculty evaluation and reward decisions to a single area, however, discounts the valuable work of a diversified faculty. This very diversity and range of expertise enhances the reputation of an institution and enables the wise use of resources. The obligation of faculty is to provide evidence of scholarly productivity in one or more of the scholarship functions. Institutional leaders are obligated to enable that process and reward positive outcomes.

Evaluation of Faculty Performance

Evaluation of faculty performance is intended to promote quality improvement. The focus of faculty performance evaluation is guided by the philosophy, mission, and goals of the parent institution and the school or division in which the nursing program is housed. Faculty evaluations may be structured against specific job descriptions related to classroom or clinical teaching assignments and include expectations for scholarship, and service. Junior and community colleges and some colleges and universities focus heavily on the teaching and service mission of the institution within the community it serves. Faculty evaluation reflects this emphasis. Research universities share the teaching and service missions but include an emphasis on research and scholarship as well. Colleges and universities with religious affiliations may include expectations for church-related service in faculty review policies and standards.

The policy and process for faculty performance evaluation should be clearly communicated to faculty. A common approach is to require faculty to submit a yearly assessment of their performance during the preceding year and a development plan to the immediate supervisor that is consistent with the university and department missions and the department goals. Individual faculty goals may also be part of the development plan that includes the faculty member's goals as well as those identified by the supervisor. Goals can be short term and long term and should include strategies or activities planned to fulfill the goals and a timeline for completion. The goals and activities are not just related to teaching but may also be related to acquiring tenure and promotion. Periodic meetings with the faculty to review progress on development goals should be conducted by the supervisor or administrator.

The faculty member is expected to provide a self-evaluation at the end of the academic year that documents how performance and development goals were attained, what barriers blocked achievement of goals, and how these barriers will be overcome in the future so that performance will be improved. A portfolio process may also be used, in which the faculty member includes the development plan, self-evaluation, copies of student course evaluations, examples of scholarly work and service, or other artifacts that demonstrate faculty productivity. During the annual performance review, the supervisor reviews the faculty member's portfolio and provides written feedback on the faculty member's progress in fulfilling the job description and expectations. Depending on the processes used throughout the institution, performance evaluation may be done using standard forms with numerical rating scales. The use of standardized forms provides the opportunity to consistently analyze faculty performance across the unit and determine whether the faculty demonstrates development needs in any one particular area. For example, if a number of new faculty are not performing well on a certain measure, additional orientation or training may be needed.

Peer review provides another component for the evaluation of faculty performance. Promotion and tenure review is a well-established form of peer review already in place in most institutions of higher learning. The criteria for the evaluation are developed by faculty and implemented through a faculty committee. Committee reviews usually are composed of both formative and summative evaluation procedures. A common practice is to review faculty at the midpoint of the probationary period, usually in the third year of appointment. A formative review may occur at regular intervals before the summative tenure review is conducted. Formative reviews allow the committee to provide advice to individual faculty members in preparation for the summative review that occurs near the end of the probationary period, usually the sixth year after initial appointment. In larger institutions, a primary committee of peers at the school or division level may do the initial review of a faculty member's final tenure portfolio, along with their recommendation regarding promotion or tenure, before it is forwarded to administration and a campus committee of peers and colleagues for further review.

Final recommendations are submitted to institutional administration, the board of trustees, or other institutional governing body for final approval. Variations on this theme relate to the unique features of a given institution.

A common problem in higher education, especially in research intensive universities, is the lack of evaluation plans and criteria for all classifications of faculty. Although the criteria and processes for promotion and tenure of tenure-track faculty are usually in place and subject to ongoing review and refinement, such criteria do not always exist for others beyond the routine annual review. Some schools have non–tenure-track faculty serving in lecturer, scientist, or clinical appointments who would benefit from the same careful delineation of criteria for systematic review of their roles consistent with their job descriptions and productivity expectations. Boyer's model of scholarship and the six attributes for evaluation may provide a consistent approach to performance review for non–tenure-track faculty (Wood et al., 1998). Another group of faculty that requires evaluation and the opportunity to grow and develop is the part-time faculty cohort. Increasingly, expectations for annual review of part-time faculty with reappointment are contingent on favorable reviews. Adaptation of the tenure-track evaluation format can provide direction to create similar evaluative processes for non–tenure-track and part-time faculty.

External factors may influence elements of faculty evaluation. For example, external bodies such as state legislatures and education commissions may establish standards for accountability that must be met by all higher education programs in the state. A common example is in the teaching component of the faculty role. There are often mandates for faculty workload in terms of credit hours or classes taught. There are multiple ways to address this standard. Whatever productivity model is used, certain general standards apply. Faculty workloads should be designed to meet the mission and goals of the parent institution and the school or division and include those elements of the professional role of faculty emphasized by the institution (teaching, service, research). Although equity of workload expectations is an important standard, so is the flexibility to negotiate assignments to meet the needs of the school. Box 26-8 provides a summary of the elements associated with evaluation of the faculty.

BOX 26-8 Elements of Faculty Evaluation

- Faculty members are qualified and sufficient in number to accomplish the mission, philosophy, and expected outcomes of the program.
- Faculty receive orientation that prepares them to be successful.
- Faculty receive adequate support for professional development.
- Faculty achievements in scholarly activity support program effectiveness and the mission of the university.
- Evaluation of faculty performance promotes quality improvement.
- Aggregate and individual faculty outcomes demonstrate program effectiveness.

Evaluation of Learning Resources

Classroom and laboratory facilities need to provide an effective teaching and learning environment to support program effectiveness. A review of instructional space includes evaluation of support space and a determination of whether classrooms are of sufficient size, number, and comfort to facilitate teaching and learning. Support space might include a learning resource center, a simulation laboratory, a computer cluster, and storage for instructional equipment and supplies. Additional support space may include lounges for students, staff, and faculty. In addition, office space and equipment, as well as conference rooms and space to support faculty teamwork and research, are needed. Faculty need to have individual offices that have floor-to-ceiling walls to provide privacy for counseling, sensitive advisement, and evaluation conferences. Beyond these basic elements, space requirements are dictated by the mission and goals of the program. The space available should be congruent with the productivity expected of those who use the space, equipment, and supplies. This element is often reviewed through surveys of faculty, students, and staff. Another component of this review is documentation of holdings. It is important not only to have space and equipment needed to accomplish the mission and program goals but also to know where it is located and how well it is maintained.

Clinical facilities should be evaluated to determine their effectiveness in providing appropriate learning experiences in relation to the mission and goals of the program. This evaluation includes consideration of the patients served by the facility. It is important to assess whether the patient population profile is consistent with the learning objectives of the program and whether the number of patients is sufficient to support the student population. It is equally important for the standard of care provided by the institution to be of high quality so that students will be socialized to high standards. One measure of quality is the accreditation of the facility. Another is the expert judgment of the faculty members who review the facility. The willingness of staff to interact with students in a facilitative manner is important, as is the skill of staff as role models. It is important to know how many other student groups are using the same facility and units within the facility and how easily reservations for these areas can be scheduled. Any special restrictions or requirements may also influence decisions about use of the facility.

Evaluation of the clinical experience may also include review of agency contracts. These contracts should be filed in a central location and should be reviewed on a regular schedule. The conditions of the agreement should be spelled out, and some standards must be met. For example, all contracts should include the process and time frame for canceling or discontinuing the contract with a clause that allows any students scheduled for that facility to complete the current course of study. It is also important that faculty maintain control of student assignments and evaluations within the framework of the agreed-on restrictions and regulations. A review of contracts by legal counsel will ensure that expert judgment has been applied to the legal parameters of the contract.

Some schools have developed and implemented faculty-run clinics that also serve as learning sites for students. Reviews and contracts related to student learning in these clinics should be subject to the same evaluation as any other facility under consideration.

Instructional Technology

Information and instructional technology must be up to date and support the achievement of program goals. Productivity is directly related to the technology available to students and faculty, which enables them to meet their responsibilities and to create a dynamic learning environment. Outcome measures can be specifically stated in this area. For example, one might state that increasing numbers of faculty incorporate virtual simulations into teaching methods until all faculty use virtual experiences to enhance student learning. Another outcome measure might state that virtual technology will be integrated throughout curricula by a stated target date. Assessment of virtual lab usage that includes frequency of use and type of learning experiences from simple to complex simulations can be completed. Faculty and student satisfaction with the virtual lab is another effective outcome measure. Technology needs should be linked broadly to the mission and goals of the school and specifically to the teaching, scholarship, and learning needs of faculty and students.

Also, an assessment of student and faculty skills in the use of information technology at the time of admission or employment should be included. These data provide information for student and faculty development opportunities in the use of both software and hardware in the school itself and in resource facilities such as the library or a computer laboratory. Exciting advances have been made in instructional technology available for the teaching and learning of skills in nursing, but they require planning for availability of the equipment and software and preparation of faculty and students to use these resources. Creating a collaborative relationship with the information system's personnel is necessary to ensure an effective, ongoing dialogue between users of technology (faculty and students) and personnel who maintain the technology equipment.

Distance Education

Distance education is becoming more common in higher education and in nursing education. Distance education, in the context of course credit hour allocation and program review, is defined by various national and state commissions of higher education. In one state, a course is considered to be offered at a distance if 80% of the course content is offered at a distance and a program is considered to be offered at a distance if 80% of the program requirements are offered at a distance (Definitions of Distance Education (courses, programs and students) for SIS Coding and Compliance Review and Reporting Credit Hour Allocation, 2013). Mixed or blended models can also be found where learners use printed and electronic materials and come together face-to-face at specific intervals in addition to the online or distance component.

When a program uses distance education for part or all of course delivery, the influence of this delivery mode on program outcomes, teaching–learning practices, and the use of technology and the teaching and learning quality that results must be considered in evaluation. Methods of data collection may need modification for distance education programs. Because students are not on-site, creative methods such as the use of video and portfolios may be needed to assess student learning. Different instructional strategies that are interactive and creative are needed. Recruitment and retention of students require special consideration in distance education because some students may lack the motivation or technological competence to be successful. Other aspects of program implementation that need special consideration for distance education include faculty development and support, student orientation and instruction on how to learn on-line, and learning resources and support services. The appropriate technology, especially Internet delivery modes, and user support must be available to sustain distance education. Costs associated with distance education should be considered in the financial analysis. (See also Chapter 21.)

Library Resources

Library resources must be sufficient to support the programs of learning offered by the institution and the school. Issues of concern in this evaluation include the holdings (books and journals), services, and rates of use. Faculty, students, and librarians are important stakeholders in this review, and each cohort often has a very different perception when the same questions are asked. There is controversy about the relative importance of on-site holdings and access to holdings through interlibrary loan and online databases. Clearly, a core collection of holdings is crucial to students and faculty.

Various standards are used to measure the adequacy of library holdings. Some schools use published source lists as standards for library holdings. The *American Journal of Nursing* list of resources, based on an annual review of books, is often used as a standard. Some schools consider it important to include any required textbooks and required readings in the library holdings, at least at the undergraduate level. Graduate programs may require more extensive databases with access to more materials than undergraduate programs because of the scope of reading expectations. Faculty task forces are often assigned to review library holdings in relation to graduate education in specialty majors. Comparisons with the holdings of peer institutions with similar programs are sometimes used in these reviews. Some programs rely on the expertise of the faculty on the task force. Still others survey all faculty in the major for lists of holdings they consider to be critical. The aggregate becomes a point of reference for the review.

Library services are as important as the holdings and are usually assessed by a survey method. Evaluation of library services should occur on a consistent basis. Librarians, students, and faculty may indicate their views about services offered and the effectiveness of those services. Surveys may be internally developed and provide very specific information about library services. For example, an internal survey may review the interlibrary loan system to determine both satisfaction and levels of use related to the time frame for borrowing materials. This may be measured against an established goal, such as an average time of 1 week to secure a book. In addition to the quantitative data, an opportunity to comment on the best features and areas of concern related to library holdings and services often provides valuable qualitative data. Some libraries maintain specific use data by school or division. Others do not but can estimate whether a given group of students use the library facilities less, the same, or more than other students. Some libraries have very liberal hours and some do not. This may become an evaluation question, depending on the context.

Most libraries are able to make effective use of technology. The Internet provides access to a wide variety of resources and access to full-text articles and copying services. This type of information, ubiquitous because of the Internet, brings new opportunities and challenges to provision of information resources to students over a wide geographic area. Those who make use of this opportunity will establish specific criteria for evaluation geared to access. It is important to identify and review the databases available to faculty and students and methods used to orient them to the use of this service. Box 26-9 provides a summary of the elements associated with evaluation of learning resources.

BOX 26-9 Evaluation of Learning Resources

- Classroom and laboratory facilities provide an effective teaching and learning environment.
- Clinical facilities provide effective learning experiences.
- Information and instructional technology is up to date and supports achievement of program goals.
- Library services and holdings are comprehensive and meet needs of students and faculty.

Evaluation of Administrative Effectiveness, Structure, and Governance

The qualifications and leadership skills of program administrators are important to program effectiveness. Formal evaluation of administrators should occur annually or at regularly specified intervals. The specific evaluation of the administrator may include the extent to which the administrator guides the establishment of a clear mission and goals for the unit and the effectiveness with which the administrator represents the department or school, both internally and externally, and contributes to the reputation of the unit within and beyond the institution. Attention should be focused on the administrator's ability to raise funds and to allocate the budget in a fair and effective manner. Evidence of integrity and collegiality is an issue of concern, as are the leadership qualities of conflict resolution, decision making, motivation, and interpersonal skills.

Regardless of the university size and focus, evaluation of administrative effectiveness should be a collaborative process in which faculty members participate. Faculty members should have the opportunity to provide evaluative feedback on the performance of administrative faculty. This collaborative process can be replicated at various levels within the nursing school and the institution. For example, the responsibility for the evaluation of the nursing department chair may rest with the dean of the school; however, information from faculty members should be considered in that evaluation. This process may be repeated to the level of the vice president for academic affairs who evaluates the dean and in turn receives evaluation feedback from the faculty. At all levels, input from supervisors and subordinates is taken into consideration as the faculty or administrator writes his or her own self-evaluation, identifying strengths, plans for improvement, and goals for the upcoming year. In addition to defining the appropriate process for performance review, faculty and administrators should reflect on the effectiveness of the process, including the utility of evaluation forms and the usefulness of evaluation in improving performance.

The use of standard assessment tools, such as those provided by the IDEA Center for the evaluation of department chairs and deans, is another means of obtaining feedback on administrative effectiveness. The advantage of these standardized tools is that they provide the opportunity to compare administrative performance with national benchmarks. The disadvantage of this approach is the cost.

In addition to effective leadership, the structure and governance of the department must provide effective means for communication and problem solving. Bylaws and written policies are two mechanisms for promoting effective department governance. The nursing school's bylaws should be examined for congruence with the constitution and bylaws of the larger institution and the structures included to facilitate faculty governance in relation to academic authority. For example, it is useful to do a comparative analysis of standing committees and the mission and goals of the school. Are the standing committees configured to address major issues related to faculty affairs, student affairs, curriculum, budget, and major thrusts of the mission? In universities with a school of law, consultation is often readily available to review the fit of the bylaws with parliamentary rules and congruence checks.

The extent to which stakeholders are included in the committee structures delineated in the bylaws is important as well. For example, are students represented on appropriate committees and how are voting privileges defined? Whether the established mechanisms actually function in the manner described is another issue for evaluation. Minutes of all standing committees should be filed in a central location. These minutes should reflect membership, agenda items, salient discussions, and a precise statement of decisions made and actions taken. It is useful for evaluation follow-up to designate membership annually in the minutes of the first meeting of each committee. After each name, there should be an indicator of representation (e.g., faculty, student, alumni, consumer). In this way, one can track whether stakeholders indicated in the bylaws are in fact represented on designated committees. Representation is an intended means of integration of stakeholders, but attendance and participation are indicators of actual participation. Therefore attendance should be recorded for each meeting. Accreditation teams may review minutes for these elements and often track membership participation and decisions. Including tracking data is important. For example, the reviewer should state how decisions and documents are channeled for final decision making. If a curriculum committee recommendation was forwarded to the faculty council for deliberation and action, the date it was forwarded should be included. The minutes of the faculty council can then be tracked to ensure that the decision item moved forward in a timely fashion and what decision was made. Accurate record keeping facilitates evaluation tracking.

Policies should be evaluated for their effectiveness in supporting and guiding communication and decision making relevant to program implementation. Policies should be organized in a manual or file and should be available to all to whom they apply. Many schools provide all new faculty with an electronic or written policy manual and send updates to the manual on a regular basis. Students usually receive information related to relevant policies at an appropriate time. For example, some policies are included in the school catalogue. Policies related to specific courses are usually included in course materials. An investigation of how policies are disseminated to those affected by the policies should be a part of the evaluation of policies. A mechanism should be in place to let the appropriate constituents know about changes in policies. Policies should be reviewed annually and updated regularly. The approval documentation that should be present on every policy will demonstrate that all stakeholders had input into their development and approval. Minutes of meetings of appropriate bodies will provide evidence of discussion and action by the stakeholders. Policies need to be clearly stated and widely communicated. Evidence that policies are not followed is cause for analyzing reasons and intervening accordingly. Box 26-10 highlights elements for evaluation of administrators, organizational structure, and governance.

BOX 26-10 Evaluation of Administrators, Organizational Structure, and Governance

- Qualifications and skills of program administrators enhance program effectiveness.
- The structure and governance of the department provides effective means for communication, decision-making, and problem solving.
- Nursing faculty participate actively in the university governance system.
- There is an adequate number of qualified staff and professional personnel to support program effectiveness.

Evaluation of Fiscal Resources

Program effectiveness depends on the availability of adequate fiscal resources. The budget of the nursing unit (school or department) should be reviewed in relation to personnel, equipment and supplies, travel, and infrastructure. As a starting point, personnel salaries are reviewed in terms of supply and demand and against guidelines for faculty and staff salaries at the university and also regionally and nationally. For example, one may have indicated a desired mix of faculty to meet the mission and goals, but that mix depends on the fiscal ability to recruit and attract faculty to meet the mix outcome expectation. If a large percentage of the personnel budget is targeted for part-time faculty, it may be difficult to convert to full-time positions at a desired level to meet broad educational goals in terms of teaching, scholarship, and service. The data gathered in the comparative analysis of salaries noted previously will also have implications for the budget review. If salaries need to be upgraded or compression issues exist, there will be a need for a review of alternatives available to meet competing needs for fiscal support.

As technology advances, it becomes increasingly important to identify fiscal support for its use beyond the usual physical environment considerations noted in the physical space section. Although internal and external sources may be found for the acquisition of such technology, funding for maintenance and upgrading is an issue that requires attention. Many programs have received grants for technology hardware only to find that the monies for software, upkeep, and upgrading are not available in the budget. Careful record keeping provides a database for projecting future needs in this area, as well as the cost–benefit evaluation of technology. Decisions must be made regarding the technology that will provide the greatest return for the investment involved. These data also provide supportive evidence when one goes in search of additional funding. Solid data make a stronger case than a wish list. Future acquisitions may depend in part on the data available about the effective use of existing technology. This is a multiple stakeholder issue.

Maintenance and extension of infrastructure needs require careful documentation as well. Records of such basic issues as heating, lighting, and telephone service provide trend data for projecting future needs. The need for building maintenance and expansion for new programs must be documented; requesting funds without data will ultimately result in the need to make choices that may not be well grounded.

Funding for faculty development is important to faculty growth. Input from administration and faculty is needed to target the funds based on the mission and goals of the school and department. For example, if increased scholarship productivity is a goal, a percentage of this budget might be targeted for attending research conferences and giving presentations. A percentage might be targeted for conferences and presentations related to teaching and learning to advance excellence in teaching. Some schools designate some funds to enable students to participate in scholarly conferences or to present papers based on their student research efforts. Evaluation requires a review of the use of the monies for the designated purposes and follow-up in some cases to determine what benefit accrued to the school from the individual's activities funded by the school. Some schools indicate the amount any one person can receive in a specified period and monitor this as an evaluation measure to foster equity.

Fiscal resources may also depend on the ability of the nursing school to seek and secure external funding. The size and nature of the parent institution and the school or division will guide outcome expectations in this area. Increasingly, schools are pressed to obtain external funding for programs and scholarship efforts. The sources of stable funding also influence this area. State schools have, in the past, assumed that they would receive their funding in thirds from the state, from tuition, and from external funding. State appropriations are decreasing in most states, and efforts are being made to control increases in tuition and fees to offset this loss. As a result there is a greater need to establish clear goals for external funding and to measure progress in this area. Stated goals may be somewhat broad or very specific. For example, some schools may simply indicate that there will be evidence of increased external funding reviewed on an annual basis. In this scenario, any increase is evidence of success. Other schools may set specific goals such as indicating the percentage of increase expected every 1 or 2 years or a 5-year goal of an increase at a stated level with annual targets to achieve the long-term goal. Others indicate specifically where the increases should occur. For example, some schools indicate a desire to increase funding from specific sources such as the National Institutes of Health. These measures provide specific evaluation targets. Trend data over 5- and 10-year periods are useful for analysis of progress over time and as a database for future goals.

Another issue related to fiscal resources is development monies. Often resources must be provided to establish a fundraising program from which returns are expected. For example, many schools support a "friends of (discipline)" advisory group gathered to enable fundraising campaigns. The goals of the fundraising should be specified. Some believe that giving is more likely to occur when a specific project that is valued by potential donors is identified. Certainly, a percentage of monies should be designated to be used at the discretion of the school to advance goals, but targeted funding is also critical to success. Evaluation includes measuring the cost of the fundraising effort against resulting gains. Trend data are critical to this area. It is important to know not only the amount of giving but also the sources of those gifts and the relationship of those sources to marketing efforts.

Many schools have targeted financial incentive projects to encourage donors to engage in the educational mission. Examples include endowed chairs, centers of excellence, technology initiatives, faculty and student recognition programs, library enhancement, and programs for curricular innovations. Evaluation of the success of these initiatives reaches beyond the mere counting of dollars received. It should include the congruence of the initiative to the stated mission and goals, trend data with indicators of performance outcomes for the investment, comparisons with peer institutions, and analysis of the worth of the initiative in meeting the stated goals for that initiative.

The sources of funding are important for review as indicators for future efforts as well. Some schools have relied exclusively on alumni as a source for development monies. Others reach out to corporations and special interest groups. In nursing, for example, hospitals have often provided funding for initiatives of interest to future human resources. They are more likely to continue their interest if evaluation reports are created indicating the efficient and effective use of the monies provided. One of the elements of evaluation often overlooked in this area is the mechanism to inform donors of the outcomes achieved as a result of their generosity. This alone may affect future giving.

Another source of data for analysis and decision making is a review of the goals of funding groups and state initiatives that may have attached funding. When the goals and initiatives of external agencies are congruent with the mission and goals of the school, this may provide opportunities to apply for funds that will contribute to the desired outcome of increased external funding. These data are usually available through the parent institution, library searches, professional organizations, the office of research and development, or direct contact with the funding group.

Regardless of the sources of funding, nursing programs, like others in higher education, are facing greater expectations to be cost-effective. As colleges and universities face the need to increase quality and strengthen academic reputation, they also face state and national calls for financial accountability. Because academic programs are the primary driver of costs, it is logical that institutions of higher education examine the cost-effectiveness of academic programs. Dickeson (2010) proposed a process to prioritize academic programs by conducting a simultaneous review of programs using a common set of criteria to determine which programs are most effective, efficient, and central to the mission. The outcome of program prioritization is the strategic allocation of resources and may involve closure of less productive programs to move resources to more productive programs. Nursing schools may find themselves participating in institutional program prioritization projects in the near future. Large nursing schools with multiple nursing programs may need to conduct a school-based prioritization project to determine resource allocation among nursing programs.

An adequate number of qualified staff and professional personnel is necessary to support program effectiveness. For faculty to meet the expectations of teaching, scholarship, and service, the support personnel available to them is critical. The nature of the institution and the mission and goals also influence the standards set in this area. Nursing schools with graduate programs, for example, consider the number of graduate assistants and research assistants to be an issue of importance, and in some cases computer programmers and statisticians may be important to goal achievement.

The level of clerical and professional staff is important to all program levels. Faculty-to-staff ratios and satisfaction surveys to elicit administration, faculty, and staff perceptions about the quality of this support provide baseline data for this review. The analysis of these data may suggest the need for further data to complete a full analysis.

Many institutions of higher education have central evaluation tools and processes for the evaluation of professional and clerical staff. Others rely on school or departmental evaluation. Still others supplement the central evaluation process with unit-specific efforts. The scope of staff under review will vary widely according to the size and complexity of the school. In any event, the evaluation should focus on the job descriptions and expectations of the individuals under review and the extent to which the job responsibilities are met in terms of efficiency and effectiveness. As with all other areas of evaluation, the process should include feedback on strengths and areas for growth; the establishment of goals for growth should be appropriate to the evaluation findings. All subsequent evaluations include a review of progress toward the stated goals. A common problem encountered in staff evaluation is the finding that the role of the staff member has drifted, because of changing circumstances, from the job description. This may create tensions that negatively affect evaluation. It is therefore necessary to include a periodic review of the job description for congruence with ongoing expectations. Revisions should occur as needed and as a collaborative effort between the staff member and the appropriate supervisor.

Box 26-11 provides a summary of the elements associated with evaluation of fiscal resources.

> *BOX 26-11* **Elements of Evaluation of Fiscal Resources**
>
> - Faculty and staff salaries are commensurate with institutional, regional, and national salary guidelines.
> - Budget supports technology and instructional innovations.
> - There are fiscal resources to recruit and develop faculty and staff.
> - There is a plan to raise funds from external sources, foundations, alumni, and friends.

Evaluation of Partnerships and Relationships with External Agencies

Program effectiveness is influenced by the relationship of the nursing program with outside agencies. For example, partnerships and collaborative arrangements with health care agencies are essential to providing needed educational experiences for students. One method of facilitating these relationships is establishing an advisory board that can provide a direct communication link with these important stakeholders. The composition of the advisory board should be evaluated to determine that its membership is appropriate. The purpose and functions of the advisory board should be communicated to members and reviewed periodically for clarity. Effectiveness of the board's function can be determined by surveying board members and nursing faculty regarding their perception of the board's effectiveness in fulfilling its purpose.

Many nursing programs have agreements with other educational institutions that provide mobility pathways for students to complete upper-level degrees. An articulation agreement may define special admissions policies and the type of transfer credits that will be accepted between a community college and a university. For example, an articulation agreement may involve the admission of students in an associate degree program to a baccalaureate degree program while they are enrolled in the associate degree program. The effectiveness of these articulation agreements and mobility plans can be evaluated by having both institutions review the transfer admission criteria for appropriateness. The nursing program accepting students should conduct a periodic audit of the transcript evaluation process to ensure that transcripts are being accurately evaluated. The final test of the effectiveness of an articulation agreement is an examination of enrollment and various outcomes. Does the agreement support enrollment goals? Are students in the mobility program successful? Comparison of progression, retention, and completion rates of the students in the mobility program with those of students in a more traditional program will provide baseline data from which to determine the effectiveness of the articulation program. Box 26-12 provides a summary of the elements to consider when evaluating partnerships and relationships with external agencies associated with evaluation of the interorganizational dimension.

> *BOX 26-12* **Evaluation of Partnerships and External Agencies**
>
> - Advisory board and other communities of interest provide effective communication links with important stakeholders to support program improvements and quality.
> - Articulation and other collaborative agreements are mutually beneficial and written agreements meet requirements of both parties' organization.

Evaluating Student Support Services

The evaluation plan also includes elements of evaluating student support services prior to admission, while matriculating, and after graduation. If the program's relationship with prospective students is not satisfactory, students will be discouraged from pursuing admission. A positive relationship with prospective students begins when students receive current and accurate information about the program. Because of the cost of higher education, prospective students need accurate information about financial aid. Transcript evaluation needs to be accurate and performed in a timely manner for all transfer students. New student registration should be run efficiently and provide a welcoming atmosphere. The admission and registration process should occur efficiently in as little time and hassle as possible. Universities may lose students if there is frustration because of being sent from one place or person to another to get admitted and enrolled. After students are admitted and registered, they will need orientation to the nursing program. Orientation should provide information about nursing program policies, especially requirements for admission into clinical courses and academic progression policies.

Activities at program completion may influence the satisfaction of students and their ongoing relationship as alumni, as well as success in achieving terminal outcomes. The nursing school may offer special workshops in preparing students for licensure examinations. Career services may provide assistance in résumé preparation and job searches.

Academic advising is an important factor in program effectiveness and influences student success from program entry through completion. Some institutions use staff-level student advisers to assist students with registration and ongoing advisement, whereas others assign students to faculty advisers. Programs to educate faculty in effective advising should be evaluated for their utility. Further analysis of advising effectiveness can be determined by surveying students regarding their level of satisfaction with advising. As a component of the advising system, academic advising records are created when a student enters the program. These records should provide a thorough and objective record of student advisement. An audit of student files may be done to determine that files are set up correctly and maintained accurately through program completion.

Other aspects of the immediate environment that influence program success include housing, health services, student academic support services, business office and registrar, and co-curricular activities. One method of evaluating these functions is through student satisfaction surveys. One survey commonly used to assess the engagement of students in support services and activities on campus is the National Survey of Student Engagement (Indiana University School of Education Center for Postsecondary Research, 2014). This survey examines student engagement in effective educational practices by measuring the amount of time students spend on educationally related activities and how institutions organize the curriculum and on-campus activities to encourage student participation in campus activities. Results are provided at an institutional level, and comparisons are made with national norms.

Box 26-13 provides a summary of the elements associated with evaluation of student support services

BOX 26-13 Evaluation of Student Support Services

- Prospective students receive current and accurate information about program options, admission criteria, and financial aid.
- Student recruitment plans support admission for a diverse population of students.
- Transcript evaluation is accurate and performed in a timely manner for all transfer students.
- New student registration is run efficiently and provides a welcoming atmosphere.
- Students receive adequate orientation to the program.
- Services are in place to support an academically, linguistically, and culturally diverse group of students.
- Academic advising is effective.
- Advising records are accurate and maintained from program entry through program completion.
- Support for student learning is adequate.
- Students receive final preparation after program completion for licensure examinations.

Outcome Evaluation

The purpose of outcome evaluation is to determine how well the program has achieved the expected outcomes. This step of the evaluation plan may be integrated into the final semester courses or may be applied at exit and during alumni and employer follow-up studies. For each of the outcomes, a simple model provides a framework for assessment and evaluation. The behavior of interest must be clearly defined and the attributes of that behavior must be delineated with benchmarks set. Faculty must then determine what measures will be used to assess the behavioral attributes with rationale for the selected measures. Finally, faculty must demonstrate how the data from such assessment and evaluation measures have been used to develop, maintain, or revise curricula. To achieve this final objective for outcome evaluation, it must be placed within the context of overall program evaluation. Outcomes assessment in isolation will not provide adequate direction for program revision. Nevertheless, outcome evaluation is critical in that it may be the primary measure by which external stakeholders judge the merit of the program.

Student Outcomes

Student outcomes are measured at multiple levels in the program of learning. Student learning outcomes deal with attributes of the learner that demonstrate achievement of program goals. Examples include critical thinking, communication, and therapeutic interventions. Other areas of measurement of learner outcomes occur at the course, clinical practice, and classroom levels. This level of outcome measurement is discussed in detail in Chapters 23 through 25. Assessment of learner outcomes at the broad program level usually involve aggregate data designed to examine general measures of learner success. At this level, one can communicate to the public the extent to which one is preparing well-educated and competent practitioners to meet the human resource needs of the community.

Of particular interest are the graduation and retention rates in each program within the school. A clear understanding of the graduation and retention rates will influence decisions about recruitment and retention methods in the future. The state is interested in the graduation rate from the perspectives of human resource flow and as a measure of return on investment in the educational program. Tracking graduation rates is a measure of the productivity of a program and may provide information about the program itself. A low graduation rate or high attrition rate can indicate problems with admission criteria, the curriculum, or teaching effectiveness and mentoring of students. It is useful to track the absolute attrition of individuals over time, as well as to document the number of graduates compared with the number of program entrants by graduation year. This allows the program to track students who are readmitted and who eventually graduate. In programs with high numbers of adult students, there may be a larger number of students who leave the program because of family problems or job-related issues. They may return and graduate at a later date. Thus a given class, when defined by the admission enrollment, may have a lower attrition rate than a class defined by numbers admitted and numbers graduated in a defined expected time span for program completion

Many programs use the pass rate on national licensing examinations or certification examinations as a measure of program success. The number of graduates licensed or certified to practice in a given area is seen as a measure of production of qualified human resources. Pass rates that are lower than the benchmark set by the school or set by approval or accreditation bodies may be an indication of an issue in the nursing program such as problems with the curriculum. However, variables other than the program of learning, such as individual preparation or test anxiety, may also influence a graduate's performance on the examination. Certainly, a school should be concerned if the pass rate falls below reasonable norms, and additional assessment measures should be initiated to attempt to determine what issues may be involved and what might be done to improve those concerns. There may be issues involved that are not under the control of the nursing program.

Employment rate is an aggregate measure of product demand. The extent to which the graduates are able to find employment may provide both marketing data and a broad measure of employer satisfaction with the product a program produces. Less information may be gleaned in a tight market in which demand exceeds supply. When the demand is high, employment rates may be more an indication of need than selective employment based on the quality of the applicant. When the supply exceeds the demand, the specific applicants the employer selects may provide stronger data. If the graduates of a given program are not in demand or are not marketable, the nursing program should be evaluated to determine if the reason for the decreased marketability is related to the quality of the graduate and the curriculum. Obtaining data from potential and current employers may be useful. Ultimately, the viability of the program may be questioned.

Employer Outcomes: Graduate Employment Rates and Satisfaction

Employer surveys may provide a means to determine the extent to which the consumer believes the graduate of the program has the skills necessary to meet employment expectations. Feedback from employers provides useful data for program review. It is difficult to obtain good response rates from employer surveys. Brevity and ease of completion are key to a high response rate. This is of particular importance during a time of work redesign and increasing demands on the time of employers in health care. Extensive survey tools designed for each program with long lists of questions about skills to which the individual is asked to respond are less likely to be completed. Respondents are more likely to reply to fewer questions that have been well developed to provide useful information. Other avenues for gathering data may be useful such as focus groups made up of employers.

Gathering data related to several areas are of particular interest. Brief demographic information about the nature of the agency is helpful in learning which settings use the program graduates. Expressed concerns or commendations may be specific to a given setting. Whether the employer hires graduates of the program and to what extent are other areas of interest. It is useful to know whether an employer would hire more graduates of the program if they were available. When questions about satisfaction with particular abilities are asked, it is helpful to state them in broad terms rather than providing the traditional laundry list of individual skills. For example, data about satisfaction may be linked to the extent to which an employer believes the graduates of the program are able to problem-solve, think critically, resolve conflicts, communicate effectively, use resources efficiently, and perform essential psychomotor skills safely. These and other broad classifications of behaviors can be selected on the basis of program outcome expectations. Provision of space for comments allows for the addition of qualitative information and the opportunity to identify any specific areas of concern.

Another issue in many employer surveys is the identification of which stakeholders are in the best position to respond to particular questions. Although an administrator may be able to respond more quickly and accurately to demographic questions and inquiries about the number of graduates employed, he or she may not be in the best position to respond to questions about the skills and abilities of graduates. The administrator may respond according to perceptions based on factors other than direct observation. Some employers delegate completion of the survey. Therefore it is helpful to request information about the respondent in the cover letter that accompanies the survey. For example, one might ask for the title of the respondent as a guide for determining how likely he or she is to be in a position of interacting directly with graduates. Some schools send employer surveys to graduates

BOX 26-14 Example: Employer Survey

To improve the quality of our academic nursing program, your thoughtful and honest responses to this survey are very important to us. Darken the oval that corresponds to your response.

Section I: Program Goals	**Poor**	**Fair**	**Good**	**Excellent**
1. Example program goal #1: Value …	0	0	0	0
2. Example program goal #2: Communicate …	0	0	0	0

Section II: Components of Program Goals	**Poor**	**Fair**	**Good**	**Excellent**
3. Example: Manages an environment that promotes clients' self esteem, dignity, safety, and comfort.	0	0	0	0
4. Example: Establishes and maintains effective communication with clients, families, significant others, and health team members.	0	0	0	0
5. Example: Promotes continuity of client care by utilizing appropriate channels of communication external to the organization.	0	0	0	0

Section III: Overall Satisfaction with ASN Nursing Program	**Poor**	**Fair**	**Good**	**Excellent**
6. My overall satisfaction with this employee is:	0	0	0	0

Other Examples of Employer Survey Questions:

7. What is your primary source of information about this graduate?
8. What are your recommendations for strengthening this nursing program?
9. What suggestions do you have to facilitate transition into the professional role?
10. What changes in the health care environment will affect the educational preparation of future graduates?
11. Other comments: Survey completed by: ____ Position ____

and request that they forward the surveys to their immediate supervisors for completion. This practice is problematic in that it usually results in a low return rate and a completed survey often reflects a respondent's reaction to an individual graduate rather than the aggregate of program graduates he or she has observed. Box 26-14 provides an example of an employer survey and sample questions.

Another method of obtaining ongoing feedback about the graduates of a program is to establish an advisory committee of consumers from agencies that typically employ program alumni. Such committees often provide advice and counsel on multiple matters, but satisfaction with the product and advice about the changing needs of the marketplace are traditional agenda items for such a group.

Alumni Evaluation: Employment Rates and Profile

There are multiple avenues for obtaining alumni data. One approach is to survey students who are about to become alumni. The exit survey is a method of determining product satisfaction with a program just completed. At this point, students' perceptions are fresh in their minds. Through the exit survey, it is possible to learn which students have found employment at the time of graduation, follow up on entry data collected for comparison purposes, and identify students' perceptions about the strengths and weaknesses of the program they have just completed. An online survey generally has a higher return rate than a survey sent through the regular mail. The exit survey is usually done within 10 days of graduation and has the advantage of a higher return rate than surveys sent at a later time. A disadvantage is that the exiting students may not have had an opportunity to apply their education in a work setting, which may change their perceptions.

Another method commonly used for exit data is the focus group. A focus group provides an opportunity for a representative group of students in the graduating classes to reflect in more detail about their experiences. Selection of the moderator is important to the collection of rich and valid insights (Nestel et al., 2012; Wilson et al., 2013).

A first concern is that the moderator be skilled in group process and listening. The moderator should have several questions prepared to guide the group discussion yet be able to respond to and facilitate group discussion when other relevant issues emerge. In an end-of-program focus session, more open-ended questions encourage free-flowing responses and invite the participants to provide the amount of information they wish. If specific types of information are desired, the questions may be more structured. The more structured the question, the more reliable the data, but the trade-off may be less richness of data. One may find it useful to begin with open and broad questions and follow up with more structured questions as the discussion unfolds.

If the focus group is conducted by someone the students view as a neutral person and if that person is able to facilitate equally the expression of opposing points of view, the participants are more likely to be open in their comments and the content is likely to be more valid. Focus groups have the advantage of providing qualitative data in more detail than is usually obtained in a written survey, but they have the disadvantage of being a representative group that may or may not provide the range of data that a full group survey would provide. Use of both a survey and a focus group may resolve this issue, but students may be reluctant to participate in more than one end-of-program evaluation effort when they are in the process of final examinations and end-of-semester evaluations. Timing is important in this effort.

Alumni surveys may be conducted at regular intervals to obtain long-term data about the products of an educational program. Data can be collected in a nonthreatening way and they are relatively inexpensive to administer. When such surveys are conducted depends on the data desired, the size and complexity of programs in the school, and the cost–benefit ratio of the survey effort. It is common to complete at least 1-year and 5-year surveys. The information sought depends on the level of the program and the outcome measures for which data are sought. Alumni surveys can involve the use of a tool developed by the nursing program or can be done using a standardized tool such as that developed by Educational Benchmarking, Inc. The advantage to a standardized tool is the ability to make comparisons to other schools nationwide and to accreditation standards. One approach is to provide a two-part survey in which one part is devoted to broad outcome measures and the graduates' perceptions of their general education experience on the campus. Questions on this survey may relate to perceptions about the extent to which they acquired skills such as critical thinking and effective written and oral communication; gained an understanding of different cultures and philosophies; and developed a sense of values and ethical standards, leadership skills, an appreciation of the arts, an ability to view events and phenomena from different perspectives, and an understanding of scientific principles and methods. One can also learn about the alumni's view of services available across the campus and opportunities to interact with students and faculty across disciplines. An advantage to this survey is the opportunity to compare the responses of students across disciplines to determine relative experiences and perceptions.

The second component of an alumni survey is usually discipline specific. In addition to general demographic data, the survey seeks information about positions held (title, location, population served, salary), the extent to which alumni believe they were prepared to practice according to the program outcomes, their general satisfaction with the program and activities related to scholarship such as publications, presentations, certifications, and entering advanced educational programs. Graduate programs find data related to the scholarship of alumni to be particularly valuable.

When surveys are conducted, the questions should be considered carefully in terms of data that will be used in decision making. If surveys are concise and questions are clearly stated, responses are more likely to be received. As a general rule, response rates will be improved if the survey does not exceed four pages. A high response rate increases the credibility of the data in reflecting the perspectives of the population surveyed. The survey can be sent through regular mail or online. Online surveys have better response rates and are cheaper to send. It is sometimes helpful to follow up with a paper survey after an online survey has been sent. With the volume of e-mails sent, the message may be lost or ignored. Follow-up of nonrespondents via e-mail or paper is helpful in increasing response rates (Grava-Gubis & Scott, 2008). Either way, the cover letter is an important element of the survey. The letter should be concise yet spell out the importance of the data to the educational program and the value placed on the input received from graduates. The more personalized the letter and the more professional the survey tool, the more likely it is that alumni will respond. The letter should also include a statement about confidentiality and the use of pooled or aggregate data in reports of survey findings to protect the anonymity of the respondents. Although it is useful to have several open-ended questions to obtain qualitative data, the simpler the tool is to complete, the more likely it is that respondents will complete the task. Well-designed questions, for which the respondent can check or circle an item or provide a number as a response, are more likely to be answered. Multiple mailing is another method of improving the return rate. There are several opinions about the best mailing sequence. One method is to send a second mailing or e-mail within 2 to 3 weeks of the first, with a second survey tool included in case the first mailing has been misplaced. If the survey is being sent through regular mail and cost is an issue, a reminder card may suffice. A third mailing in the form of e-mail or a postcard should occur between 10 days and 3 weeks after the second mailing, depending on the nature of the survey. Rewards can sometimes help with response rates. A small monetary reward or an opportunity to be entered into a lottery are commonly used strategies (Grava-Gubis & Scott, 2008).

Box 26-15 provides an example of an alumni survey and sample questions.

Box 26-16 provides a summary of the elements associated with outcomes evaluation.

Improving Program Outcomes

For the purpose of determining how to improve the program's outcomes, faculty first must review each variable that contributes to program success. These can include:

1. Qualifications of students admitted to the program
2. Definition and implementation of progression policies
3. Quality of the curriculum
4. Quality of instruction
5. Evaluation methods used to determine students' knowledge, skills, and abilities
6. Student preparation for employment and employer satisfaction.

The program evaluation plan should be reviewed at regular intervals to determine that each of these variables are examined as a part of the program evaluation plan. A similar process should be followed for all program outcomes. Mapping the relationship between and among variables may help to clarify the role each variable has in influencing outcome achievement.

BOX 26-15 Example: Alumni Survey

As a graduate of our nursing program, you are especially qualified to tell us what works well and what does not. We would like your input and would appreciate any suggestions that you might have. Would you please take a few minutes and complete this survey. The survey is completely anonymous.

Darken the oval that corresponds to your response.

Section I: Perceptions of Attainment of Program Goals. Indicate How Well the Program Prepared You to Fulfill the Following Program Goals.	**Poor**	**Fair**	**Good**	**Excellent**
1. Sample program goal #1: Integrate ...	0	0	0	0
2. Sample program goal #2: Utilize ...	0	0	0	0
3. Sample program goal #3: Synthesize ...	0	0	0	0

Section II. Satisfaction with Nursing Courses. Indicate How Well Each Course Contributed to Your Attainment of Program Goals.	**Course Not Taken—Does Not Apply**	**Poor**	**Fair**	**Good**	**Excellent**
4. Sample Course A	0	0	0	0	0
5. Sample Course B	0	0	0	0	0
6. Sample Course C	0	0	0	0	0

Section III: Overall Satisfaction with BSN Nursing Program		**Poor**	**Fair**	**Good**	**Excellent**
7. My overall satisfaction with the Nursing Program at University of A.	0	0	0	0	0

Additional Example Survey Questions:

8. What semester and year did you graduate or complete your program at University A?
9. What I liked best about my program was:
10. One thing I believe should be changed is:
11. What suggestions do you have to facilitate transition from the student role to professional practice?
12. Additional Comments

Potential variables should be reviewed annually and added to the evaluation plan as needed. Intervening variables may be identified through literature review, program evaluation reports, or internal studies. All variables need to be evaluated at some point in the program evaluation plan. Analysis of these variables will help to define where to make program improvements so that benchmarks can be met.

Internal Program Evaluation

Some universities require programs to undertake an internal evaluation or review of their programs. The purpose of many of these program evaluations is to assess and improve the quality of programs and whether or not they are helping to accomplish the university's mission. The questions to be answered include (1) How well are we doing what we say we are doing? (2) How do we support student learning? (3) How well are the academic programs relating to each other; and (4) Is the university fulfilling its mission and achieving its goals? This process informs the university about successes and weaknesses in the programs so that improvements can be made. The assessments are generally made in a rotation so that each program is reviewed at a specific interval.

The process usually calls for a written, evidence-based self-study. The information is reviewed

BOX 26-16 Elements of Outcomes Evaluation

- Students achieve all program goals and outcomes by graduation.
- Students achieve all technical competencies by graduation.
- The program has defined a benchmark for graduation rates.
- The program has defined a benchmark for first-time NCLEX passage rates and certification rates as appropriate.
- The program has defined a benchmark for employment rates.
- Students are satisfied with the overall quality of the program.
- Employers are satisfied with the performance of graduates.
- Other potential outcomes are identified and evaluated

NCLEX, National Council Licensure Examination.

by a team from outside the department and at least one representative from the profession who is external to the school who can be objective reviewers. The reviewers are responsible for synthesizing and making judgments about the program quality. Those judgments then lead to a list of recommendations for improvement. The availability of resources to accomplish the goals and recommendations is assessed along with the involvement of campus administrators, faculty, and the community in the program and its evaluation.

Although each institution may have a different process, many regional accrediting bodies require that institutions of higher learning conduct internal program evaluations (Middle States Commission on Higher Education, 2014).

Comprehensive Program Evaluation

Overall program evaluation provides the opportunity to examine the program in its entirety and to make revisions to improve its effectiveness. Program evaluation seeks to ensure that program improvement occurs as a result of a comprehensive program evaluation.

A comprehensive program evaluation plan should be developed and written and should include the following questions:

1. What areas should be evaluated?
2. How often should the evaluation occur?
3. Who is responsible for collecting and analyzing the data?
4. Who is responsible for making decisions based on the data?
5. What benchmarks is the program setting to show quality?

The areas to be evaluated include any potential intervening factors and should designate what data will be collected and how the data will be collected. The accreditation standards are often used as a framework to help define intervening factors and demonstrate that the standards are met. The evaluation plan should also be reviewed at regular intervals for completeness.

The time frame for evaluation of each area should be set. For example, the mission and goals of the program may not need to be evaluated often. A cycle of every 3 or every 5 years may be often enough for something so all-encompassing that changing it would only occur very carefully. However, graduation rates and National Council Licensure Examination—Registered Nurse (NLCEX–RN) pass rates need to evaluated annually.

Someone should be designated as responsible for the data collection, analysis, and decision making related to each item in the evaluation plan. Things tend to be overlooked unless someone takes responsibility. The responsibility will lie with a committee or a person associated with a position. For example, evaluation of faculty often lies with the dean, whereas evaluation of the curriculum lies with the faculty or a faculty committee such as a curriculum committee.

Setting benchmarks provides a goal for which to aim. It is a quality designation that allows you to determine progress toward attainment of the goal. They should be set fairly high but not at an unattainable level. They should be reviewed at regular intervals and altered as appropriate. Examining other schools nationwide and trend data for some benchmarks may help faculty set the benchmark. For example, it may be unreasonable to set 100% pass rate as a benchmark for NCLEX–RN. However, after examining trend data you may decide that 90% is an attainable benchmark that demonstrates quality.

Once the evaluation plan is developed, it should be implemented correctly. Identifying evaluation activities called for in the plan by responsible parties at the beginning of the academic year will help to ensure that evaluation activities are completed. Entering the program evaluation plan into an electronic spreadsheet or database may assist faculty in determining responsible parties, activities, and time frames allowing the plan to be sorted on these categories. Preparation of a year-end report with all completed forms and data sets will help track implementation of evaluation activities.

A record of the data collected, the analysis of the data, decisions made related to the data, and program changes resulting from evaluation activities should be maintained. Analysis of the data may not always result in change. The ultimate decision may be to gather data for another year or to maintain what exists and reevaluate. But any decision should be reported.

Actions taken to improve program quality can be summarized in a yearly report. This report will serve as a permanent record of the utility of the evaluation plan in bringing about program improvements. Faculty may want to review these summary reports, discuss strengths and limitations of the plan, and propose changes to improve the plan's effectiveness after they have reviewed year-end reports. Questions that will help guide this review include the following: "Does the plan provide information when it is needed for decision making?" "Do the faculty trust the information provided by evaluation strategies?"

Another important factor in the plan's effectiveness is the reliability and validity of evaluation tools. Reliability refers to the accuracy of measurement. Validity means that evaluation tools measure what they intend to measure. Internally developed measurement tools should be evaluated for reliability and validity at the time of their development. If faculty are unable to demonstrate reliability and validity of evaluation tools, they will not be able to trust the results of program evaluation activities. In addition, data need to be appropriately aggregated and trended over time to support decision making. Faculty should be cautious about making decisions based on limited data.

The evaluation of any education program is context specific. Consequently, the results of program evaluation may not be generalized to other programs. Nevertheless, nursing faculty should report successful strategies in program evaluation in the nursing literature. Nursing faculty across the nation may benefit from program evaluation research studies, such as those that report successful assessment strategies or provide insight about intervening variables for common program outcomes.

Box 26-17 provides a summary of the elements associated with comprehensive program evaluation.

BOX 26-17 Elements of Comprehensive Program Evaluation

- Assessment strategies are reliable and valid.
- Evaluation activities provide meaningful data for program improvement.
- The evaluation plan is reviewed and modified to improve its effectiveness.
- The evaluation plan is implemented as written decisions are made and changes implemented related to the data collected.

Accountability for Program Evaluation

Responsibility for development and implementation of the program evaluation plan rests with the nursing administration and faculty. The process for development and implementation may vary across nursing schools, depending on such factors as the number of faculty in the nursing school and the institutional resources available to support the evaluation. In some schools, an evaluator position is created to manage program evaluation practices, including the development and implementation of the program evaluation plan. An office of evaluation may be necessary in large schools, providing support staff to coordinate data collection at multiple levels. A common approach in small- and moderate-sized nursing schools is to appoint a standing committee of faculty who provide leadership and coordination of evaluation efforts. Regardless of the plan, the nursing faculty must determine accountability for each element of the evaluation plan. Without clear accountability and firm time frames, it is easy for evaluation efforts to get lost in the press of daily demands on faculty and administration.

Another issue of concern is the reporting and recording of evaluation data. Information is of little value to decision making unless it is channeled to those who are responsible for making decisions. Careful attention to this issue not only increases the likelihood that decisions will be based on actual data but also facilitates analysis of the value of the data. Evaluation data also serve as a rich resource when responses to external reports and accreditation expectations are required. One of the dangers is data overload. Because data are used for making decisions, it is best to determine what information is necessary and what is interesting but not important. Over time, a goal of evaluation is to streamline the amount of data collected. Asking questions such as "Why do we need these data or information?" and "How will these data or information assist in making decisions for improvement?" will assist in eliminating data overload.

The location of evaluation information is also important. Access to the information increases the likelihood of its use. An official location for evaluation reports ensures that they can be found when they are needed. Advances in technology have made the development of computer databases an important source of information that can be accessed by multiple stakeholders from a central location or file server.

Finally, the outcome of evaluation efforts in terms of creating change is an element that is sometimes omitted in record keeping. Accrediting bodies are as concerned about the actions that result from analysis of evaluation data as they are that a plan is in place. The best plan loses value if it does not create change when a need for intervention is indicated by the data.

Summary

Program evaluation is a comprehensive and complex process. Use of a systematic approach to program evaluation increases the likelihood that all program elements will receive appropriate attention and that evaluation activities will lead to program improvement. This chapter provided an overview of the evaluation process and its use as a guide for improvement for nursing education programs. The program evaluation plan serves as a road map to ensure that program evaluation activities are appropriately implemented. Development and implementation of a carefully designed program evaluation plan will support continuous quality improvement for nursing education programs.

REFLECTING ON THE EVIDENCE

1. What are the advantages and disadvantages of program evaluation?
2. What is the connection between program evaluation and accreditation standards?
3. How can program administrators minimize the challenges of implementing a program evaluation plan?
4. How can a systematic program evaluation be used in new program development?
5. What is the process for developing and implementing a comprehensive evaluation plan?

REFERENCES

Aguilar, A., Stupans, I., Scutter, S., & King, S. (2013). Towards a definition of professionalism in Australian occupations therapy: Using the delphi technique to obtain consensus on essential values and behaviours. *Australian Occupational Therapy, 60*, 206–216. http://dx.doi.org/10.111/1440-1630, 12017.

American Association of Colleges of Nursing. (2013). *AACN annual report*. Retrieved from, www.aacn.nche.edu.

American Association of Colleges of Nursing (AACN). (2014). *2013–2014 salaries of instructional and administrative nursing faculty in baccalaureate and graduate programs in nursing*. Retrieved from, http://www.aacn.nche.edu.

American Nurses Association. (2010). *Nursing: Scope and standards of practice*. Retrieved from, http://www.nursing world.org.

Association of American Colleges and Universities. (2002). *Greater expectations: A new vision for learning as a nation goes to college*. Washington, DC: Author.

Bloom, B. S. (1956). *Taxonomy of educational objectives: The classification of educational goals, Handbook I, Cognitive domain*. New York: McKay.

Boyer, E. L. (1990). *Scholarship rediscovered: Priorities of the professorate*. Princeton, NJ: The Carnegie Foundation for the Advancement of Teaching.

Breckenridge, D. M., Wolf, Z. R., & Roszkowski, M. J. (2012). Risk assessment profile and strategies for success instrument: determining prelicensure nursing students' risk for academic success. *Journal of Nursing Education*, (3), 160–166.

Brown, T., Bourke-Taylor, H., & Williams, B. (2012). Curriculum alignment and graduate attributes: Critical elements in occupational therapy education. *British Journal of Occupational Therapy, 75*(4), 163.

Brown, J. F., & Marshall, B. L. (2008). Continuous quality improvement: An effective strategy for improvement of program outcomes in a higher education setting. *Nursing Education Perspectives, 29*(4), 205–211.

Carey, E. C., & Weissman, D. E. (2010). Understanding and finding mentorship: A review for junior faculty. *Journal of Palliative Medicine, 13*(11), 1373–1379.

Chen, H. (1990). *Theory driven evaluation*. Newbury Park, CA: Sage.

College and University Professional Association for Human Resources. (2014). *2013–14 faculty in higher education salary survey*. Retrieved from, www.cupa-hr.org.

Commission on Collegiate Nursing Education (CCNE). (2013). *Standards for accreditation of baccalaureate and graduate nursing education programs*. Retrieved from, http://www.aacn.edu/accreditation.

Cronenwett, L., Sherwood, G., & Gelmon, S. B. (2009). Improving quality and safety education: The QSEN learning collaborative. *Nursing Outlook, 57*(6), 304–308.

Danielson, C. (2012, November). Observing classroom practice. *Educational Leadership*, 32–37.

Definitions of Distance Education [Courses, Programs and Students] for SIS Coding and Compliance Review and Reporting Credit Hour Allocations, (2013). Indiana University Office of Online Education and Student Services and Systems. retrieved from http://online.iu.edu/_assets/docs/definitions0913.pdf.

Dickeson, R. C. (2010). *Prioritizing academic programs and services: Reallocating resources to achieve strategic balance*. San Francisco: Jossey-Bass.

Ewell, P. T. (1985). *Introduction to assessing educational outcomes: New directions for Institutional research*. San Francisco: Jossey-Bass.

Glennon, C. D. (2006). Reconceptualizing program outcomes. *Journal of Nursing Education, 45*(2), 55–58.

Grava-Gubis, I., & Scott, S. (2008). Effects of various methodologic strategies: Survey response rates among Canadian physicians. *Canadian Family Physician, 54*(10), 1424–1430.

Indiana University School of Education. (2014). *National Survey of Student Engagement*. Retrieved from, www.nsse.iub.edu.

Institute of Medicine (IOM). (2011). *The future of nursing: Leading change, advancing health*. Washington, D.C.: The National Academies Press.

Johnson, T. D., & Ryan, K. E. (2000). A comprehensive approach to the evaluation of college teaching. In K. Ryan (Ed.), *Evaluation of teaching in higher education: A vision for the future* (pp. 109–123). San Francisco: Jossey-Bass.

Lunenburg, F. C. (2011). Curriculum development: Deductive models. *Schooling, 2*(1), 1–17.

Merritt, B. K., Blake, A. I., McIntyre, A. H., & Packer, T. (2012). Curriculum evaluation: Linking curriculum objectives to essential competencies. *Canadian Journal of Occupational Therapy, 79*(3), 175–180.

Middle States Commission on Higher Education. (2014). *Accreditation criteria*. Retrieved from, www.msche.org.

National League for Nursing Commission on Nursing Education Accreditation (2015). Retrieved from, http://www.nln.org/accreditation-services/the-nln-commission-for-nursing-education-accreditation-(cnea).

National Organization of Nurse Practitioner Faculties. (2012). *Criteria for evaluation of nurse practitioner programs*. Retrieved from, http://www.nonpf.com.

Nestel, D., Ivkovic, A., Hill, R. A., Warrens, A. N., Paraskevas, P. A., McConnell, J. A., et al. (2012). Benefits and challenges of focus groups in the evaluation of a new Graduate Entry Medical Programme. *Assessment & Evaluation in Higher Education, 37*(1), 1–17.

Newton, S. E., Smith, L. H., Moore, G., & Magnan, M. (2007). Predicting early academic achievement in a baccalaureate nursing program. *Journal of Professional Nursing, 23*, 144–149.

Reig, S. A. (2007). Classroom assessment strategies: What do students at risk and teachers perceive as effective and useful? *Journal of Instructional Psychology, 34*(4), 214–225.

Rui, N., & Feldman, J. M. (2012). IRR (inter-rater reliability) of a COP (classroom observation protocol)—A critical appraisal. *US-China Educational Review, B, 3*, 305–315.

Sauter, M. K. (2000). *An exploration of program evaluation in baccalaureate nursing education*. (Unpublished doctoral dissertation), Bloomington, IN: Indiana University School of Nursing.

Scriven, M. (1991). Prose and cons about goal-free evaluation. *American Journal of Evaluation, 12*(55), http://dx.doi.org/10.1177/109821409101200108.

Sellers, S. C., & Haag, B. A. (1993). A nursing textbook evaluation instrument for multicultural, nonsexist concepts. *Journal of Nursing Education, 22*(6), 270–272.

Stravropoulou, A., & Stroubouki, T. (2014). Evaluation of educational programmes—the contribution of history to modern evaluation thinking. *Health Science Journal, 8*(2), 193–204.

Stufflebeam, D. L. (2003, October 3). The CIPP model for evaluation. Paper presented at the 2003 Annual Conference of the Oregon Program Evaluation Network (Open). Portland, Oregon, October 3, 2003.

Tyler, R. W. (1949). *Basic principles of curriculum and instruction*. Chicago, IL: University of Chicago Press.

Willett, T. G., Marshall, K. C., Broudo, M., & Clarke, M. (2007). TIME as a generic index for outcome-based medical education. *Medical Teacher, 29*, 655–659.

Wilson, M. W., Morreale, M. K., Waineo, E., & Balon, R. (2013). The focus group: A method for curricular review. *Academic Psychiatry, 37*(4), 281–282.

Wood, S. O., Biordi, D. L., Miller, B. A., Poncar, P., Snelson, C. M., Banks, M. J., et al. (1998). Boyer's model of scholarship applied to a career ladder for nontenured nursing faculty. *Nurse Educator, 23*(3), 33–40.

27 The Accreditation Process*

Michael J. Kremer, PhD, CRNA, FNAP, FAAN
Betty J. Horton, PhD, CRNA, FAAN

Accreditation is an ongoing, voluntary process that has existed in the United States for more than 100 years and is pursued by nursing programs to ensure the quality of those programs. Through the accreditation process, nursing programs are held accountable for establishing appropriate program outcome measures and designing effective evaluation systems for measuring program outcomes. This process promotes continuous quality improvement as nursing programs strive to meet their educational goals. The Accreditation Commission for Education on Nursing (ACEN) and the Commission on Collegiate Nursing Education (CCNE) are two accreditation agencies for nursing education programs. Each agency has been recognized by the U.S. Department of Education (USDE) and is dedicated to maintaining quality nursing programs. At this writing, the National League for Nursing (NLN) is developing another nursing education program accreditation agency, the NLN Commission for Nursing Education Accreditation (NLN CNEA), which is in the process of seeking USDE recognition.

Accreditation and regulation are two distinct, independent entities. State boards of nursing regulate nursing education and practice. The state boards of nursing develop rules and regulations designed to protect the health, safety and welfare of the public. Consistent with this mission, nursing programs must comply with the administrative codes of state boards of nursing and submit annual reports addressing compliance with state regulatory standards. A nursing program may lose its accreditation status and remain operational, because accreditation agencies lack the authority to close a program. However, state boards of nursing have the statutory authority to close nursing programs under their jurisdiction that do not comply with the criteria as stated in the administrative code.

This chapter provides an overview of the accreditation process for nursing programs. The chapter discuses elements of the accreditation process for nursing programs, including preparation of the self-study document, use of consultants, and the on-site visit.

Overview of the Accreditation Process

Accreditation is "a process of external quality review created and used by higher education to scrutinize colleges, universities and programs for quality assurance and quality improvement" (Eaton, 2012, p. 1). Accreditation provides evidence of quality education to stakeholders including students, families, and the general public. The linkage of quality and accreditation enhances funding opportunities in the public and private sectors and enhances employment opportunities for graduates of accredited programs. Accreditation facilitates the transfer of academic credits between institutions. Graduation from an accredited nursing program is an admissions requirement for many graduate programs.

External review of accreditation agencies is provided through USDE recognition as well as through the Council for Higher Education Accreditation (CHEA). The U.S. Secretary of Education is required by law to publish a list of recognized accrediting agencies that are considered to be reliable authorities as to the quality of postsecondary education provided by the institutions and programs they accredit. In addition to meeting quality criteria,

*The authors acknowledge the work of Marsha Howell, DNS, RN, CNE, FAAN, in the previous edition of the chapter.

agencies that successfully complete the application process must meet criteria unrelated to quality, such as demonstrating a link to funding programs administered by the USDE or other federal agencies. CHEA is a nongovernmental association that includes thousands of degree-granting colleges and universities. CHEA provides recognition for institutional and programmatic accrediting agencies. CHEA's recognition process focuses on the quality of regional accreditors that accredit 2- and 4-year public and private colleges and universities; national faith-related accreditation agencies, which accredit nonprofit, degree-granting, religious or doctrine-based institutions; national career related accreditors, which review single-purpose, for-profit, career-based institutions, and programmatic accreditors for specific programs and professions (Eaton, 2012; USDE, n.d.).

Categories of Accrediting Agencies

There are different categories of accrediting agencies, including institutional and programmatic. Institutions that house nursing programs may also possess regional institutional accreditation. Regional accreditors accredit institutions and are responsible for setting standards and monitoring compliance with those standards by the college or university as a whole. Regional accrediting organizations recognized by CHEA have standards and processes that "are consistent with the academic quality, improvement and accountability expectations that CHEA has established" (Council for Higher Education Accreditation [CHEA], 2010). CHEA-recognized regional accreditation organizations include the Higher Learning Commission, the Middle States Commission on Higher Education, the New England Association of Colleges and Schools Commission on Institutions of Higher Education, the Southern Association of Colleges and Schools Commission on Colleges, the Western Association of Schools and Colleges Accrediting Commission for Community and Junior Colleges, and the Western Association of Schools and Colleges Senior College and University Commission (http://www.chea.org/Directories/regional.asp).

Programmatic accreditation agencies are discipline-specific and accredit programs and professional schools such as nursing, law, and engineering. The programmatic accreditation agencies for nursing programs are ACEN and CCNE plus the emerging NLN CNEA. In addition to these entities, there are advanced practice nursing accrediting agencies including the Council on Accreditation of Nurse Anesthesia Educational Programs (COA) and the Accreditation Commission for Midwifery Education (ACME).

Some accreditation agencies serve as a "gatekeeper" for federal funds awarded to institutions and programs in the form of student aid. Grants and loans authorized under Title IV of the Higher Education Act are the major source of federal student aid. Students who want federal (and sometimes state) grants and loans need to attend a college, university, or program that is accredited and recognized by the USDE for this purpose. In this regard, a USDE-recognized accreditation agency is considered a "gatekeeper" for federal funds.

Most nursing students access federal funds through regionally accredited universities that conduct nursing programs. Other students who attend hospital-based or freestanding institutions, not associated with regionally accredited universities, rely on approved USDE category 3 programmatic accrediting agencies to obtain Title IV funds (United States Department of Education, USDE, 2014). Category 3 accrediting agencies must meet specific regulations, including provisions to be separate and independent from parent professional organizations. ACEN, COA, and ACME are recognized by USDE as Category 3 agencies, which allow the qualified programs accredited by these agencies to participate in Title IV programs. The nursing program accreditors CCNE and NLN CNEA are considered to be Category 2 accrediting agencies, and as such, do not serve as Title IV gate keepers for federal student aid, instead relying upon the institution's accreditation by a USDE recognized institutional accrediting Title IV gate keeper to serve that purpose.

Accreditation Models

The accreditation process model practiced by most accrediting agencies is a combination of a self-study and an on-site visit by a team of peer evaluators. The self-study is a document that provides a systematic and thorough examination of a program and its components as related to its stated mission and expected outcomes. The self-study provides evidence for program compliance with the standards and criteria of the accreditation agency. The self-study document is reviewed by peer evaluators including faculty members, administrators, and practitioners within the stated profession. An on-site visit is conducted by peer evaluators to verify, clarify, and amplify the content of the self-study. The peer evaluators submit a report to the accreditation agency that addresses programmatic compliance with accreditation standards based on information obtained through the self-study and on-site visit. The decision-making body of the accreditation agency is composed of elected representatives who make the final decision to grant accreditation or reaccreditation, deny accreditation, or place the program on probation. Accreditation agencies publish lists of accredited institutions and programs on their websites.

The focus of the accreditation process is similar across accreditation organizations. The basic components addressed in institutional or programmatic accreditation include:

- Measurable program outcomes
- Curricula
- Faculty
- Qualified students
- Student support services
- Quality and adequate resources
- Qualified administration
- Policies and procedures
- Formal complaint mechanism
- Systematic program evaluation plan

Nursing Programmatic Accreditation Agencies

At this writing, ACEN and CCNE serve as the two accrediting bodies for nursing programs in the United States. NLN CNEA, established in 2013, is in the process of seeking USDE recognition, and will serve as the third nursing program accreditation agency in the United States. A summary of each agency and their standards, criteria, and processes are summarized in this section, but the reader is advised to review each agency's web site for updated information.

Accreditation Commission for Education on Nursing (ACEN)

In 1997, the NLN approved the creation of the National League for Nursing Accreditation Commission (NLNAC) as an accrediting entity. In 2014 the NLNAC changed its name to the ACEN. The mission of ACEN is to support nursing education and practice as well as the public through accreditation. ACEN defines *accreditation* as "a voluntary, self-regulatory process by which non-governmental associations recognize educational institutions or programs that have been found to meet or exceed standards and criteria for educational quality" (Accreditation Commission for Education in Nursing [ACEN], 2013). ACEN provides accreditation for nursing programs ranging from practical, diploma, associate, baccalaureate, master's, post-master's certificate, to clinical doctorate programs. ACEN serves as a Title IV gatekeeper for federal funds for those nursing programs that do not possess regional accreditation and is recognized by CHEA.

ACEN is governed by a 15-member Board of Commissioners composed of individuals representing nursing education (nine commissioners), service (three commissioners), and the public sector (three commissioners). The ACEN chief executive officer reports to the Board of Commissioners. ACEN operations are supported by professional, administrative, and support staff; program evaluators; and committees.

ACEN program evaluators, or peer reviewers, participate as site visitors, evaluation review panel members, and appeal panel members. Program evaluators must meet defined criteria related to their educational preparation, nursing education expertise, and professional service in addition to attending regularly scheduled program evaluator professional development sessions. Expectations for program evaluators include maintaining confidentiality related to programs visited and recommendations made as a result of the self-study and on-site visit. ACEN site visit policies and procedures are published in the ACEN Accreditation Manual (Accreditation Commission for Education in Nursing, 2013).

ACEN Standards and Criteria

There are six ACEN accreditation standards and related criteria for each standard (Accreditation Commission for Education in Nursing, 2013). ACEN standards and criteria are published for every type of program accredited by ACEN, including the clinical doctorate, master's and post-master's certificate, baccalaureate, associate, diploma, and practical. The accreditation standards address mission, administrative capacity, faculty and staff, students, curriculum, resources, and outcomes. An Accreditation Manual Supplement for International

Programs is also available (Accreditation Commission for Education in Nursing, 2013). There is an ongoing assessment of the adequacy of these standards and criteria with a full review conducted every five years.

ACEN requires programs to be in compliance with all accreditation standards to receive initial accreditation and in substantial compliance with standards to receive continued accreditation. Nursing programs are expected to provide a summary of program strengths, areas needing development, and an action plan based on the standards and criteria. ACEN offers self-study forums for nursing programs beginning the accreditation or reaccreditation process. The focus of the forums is an overview of the accreditation process and writing a self-study.

ACEN Accreditation Process

ACEN follows the accreditation model discussed earlier in the chapter. A four-step process is used that includes a self-study report, an on-site visit, review of submitted materials by the evaluation panel, and a final decision by the Board of Commissioners (Accreditation Commission for Education in Nursing, 2013). The on-site visit is performed by site visitors composed of professional peers in education and practice. The team of site visitors looks for congruence between the self-study and their assessment of the program. The report of the on-site visitors is submitted to ACEN and a copy is sent to the nursing program administrator, who has 2 weeks to review the report and clarify any factual errors on a response form. The final draft of the report is sent to the on-site visitors and the nursing program administrator. The next step in the process is review of the report by the evaluation review panel. This body validates the report of the on-site review team and determines if evidence demonstrates compliance with the accreditation standards and criteria. The review panel is appointed by the ACEN Board of Commissioners and one of the commissioners serves as a member of the review panel. The nursing program administrator may attend the meeting of the evaluation review panel in person or via conference call. A recommendation from the evaluation review panel is made to the ACEN Board of Commissioners, which has the sole authority for determining the accreditation status of nursing program applicants.

Initial Accreditation and Continuing Accreditation

Nursing programs that seek initial ACEN accreditation must comply with its current policies and procedures, which are available at www.acenursing.org and are subject to change. Current requirements stipulate that the chief executive officer of the college or university initiates the process and authorizes ACEN to begin the accreditation process. ACEN assigns the nursing program a mentor to facilitate the self-assessment process. The nursing program applies for candidacy status by submitting state board of nursing approval documentation, fees, and information related to the faculty members, curriculum, and resources. Once candidacy status is established, the nursing program has 2 years to complete the accreditation process. The nursing program must be in compliance with all accreditation standards and criteria to receive initial accreditation. Failure to comply with accreditation standards and criteria may result in denial of accreditation. Programs are reviewed again by ACEN 5 years following receipt of initial accreditation (Accreditation Commission for Education in Nursing, 2013).

Nursing programs that seek continuing accreditation must be in compliance with all ACEN standards and criteria to receive an accreditation term of 8 years. Shorter terms of accreditation and various sanctions are imposed, depending on the type and number of citations, for programs that do not fully comply (Accreditation Commission for Education in Nursing, 2013). Nursing programs that face possible denial or revocation of accreditation can appeal those decisions. ACEN policy provides a 30-day timeframe to initiate the appeal of an adverse accreditation decision. An appeal panel reviews all pertinent materials, including any documentation relevant to the adverse accreditation decision and testimony presented at an appeal hearing where representatives of the nursing program, including the program administrator, may present evidence. The decision of the appeal panel may range from affirmation of the adverse decision, to reversal of the decision, or remanding the decision to the Board of Commissioners. All ACEN accreditation decisions are made available to the USDE, state boards of nursing, and the public. The ACEN website (www.acenursing.org) provides extensive information to guide nursing programs in every aspect of the accreditation process.

Commission on Collegiate Nursing Education

In 1998 the Nursing Education Accreditation Commission (NEAC) was created by the AACN for the sole purpose of accrediting baccalaureate and higher-degree nursing programs, including MSN and DNP program. The NEAC was subsequently renamed the *Commission on Collegiate Nursing Education.* In 2000 CCNE received initial USDE recognition. CCNE strives to be mission-driven with foci including innovation, autonomy, and creativity. The CCNE is autonomous from the AACN. Its mission is to serve as "an autonomous accrediting agency, contributing to the improvement of the public's health." CCNE provides accreditation for baccalaureate and higher-degree programs in nursing, including master's of science in nursing (MSN), doctorate in nursing practice (DNP) and post-baccalaureate nurse residency programs. Doctor of Philosophy (PhD) programs are accredited by regional accreditation agencies. CCNE is the autonomous accreditation agency of the American Association of Colleges of Nursing (AACN). CCNE does not provide Title IV gatekeeping functions for the programs it accredits. The Commission serves the public interest by assessing and identifying programs that engage in effective educational practices. "As a voluntary, self-regulatory process, CCNE accreditation supports and encourages continuing self-assessment by nursing programs and supports continuing growth and improvement of collegiate professional education and post-baccalaureate nurse residency programs" (Commission on Collegiate Nursing Education, 2009a, para. 1).

The CCNE accreditation process is based on its core values:

- Foster trust in the process, in CCNE, and in the professional community.
- Focus on stimulating supporting continuous quality improvement in nursing education programs and their outcomes.
- Be inclusive in the implementation of its activities and maintain openness to the diverse institutional and individual issues and opinions of the interested community.
- Rely on review and oversight by peers from the community of interest.
- Maintain integrity through a consistent, fair, and honest accreditation process.
- Value and foster innovation in both the accreditation process and the programs to be accredited.
- Facilitate and engage in self-assessment.
- Foster an educational climate that supports program students, graduates, and faculty in their pursuit of lifelong learning.
- Maintain a high level of accountability to the public served by the process, including consumers, students, employers, programs, and institutions of higher education.
- Maintain a process that is both cost-effective and cost-accountable.
- Encourage programs to develop graduates who are effective professionals and socially responsible citizens.
- Ensure autonomy and due process in its deliberations and decision-making processes.

CCNE is governed by a 13-member Board of Commissioners that is composed of 3 deans of nursing programs, 3 faculty, 2 professional consumers, 2 public consumers, and 3 practicing nurses. The CCNE executive director reports to the CCNE Board of Commissioners. The CCNE infrastructure also includes staff and standing committees, which include the Accreditation Review, Budget, Nominating, Report Review, and Hearing Committees. CCNE staff members report to the director and assistant director and are responsible for supporting all board and standing committee activities as well as administration of accreditation processes and procedures.

The CCNE site evaluators are nursing faculty members, administrators, and practicing nurses. Each on-site reviewer completes CCNE evaluator training. Site evaluators are expected to maintain confidentiality at all times regarding the accreditation process. Individuals selected as CCNE accreditation team leaders attend training for leading on-site visits. Resources for on-site evaluators are found on the CCNE website: www.aacn.nche.edu/accreditation/EvalResourceBG.htm.

CCNE Standards, Key Elements, and Elaborations

Four CCNE standards with 23 key elements address mission and governance, institutional commitment and resources, curriculum, and teaching–learning practices. These standards address expected institutional performance and the key elements provide direction in meeting the overall standard. The rationale for providing key elements is to provide nursing programs with the opportunity to interpret each key element at the broadest level, allowing for creativity and innovation. Elaborations are provided for each key element and are used to help clarify and interpret each key element. At the end of each standard is a list of possible supporting documentation for the self-study and on-site visit that can be used to demonstrate compliance with the standard. During the programmatic self-assessment process in preparation for an accreditation review, nursing programs are expected to address strengths, challenges, and an action plan for each standard, noting evidence of the ongoing improvement process in action. CCNE provides self-study workshops and accreditation updates throughout each year to educate nursing programs about the CCNE accreditation process.

Nursing programs that possess CCNE accreditation or those that are in the process of seeking accreditation are required to use the professional standards and guidelines developed by the AACN. Programs can also use professional standards in addition to the AACN Essentials, such as the Criteria for Evaluation of Nurse Practitioner Programs (Criteria for Evaluation of Nurse Practitioner Programs, AACN, 2012). Each program type has a specific set of "essentials" that guide the nursing program and its curriculum. These curricular essentials outline the expected outcomes needed for graduates of specific programs. For example, *The Essentials of Baccalaureate Education for Professional Nursing Practice* (American Association of Colleges of Nursing, 2008) are incorporated in CCNE-accredited baccalaureate programs and specify the competencies needed in a baccalaureate graduate. AACN also promulgates essentials for MSN and DNP education.

CCNE Accreditation Process

The CCNE accreditation process is similar to that used by other accreditation agencies. Commission on Collegiate Nursing Education (CCNE) (2009) identified a six-step accreditation process. The nursing program develops a self-study report that it uses to perform a self-assessment of how its program meets the CCNE standards and key elements. An on-site visit is conducted, during which a peer evaluation team validates the self-study findings. The peer evaluators are described as a fact-finding team. The evaluators prepare a report that describes whether the program complies with CCNE accreditation standards and the related key elements for each standard. The report of the evaluation team is sent to the nursing program and the administrator has the opportunity to respond to the report and clarify any areas in question.

The CCNE Accreditation Review Committee (ARC) reviews the self-study, the report of the evaluation team and the response of the program to the team report. The ARC makes a recommendation to the CCNE Board of Commissioners regarding accreditation. The CCNE Board of Commissioners reviews the ARC recommendation and decides whether to grant initial or continuing approval, deny approval, or withdraw accreditation of the program. The Board of Commissioner periodically reviews nursing programs between accreditation visits to monitor continued compliance with the standards (www.aacn.nche.edu/ccne-accreditation/standards-procedures-resources/overview).

Initial and Continuing Accreditation

CCNE policies and procedures are available on the agency website: www.aacn.nche.edu/ccne-accreditation/standards-procedures-resources/overview. Current requirements mandate that the chief executive officer of the sponsoring institution and the chief nursing administrator begin the process for initial CCNE accreditation through request of program applicant status from CCNE. The nursing program must demonstrate that the sponsoring institution is accredited, and that approval from the state board of nursing has been obtained. Applicant programs must show that they have the potential to meet the accreditation standards and pay the necessary fees. Once applicant status is received, the nursing program has 2 years to complete the accreditation process, including development of a self-study document and scheduling an on-site visit. Nursing programs that receive initial CCNE accreditation are reviewed again 5 years after initial accreditation has been granted. A progress improvement report is submitted at the midpoint of the 5-year accreditation term. Nursing programs that do not comply with CCNE accreditation standards do not receive accreditation recognition from CCNE.

Nursing programs that seek reaffirmation of their CCNE accreditation are required to contact the agency 12 to 18 months prior to the planned on-site visit. The chief nursing administrator sends a letter of intent for reevaluation and possible dates for the on-site visit. A 10-year term of continuing accreditation is granted by the CCNE Board of Commissioners for nursing programs found to be in compliance with all CCNE accreditation standards. CCNE reaffirms the accreditation of these programs based on the self-study and report of the on-site visit. Nursing programs that are found out of compliance with CCNE accreditation standards may have their accreditation withdrawn. Programs have the opportunity to "show cause" as to why withdrawal of CCNE accreditation should not occur by responding to the concerns of the Board of Commissioners regarding lack of compliance. There is a specified time frame during which a program can initiate a "show cause" action with CCNE. CCNE accreditation decisions are communicated to USDE, other applicable institutional accreditation agencies and the public, if applicable. Nursing programs that face denial or revocation of accreditation can appeal the decision per CCNE procedures. Nursing programs have 10 days to begin the appeal process after receiving notification of an adverse accreditation decision. A Hearing Committee is appointed by the chair of the CCNE Board of Commissioners. The purpose of the committee is to review all written evidence and oral testimony provided during the appeal process. During the appeal process, the appellant nursing program bears the burden of proof. The Hearing Committee submits a written recommendation to the Board of Commissioners to affirm the adverse accreditation decision or to remand the action for reconsideration by the Board of Commissioners. Information about all aspects of the CCNE accreditation process is located on the AACN website: www.aacn.nche.edu.

National League for Nursing Commission for Nursing Education Accreditation (NLN CNEA)

The NLN established a new autonomous accreditation division in September 2013 by vote of the NLN membership, in response to requests for additional program accreditation options within the nursing profession. The NLN CNEA will provide accreditation for all types of nursing programs including practical/vocational, diploma, associate, baccalaureate, master's, post-master's certificate, and clinical doctorate programs. The NLN CNEA will not provide Title IV gatekeeping functions. Information about the NLN CNEA can be found at their web site, http://www.nln.org/cnea.

As its mission, the NLN CNEA:

> promotes excellence and integrity in nursing education globally through an accreditation process that respects the diversity of program mission, curricula, students, and faculty; emphasizes a culture of continuous quality improvement; and influences the preparation of a caring and competent nursing workforce" (NLN CNEA, 2015).

NLN CNEA incorporates the NLN's organizational core values of caring, diversity, integrity, and excellence throughout the accreditation services that it provides.

NLN CNEA is governed by a 15-member Board of Commissioners that is composed of nurse educator representatives (10); nursing practice representatives (3); and public representatives (2). The NLN CNEA executive director reports to the NLN CNEA Board of Commissioners. NLN CNEA staff members report to the executive director and are responsible for supporting all board and standing committee activities as well as administration of accreditation processes and procedures.

NLN CNEA Standards and Accreditation Process

There are five NLN CNEA standards with accompanying quality indicators and interpretative guidelines. The five standards are related to mission, governance, and resources; faculty; students; curriculum and teaching, learning, and evaluation processes; and program outcomes, and are based upon a model of continuous quality improvement. As of this writing, the quality indicators and interpretive guidelines are in the process of being finalized by the NLN CNEA Board of Commissioners. The proposed standards can be found at http://www.nln.org/cnea. The policies and processes that will govern the NLN CNEA accreditation processes are under development and can be found on the NLN CNEA website. NLN CNEA anticipates beginning to accredit nursing programs in 2016.

Steps in the Nursing Program Accreditation Process

Preparation for the programmatic accreditation process should begin 1 to 3 years prior to the planned visit for nursing programs seeking initial or continued accreditation to have sufficient time to ensure that all elements of the accreditation process have been completed. This preparation time may vary based on the number of internal programs to be accredited within the overall nursing program. For example, a nursing program may have baccalaureate, MSN, and DNP degree options to be reviewed for accreditation. Other institutions may have only one nursing program, such as an associate or baccalaureate degree program.

A systematic program evaluation needs to be conducted that addresses all aspects of the nursing program with specified measurable performance indicators and benchmarks along with appropriate measurement tools, data analysis, and dissemination of findings (see Chapter 26). Examples of areas to be addressed include aggregate measures such as achievement of program outcomes; quality of instruction and resources for learning; and overall satisfaction with the program by students, alumni, faculty, and employers. Nursing programs need to have mechanisms for tracking data to support program outcomes, including program completion and graduation rates, licensing and certification examination pass rates, alumni and employer satisfaction, and graduate employment. Institutional assessment plans, including databases, analysis, and dissemination of assessment findings facilitate the work of program evaluation. Programs will be expected to collect, trend, and analyze these data during a specified period (e.g., 3 years of aggregate data).

Professional standards and guidelines need to be reflected in the program and its components. These standards and guidelines serve as building blocks for the nursing curriculum and must be consistent with the mission, goals, and expected outcomes of the program. Professional standards and guidelines are developed by professional nursing and specialty organizations, state regulatory agencies, and nationally recognized accreditation organizations. ACEN, CCNE, and NLN CNEA support the use of professional nursing standards and expect that nursing programs can demonstrate how these standards are used within the curriculum and their consistency with overall program outcomes. Although CCNE requires certain AACN professional standards based on program type, nursing programs have the opportunity to use other professional standards in addition to those required. Table 27-1 lists examples of professional standards and guidelines.

Preparing the Self-Study Report

One of the first steps in preparing the self-study document is agreement on the type of structure and approach to be used when writing the report. This can vary by institution, but the faculty and administration need to agree on structure and approach so that the self-study authors operate within a common framework. Various approaches can be used to create the self-study, such as matching individual standards to specific standing committees

TABLE 27-1 Examples of Professional Standards and Guidelines

Adult-Gerontology Acute Care Nurse Practitioner Competencies (AACN, 2012).

Adult-Gerontology Clinical Nurse Specialist Competencies (AACN, 2010).

Adult-Gerontology Primary Care Nurse Practitioner Competencies (AACN, 2010).

Criteria for Evaluation of Nurse Practitioner Programs (National Task Force on Quality Nurse Practitioner Education, 2012).

Educational Standards and Curriculum Guidelines for Neonatal Nurse Practitioner Programs (National Association of Neonatal Nurses [NANN], 2009).

National League for Nursing (NLN) Outcomes and Competencies for Graduates of Practical/Vocational, Diploma, Associate Degree, Baccalaureate, Master's, Practice Doctorate and Research Doctorate Programs in Nursing (NLN, 2009).

National Association for Practical Nurse Education and Service (NAPNES) Standards of Practice for Licensed Practical/Vocational Nurses (NAPNES, 2004).

Nurse Practitioner Core Competencies (National Organization of Nurse Practitioner Faculties [NONPF], 2012).

Population-Focused Nurse Practitioner Competencies (Family/Across the Lifespan, Neonatal, Pediatric Acute Care, Pediatric Primary Care, Psychiatric-Mental Health, Women's Health/Gender-Related (NONPF Population-Focused Competencies Task Force, 2013).

The Essentials of Baccalaureate Education for Professional Nursing Practice (AACN, 2008).

The Essentials of Master's Education for Advanced Practice Nursing (AACN, 1996).

The Essentials of Doctoral Education for Advanced Nursing Practice (AACN, 2006).

Criteria for Evaluation of Nurse Practitioner Programs (National Task Force on Quality Nurse Practitioner Education, 2008).

Nursing: Scope and Standards of Practice (ANA, 2010).

Case Management Society of America (CMSA) Standards of Practice for Case Management (CMSA, 2010).

Core Competencies for Interprofessional Collaborative Practice (Interprofessional Education Collaborative Expert Panel, 2011).

Domains and Core CNS Competencies (NONPF, 2010).

Emphasizing the Older Adult in Nurse Practitioner Curriculum (NONPF, 2008).

National Association of Clinical Nurse Specialties Core Practice Doctoral Competencies (2009)

National Association of Neonatal Nurse Practitioners (2010).

NLN Core Competencies for Nurse Educators (NLN, 2012).

NLN Hallmarks of Excellence (NLN, 2004).

Practice Doctorate Nurse Practitioner Entry-Level Competencies (NONPF, National Panel for NP Practice Doctorate Competencies, 2006).

Quad Council Competencies for Public Health Nursing (2013).

Standards for Accreditation of Nurse Anesthesia Educational Programs (COA, 2014).

Standards for Accreditation of Nurse Anesthesia Programs—Practice Doctorate.

for development of first drafts, assignment of one or two faculty members to write the self-study, assignment of faculty teams to write each standard, hiring a professional writer, or developing a self-study steering committee composed of individuals who represent all internal programs and administration. Each representative on the steering committee heads up a writing team of faculty. It is helpful to identify faculty with expertise in writing and editing with strategic placement of these individuals on specific teams.

Regardless of the approach used to develop a self-study, faculty members must be knowledgeable about and invested in the self-study process and kept abreast of progress on the document. For example, accreditation can be a recurring faculty meeting agenda item. An author and editor with responsibility for the final self-study draft needs to be identified. This individual can ensure that the document is comprehensive, clear, and concise. The author with final draft responsibility can perform a comprehensive review of the document, removing erroneous materials, deleting content that is duplicated, and ensuring that each standard has been adequately and accurately addressed.

All faculty need to be conversant with the self-study document and how accreditation standards and criteria have been addressed. If outside consultants have been involved in the development of the self-study, it is especially important for faculty to familiarize themselves with its content so that they can respond accurately to questions from on-site reviewers, providing clarification where necessary.

The development of a timeline for completion of the accreditation self-study document and planning of the on-site visit is crucial. Adequate time must be provided to perform a self-review and self-assessment of all components of the nursing program, complete the self-study process, and write the self-study document. If adequate time is allowed for self-study development, there is less pressure on the involved faculty and staff, resulting in a comprehensive and well-written document.

During the self-study process it is not desirable to make any major programmatic changes. Major programmatic changes have the potential to change the focus of faculty members from self-review, self-assessment, and self-study development to implementation of the proposed change. The need for major changes may become apparent during the self-study process and can be identified as such.

The self-study timeline is created by working backward and beginning with the possible dates for the on-site visit. Necessary events to include in the timeline are the due dates for drafts of each standard; faculty meetings to discuss standards both during self-study development and in preparation for the on-site visit; documentation of program improvement and program outcomes; finalizing the self-study; setting a mock site visit date with an external consultant; development of due dates for printing and binding self-study copies for faculty, administration, and visitors; preparation of the resource room; and finalizing the agenda for the site visit. The program may choose to rely more on digital versions of the self-study and supporting documents that can be housed on a secure network drive or flash drives, with backup hard copies.

Correct interpretation of the accreditation standards is important during development of the self-study document and sets the stage for a successful on-site review. Each of the nursing accreditation agencies provides self-study workshops, webinars, and forums for faculty to attend that provide important information related to interpretation of each standard, clarifying any areas of confusion and providing examples of evidence to support fulfillment of each criterion. Faculty members who write self-studies need to understand the importance of addressing the involved accreditation standards. Narrative statements need supporting documentation that provides evidence of how the program meets criteria. The identification of program strengths, challenges and areas needing development, along with an action plan, provides evidence for the program evaluators that an overall commitment to continuous quality improvement exists.

It is helpful to have faculty members who serve as on-site accreditation reviewers who can be used as internal consultants during the creation of the self-study. These individuals can provide valuable insights into the development and organization of the self-study document.

Providing evidence of how accreditation standards are met is an important aspect of the self-study. Use of data for quality improvement helps self-study authors maintain their focus on quality while performing a thorough programmatic assessment. The visiting evaluation team needs a clear, concise picture of the program.

The self-study team needs to demonstrate in the self-study document that programs use assessment data to close "feedback loops." Narrative self-study statements need supporting documentation that evidence how criteria are met. Documentation is needed on-site, but the self-study is strengthened when reviewers are provided with tangible examples of how accreditation criteria are met. For example, evaluations for a particular course may not consistently meet programmatic benchmarks. If the evaluation data are used to bring about change, such as modified content delivery methods, or inclusion of new instructors, this supports use of evaluation data to close the feedback loop. If evaluative data are collected and not used in decision-making processes, the feedback loop is not closed. Data-based programmatic decision making should be reflected in self-study responses to specific criteria as well as in the supporting documentation for the self-study.

Supporting documents that reflect compliance with specific criteria include committee, course, and faculty organization minutes, including the committee and course name and meeting dates. To the extent that these documents reflect use of assessment data to close feedback loops, the program can demonstrate a commitment to quality improvement. Referencing other conducting organization information such as the catalogue, including page numbers and data sources, facilitates a concise programmatic review. The use of tables, charts, and graphs is recommended wherever possible. Essential tables and figures should be placed in the body of the self-study. Documents such as the strategic plan, curriculum evaluation system, and organizational chart should be appropriately referenced and placed in the appendices, where page limitations are not as much of an issue.

An external consultant who is knowledgeable about the involved accreditation, standards, policies, and procedures of the accreditation agency that will be making the on-site visit can be instrumental in completion of the self-study document and in preparation for the on-site visit. The external consultant can review the self-study document in detail and offer objective recommendations for improvement. During a mock on-site visit, the external consultant can provide opportunities for faculty and administration to engage in a simulated accreditation visit. This allows faculty and administration to practice their responses to questions that might be asked during the actual on-site visit. The mock visit can help faculty identify their knowledge strengths and areas needing further development related to the self-study content. A mock on-site visit can alert faculty about which faculty members are better suited for responding to certain types of questions. The simulated visit shows faculty the importance of preparation, including each faculty member knowing the accreditation standards and program responses as well as engaging with the on-site evaluators during the site visit. During the mock visit, faculty members should be reminded to respond with short answers and use examples to further clarify their points.

The self-study document should be neatly formatted and easily accessible. The self-study narrative and supporting documents should be professionally printed to ensure an overall attractive appearance. The ability of readers to move from standard to standard and from standard to specific supporting tables and appendices without difficulty is important to on-site evaluators and reviewers. The use of printed tab dividers between each standard and for each appendix helps ensure accessibility of materials. Providing a detailed table of contents and list of all tables and appendices aids in ease of reading and decreases the time needed to search for specific documents.

If the self-study and supporting documents are provided in digital format to the on-site reviewers, the program can use hyperlinks in the narrative so that readers can easily access online reference documents. Program files such as course and faculty evaluations and faculty CVs can also be provided in electronic form for reviewers.

An example of a response to CCNE Standard I-A is presented in Box 27-1. This example is conceptual and not prescriptive, as various strategies may be employed to address the compliance of a program with accreditation criteria.

The On-Site Visit

The purpose of the on-site visit is to provide the evaluation team with the opportunity to verify, clarify, and amplify information provided in the self-study document. During the on-site visit, accreditation reviewers assess the compliance of the program with accreditation standards and learn how the nursing program uses assessment data for quality improvement purposes. The evaluation team accomplishes its purpose by conducting interviews with the communities of interest, including faculty members, students, central administration,

BOX 27-1 Example of a CCNE Self-Study Response

I-A. The mission, goals and expected program outcomes are:

- Congruent with those of the parent institution.
- Consistent with relevant professional nursing standards and guidelines for the preparation of nursing professionals.

Elaboration: The program's mission statement, goals, and expected program outcomes are written and accessible to current and prospective students, faculty, and other constituents. Program outcomes include student outcomes, faculty outcomes, and other outcomes identified by the program. A mission statement may relate to all nursing programs offered by the nursing unit or specific programs may have separate mission statements. Program goals are clearly differentiated by level when multiple degree/certificate programs exist. Student outcomes may be expressed as *competencies, objectives, benchmarks,* or other terminology congruent with institutional and program norms.

The program identifies the professional nursing standards and guidelines it uses. CCNE requires, as appropriate, the following professional nursing standards and guidelines:

- The Essentials of Baccalaureate Education for Professional Nursing Practice (American Association of Colleges of Nursing [AACN], 2008)
- The Essentials of Master's Education in Nursing (AACN, 2011)
- The Essentials of Doctoral Education for Advanced Nursing Practice (AACN, 2006)
- Criteria for Evaluation of Nurse Practitioner Programs (National Task Force on Quality Nurse Practitioner Education [AACN], 2012)

A program may select additional standards and guidelines.

A program preparing students for certification incorporates professional standards and guidelines appropriate to the role/area of education.

An APRN education program (degree or certificate) prepares students for one of the four APRN roles and at least one population focus, in accordance with the Consensus Model for APRN Regulation: Licensure, Accreditation, Certification, and Education, AACN (July, 2008).

PROGRAM RESPONSE

School of Nursing Mission and Vision. The School of Nursing (SON) mission is to *promote and protect the health of the public by preparing future leaders in nursing practice, education and research.* This mission is consistent with that of the University and shares the common themes of education, research, and quality health care.

The SON mission is written, public, and accessible to current and prospective students and faculty through the SON Handbook (Available in the Resource Room) and to other constituents through the SON website under Facts About the School. The mission statement was revised earlier this year to more accurately describe the direction of the SON.

Central to our mission is the vision that the SON will be an academic leader in nursing education through innovation and excellence in nursing practice, education, and research. The strategic priorities of the SON include:

- Develop future generations of leaders in education, practice, research, and policy.
- Create new knowledge and apply it to practice.
- Lead in the transformation of the health care system so that nurses will practice to the fullest extent of their education and training.
- Understand and participate in health care policy development.
- Collaborate effectively with other health care professions in learning and practice.
- Ensure that SON activities are aligned with University goals.
- Engage with community partners to improve health care.

DIFFERENTIATION AMONG PROGRAM GOALS

The SON *prepares future leaders in nursing practice* by educating nurse leaders and practitioners whose practice is client-centered and evidence-based. Program goals describe our graduates and clearly differentiate among each of the program levels.

- The Clinical Nurse Leader (MSN) program prepares graduates as generalist nurses with a focus on practice and clinical leadership at the micro-system level.
- The Doctor of Nursing Practice (DNP) program prepares graduates to effect change through evidence-based decision making, outcomes management, and health policy improvements for diverse populations in a variety of settings. The DNP program includes BSN to DNP and MSN to DNP options that include preparation as APRNs (nurse anesthetists, clinical nurse specialists, nurse practitioners) in one of five population foci (adult-gerontology, family/individual across the lifespan, neonatal, pediatrics, and psychiatric-mental health); Advanced Public Health Nurses (APHN), Systems Leaders, and Leaders to Enhance Population Health Outcomes.
- The postgraduate certificate program prepares graduates who seek advanced knowledge and skills and acquire certification to function as APRNs in one of four population foci: adult-gerontology, pediatrics, neonatal, or psych/mental health.
- The Doctor of Philosophy in Nursing Sciences (PhD) prepares clinical researchers who contribute to the scientific basis of care provided to individuals across the lifespan.

BOX 27-1 Example of a CCNE Self-Study Response—cont'd

Expected student outcomes are described as terminal objectives that are specific to each program level. Cognitive outcomes that are common to all programs include knowledge of core concepts, analytic thinking, evidence-based decisions, outcomes assessment, and nursing roles. Psychomotor outcomes are reflected in the clinical evaluation tools and are role-specific. Affective outcomes include advocacy, autonomy, human dignity, and integrity. The DNP terminal objectives were revised in 2010 in concert with the transition of advanced specialty programs to the DNP level.

PROFESSIONAL STANDARDS THAT GUIDE OUR EDUCATIONAL PROGRAMS

All programs offered by the SON are based on national nursing standards developed by AACN. The Doctor of Nursing Practice incorporates the *AACN Essentials of Doctoral Education for Advanced Nursing Practice.* The course approval process that is described under Standard III requires that course directors submit evidence of the alignment between terminal objectives, course objectives, curricular threads, course content, learning activities and the *AACN Essentials*, NONPF-DNP Core Domains and/or NACNS Core Competencies. The alignment between DNP terminal objectives, AACN *Essentials of Doctoral Education for Advanced Nursing Practice* and NONPF Core Competencies are found in Appendix X.

APRN tracks, including the BSN to DNP, MSN to DNP and postgraduate certificate options, also incorporate the *Criteria for Evaluation of Nurse Practitioner Programs* (National Task Force on Quality Nurse Practitioner Education, 2012). APRN tracks prepare students for one of our four APRN roles in at least one population focus in accordance with the *Consensus Model for APRN Regulation: Licensure, Accreditation, Certification and Education* (Advanced Practice Registered Nurse [APRN] Consensus Work Group, 2008). This is further described in Key Element I-B and is evident in current curricular descriptions under Standard III.

In addition, each of the clinical tracks that prepares APRNs and community/public health specialists includes competencies specific to each specialty area: *Nurse Practitioner Core Competencies* (NONPF, 2012); *Population-Focused Nurse Practitioner Competencies* (Family/Across the Lifespan, Neonatal, Pediatric Acute Care, Pediatric Primary Care, Psychiatric-Mental Health, Women's Health/Gender-Related) (NONPF Population-Focused Competencies Task Force, 2013); *Adult-Gerontology Acute Care Nurse Practitioner Competencies* (AACN, 2012); *Adult-Gerontology Primary Care Nurse Practitioner Competencies* (AACN, 2010); *Standards for Accreditation of Nurse Anesthesia Educational Programs* (COA, 2012); National Association of Neonatal Nurse Practitioners (2010); Quad Council Competencies for Public Health Nursing (2013); *National Association of Clinical Nurse Specialties Core Practice Doctoral Competencies* (2009); *Practice Doctorate Nurse Practitioner Entry-Level Competencies* (NONPF, National Panel for NP Practice Doctorate Competencies, 2006); *Core Competencies for Interprofessional Collaborative Practice* (Interprofessional Education Collaborative Expert Panel, 2011); *Domains and Core CNS Competencies* (NONPF, 2010); *Emphasizing the Older Adult in Nurse Practitioner Curriculum* (NONPF, 2008); *Adult-Gerontology Clinical Nurse Specialist Competencies* (AACN, 2010); and *Educational Standards and Curriculum Guidelines for Neonatal Nurse Practitioner Programs* (NANN, 2009). Copies of professional standards are available in the Resource Room.

Upon successful completion of the APRN and postgraduate certificate programs, graduates are eligible for certification by the American Nurses Credentialing Center, Pediatric Nursing Certification Board, National Board for Certification and Recertification of Nurse Anesthetists, American Academy of Nurse Practitioner Certification Programs and the National Certification Corporation.

clinical agency representatives, alumni, employers, and any other program stakeholders. The leader of the evaluation team and nursing program administrator jointly determine the agenda for the on-site accreditation visit.

The evaluation team will have a designated area called the resource room where a hard copy of the self-study and supporting documents are housed. This area will serve as the "home base" for the evaluation team during the on-site visit.

Preparing for the On-Site Visit

Careful preparation for the on-site visit helps ensure that the evaluation team has access to necessary documents and to create a positive and pleasant climate for the evaluation team members and the nursing program. The nursing program administrators will develop a draft agenda that will be sent to the team leader or chair of the evaluation team for their final approval. It is not unusual for this approval process to go through multiple iterations prior to finalization. During the development of the agenda, meeting times need to be designated for the evaluation team members to interview individuals and groups including the president, provost, clinical agencies, and alumni. It is important to inform the communities of interest for the program about the accreditation visit in a timely manner so that scheduling will be manageable. Typically letters are sent by the chief nurse administrator to the members of the communities of interest that include the on-site visit dates and agenda, as well as inviting these individuals or groups to submit comments about the nursing program. Notices are placed on websites and in college publications, are announced in class, and are distributed electronically through learning management systems and e-mail lists. Information about public meetings related to the accreditation visit can be placed in local media, including newspapers and radio.

The on-site visit agenda should reflect meeting times for the following individuals, groups, and sites to be visited: central administration, including the president and provost; key individuals on campus, such as the deans of the graduate school, libraries, and distance education, if applicable, as well as the registrar and chief financial officer; students, faculty, alumni, and clinical agency representatives; and clinical and classroom sites. Transportation to and from meetings and clinical sites needs to be finalized based on the agenda.

Faculty members and clinical site leadership need to be notified if the evaluation team will be visiting their clinical sites. Finally, there needs to be ample blocks of time designated for the evaluation team to spend in the resource room. Time for breaks between meetings should be included in the agenda for the on-site review. While planning the agenda events may occur several months in advance, it is a good practice to confirm the agenda with all stakeholders a week or two before the actual visit.

Preparing the Resource Room

Because the resource room will be considered the "home base" for the evaluation team, it should be equipped in a manner that will meet the needs of the evaluation team. There should be tables and chairs; computers and a printer; office supplies such as pens, pencils, and sticky notes; and a listing of all exhibits available for review. It is also good to have water, soft drinks, and snacks available for the team. Everything should be easily accessible to the evaluation team. One approach for effective resource room preparation is assignment of specific faculty members to this area. These faculty members would be responsible for ensuring that all documents are labeled and correctly placed in the resource file. The resource file should be categorized according to standards and criteria or key elements. One recommendation is to make multiple copies of short documents such as minutes, highlight the information cited in the self-study, and place a copy in each criterion or key element file where the minutes show support within the self-study. This allows more than one accreditation team member to simultaneously access the information.

The resource file should contain documents including examples of student work, course syllabi, course schedules, faculty teaching assignments, faculty vitae and accomplishments, evaluation responses from all sources, minutes cited in the self-study that demonstrate utilization of data to close feedback loops, student complaints and grievances, and letters from members of the community of interest for the program. On-site reviewers may want to review the files of students or faculty members who have submitted complaints or grievances to evaluate the application of due process for these appellants. Evidence of aggregate data tracking, including NCLEX and certification examination pass rates and employment rates should be available in the resource room for the evaluation team to view. The resource room should also contain documents related to the most recent reviews by other external agencies, including the regional accreditor and the state board of nursing.

Many nursing programs use information technology, including learning management systems, for document management and delivery of course content. Resource rooms may incorporate digital resources. For example, on-site reviewers may be provided with access to internal data sources such as a password-protected shared drive where accreditation documents are housed. External services such as Dropbox and Google Drive are web-supported file sharing options. Document management systems such as Dokmee and FileHold allow users to centralize documents securely online and ensure that current versions of software are used (Capterra, 2014; Thompson & Bovril, 2011).

Some programs may elect to use a hybrid approach to documents available in the resource room; some documents, such as the self-study and college and university catalogs, may be made available in both hard copy and electronic format, and other files, such as course and instructor evaluations, made available digitally. Site team evaluators may be provided with flash drives that contain all accreditation-related documents, or temporary access to password-protected shared drives or learning management systems where accreditation-related documents are stored. The self-study narrative can provide direct links to online supporting documentation through the use of hyperlinks.

Use of digital documents in the resource room decreases the amount of hard copy documents required. This decreases resource use, including copying and binding time and paper consumption, and saves space. Digital documents, including the self-study and supporting evidence, are advantageous to reviewers because the need to transport weighty hard copy documents is obviated and accreditation-related documents can be viewed from any computer work station (Thompson & Bovril, 2011).

All nursing accrediting agencies provide information about documents that should be available in the resource room during accreditation visits on their respective websites. See ACEN (www.acenursing.org/accreditation-manual/), CCNE (www.aacn.nche.edu/accreditation/pdf/advice.pdf), and NLN CNEA (http://www.nln.org/cnea).

Decision-Making Process by the Accreditation Organization

All accrediting agencies follow similar steps in their decision-making processes, which are in part regulated by the USDE. The processes of these agencies include the following steps:

- A peer evaluation team submits a report to the accreditation agency based on compliance with the accreditation standards as demonstrated in the self-study document and verified through the on-site visit.
- The chief nursing administrator of the nursing program has the opportunity to respond to the report of the evaluation team.
- The report of the evaluation team, response of the nursing program to the report, and the self-study document are sent to the review panel of the accreditation agency. The review panel makes a recommendation regarding the accreditation decision.
- The recommendations of the review panel and all relevant materials are sent to the Board of Commissioners, which makes the final decision on whether to grant, reaffirm, deny, or withdraw accreditation.
- The final accreditation decision is communicated to the USDE, the parent institution, and appropriate accreditation and regulatory agencies.

Each accreditation agency has an appeals process that the nursing program may choose to pursue based on an adverse accreditation decision. There is a prescribed timeframe during which appeals of an accreditation decision may be generated. The appellant program may incur additional fees associated with submission of an appeal.

Summary

Accreditation is a voluntary activity that has a 100-year history in the United States. In other countries, governments frequently provide oversight of educational institutions. Privately operated U.S. accreditation agencies provide quality assurance and quality improvement for their accredited programs and institutions. They also can serve as gatekeepers for accredited programs and institutions to access programs administered by the USDE or other federal agencies, including student financial aid programs. Accreditation agencies that are recognized by federal and state governments are considered to be reliable authorities on academic quality (Association of Specialized and Professional Accreditors [ASPA], 2007; Council for Higher Education Accreditation, CHEA, 2010; COA, 2014).

Accreditation is a peer process that involves granting of public recognition to an institution or specialized program by a private, nongovernmental agency. Granting of accreditation indicates that the institution or program meets or exceeds nationally established standards for acceptable educational quality. Institutions or specialized programs are evaluated based on their own stated purposes if those purposes are educationally appropriate, meet accreditation standards, and fall within the recognized scope of the accreditation agency (ASPA, 2007; Council for Higher Education Accreditation, CHEA, 2010; COA, 2014).

Accreditation exists to ensure quality assessment and to assist with quality improvement. Accreditation can apply to institutions or programs, whereas certification and licensure are related to individuals. Accreditation does not ensure the quality of individual graduates, but provides reasonable assurance of the context and quality of the education that is offered (ASPA, 2007; Council for Higher Education Accreditation, CHEA, 2010; COA, 2014).

Accreditation is of benefit to the public for these reasons:

- Reasonable assurance of the external evaluation of a program and its conformity with general expectations in the professional field
- Identification of programs that have voluntarily undertaken explicit activities directed at quality improvement
- Improvement in the professional services available to the public, resulting from evidence-based program requirement modifications
- Less need for intervention by public agencies in educational program operations because private accreditation provides resources for quality assessment and quality improvement

Students benefit from these aspects of accreditation:

- Reasonable assurance that the educational activities of an accredited program are satisfactory and meet student needs
- Facilitation of academic credit transfer between programs and institutions
- Provides a uniform prerequisite for entering the profession
- Establishes eligibility to seek Title IV financial aid and other federal and state programs

Programs benefit from accreditation through these mechanisms:

- Accreditation provides a stimulus for self-directed improvement
- The accreditation agency may provide peer review and counsel
- The reputation of the program is enhanced because it is accredited
- Accreditation may be a mechanism that provides eligibility for selected governmental funding programs and private foundation grants

Professions benefit from accreditation in that it provides:

- A means for participation of practitioners to establish requirements for professional education
- A contribution to professional unity through bringing together practitioners, educators, students, and the communities of interest in an activity that improves professional preparation and practice (ASPA, 2007; Council for Higher Education Accreditation, CHEA, 2010; COA, 2014).

Successful completion of the accreditation process is a significant achievement for all nursing programs. The components of self-review and self-assessment should be viewed as ongoing rather than sporadic. Achievement of accreditation demonstrates programmatic commitment to quality assessment and quality improvement.

With the existing agencies of ACEN and CCNE and the emerging NLN CNEA, most nursing programs will have the option to choose from among the three program accrediting agencies. Baccalaureate and higher degree programs will be able to choose to seek accreditation from ACEN, CCNE, or NLN CNEA. Associate degree, diploma, and practical/vocational nursing programs seeking accreditation will be able to choose from ACEN or NLN CNEA. If the programs require program accreditation for Title IV funding authorization, ACEN will remain the nursing accrediting agency of choice. Achieving accreditation from any of the three nursing program agencies is considered a mark of program quality.

Although faculty members may view the accreditation process as tedious and time consuming, it is an opportunity for programmatic improvement. Accreditation agencies provide detailed guidelines for nursing programs to use in their pursuit of initial and continuing accreditation.

REFLECTING ON THE EVIDENCE

1. How can technology be used to advance the accreditation process?
2. Are there other accreditation models that may streamline the accreditation process?
3. Based on your experience with the accreditation process, what are some recommendations for better engagement of faculty in the accreditation process, particularly new or junior faculty?

REFERENCES

Accreditation Commission for Education in Nursing (ACEN). (2013). *ACEN accreditation manual.* Retrieved from, www.acenursing.org.

American Association of Colleges of Nursing. (2008). *The essentials of baccalaureate education for professional nursing practice.* Author.

American Association of Colleges of Nursing. (2012). Retrieved from, http://www.aacn.nche.edu/education-resources/evalcriteria2012.pdf.

Association of Specialized Professional Accreditors. (2007). Retrieved from, http://www.aspa-usa.org/.

Capterra. (2014). *Top document management software products.* Retrieved from, http://www.capterra.com/document-management-software/.

Case Management Society of America. (2010). *Standards of practice for case management.* Retrieved from, www.cmsa.org.

Commission on Collegiate Nursing Education (CCNE). (2009). *CCNE mission statement and goals.* Retrieved from, www.aacn.nche.edu.

Council for Higher Education Accreditation (CHEA). (2010). Retrieved from, www.chea.org.

Council on Accreditation of Nurse Anesthesia Educational Programs. (2014). Retrieved from http://home.coa.us.com/Pages/default.aspx.

Criteria for Evaluation of Nurse Practitioner Programs. (2012). *American Association of Colleges of Nursing.* Retrieved from, http://www.aacn.nche.edu/education-resources/evalcriteria2012.pdf.

Eaton, J. (2012). *An overview of U.S. accreditation.* Washington, D.C.: Council for Higher Education Accreditation.

National Association for Practical Nurse Education and Service (NAPNES). (2004). *NAPNES standards of practice for licensed practical/vocational nurses.* Retrieved from, www.napnes.org.

National Task Force on Quality Nurse Practitioner Education. (2008). *Criteria for evaluation of nurse practitioner programs: A report of the national task force on quality nurse practitioner education.* Retrieved from, www.aacn.nche.edu.

National League for Nursing Commission on Nursing Education Accreditation. (2015). Retrieved from, http://www.nln.org/accreditation-services/the-nln-commission-for-nursing-education-accreditation-(cnea).

Thompson, C., & Bovril, C. (2011). Information technology as a tool to facilitate the academic accreditation process. *Nurse Educator, 36*(5), 192–196.

United States Department of Education (USDE). (2014). *Accreditation FAQs.* Retrieved from, www.ope.ed.gov/accreditation/FAQ/Accr.aspx.

Index

Note: Page numbers followed by *b* indicate boxes, *f* indicate figures and *t* indicate tables.

G

H

T

U

V

W